Essentials of Sports Nutrition

Essentials of Sports Nutrition

Editor: Peyton Turner

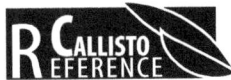

R CALLISTO REFERENCE

www.callistoreference.com

Callisto Reference,
118-35 Queens Blvd., Suite 400,
Forest Hills, NY 11375, USA

Visit us on the World Wide Web at:
www.callistoreference.com

ISBN: 978-1-63239-897-0 (Hardback)

The publisher's policy is to use permanent paper from mills that operate a sustainable forestry policy. Furthermore, the publisher ensures that the text paper and cover boards used have met acceptable environmental accreditation standards.

Trademark Notice: Registered trademark of products or corporate names are used only for explanation and identification without intent to infringe.

Printed in the United States of America.

Cataloging-in-Publication Data

Essentials of sports nutrition / edited by Peyton Turner.
    p. cm.
Includes bibliographical references and index.
ISBN 978-1-63239-897-0
1. Athletes--Nutrition. 2. Sports--Physiological aspects.3. Nutrition. 4. Athletes--Health and hygiene.
I. Turner, Peyton.
TX361.A8 E87 2017
613.7--dc23

Table of Contents

Permissions

List of Contributors

Index

Preface

This book has been an outcome of determined endeavour from a group of educationists in the field. The primary objective was to involve a broad spectrum of professionals from diverse cultural background involved in the field for developing new researches. The book not only targets students but also scholars pursuing higher research for further enhancement of the theoretical and practical applications of the subject.

Sports nutrition refers to the study of food and nutrition in relation to sports and athletic performance. It incorporates the study of various vitamins, minerals, diets, supplements and organic substances that strengthen the body of the sports persons and enhances their performance. Sports nutrition plays a crucial role in the sports like weight lifting, bodybuilding, swimming, rowing, running, cycling, etc. This book traces the progress of this field and highlights some of its key concepts and applications. Different approaches, evaluations, methodologies and advanced studies on sports nutrition have been included in this text. Students, researchers, experts and all associated with this subject will benefit alike from the book. It is a vital tool for all researching or studying sports nutrition as it gives incredible insights into emerging trends and concepts.

It was an honour to edit such a profound book and also a challenging task to compile and examine all the relevant data for accuracy and originality. I wish to acknowledge the efforts of the contributors for submitting such brilliant and diverse chapters in the field and for endlessly working for the completion of the book. Last, but not the least; I thank my family for being a constant source of support in all my research endeavours.

Editor

Effects of protein type and composition on postprandial markers of skeletal muscle anabolism, adipose tissue lipolysis, and hypothalamic gene expression

Christopher Brooks Mobley[1], Carlton D Fox[1], Brian S Ferguson[1], Corrie A Pascoe[1], James C Healy[1], Jeremy S McAdam[1], Christopher M Lockwood[2] and Michael D Roberts[1*]

Abstract

Background: We examined the acute effects of different dietary protein sources (0.19 g, dissolved in 1 ml of water) on skeletal muscle, adipose tissue and hypothalamic satiety-related markers in fasted, male Wistar rats (~250 g).

Methods: Oral gavage treatments included: a) whey protein concentrate (WPC, n = 15); b) 70:30 hydrolyzed whey-to-hydrolyzed egg albumin (70 W/30E, n = 15); c) 50 W/50E (n = 15); d) 30 W/70E (n = 15); and e) 1 ml of water with no protein as a fasting control (CTL, n = 14).

Results: Skeletal muscle analyses revealed that compared to CTL: a) phosphorylated (p) markers of mTOR signaling [p-mTOR (Ser2481) and p-rps6 (Ser235/236)] were elevated 2–4-fold in all protein groups 90 min post-treatment (p < 0.05); b) WPC and 70 W/30E increased muscle protein synthesis (MPS) 104% and 74% 180 min post-treatment, respectively (p < 0.05); and c) 70 W/30E increased p-AMPKα (Thr172) 90 and 180-min post-treatment as well as PGC-1α mRNA 90 min post-treatment. Subcutaneous (SQ) and omental fat (OMAT) analyses revealed: a) 70 W/30 W increased SQ fat phosphorylated hormone-sensitive lipase [p-HSL (Ser563)] 3.1-fold versus CTL and a 1.9–4.4-fold change versus all other test proteins 180 min post-treatment (p < 0.05); and b) WPC, 70 W/30E and 50 W/50E increased OMAT p-HSL 3.8–6.5-fold 180 min post-treatment versus CTL (p < 0.05). 70 W/30E and 30 W/70E increased hypothalamic POMC mRNA 90 min post-treatment versus CTL rats suggesting a satiety-related response may have occurred in the former groups. However, there was a compensatory increase in orexigenic AGRP mRNA in the 70 W/30E group 90 min post-treatment versus CTL rats, and there was a compensatory increase in orexigenic NPY mRNA in the 30 W/70E group 90 min post-treatment versus CTL rats.

Conclusions: Higher amounts of whey versus egg protein stimulate the greatest post-treatment anabolic skeletal muscle response, though test proteins with higher amounts of WPH more favorably affected post-treatment markers related to adipose tissue lipolysis.

Keywords: Whey protein, Egg protein, Hydrolyzed protein, Muscle protein synthesis, Lipolysis

* Correspondence: mdr0024@auburn.edu
[1]School of Kinesiology, Molecular and Applied Sciences Laboratory, Auburn University, 301 Wire Road, Office 286, Auburn, AL 36849, USA
Full list of author information is available at the end of the article

Background

Dietary whey protein has numerous well-known health benefits. For instance, whey protein feeding has been shown to acutely increase postprandial muscle protein synthesis (MPS) in rodents [1,2] and humans [3,4], whereas chronic whey protein supplementation has been shown to consistently increase muscle mass with exercise training [5-7]. Acute whey protein feeding has also been shown to reduce appetite 90–180 min following low-dose ingestion [8-10] by potentially affecting anorectic hormone and hypothalamic mRNA expression patterns [11,8,9]. Chronic whey protein supplementation has also been shown to reduce adiposity in rodents and humans [12-14,5]; an effect which may be explained by an increased expression of adipose tissue lipolysis-related gene expression patterns following chronic supplementation [12], an increase in protein-induced thermogenesis (reviewed in [15]), and/or a consistent reduction in food intake given its satiety-stimulatory effects as discussed above.

More recent data has focused on the potential health benefits of hydrolyzed dietary proteins. In short, commercial hydrolysis of different dietary protein sources is thought to [16-18]: a) expedite the digestion of amino acids via 'pre-digestion' thus increasing their postprandial bioavailability; and b) liberate bioactive peptides that are able to exhibit physiological responses that otherwise would be diminished from consuming intact protein sources. Indeed, in vivo [19,20] and in vitro [21] evidence suggests that hydrolyzed whey or native whey protein increases the activation of postprandial intramuscular insulin signaling markers. Putative bioactive peptides from whey protein hydrolysates (WPH) have also been shown to exhibit insulin secretagogue properties versus intact whey protein [22,23]. Likewise, we have recently demonstrated that acute WPH feeding in rats increases the appearance of di- and oligopeptides as well as numerous lipolysis-related serum markers (i.e., epinephrine, glycerol and numerous free fatty acids) compared to an isonitrogenous WPC feeding condition [18]. Thus, it is of interest to further examine how WPH versus WPC ingestion differentially affects various physiological systems.

Widespread interest has also surrounded the positive health benefits of dietary egg protein due to its high essential amino acid (EAA) content and high digestibility [24]. Similar to whey protein, egg protein feeding in rats has been found to significantly increase postprandial MPS [1]. Likewise, one report suggests that bioactives isolated from egg protein down-regulate serum myostatin (MSTN) [25]; an effect which may enhance skeletal muscle hypertrophy with chronic supplementation. However, unlike the aforementioned whey protein research, there is a paucity of data regarding the physiological effects of dietary egg protein on other tissues (i.e., adipose tissue and the hypothalamus), though there is some evidence to suggest that egg-based breakfast meals can increase satiety post-ingestion [26] and cause weight loss in overweight individuals over the long-term [27].

Given the widespread interest regarding the physiological effects of dietary whey and egg proteins, as well as hydrolyzed versus intact protein forms, the purpose of this study was to examine how different solutions of extensively hydrolyzed whey and egg albumin protein (EPH) blends, in combination with a standardized blend of cow colostrum and egg yolk extract acutely affect post-prandial markers of skeletal muscle anabolism, adipose tissue lipolysis and thermogenesis, and hypothalamic mRNA expression patterns in rodents. Treatments included: 300 human equivalent mg of bovine colostrum and egg yolk extract (0.0057 g protein rat dose) in addition to 10 human equivalent g protein dose (0.19 g protein rat dose) of, a) high-dose WPH + low-dose EPH (70 W/30E); b) equal doses of both WPH and EPH (50 W/50E); and c) low-dose WPH + high-dose EPH (30 W/70E). An isonitrogenous amount of intact whey protein concentrate (WPC) was also fed to a fourth group of rats as a positive feeding control, and 1 ml of water with no protein was fed to a fifth group of rats as a fasting control (CTL). Based upon the aforementioned literature, we hypothesized that all protein treatments would similarly increase postprandial markers of skeletal muscle anabolism as well as satiety-related hypothalamic markers relative to CTL. We also hypothesized that higher proportions of whey protein (i.e., WPC and 70 W/30E) would induce larger increases in adipose tissue lipolysis markers relative to other feeding groups; though we also hypothesized that the hydrolysates would outperform the WPC on markers of muscle anabolism, adipose tissue lipolysis and satiety.

Experimental methods

Animals and feeding protocols

All experimental procedures described herein were approved by Auburn University's Institutional Animal Care and Use Committee. Male Wistar rats (~250 g) approximately 8–9 weeks old were purchased from Harlan Laboratories and were allowed to acclimate in the animal quarters for 5 days prior to experimentation. Briefly, animal quarters were maintained on a 12 h light: 12 h dark cycle, at ambient room temperature, with water and standard rodent chow (18.6% protein, 44.2% carbohydrate, 6.2% fat; Teklad Global #2018 Diet, Harlan Laboratories) provided to animals *ad libitum*.

The day prior to acute protein feeding experiments, food was removed from home cages resulting in an 18 h overnight fast. The morning of experimentation, animals were removed from their quarters between 0800–0900, transported to the Molecular and Applied Sciences Laboratory and were allowed to acclimate for approximately 3–5 h. Thereafter, rats were administered either WPC, 70 W/30E,

50 W/50E, 30 W/70E at a human equivalent (eq.) dose of 10 g protein (0.19 g protein rat dose) dissolved in 1 ml of tap water via gavage feeding. Doses were calculated per the species conversion calculations of Reagan-Shaw et al. [28], whereby the human body mass for an average male was assumed to be 80 kg. The group of non-fed CTL rats was gavage-fed 1 ml of tap water. Dietary components of each test protein solution are presented in Table 1.

Of note, We examined how graded doses of WPC in solution (0.19, 0.37, and 0.93 g protein) stimulated MPS and Akt-mTOR markers 90 min post-gavage in order to

Table 1 Contents of each protein per the 0.19 g protein dose of each respective protein

Amino Acid	70 W/30E (mg)	50 W/50E (mg)	30 W/70E (mg)	WPC (mg)
Alanine	10	10	10	9
Arginine	8	8	9	6
Aspartic Acid	21	20	19	22
Cysteine	5	5	5	4
Glutamic Acid	31	29	26	34
Glycine	4	5	5	4
Histidine*	4	4	4	4
Isoleucine*†	11	11	10	12
Leucine*†	20	19	17	23
Lysine*	17	15	14	19
Methionine*	5	5	6	4
Phenylalanine*	8	9	9	7
Proline	12	11	9	17
Serine	12	12	11	12
Threonine*	11	10	9	12
Tryptophan*	3	3	3	3
Tyrosine	7	7	7	6
Valine*†	12	12	12	11
*Total EAAs**	*92*	*87*	*83*	*95*
Total BCAAs†*	*43*	*41*	*38*	*46*
M.W.	70 W/30E	50 W/50E	30 W/70E	WPC
(kDa)	(%)	(%)	(%)	(%)
<1.0	40	39	40	0
1.0 - 5.0	23	22	23	7
5.0 - 10.0	6	6	6	11
>10.0	30	32	32	82

As stated in the methods, rats were administered either WPC, 70 W/30E, 50 W/50E, or 30 W/70E at a human equivalent (eq.) dose of 10 g protein (equaled a true dose of 0.191 g of protein) dissolved in 1 ml of water via gavage feeding. While not stated in the methods, total protein was determined using the Dumas (N x 6.38) test method. Furthermore, amino acid concentrations (g/100 g) were determined using liquid chromatography. Finally, molecular weight (M.W.) distribution was determined by high-performance liquid chromatography size exclusion (HPLC-SEC), on an Agilent 1290 Infinity Quaternary LC System w/ TOSOH TSKgel G2000SW 7.5 mm ID × 30 cm (10 μm) column at a wavelength of 205 nm. Symbols: * indicates an essential amino acid; † indicates a branched chain amino acid (BCAA).

determine an optimal dose that adequately elicited a post-prandial physiological response. These preliminary results demonstrated that 10 human eq. g of WPC (0.19 g protein) increased markers of mTOR activation and MPS 90 min post-gavage, and this generally was equal to the 19 human eq. g (0.37 g protein) and 48 human eq. g (0.93 g protein) doses (Additional file 1: Figure S1). Thus, given that the 10 human eq. g of WPC (0.19 g protein) elicited similar anabolic responses compared to higher doses, we opted to use the 10 human eq. g (0.19 g) dose for each test protein. While this dose is not typically associated with the optimal human MPS response to protein ingestion (i.e., 20–40 g), it should be noted that the species conversion calculations of Reagan-Shaw et al. is a basis to dose rats relative to humans and, alternatively, these human eq. dosages should not be viewed in absolute terms when comparing species (i.e., 10 human eq. g appears to elicit an anabolic response in rats whereas 20–40 g in humans is needed).

The gavage feeding procedure involved placing the animals under light isoflurane anesthesia for approximately 1 min while gavage feeding occurred. Following gavage feeding, rats were allowed to recover 90 or 180 min prior to being euthanized under CO_2 gas in a 2 L induction chamber (VetEquip, Inc., Pleasanton, CA, USA). Animals that were sacrificed 180 min post-treatment were injected intraperitoneally with puromycin dihydrochloride (5.44 mg in 1 ml of diluted in phosphate buffered saline; Ameresco, Solon, OH, USA) 30 min prior to euthanasia in order to determine skeletal muscle protein synthesis via the surface sensing of translation (SUnSET) method described in detail elsewhere [29]. Of note, with the SUnSET method MPS is determined through the incorporation of puromycin into actively synthesized proteins given that it is a structural analogue of aminoacyl-transfer RNA; specifically tyrosyl-tRNA. It should also be noted that the SUnSET method is an alternative method for measuring MPS compared to radioactive isotope (e.g. ^{3}H-phenylalanine or ^{35}S-methionine), or stable isotope (e.g.^{15}N-lysine, ^{13}C-leucine or [ring-^{13}C6]-phenylalanine) tracers. Goodman et al. [29] compared the SUnSET method to a ^{3}H-phenylalanine flooding method in *ex vivo* plantaris muscle preparations isolated from animals that had undergone synergist ablation. Remarkably, these authors determined that MPS rates increased 3.6-fold as determined by the SUnSET method and 3.4-fold as determined by the tracer method; a finding which proves the reliability of this method in detecting sensitive changes in MPS.

Immediately following euthanasia, whole blood was removed via heart sticks using a 21-gauge needle and syringe, placed in a serum separator tubes, and processed for serum extraction via centrifugation at 3,500 × *g* for 5 min. Serum was aliquoted into multiple 1.7 ml microcentrifuge tubes for subsequent biochemical assays and then frozen for later analysis. Approximately two 50 mg pieces of mixed gastrocnemius muscle was harvested using standard dissection techniques and placed in homogenizing buffer [Tris base; pH 8.0, NaCl, NP-40, sodium deoxycholate, SDS with added protease and phosphatase inhibitors (G Biosciences, St. Louis, MO, USA)] and Ribozol (Ameresco) for immunoblotting and mRNA analyses, respectively. Approximately two 50 mg pieces of subcutaneous adipose tissue (SQ) from the inguinal crease was harvested and placed in the aforementioned Tris base homogenizing buffer and Ribozol for immunoblotting and mRNA analyses, respectively. Due to tissue limitations, only one 50 mg piece of omental adipose tissue (OMAT) was harvested and placed in the aforementioned Tris base homogenizing buffer for immunoblotting. Finally, removal of the hypothalamus was performed per the methods similar to those previously employed [30]. Briefly, brains were removed and rinsed in 1x phosphate buffered saline. Brains were then placed posterior side up in a 1.0 mm acrylic sectioning apparatus (Braintree Scientific, Braintree, MA, USA) and a 2.0-mm coronal slice of each brain was made between Bregma-1.6 and-1.8 mm. Coronal slices were immediately placed on an ice-cooled stage and two bilateral punches (2.0 mm diameter) were made to capture the hypothalamus. Tissue was immediately placed in Ribozol and stored at-80°C until RNA isolation.

Gastrocnemius muscle, SQ and OMAT samples placed in Tris base homogenizing buffer were homogenized using a 1.7 ml tube using a tight-fitting micropestle, insoluble proteins were removed with centrifugation at $500 \times g$ for 5 min at 4°C, and supernatants were assayed for total protein content using a BCA Protein Assay Kit (Thermo Scientific, Waltham, MA, USA) prior to immunoblotting sample preparation. Muscle, SQ, and hypothalamus samples placed in Ribozol were subjected to total RNA isolation according to manufacturer's instructions, and concentrations were performed using a NanoDrop Lite (Thermo Scientific) prior to cDNA synthesis for mRNA analyses. Extra gastrocnemius muscle and SQ fat not processed during dissections were flash-frozen in liquid nitrogen and stored at-80°C for later potential analyses.

Directed Akt-mTOR phosphoproteomics

The PathScan® Akt Signaling Antibody Array Kit (Chemiluminescent Readout; Cell Signaling, Danvers, MA, USA) containing glass slides spotted with antibodies was utilized to detect phosphorylated proteins predominantly belonging to the Akt-mTOR signaling network.

The kit assays p-Akt (Thr308), p-Akt (Ser473), p-rps6 (Ser235/236), p-AMPKα (Thr172), p-Pras40 (Thr246), p-mTOR (Ser2481), p-GSK-3α (Ser21), p-GSK-3β (Ser9), p-p70s6k (Thr389), p-p70s6k (Thr421/Ser424), p-BAD (Ser112), p-PTEN (Ser380), p-PDK1 (Ser241), p-ERK1/2 (Thr202/Tyr204), p-4E-BP1 (Thr37/46). However,

we specifically analyzed p-Akt (Ser473), p-rps6 (Ser235/236), p-AMPKα (Thr172), p-mTOR (Ser2481), p- p-p70s6k (Thr389), and p-4E-BP1 (Thr37/46) in order follow a 'linear' analysis in Akt-mTOR signaling. Briefly, gastrocnemius homogenates were diluted to 0.5 µg/µl using cell lysis buffer provided by the kit and assayed according to manufacturer's instructions. Slides were developed using an enhanced chemiluminescent reagent provided by the kit, and spot densitometry was performed through the use of a UVP Imager and associated densitometry software (UVP, LLC, Upland, CA, USA). The calculation of each phosphorylated target was as follows:

(Density value of the target − negative control)/summation of all density values for the sample.

It should be noted that this high throughput antibody chip array for muscle phosphorylation markers was used rather than single antibodies due to resource constraints. Notwithstanding, and as discussed in the results section, the results presented herein are in agreement with past literature showing that protein feeding affects numerous targets on the aforementioned antibody array chip. Furthermore, our preliminary WPC graded-dose feedings show an increase in Akt-mTOR markers across multiple doses relative to fasting rats (Additional file 1: Figure S1). We have also internally tested this array on exercised rat muscle as well as C2C12 cell culture lysates deprived of or treated with L-leucine, and have produced reproducible results commensurate with prior literature examining these markers (i.e., increased activation of mTOR markers which parallel increases in MPS; *unpublished observations*).

Western blotting

As mentioned prior, the SUnSET method was employed in order to examine if different dietary protein blends differentially affected MPS. Briefly, 2 µg/µl gastrocnemius Western blotting preps were made using 4x Laemmli buffer. Thereafter, 20 µl of prepped samples were loaded onto pre-casted 4–20% SDS-polyacrylamide gels (C.B.S. Scientific Company, San Diego, CA, USA) and subjected to electrophoresis (200 V @ 75 min) using pre-made 1x SDS-PAGE running buffer (C.B.S. Scientific Company). Proteins were then transferred to polyvinylidene difluoride membranes, and membranes were blocked for 1 h at room temperature with 5% nonfat milk powder. For muscle samples, mouse anti-puromycin IgG (1:5,000; Millipore) was incubated with membranes overnight at 4°C in 5% bovine serum albumin (BSA), and the following day membranes were incubated with anti-mouse IgG secondary antibodies (1:2,000, Cell Signaling) at room temperature for 1 h prior to membrane development described below. Thereafter, membranes were stripped of antibodies via commercial stripping buffer (Restore Western Blot Stripping Buffer, Thermo Scientific), membranes were incubated with rabbit anti-beta-actin

(1:5,000; GeneTex, Inc., Irvine, CA, USA) as a normalizer protein overnight at 4°C in 5% BSA, and the following day membranes were incubated with anti-rabbit IgG secondary antibodies (1:2,000, Cell Signaling) at room temperature for 1 h prior to membrane development.

SQ and OMAT samples were assayed with rabbit anti-phospho-hormone sensitive lipase [p-HSL (Ser563) IgG (1:1000; Cell Signaling)] overnight at 4°C in 5% BSA. The following day membranes were incubated with anti-rabbit IgG secondary antibodies (1:2,000, Cell Signaling) at room temperature for 1 h prior to membrane development. Membranes were stripped, incubated with rabbit glyceraldehyde 3-phosphate dehydrogenase (GAPDH; 1:5,000; GeneTex) overnight at 4°C in 5% BSA, and the following day were incubated with anti-rabbit IgG secondary antibodies (1:2,000, Cell Signaling) at room temperature for 1 h prior to membrane development.

Membrane development was performed using an enhanced chemiluminescent reagent (Amersham, Pittsburgh, PA, USA), and band densitometry was performed through the use of a UVP Imager and associated densitometry software (UVP, LLC, Upland, CA, USA).

Real-time RT-PCR

RNA from each tissue (500 ng of hypothalamus RNA and 1 μg of gastrocnemius and SQ RNA) were reverse transcribed into cDNA for real time PCR analyses using a commercial cDNA synthesis kit (Quanta Biosciences, Gaithersburg, MD, USA). Real-time PCR was performed using SYBR-green-based methods with gene-specific primers [MSTN, Mighty/Akirin-1, Myosin Heavy Chain 4 (Myhc4), p21Cip1, Atrogin-1, MuRF-1, GLUT-4, Insulin-like growth factor-1ea (IGF-1Ea), proopiomelanocortin (POMC), neuropeptide Y (NPY), agouti-related protein (AGRP), leptin receptor (LEPR), peroxisome proliferator-activated receptor gamma co-activator 1-alpha (PGC-1α), uncoupling protein 3 (UCP3), carnitine palmitoyltransferase 1b (CPT1B), beta-2 microglobulin (B2M), and beta-actin] designed using primer designer software (Primer3Plus, Cambridge, MA, USA). The forward and reverse primer sequences are as follows: [MSTN: forward primer 5′-ACGCTACCACG-GAAACAATC-3′, reverse primer 5′-CCGTCTTTCATG GGTTTGAT-3′; Mighty/Akirin-1: forward primer 5′-TTTGATCTTGGGGATTCTGG-3′, reverse primer 5′-GCCTGGAAACAGTCCCTGTA-3′; p21Cip1: forward primer 5′-AGCAAAGTATGCCGTCGTCT-3′, reverse primer 5′-ACACGCTCCCAGACGTAGTT-3′; Atrogin-1: forward primer 5′-CTACGATGTTGCAGCCAAGA -3′, reverse primer 5′- GGCAGTCGAGAAGTCCAGTC-3′; MuRF-1: forward primer 5′-AGTCGCAGTTTCGAAG-CAAT-3′, reverse primer 5′-AACGACCTCCAGACATG-GAC-3′; GLUT-4: forward primer 5′-GCTTCTGTTGCC CTTCTGTC-3′, reverse primer 5′-TGGACGCTCTCTTT

CCAACT-3′; IGF-1Ea: forward primer 5′-TGGTGGACG CTCTTCAGTTC-3′, reverse primer 5′-TCCGGAAGCA ACACTCATCC-3′; POMC: forward primer 5′-GAAG GTGTACCCCAATGTCG-3′, reverse primer 5′-CTTCT CGGAGGTCATGAAGC-3′; NPY: forward primer 5′-AG AGATCCAGCCCTGAGACA-3′, reverse primer 5′-AAC-GACAACAAGGGAAATGG-3′; AGRP: forward primer 5′-CGTGTGGGCCCTTTATTAGA-3′, reverse primer 5′-CAGACCTTCTGATGCCCTTC-3′; LEPR: forward primer 5′-CTGGGTTTGCGTATGGAAGT-3′, reverse primer 5′-CCAGTCTCTTGCTCCTCACC-3′; PGC-1α: forward primer 5′-ATGTGTCGCCTTCTTGCTCT-3′, reverse primer 5′-ATCTACTGCCTGGGGACCTT-3′; UCP3: forward primer 5′-GAGTCAGGGGACTGTGGAAA-3′, reverse primer 5′-GCGTTCATGTATCGGGTCTT-3′; CPT1B: forward primer 5′-CCCAGTTCTGAGACCAGCTC-3′, reverse primer 5′-TAGGCACCTAAGGGCTGAGA-3′; B2M: forward primer 5′-CCCAAAGAGACAGTGGGTGT-3′, reverse primer 5′-CCCTACTCCCCTCAGTTTCC-3′; beta-actin: forward primer 5′-GTGGATCAGCAAGCAGGAG T-3′, reverse primer 5′-ACGCAGCTCAGTAACAGTCC-3′] and SYBR green chemistry (Quanta). Primer efficiency curves for all genes were generated and efficiencies ranged between 90% and 110%, and melt curve analyses demonstrated that one PCR product was amplified per reaction.

SQ cAMP determination

Frozen SQ samples were subjected to 3′–5′-cyclic adenosine monophosphate (cAMP) assays using a rat-specific spectrophotometric commercial assay (R&D Systems, Inc., Minneapolis, MN, USA). Briefly, approximately 50–100 mg of tissue was homogenized in 500 μl of 0.1 N HCl. Samples were subjected to 10 min of centrifugation at 10,000 × g at 4°C, and neutralized with 50 μl of 1 N NaOH. Samples were then diluted 2-fold with the assay diluent provided, and cAMP concentrations were determined according to the manufacturer's recommendations.

Serum analyses

Serum samples were assayed for lipolysis markers including free fatty acids (FFAs) as well as epinephrine (EPI) and norepinephrine (NorEPI) using rat-specific spectrophotometric commercial assays according to the manufacturer's recommendations (FFAs: Abcam, Cambridge, MA, USA; EPI/NorEPI: Abnova, Taipei City, Taiwan). Serum samples were also analyzed for triiodothyronine (T3) using a rat-specific spectrophotometric commercial assay according to the manufacturer's recommendations (Abnova).

Statistics

All data are presented in figures and tables as means ± standard error values. Given that each post-treatment time point were comprised of independent groups of rats, statistical comparisons were performed using one-way ANOVAs, and statistical significance was set at $p < 0.05$ (SPSS v 22.0, IBM, Armonk, NY, USA). When between-group significance was obtained, a Fisher's LSD *post hoc* test was performed in order to determine specific between-group comparisons.

Results

A higher proportion of whey protein versus egg protein elicits the most favorable postprandial anabolic response

mTOR pathway targets were assayed in order to determine how each protein source affect post-prandial Akt-mTOR signaling substrates which, when activated, lead to increases in MPS. p-mTOR (Ser2481) was approximately 2-to-3-fold greater for protein-fed versus CTL rats 90 min post-gavage (WPC vs. CTL $p = 0.006$, 70 W/30E vs. CTL $p = 0.005$, 50 W/50E vs. CTL $p < 0.001$, 30 W/70E $p = 0.022$; Figure 1a), though it only remained significantly elevated in the 70 W/30E group 180 min post-gavage compared to CTL rats ($p = 0.010$; Figure 1a). p-p70s6k (Thr389) was significantly elevated approximately 2-fold in 70 W/30E and 50 W/50E versus CTL rats 90 min post-feeding (70 W/30E vs. CTL $p = 0.011$, 50 W/50E vs. CTL $p = 0.007$; Figure 1b), and this marker remained significantly elevated in 70 W/30E versus CTL rats 180 min

post-feeding (~1.9-fold, $p = 0.020$; Figure 1b). p-rps6 (Ser235/236) was approximately 2.8-to-4-fold greater for protein-fed versus CTL rats 90 min post-gavage (WPC vs. CTL $p < 0.001$, 70 W/30E vs. CTL $p < 0.001$, 50 W/50E vs. CTL $p < 0.001$, 30 W/70E $p = 0.003$; Figure 1c), and this marker remained 2.7-to-2.9-fold elevated 70 W/30E and 50 W/50E versus CTL rats 180 min post-feeding (70 W/30E vs. CTL $p = 0.002$, 50 W/50E vs. CTL $p = 0.007$; Figure 1c). Interestingly, except for the 30 W/70E group, all protein-fed groups presented statistically 30–50% lower p-4E-BP1 (Thr37/47) values 90 min (WPC vs. CTL $p < 0.001$, 70 W/30E vs. CTL $p = 0.003$, 50 W/50E vs. CTL $p < 0.001$, 30 W/70E $p = 0.064$; Figure 1d) and 180 min (WPC vs. CTL $p = 0.036$, 70 W/30E vs. CTL $p = 0.009$, 50 W/50E vs. CTL $p < 0.011$, 30 W/70E $p = 0.107$; Figure 1d) post-feeding versus CTL rats. MPS levels were higher in WPC and 70 W/30E versus CTL rats 180 min post-feeding (WPC vs. CTL $p = 0.007$, 70 W/30E vs. CTL $p = 0.032$; Figure 1e), though there was no statistical differences between protein feeding groups.

Select gastrocnemius mRNAs related to skeletal muscle hypertrophy are differentially affected by protein type

While transient gene expression patterns in response to feeding provide limited information, mRNA expression

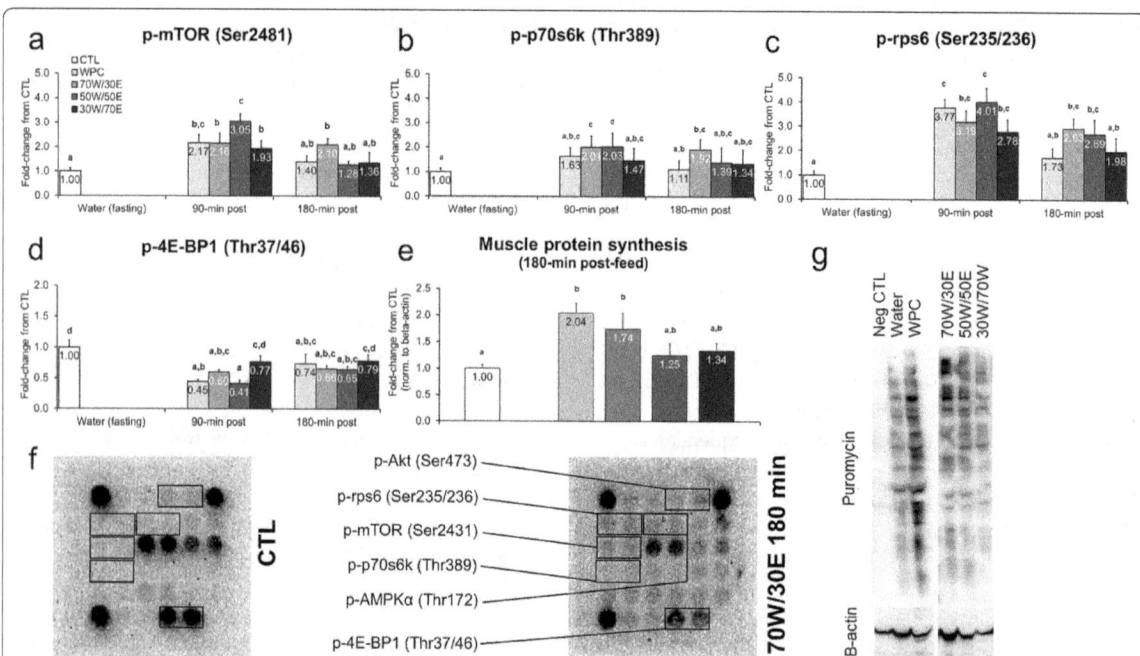

Figure 1 Effects of different protein feedings on skeletal muscle anabolism markers. Legend: Effects of each protein on gastrocnemius p-mTOR (Ser2481) (**panel a**), p-p70s6k (Thr389) (**panel b**), p-rps6 (Ser235/236) (**panel c**), p-4E-BP1 (Thr37/46) (**panel d**), and muscle protein synthesis (MPS) (**panel e**). Data are presented as means ± standard error (CTL n = 12–14 per bar, protein groups n = 6–8 per bar). One-way ANOVAs with a Fisher's LSD *post hoc* test were performed and significant between-feeding differences are represented with different superscript letters ($p < 0.05$). **Panel f**: Example digital images of Akt-mTOR substrates of CTL rats and 70 W/30E-fed rats 180 min post-gavage. **Panel g**: Representative digital images of puromycin integration into muscle protein (SUnSET determination of MPS).

patterns of anabolic genes are a putative index regarding whether or not a particular protein source may have a potential impact on long-term anabolism. MSTN mRNA increased in the 30 W/70E group versus fasting rats 90 min post-feeding (p < 0.001; Figure 2a), and 30 W/70E and 50 W/50E increased MSTN mRNA 180 min post-feeding versus CTL rats (30 W/70E p = 0.003, 50 W/50E p < 0.001; Figure 2a). Mighty/Akirin-1 mRNA, which is transcriptionally down-regulated by MSTN [31] and is related to muscle hypertrophy [32], was similar between groups 90 min post-treatment but: a) was greater in the WPC and 70 W/30E groups 180 min post-treatment compared to 50 W/50E rats (WPC vs. 50 W/50E p = 0.001, 70 W/30E vs. 50 W/50E p = 0.001; Figure 2b); and b) was greater in the WPC, 70 W/30E and 30 W/70E groups 180 min post-treatment compared to CTL rats (WPC vs. CTL p < 0.001, 70 W/30E vs. CTL p < 0.001, 30 W/70E vs. CTL p = 0.046; Figure 2b). p21Cip mRNA, which is a gene potentially related to skeletal muscle hypertrophy [33], remained similar between CTL and all protein-fed groups 90 min post-feeding (Figure 2c). However, p21Cip mRNA generally increased 3–4-fold in all protein groups 180 min post-treatment versus CTL rats and 90 min post-treatment values (WPC vs. CTL p = 0.005, 70 W/30E vs. CTL p = 0.001, 50 W/50E p < 0.001, 30 W/70E vs. CTL p = 0.004; Figure 2c). Atrogin-1 mRNA remained unaltered 90 min post-feeding in all protein groups compared to CTL rats, but increased in the 70 W/30E 180 min post-feeding versus CTL rats (p = 0.049; Figure 2d). MuRF-1 mRNA remained unaltered 90 min post-feeding in all protein groups compared to CTL rats, but was greater 180 min post-feeding in the WPC and 70 W/30E groups versus CTL rats at this time point (WPC vs. CTL p = 0.020, 70 W/30E vs. CTL p = 0.032;

Figure 2e). No between-group differences existed for IGF-1Ea expression patterns (Figure 2f).

Select gastrocnemius metabolic-related phosphoprotein and mRNAs are differentially affected by protein type

While markers of metabolic-related signaling and gene expression in response to feeding provide limited information, these markers also provide putative index regarding whether or not a particular protein source may have a potential impact on long-term metabolic alterations within skeletal muscle. At 90 min post-feeding, WPC and 70 W/30E increased p-Akt (Ser473) compared to CTL rats (WPC vs. CTL p = 0.012, 70 W/30E vs. CTL p = 0.031; Figure 3a), though this increase returned to CTL levels 180 min post-feeding. At 90 min post-treatment, 70 W/30E and 50 W/50E increased p-AMPKα (Thr172) versus CTL rats (70 W/30E vs. CTL p = 0.033, 50 W/50E vs. CTL p = 0.013; Figure 3b), and at 180 min post-treatment 70 W/30E induced a persistent elevation in p-AMPKα (Thr172) versus CTL rats (p = 0.040; Figure 3b). 70 W/30E increased PGC-1α mRNA versus CTL rats 90 min post-treatment (p = 0.002; Figure 3c) and all other protein groups at 90 min post-treatment (70 W/30E vs. WPC p = 0.038, 70 W/30E vs. 50 W/50E p = 0.001, 70 W/30E vs. 30 W/70E p = 0.039; Figure 3c). Though statistical differences existed between treatments for GLUT-4 mRNA, fold-changes between groups were modest (~30%) and there were no clear treatment effects (Figure 3d). Finally, 70 W/30E caused a 1.7-to-2.2-fold increase in CPT1B mRNA versus CTL rats 90 min (p = 0.012; Figure 3e) and 180 min post-treatment (p < 0.001; Figure 3e) as well as other protein groups at 90 min (70 W/30E vs. WPC p = 0.025, 70 W/30E vs. 50 W/50E p = 0.001, 70 W/30E vs. 30 W/70E p = 0.047; Figure 3e) and 180 min post-treatment (70 W/30E vs. WPC p = 0.001, 70 W/30E vs.

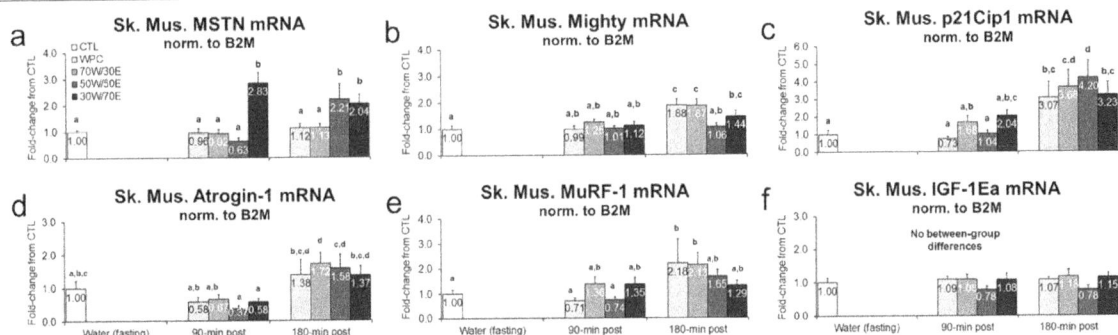

Figure 2 Effects of different proteins on post-treatment gastrocnemius hypertrophy-related mRNA expression patterns. Legend: Effects of each protein on gastrocnemius MSTN mRNA (**panel a**), Akirin-1/Mighty mRNA (**panel b**), p21Cip1 mRNA (**panel c**), Atrogin-1 mRNA (**panel d**), MuRF-1 mRNA (**panel e**), and IGF-1Ea mRNA (**panel f**). Data are presented as means ± standard error (CTL n = 12–14 per bar, protein groups n = 6–8 per bar). One-way ANOVAs with LSD *post hoc* test were performed and significant between-feeding differences are represented with different superscript letters (p < 0.05).

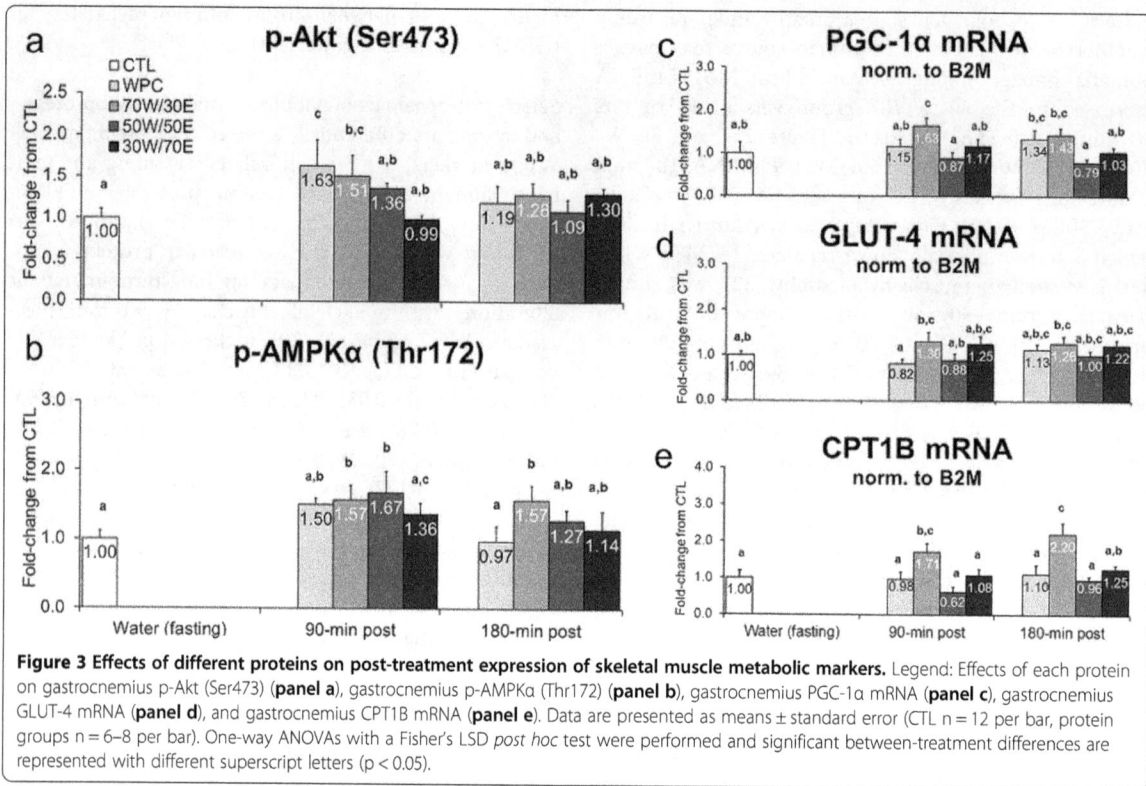

Figure 3 Effects of different proteins on post-treatment expression of skeletal muscle metabolic markers. Legend: Effects of each protein on gastrocnemius p-Akt (Ser473) (**panel a**), gastrocnemius p-AMPKα (Thr172) (**panel b**), gastrocnemius PGC-1α mRNA (**panel c**), gastrocnemius GLUT-4 mRNA (**panel d**), and gastrocnemius CPT1B mRNA (**panel e**). Data are presented as means ± standard error (CTL n = 12 per bar, protein groups n = 6–8 per bar). One-way ANOVAs with a Fisher's LSD *post hoc* test were performed and significant between-treatment differences are represented with different superscript letters (p < 0.05).

50 W/50E p < 0.001, 70 W/30E vs. 30 W/70E p = 0.005; Figure 3e).

Select lipolysis markers are differentially affected by protein type

Transient alterations in adipose tissue p-HSL and lipolytic/thermogenic gene expression patterns may provide insight into longer-term alterations that occur at the tissue level (i.e., decrements in fat mass size). Protein feeding did not alter OMAT p-HSL (Ser563) 90 min post-treatment, though WPC, 70 W/30E and 50 W/50E significantly increased this marker 3.8 and 6.5-fold, respectively, 180 min post-feeding versus CTL rats (70 W/30E vs. CTL p < 0.001, 50 W/50E vs. CTL p = 0.019; Figure 4a). Likewise, protein feeding did not alter SQ p-HSL (Ser563) 90 min post-treatment, though 70 W/30 W increased SQ p-HSL (Ser563) 3.1-fold versus CTL rats (p = 0.001; Figure 4b) and 1.9-to-4.4-fold versus all other protein groups 180 min post-treatment (70 W/30E vs. WPC p = 0.001, 70 W/30E vs. 50 W/50E p = 0.015, 70 W/30E vs. 30 W/70E p = 0.035; Figure 3e). Interestingly, 70 W/30E increased SQ cAMP 180 min post-treatment versus CTL rats (p = 0.045; Figure 4c) as well as the 30 W/70E group (p = 0.047; Figure 4c) suggesting that a high proportion of WPH in the test protein may facilitate cAMP-mediated p-HSL activation to increase

lipolysis. WPC and 70 W/30E depressed serum free fatty acids 90 min post-treatment versus CTL rats (WPC vs. CTL p = 0.012, 70 W/30E vs CTL p < 0.001; Figure 4e), but this was normalized by 180 min post-treatment. Finally, with regards to thermogenic SQ gene expression markers, 70 W/30E and 50 W/50E tended increase PGC-1α mRNA versus CTL rats 180 min post-treatment (70 W/30E vs. CTL p = 0.083, 50 W/50E vs. CTL p = 0.054; Figure 4f). Furthermore, 50 W/50E increased SQ UCP3 mRNA versus all other protein groups CTL rats 180 min post-treatment (p = 0.004–0.042; Figure 4 g).

Serum lipolysis and thermogenic hormones are minimally affected by protein type

Given that various OMAT and SQ markers of lipolysis and thermogenesis were differentially affected by different protein types, we next examined if protein feedings affected select hormone levels related to these physiological processes. There was no consistent protein feeding effect on serum catecholamines. WPC and 30 W/70E exhibited 40% lower EPI levels compared to CTL rats 90 min post-treatment (WPC vs. CTL p = 0.039, 30 W/70E vs. CTL p = 0.037; Figure 5a), and 50 W/50E exhibited 60% lower EPI levels compared to CTL rats 180 min post-treatment (p = 0.001; Figure 5a). 50 W/50E exhibited 60% lower

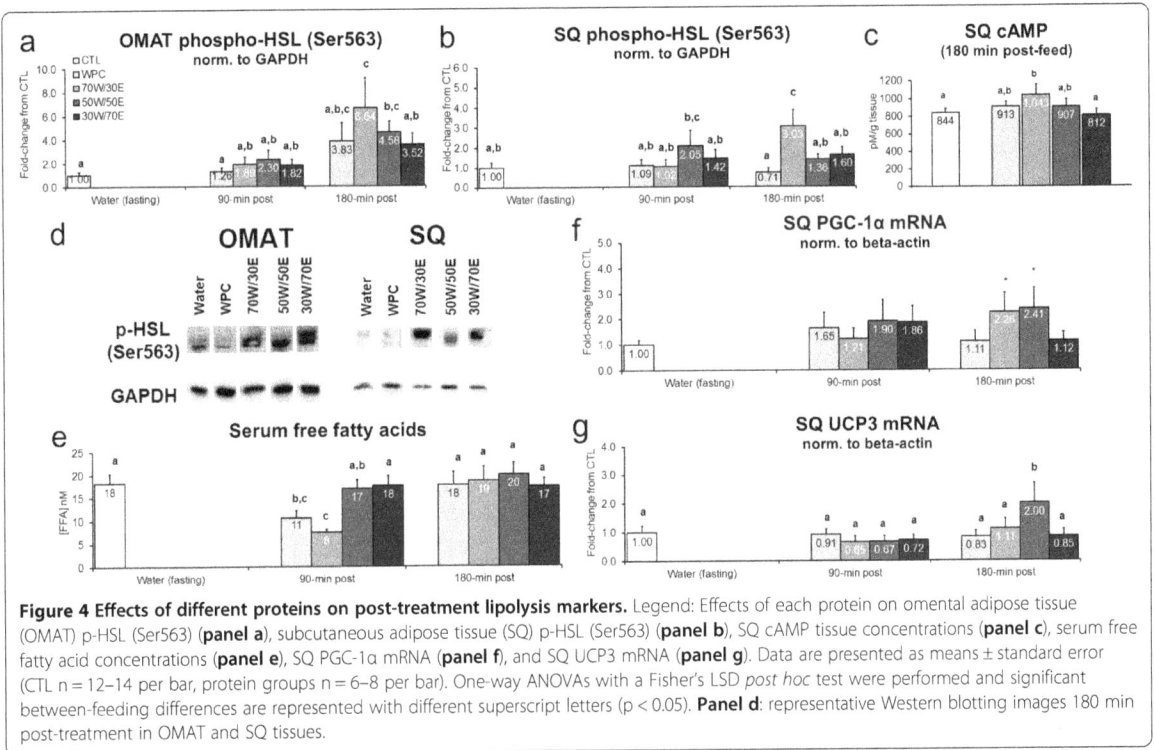

Figure 4 Effects of different proteins on post-treatment lipolysis markers. Legend: Effects of each protein on omental adipose tissue (OMAT) p-HSL (Ser563) (**panel a**), subcutaneous adipose tissue (SQ) p-HSL (Ser563) (**panel b**), SQ cAMP tissue concentrations (**panel c**), serum free fatty acid concentrations (**panel e**), SQ PGC-1α mRNA (**panel f**), and SQ UCP3 mRNA (**panel g**). Data are presented as means ± standard error (CTL n = 12–14 per bar, protein groups n = 6–8 per bar). One-way ANOVAs with a Fisher's LSD *post hoc* test were performed and significant between-feeding differences are represented with different superscript letters ($p < 0.05$). **Panel d**: representative Western blotting images 180 min post-treatment in OMAT and SQ tissues.

NorEPI values compared to compared to CTL rats 180 min post-treatment ($p = 0.006$; Figure 5b)

There was also no consistent protein feeding effect on serum T3 levels. WPC generally presented greater serum T3 levels versus other treatments 90 and 180 min post-feeding, though these values were not statistically different from fasting rats (Figure 5c). Moreover, 50 W/50E-fed rats exhibited depressed T3 levels compared to CTL rats 90 min post-feeding ($p = 0.020$; Figure 5c), though this effect was normalized by 180 min post-feeding. Similarly, 70 W/30E-fed rats presented significantly depressed T3 levels by 180 min post-feeding compared to CTL rats ($p = 0.023$; Figure 5c).

Effects of different protein feedings on hypothalamic mRNA expression patterns

Transient alterations in anorectic and orexigenic gene expression patterns could suggest that an altered satiety response occurs to different protein types. Interestingly, 70 W/30E and 30 W/70E increased hypothalamic POMC mRNA 90 min post-treatment versus CTL rats suggesting a satiety-related response may have occurred in the former groups (70 W/30E vs. CTL $p = 0.008$, 30 W/70E vs. CTL $p = 0.007$; Figure 6a). However, there was a compensatory increase in orexigenic AGRP mRNA in the 70 W/30E group 90 min post-treatment versus CTL rats ($p = 0.040$; Figure 6b). Likewise, there was a compensatory increase in

orexigenic NPY mRNA in the 30 W/70E group 90 min post-treatment versus CTL rats ($p = 0.032$; Figure 6c), and a significant increase in this marker in the 50 W/50E group 180 min post-treatment versus CTL rats ($p = 0.009$; Figure 6c). Though statistical differences existed between groups for hypothalamic LEPR mRNA, fold-changes between protein groups and CTL rats were modest and non-significant (±20–40%, $p > 0.05$; Figure 6d).

Discussion

Protein type is an important factor in acutely increasing markers of skeletal muscle anabolism

Whey and egg protein consumption has been posited to promote anabolic effects in skeletal muscle via greater post-feeding increases in serum amino acids versus other protein sources [2]. All test proteins in the current study increased the phosphorylation status of mTOR, p70s6k, and rps6 90 min post-feeding compared to CTL rats, though 70 W/30E-fed rats presented sustained elevations in phosphorylated mTOR and rps6 180 min post-feeding. These phosphorylated targets are positive effectors of MPS, and our findings are in agreement with past literature suggesting that whey and egg protein increase the phosphorylation of one or more of these intramuscular signaling markers following feeding with [19,34,20,35] or without [2,1] resistance exercise in rats and humans. However, it is intriguing that higher proportions of EPH (i.e.,

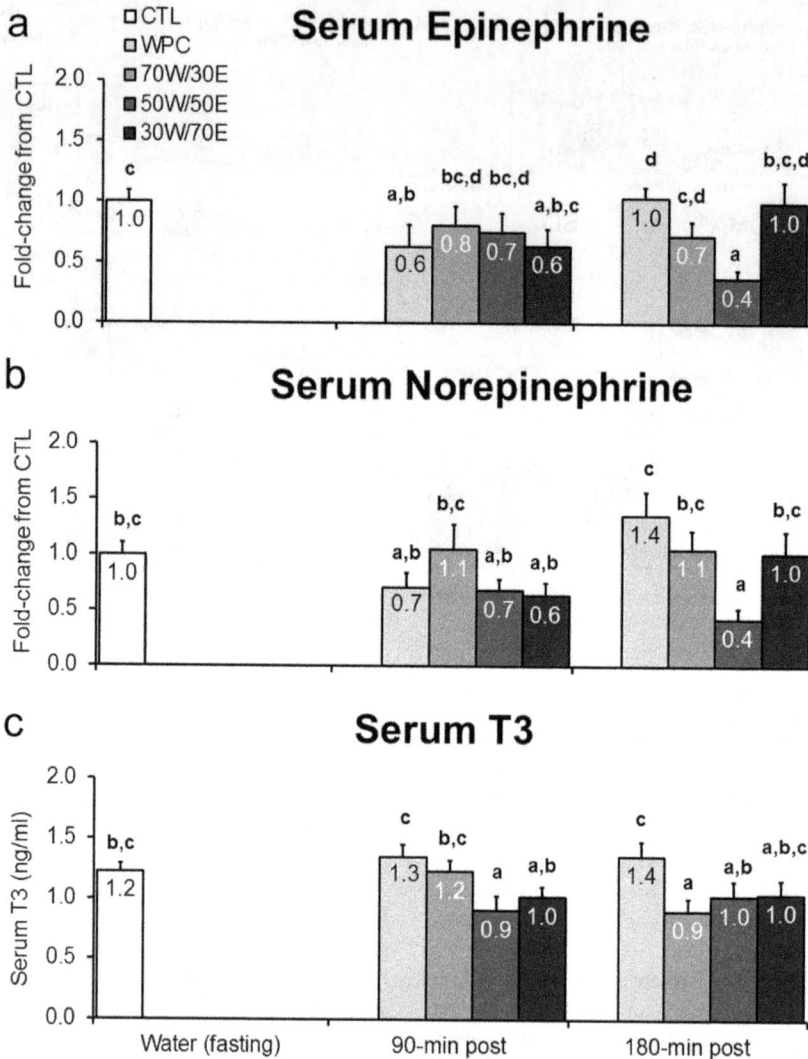

Figure 5 Effects of different proteins on post-treatment lipolytic/thermogenic hormone markers. Legend: Effects of each protein on serum epinephrine (**panel a**), norepinephrine (**panel b**), and triiodothyronine (T3) concentrations (**panel c**). Data are presented as means ± standard error (CTL n = 12–14 per bar, protein groups n = 6–8 per bar). One-way ANOVAs with a Fisher's LSD *post hoc* test were performed and significant between-treatment differences are represented with different superscript letters (p < 0.05).

50–70%) did not statistically increase MPS levels versus CTL rats. Norton et al. [1] demonstrated that a test meal containing 0.64 g of whey or egg protein similarly increases MPS 90 min post-feeding. Our study differs from the findings of Norton et al. given that: a) MPS was measured using two different methodologies; specifically we used the SUnSET method and Norton et al. used an L-^{2}H$_5$-phenylalanine tracer; b) Norton et al. measured post-feeding MPS at 90 min while we measured MPS 180 min post-feeding; and c) Norton et al. fed rats 0.64 g protein in a solid mixed-meal form while we fed rats 0.19 g of unadulterated test protein

solutions. In spite of these methodological differences, we suggest that, relative to CTL rats, a low protein dose comprised mainly of whey protein (i.e., WPC or 70 W/30E) promotes a greater post-feeding increase in MPS relative to a low dose protein solution comprised primarily of egg protein. Alternatively stated, while egg protein is a source of leucine and EAAs, it appears that whey protein is superior at stimulating MPS at lower doses in the current rodent model. While this seems contrary to the conclusions posited by Norton et al. suggesting that the high leucine content in whey and egg equally stimulate MPS, two independent human studies

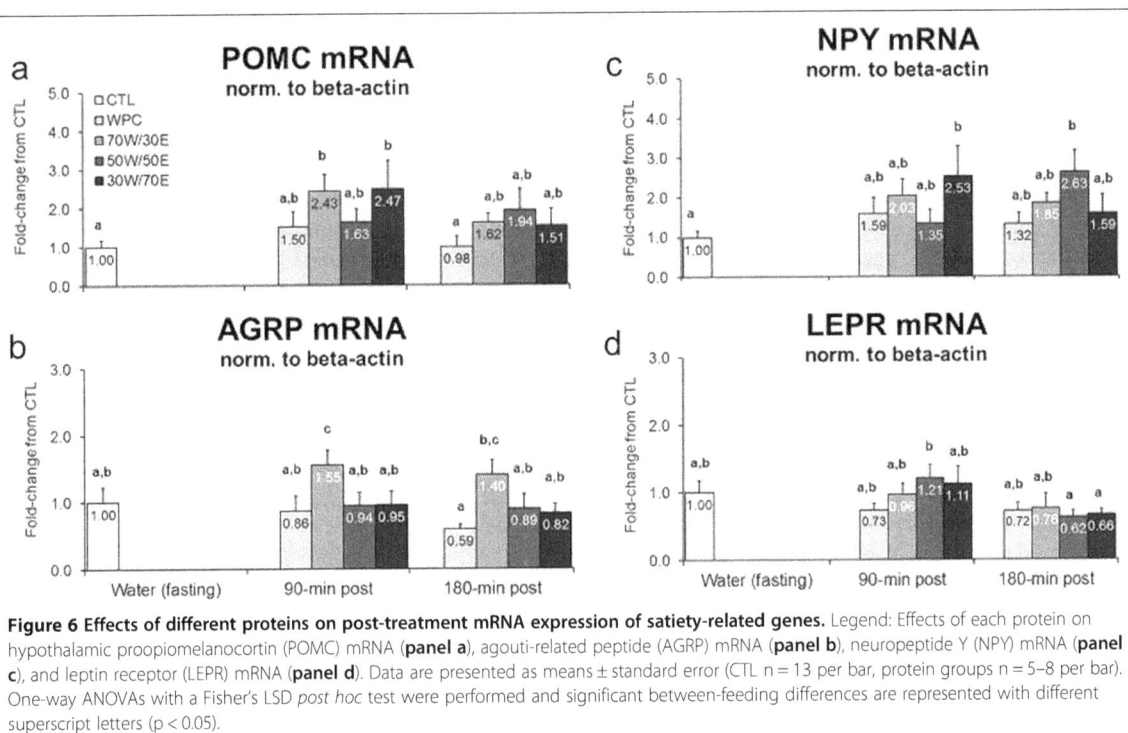

Figure 6 Effects of different proteins on post-treatment mRNA expression of satiety-related genes. Legend: Effects of each protein on hypothalamic proopiomelanocortin (POMC) mRNA (**panel a**), agouti-related peptide (AGRP) mRNA (**panel b**), neuropeptide Y (NPY) mRNA (**panel c**), and leptin receptor (LEPR) mRNA (**panel d**). Data are presented as means ± standard error (CTL n = 13 per bar, protein groups n = 5–8 per bar). One-way ANOVAs with a Fisher's LSD *post hoc* test were performed and significant between-feeding differences are represented with different superscript letters (p < 0.05).

have demonstrated that younger [36] and older subjects [37] consuming supplemental egg protein while resistance training do not experience increases in muscle mass after 8–12-week interventions. Specifically, Hida et al. [36] demonstrated that 15 g/d of egg protein supplementation in female athletes, who were engaged in a resistance training protocol, increased lean body mass by 1.5 kg, whereas a carbohydrate placebo increased lean body mass by 1.6 kg. Likewise, Iglay et al. [37] demonstrated that supplementing the diet with an additional 20 g/d of egg protein did not further increase the lean mass or skeletal muscle cross-sectional area compared to a lower protein group when both groups resistance trained for 12 weeks; of note, both groups gained roughly 1.0 kg of lean body mass.

In contrast, a recent meta-analysis examining several studies [5] clearly demonstrates that whey protein supplementation with resistance exercise is effective at increasing muscle mass in younger and older populations, and Phillips et al. [6] noted that participants engaged in 8–16 weeks of resistance exercise gain, on average, 3.0 kg of lean mass compared to 1.0 kg of lean mass gains in the placebo groups of these studies. One hypothesis deserving of future investigation is whether mammary-derived proteins, due to the inherent purpose of such proteins promoting rapid growth and development of offspring, may offer unique physiological advantages versus what can otherwise be labeled as 'nutritional protein sources' such as egg or other animal proteins. In this regard, future studies

examining why a low dose of whey protein is unique in stimulating muscle anabolism relative to other protein sources that possess a 'leucine-, BCAA-, and EAA-rich profile' are warranted.

Putative anabolic and atrogene gastrocnemius mRNA responses following different protein feedings
Akirin-1/Mighty increased approximately 90% 180 min post-feeding in the WPC and 70 W/30E groups versus CTL rats and other protein groups. Akirin-1/Mighty is a transcriptional target of MSTN that is related to controlling myotube size *in vitro* [32], and resistance exercise has been shown to transiently up-regulate Akirin-1/Mighty mRNA in rodent skeletal muscle [31]. To our knowledge, only one other recent study to date has determined that certain akirin genes are transcriptionally up-regulated in fish that were fasted 21 days and then re-fed [38]. Hence, the aforementioned study along with our current data suggests that Akirin-1/Mighty mRNA is sensitive to protein feeding, and this finding should be further examined at the mechanistic level in order to determine if whey protein affects skeletal muscle hypertrophy through increases in Akirin-1/Mighty mRNA expression.

The expression of select anabolic and catabolic-related gastrocnemius mRNAs responded differently between different treatment groups. Interestingly, higher proportions of EPH caused 90–180 min increases in MSTN mRNA versus CTL rats and/or higher proportions of whey protein.

Preliminary data in humans suggest that the consumption of fertile egg yolk powder reduces circulating MSTN levels [25]. Hence, if one or multiple putative bioactive components in egg protein extract reduce serum MSTN levels then it is possible that skeletal muscle may undergo a compensatory increase in skeletal MSTN mRNA expression to counter systemic down-regulation. Thus, while our data and other limited evidence suggests that MSTN expression is responsive to dietary egg proteins, more research is needed in order to elucidate if egg protein-induced increases in MSTN gene expression and/or signaling in skeletal muscle results in a physiological meaningful response.

All protein sources generally increased the p21Cip1 mRNA expression 180 min post-feeding compared to CTL rats suggesting that protein feeding in general regulates the expression of this gene. p21Cip1 gene expression has been theorized to promote satellite cell differentiation [39,40], though limited information suggests that p21Cip1 gene expression up-regulates protein synthesis and pathological hypertrophy in kidney epithelial cells [41]. Thus, it will be of further interest to examine if protein feeding-induced increases in skeletal muscle p21Cip1 gene expression are related to postmitotic skeletal muscle protein synthesis mechanisms.

Atrogin-1 was up-regulated in 70 W/30E-fed rats 180 min post-feeding versus CTL rats. Similarly, MuRF-1 was up-regulated in WPC-fed and 70 W/30E-fed rats 180 min post-feeding versus CTL rats. Our finding that test solutions containing predominantly whey protein increase postprandial atrogene (atrogin-1 and MuRF-1) mRNA expression is intriguing given that amino acids are thought to be anti-catabolic [42]. However, ingesting smaller protein ingestion boluses (10–20 g) have been reported to increase MuRF-1 mRNA in human skeletal muscle after resistance exercise versus a larger bolus (40 g) [43]. Thus, our finding that protein ingestion increases the mRNA expression of select atrogenes may represent a stimulation of greater muscle protein turnover rather than an increase in atrophic mechanisms.

Protein source and type as important factors in acutely affecting markers of skeletal muscle metabolism and reduced muscle catabolism

Higher proportions of whey protein in the test solutions (i.e., WPC and 70 W/30E) increased Akt phosphorylation (Ser473) 90 min post-feeding versus CTL rats. Tissue Akt phosphorylation at the Ser473 residues is a common readout for insulin signaling and sensitivity [44], and whey protein feeding following resistance exercise in humans has been shown to increase Akt phosphorylation at the Ser473 residue [19,20]. Our findings are also in partial agreement with West et al. [45] who demonstrated in humans that an EAA bolus increases skeletal muscle Akt phosphorylation (Ser473) 60 min

after feeding. As noted above, however, WPC and EPH are also a rich source of EAAs. Thus, we speculate that the increase in Akt phosphorylation in the WPC and 70 W/30E groups may have been due to the superior ability of whey protein in stimulating insulin secretion and, thus, downstream insulin signaling in skeletal muscle. While we did not measure serum insulin responses in the current study, we have previously shown that WPH feeding to rats causes a robust (>2-fold) rise in insulin 60 min post-feeding [23]. Hence, foods containing a higher proportion of whey protein may stimulate greater intramuscular insulin signaling, and future research should continue to examine if WPC or WPH feeding in acute and long-term settings can enhance insulin sensitivity in insulin-resistant subjects.

Interestingly, 70 W/30E feeding caused a 63% increase in skeletal muscle PGC-1α mRNA expression versus CTL rats, as well as a significant increase in this gene relative to all other groups 90 min post-treatment. Furthermore, rats fed 70 W/30E exhibited a significant increase in skeletal muscle CPT1B mRNA 90- and 180 min post-feeding; this being a gene which is involved with fatty acid transport to the mitochondria for fuel oxidation. Whey protein isolate has been shown to stimulate a further increase in PGC-1α mRNA expression in human skeletal muscle 6 h following cycling [46]. However, to our knowledge, this is the first study to demonstrate that a test protein containing chiefly WPH can increase post-feeding skeletal muscle PGC-1α mRNA expression independent of exercise. We posit that one potential mechanism whereby WPH stimulates the mRNA expression of PGC-1α and CPT1B is through the stimulation of AMPK activity (Figure 3a). To this end, Canto et al. [47] have demonstrated that AMPK activation increases the expression of these two genes, and this would support the hypothesis that whey protein, in particular WPH, can stimulate oxidative metabolism and mitochondrial biogenesis with long-term supplementation. This hypothesis is not unfounded given recent evidence that prolonged whey protein feeding has been shown to increase mitochondrial content and respiration in the brain [48] and liver [49]. Therefore, more mechanistic studies should examine if WPH administration increases the post-feeding expression of mitochondrial-related genes via AMPK activation and/or other mechanisms.

Effects of different proteins on post-feeding markers of lipolysis

As mentioned prior, whey protein ingestion exerts positive effects on body composition and fat mass [14,5]. Furthermore, and as mentioned previously, WPH supplementation during exercise may provide added benefit to reducing body fat versus intact/native protein sources. Despite a transient 90 min post-feeding depression in serum FFAs with 70 W/30E feeding versus CTL rats and other protein groups, 50–70% WPH protein feedings increased select markers of adipose tissue lipolysis and thermogenesis 180 min post-feeding. For instance, rats fed 70 W/30E presented increases in SQ cAMP levels as well as OMAT and SQ p-HSL (Ser563). Likewise, rats that were fed higher proportions of WPH (e.g., 70 W/30E or 50 W/50E) exhibited increases in SQ PGC-1α and UCP3 mRNA expression levels which are putative markers of adipose tissue thermogenesis [50]. Finally, 70 W/30E increased gastrocnemius CPT1B mRNA which could be suggestive of a potential long-term enhancement in fatty acid transport to the mitochondria for oxidation. Conversely, circulating catecholamine levels in response to feeding higher proportions of WPH exhibited no discernable effects. These findings are difficult to reconcile as we have previously reported that WPH increases serum EPI 30 min post-feeding versus WPC-fed and CTL rats [18]. Therefore, the 180-min post-feeding increase in lipolysis markers in the current study may be due to an earlier increase in catecholamines (i.e., within 60 min of feeding) which was not captured due to sampling time points and/or due to WPH-borne bioactives that selectively act upon adipose tissue to stimulate lipolytic mechanisms.

Of note, we measured serum T3 given that it is a well-known stimulator of thermogenesis and cellular respiration. With regards to adipose tissue lipolysis, T3 has been shown to increase adipocyte beta-adrenergic receptor which, in turn, increases lipolytic capabilities over longer-term periods [51]. Notwithstanding, there was no clear protein feeding effect on serum T3 depression, and T3 values did not seem to parallel the increased lipolysis and thermogenesis markers in rats fed 70 W/30E or 50 W/50E which refutes the potential role of thyroid hormones in facilitating this effect.

One final mechanistic explanation as to how higher proportions of WPH increased lipolysis markers is through potential tricarboxylic acid (TCA) cycle modulation. To this end, a recent study by Lillefosse et al. [52] demonstrated that chronic whey protein feeding to obese-prone rodents significantly reduced fat mass gain in response to concomitant high fat feeding. The authors suggested that whey protein feeding increases the urinary excretion of TCA substrates which are stimulators of fatty acid synthesis [53]. Alternatively stated, the ability of WPH to 'extract' TCA cycle intermediates from adipose tissue during the post-feeding period may place adipose tissue in a catabolic state thereby initiating lipolysis-related mechanisms. This is not unfounded, as we have previously noted that WPH significantly increases circulating TCA intermediates (i.e., citrate, succinate, fumarate and malate) 60 min post-feeding versus WPC-fed rats (*supplementary data* in [18]). Hence, more research is needed regarding if the depletion of TCA cycle intermediates within adipose tissue is linked to the WPH-induced lipolysis response.

Effects of different proteins on post-feeding markers of satiety

Sousa et al. [54] recently posited that, regardless of protein source, amino acids may reduce appetite via an increase in gut hormone secretion, an increase in anorexigenic POMC gene expression in the hypothalamus, and/or a reduction in orexigenic NPY gene expression in the hypothalamus. 70 W/30E and 30 W/70E increased hypothalamic POMC mRNA expression patterns 90 min post-feeding; this being a marker that favors satiety signaling in the hypothalamus [55]. However, there was a compensatory increase in the orexigenic AGRP transcript in rats fed a high proportion of WPH. Furthermore, some protein feedings induced an increased expression of hypothalamic NPY mRNA versus CTL rats which, again, suggests a potential orexigenic versus satiety response. Therefore, our mixed findings suggest that two possibilities may exist including: a) the amount of total protein fed to rats, while beneficial in stimulating skeletal muscle anabolism and adipose tissue lipolysis, was not entirely effective at initiating a satiety response; and/or b) hypothalamic signaling is so tightly regulated that a post-feeding increase in anorectic genes is countered with a compensatory increase in orexigenic genes.

Finally, it should be noted that the post-feeding effects of each protein on hypothalamic LEPR mRNA expression patterns was of considerable interest due to the central role of leptin receptor signaling in satiety. Thus, we initially hypothesized that protein-feeding induced alterations in LEPR mRNA expression may be a potential culprit in initiating longer-term body composition alterations through enhanced satiety mechanisms that have been reported to previously occur with chronic protein supplementation. To this end, McAllan et al. [11] recently performed a long-term rodent feeding study whereby C57BL/6 J mice were fed a high fat diet (HFD, 45% energy as fat) enriched with either 20% energy as casein or whey protein isolate. HFD feeding increased the hypothalamic mRNA expression of LEPR; an effect which the authors suggest may be a hallmark feature of hyperphagia and obesity development. However, mice that were co-fed whey protein isolate with the HFD presented a significant reduction in hypothalamic LEPR mRNA expression. Notwithstanding, we demonstrated no noticeable between-group differences in LEPR mRNA expression patterns which suggests that the hypothalamic expression gene is not appreciably altered after one feeding and/or LEPR gene expression may be indiscriminately regulated more so by amino acid concentration alone as opposed to specific bioactive peptides.

Conclusions

We have demonstrated that protein type provide uniquely different physiological responses over a transient postprandial time course. Specifically, and seemingly irrespective of protein type, administering higher concentrations of whey versus egg protein to healthy rodents causes: a) a greater anabolic response in rodents with regards to post-feeding MPS compared to a fasting condition; and b) an increase in intramuscular insulin sensitivity markers (i.e., Akt signaling markers and transient increases in PGC-1α mRNA expression patterns). Alternatively, the administration of higher concentrations of WPH versus EPH increases select markers of post-feeding lipolysis 3 h post-feeding. Of note, while we make assertions that whey protein forms may be more beneficial in facilitating increases in muscle mass and fat loss compared to egg protein per the current findings, the acute nature of this study is a pervading limitation of these hypotheses. Likewise, while several of tissue markers were statistically altered in response to different protein feedings, more research is needed comparing whey versus egg protein supplementation on longer-term physiologically-relevant outcomes (i.e., increases in muscle mass, decreases in fat mass, and/or alterations in satiety as suggested by our transient findings reported herein). Therefore, further research is this nutraceutical arena is warranted with regards to how protein source and type (i.e., native versus hydrolyzed), and varying combinations thereof may affect these physiological parameters in over more chronic periods and in more clinical-based populations.

Additional file

Additional file 1: Figure S1 Preliminary testing different WPC doses on post-feeding gastrocnemius phosphorylated mTOR markers and muscle protein synthesis 90 min post-treatment. Legend: data are presented as means ± standard error [CTL n = 8 per bar except for MPS where n = 3 per bar, WPC groups n = 2–3 per bar]. One-way ANOVAs with a Fisher's LSD *post hoc* test was performed; * indicates significance versus water (fasting) rats (p < 0.05). These data show that a low dose of WPC (0.19 g which is 10 human eq. g) is just as effective at stimulating most mTOR substrates and MPS levels versus moderate (0.37 g which is 19 human eq. g) and high (0.93 g which is 19 human eq. g) WPC doses. The relatively low dose (0.19 g which is 10 human eq. g) was subsequently employed for WPC, 70 W/30E, 50 W/50E and 30 W/70E comparisons.

Competing interests
Besides C.M.L., none of the authors have non-finacial and/or financial competing interests. C.M.L. is employed by 4Life, but he intellectually contributed to study design and data write-up. Therefore, all co-authors agreed that his intellectual input into this project warranted co-authorship.

Authors' contributions
CBM, CDF, BSF, CAP, JCH, JSM, CML and MDR: This person has made substantial contributions to conception and design, or acquisition of data, or analysis and interpretation of data. CBM, CML and MDR: This person primarily was involved in drafting the manuscript or revising it critically for important intellectual content. CBM, CDF, BSF, CAP, JCH, JSM, CML and MDR: This person gave final approval of the version to be published. CBM, CDF, BSF, CAP, JCH, JSM, CML and MDR: This person agrees to be accountable for all aspects of the work in ensuring that questions related to the accuracy or integrity of any part of the work are appropriately investigated and resolved. All authors read and approved the final manuscript.

Acknowledgements
The authors thank Dr. David Pascoe and Dr. Andreas Kavazis for intellectual input.

Financial Support
Funding from 4Life Research USA, LLC was used to fund the direct costs of this study, C.A.P.'s graduate assistant stipend, undergraduate technical help, and publication costs of these data.

Author details
[1]School of Kinesiology, Molecular and Applied Sciences Laboratory, Auburn University, 301 Wire Road, Office 286, Auburn, AL 36849, USA. [2]4Life Research USA, LLC, Sandy, UT, USA.

References
1. Norton LE, Wilson GJ, Layman DK, Moulton CJ, Garlick PJ. Leucine content of dietary proteins is a determinant of postprandial skeletal muscde protein synthesis in adult rats. Nutr Metab. 2012;9(1):67. doi:10.1186/1743-7075-9-67.
2. Norton LE, Layman DK, Bunpo P, Anthony TG, Brana DV, Garlick PJ. The leucine content of a complete meal directs peak activation but not duration of skeletal muscle protein synthesis and mammalian target of rapamycin signaling in rats. J Nutr. 2009;139(6):1103–9. doi:10.3945/jn.108.103853.
3. Moore DR, Tang JE, Burd NA, Rerecich T, Tarnopolsky MA, Phillips SM. Differential stimulation of myofibrillar and sarcoplasmic protein synthesis with protein ingestion at rest and after resistance exercise. J Physiol. 2009;587(Pt 4):897–904. doi:10.1113/jphysiol.2008.164087.
4. Witard OC, Jackman SR, Breen L, Smith K, Selby A, Tipton KD. Myofibrillar muscle protein synthesis rates subsequent to a meal in response to increasing doses of whey protein at rest and after resistance exercise. Am J Clin Nutr. 2014;99(1):86–95. doi:10.3945/ajcn.112.055517.
5. Miller PE, Alexander DD, Perez V. Effects of whey protein and resistance exercise on body composition: a meta-analysis of randomized controlled trials. J Am Coll Nutr. 2014;33(2):163–75. doi:10.1080/07315724.2013.875365.
6. Phillips SM, Tang JE, Moore DR. The role of milk- and soy-based protein in support of muscle protein synthesis and muscle protein accretion in young and elderly persons. J Am Coll Nutr. 2009;28(4):343–54.
7. Hulmi JJ, Lockwood CM, Stout JR. Effect of protein/essential amino acids and resistance training on skeletal muscle hypertrophy: A case for whey protein. Nutr Metab. 2010;7:51. doi:10.1186/1743-7075-7-51.
8. Sukkar SG, Vaccaro A, Ravera GB, Borrini C, Gradaschi R, Massa Sacchi-Nemours A, et al. Appetite control and gastrointestinal hormonal behavior (CCK, GLP-1, PYY 1–36) following low doses of a whey protein-rich nutraceutic. Mediterr J Nutr Metab. 2013;6:259–66. doi:10.1007/s12349-013-0121-7.
9. Diepvens K, Haberer D, Westerterp-Plantenga M. Different proteins and biopeptides differently affect satiety and anorexigenic/orexigenic hormones in healthy humans. Int J Obes (Lond). 2008;32(3):510–8. doi:10.1038/sj.ijo.0803758.
10. Luhovyy BL, Akhavan T, Anderson GH. Whey proteins in the regulation of food intake and satiety. J Am Coll Nutr. 2007;26(6):704S–12S.
11. McAllan L, Keane D, Schellekens H, Roche HM, Korpela R, Cryan JF, et al. Whey protein isolate counteracts the effects of a high-fat diet on energy intake and hypothalamic and adipose tissue expression of energy balance-related genes. Br J Nutr. 2013;110(11):2114–26. doi:10.1017/S0007114513001396.
12. Pilvi TK, Storvik M, Louhelainen M, Merasto S, Korpela R, Mervaala EM. Effect of dietary calcium and dairy proteins on the adipose tissue gene expression profile in diet-induced obesity. J Nutrigenet Nutrigenomics. 2008;1(5):240–51. doi:10.1159/000151238.
13. Pilvi TK, Korpela R, Huttunen M, Vapaatalo H, Mervaala EM. High-calcium diet with whey protein attenuates body-weight gain in high-fat-fed C57Bl/6 J mice. Br J Nutr. 2007;98(5):900–7. doi:10.1017/S0007114507764760.
14. Frestedt JL, Zenk JL, Kuskowski MA, Ward LS, Bastian ED. A whey-protein supplement increases fat loss and spares lean muscle in obese subjects: a randomized human clinical study. Nutr Metab. 2008;5:8. doi:10.1186/1743-7075-5-8.
15. Halton TL, Hu FB. The effects of high protein diets on thermogenesis, satiety and weight loss: a critical review. J Am Coll Nutr. 2004;23(5):373–85.
16. Calbet JA, MacLean DA. Plasma glucagon and insulin responses depend on the rate of appearance of amino acids after ingestion of different protein solutions in humans. J Nutr. 2002;132(8):2174–82.
17. Madureira AR, Tavares T, Gomes AM, Pintado ME, Malcata FX. Invited review: physiological properties of bioactive peptides obtained from whey proteins. J Dairy Sci. 2010;93(2):437–55. doi:10.3168/jds. 2009-2566.

18. Roberts MD, Cruthirds CL, Lockwood CM, Pappan K, Childs TE, Company JM, et al. Comparing serum responses to acute feedings of an extensively hydrolyzed whey protein concentrate versus a native whey protein concentrate in rats: a metabolomics approach. Appl Physiol, Nutr Metab =Physiologie appliquee, nutrition et metabolisme. 2014;39(2):158–67. doi:10.1139/apnm–2013–0148.

19. Kakigi R, Yoshihara T, Ozaki H, Ogura Y, Ichinoseki-Sekine N, Kobayashi H, et al. Whey protein intake after resistance exercise activates mTOR signaling in a dose-dependent manner in human skeletal muscle. Eur J Appl Physiol. 2014;114(4):735–42. doi:10.1007/s00421–013–2812–7.

20. Reitelseder S, Agergaard J, Doessing S, Helmark IC, Lund P, Kristensen NB, et al. Whey and casein labeled with L-[1–13C] leucine and muscle protein synthesis: effect of resistance exercise and protein ingestion. Am J Physiol Endocrinol Metab. 2011;300(1):E231–42. doi:10.1152/ajpendo.00513.2010.

21. Morifuji M, Koga J, Kawanaka K, Higuchi M. Branched-chain amino acid-containing dipeptides, identified from whey protein hydrolysates, stimulate glucose uptake rate in L6 myotubes and isolated skeletal muscles. J Nutr Sci Vitaminol. 2009;55(1):81–6.

22. Gaudel C, Nongonierrma AB, Maher S, Flynn S, Krause M, Murray BA, et al. A whey protein hydrolysate promotes insulinotropic activity in a clonal pancreatic beta-cell line and enhances glycemic function in ob/ob mice. J Nutr. 2013;143(7):1109–14. doi:10.3945/jn.113.174912.

23. Toedebusch RG, Childs TE, Hamilton SR, Crowley JR, Booth FW, Roberts MD. Postprandial leucine and insulin responses and toxicological effects of a novel whey protein hydrolysate-based supplement in rats. J Int Soc Sports Nutr. 2012;9(1):24. doi:10.1186/1550–2783–9–24.

24. Campbell B, Kreider RB, Ziegenfuss T, La Bounty P, Roberts M, Burke D, et al. International society of sports nutrition position stand: protein and exercise. International Society. 2007;4:8. doi:10.1186/1550–2783–4–8.

25. Colker C. Effect on serum myostatin levels of high-grade handled fertile egg yolk powder (Conference abstract). J Am Coll Nutr. 2009;28 (3).

26. Vander Wal JS, Marth JM, Khosla P, Jen KL, Dhuranthar NV. Short-term effect of eggs on satiety in overweight and obese subjects. J Am Coll Nutr. 2005;24(6):510–5.

27. Vander Wal JS, Gupta A, Khosla P, Dhuranthar NV. Egg breakfast enhances weight loss. Int J Obes (Lond). 2008;32(10):1545–51. doi:10.1038/ijo.2008.130.

28. Reagan-Shaw S, Nihal M, Ahmad N. Dose translation from animal to human studies revisited. FASEB J. 2008;22(3):659–61. doi:10.1096/fj.07–9574LSF.

29. Goodman CA, Hornberger TA. Measuring protein synthesis with sunset: a valid alternative to traditional techniques? Exerc Sport Sci Rev. 2013;41 (2):107–15. doi:10.1097/JES.0b013e3182798a95.

30. Roberts MD, Gilpin L, Parker KE, Childs TE, Will MJ, Booth FW. Dopamine D1 receptor modulation in nucleus accumbens lowers voluntary wheel running in rats bred to run high distances. Physiol Behav. 2012;105(3):661–8. doi:10.1016/j.physbeh.2011.09.024.

31. MacKenzie MG, Hamilton DL, Pepin M, Patton A, Baar K. Inhibition of myostatin signaling through Notch activation following acute resistance exercise. PLoS One. 2013;8(7):e68743. doi:10.1371/journal.pone.0068743.

32. Mobley CB, Fox CD, Ferguson BS, Amin RH, Dalbo VJ, Baier S, et al. L-leucine, beta-hydroxy-beta-methylbutyric acid (HMB) and creatine monohydrate prevent myostatin-induced Akirin-1/Mighty mRNA down-regulation and myotube atrophy. J Int Soc Sports Nutr. 2014;11:38. doi:10.1186/1550–2783–11–38.

33. Roberts MD, Dalbo VJ, Kerksick CM. Postexercise myogenic gene expression: are human findings lost during translation? Exerc Sport Sci Rev. 2011;39(4):206–11. doi:10.1097/JES.0b013e31822dad1f.

34. Farnfield MM, Carey KA, Gran P, Trenerry MK, Cameron-Smith D. Whey protein ingestion activates mTOR-dependent signalling after resistance exercise in young men: a double-blinded randomized controlled trial. Nutrients. 2009;1(2):263–75. doi:10.3390/nu1020263.

35. Farnfield MM, Breen L, Carey KA, Garnham A, Cameron-Smith D. Activation of mTOR signalling in young and old human skeletal muscle in response to combined resistance exercise and whey protein ingestion. Applied physiology, nutrition, and metabolism =. Physiol Appl Nutr Metab. 2012;37(1):21–30. doi:10.1139/h11–132.

36. Hida A, Hasegawa Y, Mekata Y, Usuda M, Masuda Y, Kawano H, et al. Effects of egg white protein supplementation on muscle strength and serum free amino acid concentrations. Nutrients. 2012;4(10):1504–17. doi:10.3390/nu4101504.

37. Iglay HB, Apolzan JW, Gerrard DE, Eash JK, Anderson JC, Campbell WW. Moderately increased protein intake predominately from egg sources does not influence whole body, regional, or muscle composition responses to resistance training in older people. J Nutr Health Aging. 2009;13(2):108–14.

38. Macqueen DJ, Kristjansson BK, Johnston IA. Salmonid genomes have a remarkably expanded akirin family, coexpressed with genes from conserved pathways governing skeletal muscle growth and catabolism. Physiol Genomics. 2010;42(1):134–48. doi:10.1152/physiolgenomics.00045.2010.

39. Hawke TJ, Jiang N, Garry DJ. Absence of p21CIP rescues myogenic progenitor cell proliferative and regenerative capacity in Foxk1 null mice. J Biol Chem. 2003;278(6):4015–20. doi:10.1074/jbc.M209200200.

40. Hawke TJ, Meeson AP, Jiang N, Graham S, Hutcheson K, DiMaio JM, et al. p21 is essential for normal myogenic progenitor cell function in regenerating skeletal muscle. Am J Physiol Cell Physiol. 2003;285(5):C1019–27. doi:10.1152/ajpcell.00055.2003.

41. Fan YP, Weiss RH. Exogenous attenuation of p21 (Waf1/Cip1) decreases mesangial cell hypertrophy as a result of hyperglycemia and IGF-1. J Am Soc Nephrol: JASN. 2004;15(3):575–84.

42. Herningtyas EH, Okimura Y, Handayaningsih AE, Yamamoto D, Maki T, Iida K, et al. Branched-chain amino acids and arginine suppress MaFbx/atrogin-1 mRNA expression via mTOR pathway in C2C12 cell line. Biochim Biophys Acta. 2008;1780(10):1115–20. doi:10.1016/j.bbagen.2008.06.004.

43. Areta JL, Burke LM, Ross ML, Camera DM, West DW, Broad EM, et al. Timing and distribution of protein ingestion during prolonged recovery from resistance exercise alters myofibrillar protein synthesis. J Physiol. 2013;591(Pt 9):2319–31. doi:10.1113/jphysiol.2012.244897.

44. Hojlund K, Glintborg D, Andersen NR, Birk JB, Treebak JT, Frosig C, et al. Impaired insulin-stimulated phosphorylation of Akt and AS160 in skeletal muscle of women with polycystic ovary syndrome is reversed by pioglitazone treatment. Diabetes. 2008;57(2):357–66. doi:10.2337/db07–0706.

45. West DW, Burd NA, Coffey VG, Baker SK, Burke LM, Hawley JA, et al. Rapid aminoacidemia enhances myofibrillar protein synthesis and anabolic intramuscular signaling responses after resistance exercise. Am J Clin Nutr. 2011;94(3):795–803. doi:10.3945/ajcn.111.013722.

46. Hill KM, Stathis CG, Grinfeld E, Hayes A, McAinch AJ. Co-ingestion of carbohydrate and whey protein isolates enhance PGC-1alpha mRNA expression: a randomised, single blind, cross over study. J Int Soc Sports Nutr. 2013;10(1):8. doi:10.1186/1550–2783–10–8.

47. Canto C, Gerhart-Hines Z, Feige JN, Lagouge M, Noriega L, Milne JC, et al. AMPK regulates energy expenditure by modulating NAD+ metabolism and SIRT1 activity. Nat. 2009;458(7241):1056–60. doi:10.1038/nature07813.

48. Shertzer HG, Krishan M, Genter MB. Dietary whey protein stimulates mitochondrial activity and decreases oxidative stress in mouse female brain. Neurosci Lett. 2013;548:159–64. doi:10.1016/j.neulet.2013.05.061.

49. Shertzer HG, Woods SE, Krishan M, Genter MB, Pearson KJ. Dietary whey protein lowers the risk for metabolic disease in mice fed a high-fat diet. J Nutr. 2011;141(4):582–7. doi:10.3945/jn.110.133736.

50. Bostrom P, Wu J, Jedrychowski MP, Korde A, Ye L, Lo JC, et al. A PGC1-alpha-dependent myokine that drives brown-fat-like development of white fat and thermogenesis. Nat. 2012;481(7382):463–8. doi:10.1038/nature10777.

51. Fain JN, Coronel EC, Beauchamp MJ, Bahouth SW. Expression of leptin and beta 3-adrenergic receptors in rat adipose tissue in altered thyroid states. Biochem J. 1997;322(Pt 1):145–50.

52. Lillefosse HH, Clausen MR, Yde CC, Ditlev DB, Zhang X, Du ZY, et al. Urinary loss of tricarboxylic Acid cycle intermediates as revealed by metabolomics studies: an underlying mechanism to reduce lipid accretion by whey protein ingestion? J Proteome Res. 2014;13(5):2560–70. doi:10.1021/pr500039t.

53. Martin DB, Vagelos PR. The mechanism of tricarboxylic acid cycle regulation of fatty acid synthesis. J Biol Chem. 1962;237:178/–92.

54. Sousa GT, Lira FS, Rosa JC, de Oliveira EP, Oyama LM, Santos RV, et al. Dietary whey protein lessens several risk factors for metabolic diseases: a review. Lipids Health Dis. 2012;11:67. doi:10.1186/1476–511X–11–67.

55. Mizuno TM, Kleopoulos SP, Bergen HT, Roberts JL, Priest CA, Mobbs CV. Hypothalamic pro-opiomelanocortin mRNA is reduced by fasting and [corrected] in ob/ob and db/db mice, but is stimulated by leptin. Diabetes. 1998;47(2):294–7.

## 2

Combined L-citrulline and glutathione supplementation increases the concentration of markers indicative of nitric oxide synthesis

Sarah McKinley-Barnard[1], Tom Andre[1], Masahiko Morita[2] and Darryn S. Willoughby[1*]

Abstract

Background: Nitric oxide (NO) is endogenously synthesized from L-arginine and L-citrulline. Due to its effects on nitric oxide synthase (NOS), reduced glutathione (GSH) may protect against the oxidative reduction of NO. The present study determined the effectiveness of L-citrulline and/or GSH on markers indicative of NO synthesis in *in vivo* conditions with rodents and humans and also in an *in vitro* condition.

Methods: In phase one, human umbilical vein endothelial cells (HUVECs) were treated with either 0.3 mM L-citrulline, 1 mM GSH (Setria®) or a combination of each at 0.3 mM. In phase two, Sprague–Dawley rats (8 weeks old) were randomly assigned to 3 groups and received either purified water, L-citrulline (500 mg/kg/day), or a combination of L-citrulline (500 mg/kg/day) and GSH (50 mg/kg/day) by oral gavage for 3 days. Blood samples were collected and plasma NOx (nitrite + nitrate) assessed. In phase three, resistance-trained males were randomly assigned to orally ingest either cellulose placebo (2.52 g/day), L-citrulline (2 g/day), GSH (1 g/day), or L-citrulline (2 g/day) + GSH (200 mg/day) for 7 days, and then perform a resistance exercise session involving 3 sets of 10-RM involving the elbow flexors. Venous blood was obtained and used to assess plasma cGMP, nitrite, and NOx.

Results: In phase one, nitrite levels in cells treated with L-citrulline and GSH were significantly greater than control ($p < 0.05$). In phase two, plasma NOx with L-citrulline + GSH was significantly greater than control and L-citrulline ($p < 0.05$). In phase three, plasma cGMP was increased, but not significantly ($p > 0.05$). However, nitrite and NOx for L-citrulline + GSH were significantly greater at 30 min post-exercise when compared to placebo ($p < 0.05$).

Conclusions: Combining L-citrulline with GSH augments increases in nitrite and NOx levels during *in vitro* and *in vivo* conditions.

Keywords: Nitric oxide, L-citrulline, L-arginine, Glutathione, Resistance exercise

Introduction

Also known as endothelium-derived relaxing factor (EDRF), nitric oxide (NO) is biosynthesized endogenously from L-arginine and oxygen, by various nitric oxide synthase (NOS) enzymes and by reduction of inorganic nitrate [1]. Cell types containing NOS have been demonstrated to be able to reutilize L-citrulline, the byproduct of NO synthesis, to L-arginine by the arginine-citrulline cycle [2]. Nitric oxide is a gaseous signaling molecule which activates soluble guanylate cyclase (sGC) in smooth muscle

cells, thereby catalyzing cyclic guanosine monophosphate (cGMP) synthesis. Intracellular cGMP serves as a cellular messenger and plays a role in a variety of biological processes, and in human blood vessels, results in vasodilation [3]. Cell types containing NOS have been demonstrated to be able to reutilize L-citrulline, the byproduct of NO synthesis, to L-arginine by the arginine-citrulline cycle [2]. An elevation in plasma L-arginine has been shown to improve endothelial function because the vascular endothelium uses NO to signal the surrounding smooth muscle to relax, thus resulting in vasodilation and increasing blood flow [4]. During exercise, vasodilation occurs as a result of various intracellular events, including the production and release of NO. However, it has recently been shown that

* Correspondence: darryn_willoughby@baylor.edu
[1]Department of Health, Human Performance, and Recreation, Baylor University, Exercise and Biochemical Nutritional Lab, 76798 Waco, TX, USA
Full list of author information is available at the end of the article

seven days of oral L-arginine supplementation at 12 g/day, while effective in elevating plasma L-arginine and NO metabolites nitrite and nitrate (NOx) after exercise, was ineffective at increasing blood flow during exercise [5].

L-citrulline has been indicated to be a second NO donor in the NOS-dependent pathway, since it can be converted to L-arginine [6]. Dietary L-citrulline supplementation has shown conflicting results regarding its effectiveness at improving exercise performance [7, 8]. Moreover, results showing favorable effects in exercise performance [8] did not assess NO status; therefore, this response cannot be related to an improvement in exercise performance. The importance of L-citrulline towards ergogenic support is based on the premise that L-citrulline is not subject to pre-systemic elimination and, consequently, could be a more efficient way to elevate extracellular levels of L-arginine. L-Citrulline can perhaps improve the effects on nitrate elimination during the course of recovery from exhaustive muscular exercise, and also serves as an effective precursor of L-arginine. It has been shown that three grams daily of oral L-citrulline supplementation for seven days elevated plasma L-arginine concentration and augmented NO-dependent signaling [9].

Glutathione is a low molecular weight, water-soluble tripeptide composed of the amino acids cysteine, glutamic acid, and glycine. Glutathione is an important antioxidant and plays a major role in the detoxification of endogenous metabolic products, including lipid peroxides. Intracellular glutathione exists in both the oxidized disulfide form (GSSG) or in reduced (GSH) state; the ratio between GSH and GSSG is held in dynamic balance depending on many factors including the tissue of interest, intracellular demand for conjugation reactions, intracellular demand for reducing power, and extracellular demand for reducing potential. In some cell types, GSH appears to be necessary for NO synthesis and NO has been shown to be correlated with intracellular GSH [10]. GSH stimulates total L-arginine turnover and, in the presence of GSH, NOS activity is increased [11]. This suggests that GSH may play an important role in protection against oxidative reaction of NO, thus contributing to the sustained release of NO. Therefore, combining L-citrulline with GSH may augment the production of NO. However, the effectiveness for oral GSH supplementation in humans, particularly in combination with L-citrulline has not been clearly delineated.

Using *in vitro* (cell culture) and *in vivo* approaches in rodents and humans, the overall purpose of this study was to determine the efficacy of L-citrulline and/or GSH supplementation towards increasing the levels of cGMP, nitrite, and NOx. We hypothesized that the combination of L-citrulline and GSH would preferentially increase the concentrations of cGMP, nitrite, and NOx levels when compared to control conditions.

Methods and procedures

L-citrulline and GSH (Setria®) used in each phase were obtained from KYOWA HAKKO BIO CO., LTD (Tokyo, Japan).

Phase 1 (*in vitro* efficacy study)

Human umbilical vein endothelial cells (HUVECs) were purchased from Clonetics (San Diego, CA, USA) and cultured in EGM-2 Bullet Kit medium (Clonetics) supplemented with 2 % fetal bovine serum (FBS) and complete endothelial growth factors at 37 ° C in humidified 5 % CO_2. The cells were seeded into twenty-four well plates 5000 cells/cm2, and sub-confluent cell monolayers were used for experiments. A subset of sub-confluent HUVECs were used as controls and the remainder were treated with either 0.3 mM L-citrulline, 1 mM GSH, or a combination of each at 0.3 mM, and incubated for 24 h. To measure nitrite production by HUVECs, the culture medium was collected and centrifuged to remove any precipitated materials. Four wells for each condition were used and nitrite concentrations of supernatants from each well were determined by high performance liquid chromatography (HPLC) (ENO-20; Eicom, Kyoto, Japan) using our previous approach [12].

Phase 2 (rodent efficacy study)

This phase of the study was conducted in accordance with the guidelines for the Institutional Animal Care and Use Committee of KYOWA HAKKO BIO CO., LTD. Twenty-three male Sprague–Dawley rats (8 weeks old; Japan SLC, Hamamatsu, Japan) were given free access to standard rat chow (CE-2, CLEA JAPAN Inc., Tokyo, Japan) and tap water in a room with controlled temperature (22 ± 2 ° C), humidity (55 ± 5 %) and a 12-h light/dark cycle. After the rats had been anesthetized with pentobarbital sodium (30 mg/kg, i.p.), a catheter was inserted into the carotid artery. Following 3 days of acclimation, the rats were randomly assigned to 3 groups and received either purified water (CON) (n = 7), L-citrulline (500 mg/kg/day) (n = 8), or a combination of L-citrulline (500 mg/kg/day) plus GSH (50 mg/kg/day) (n = 8) by oral gavage for 3 days. Blood samples were collected from the catheter at baseline and at 0, 0.25, 0.5, 1, 2, and 4 h after the last administration on Day 3. Plasma NOx (nitrite + nitrate) was measured by HPLC (ENO-20; Eicom, Kyoto, Japan) using our previous approach [12].

Phase 3 (human efficacy study)
Participants

Sixty-six apparently healthy, resistance trained [regular, consistent resistance training (i.e., thrice weekly) for at least one year prior to the onset of the study], males between the ages of 18–30 and a body mass index between 18.5–30 kg/m^2 volunteered to participate in the double-blind, randomized, placebo-controlled, parallel-groups study. Enrollment was open to men of all ethnicities. During the course of the study, six dropped out due to reasons unrelated to the study. As a result, 60 participants completed the study. The age, height, and body mass of participants in each of the four groups can be seen in Table 1. Only participants considered as low risk for cardiovascular disease and with no contraindications to exercise as outlined by the American College of Sports Medicine (ACSM) and who had not consumed any nutritional supplements (excluding multi-vitamins) one month prior to the study were allowed to participate. All participants provided written informed consent and were cleared for participation by passing a mandatory medical screening. All eligible subjects signed university-approved informed consent documents and approval was granted by the Baylor University Institutional Review Board for the Protection of Human Subjects in Research. Additionally, all experimental procedures involved in the study conformed to the ethical consideration of the Declaration of Helsinki.

Entry and familiarization session (visit 1)

Individuals expressing interest in participating in the study were interviewed on the telephone and/or e-mail to determine whether they appeared to qualify to participate in the study. Participants believed to meet eligibility criteria were then invited to attend an entry/familiarization session (visit 1). Once reporting to the lab, individuals were familiarized to the study protocol via a verbal and written explanation outlining the study design and signed an informed consent document. At this point, participants completed a medical history questionnaire and underwent a general physical examination to determine whether they met eligibility criteria. Participants also performed a muscle strength test of the elbow flexors (biceps), and were then given an appointment time to report to the laboratory for a baseline blood sample (visit 2). At this time, participants were instructed to refrain from exercise for 48 h and fast for 8 h prior to baseline blood sampling (visit 2) and post-supplementation testing at day 7 (visit 3).

Table 1 Age, height, and body mass of participants in each of the four groups

Group	Age (yrs)	Height (cm)	Body mass (kg)
PLC (n = 15)	21.80 ± 0.92	179.52 ± 2.10	83.92 ± 6.65
GSH (n = 15)	22.67 ± 0.97	179.90 ± 1.71	83.42 ± 2.92
CIT (n = 15)	21.07 ± 0.67	177.17 ± 1.55	80.46 ± 3.17
CIT + GSH (n = 15)	21.67 ± 0.56	179.03 ± 2.34	83.06 ± 2.79

Data are expressed as means ± SEM

Assessment of elbow flexor muscle strength (visit 1)

In order to determine maximum muscular strength of the elbow flexors, participants performed a one-repetition maximum (1-RM) test on the same elbow flexor machine used in the resistance exercise session based on our previous study [5]. Participants warmed up by completing 5 to 10 repetitions at approximately 50 % of the estimated 1-RM. The participant rested for 1 min, and then completed 3 to 5 repetitions at approximately 70 % of the estimated 1-RM. The weight was then increased conservatively, and the participant attempted to lift the weight for one repetition. If the lift was successful, the participant rested for 2 min before attempting the next weight increment. This procedure was continued until the participant failed to complete the lift. The 1-RM was recorded as the maximum weight that the participant was able to lift for one repetition.

Resistance exercise protocol (visit 3, day 7)

Based on our previous study [5], on day 7 participants reported to the Exercise and Biochemical Nutrition Lab at approximately 2:00 pm and performed 3 sets of 15 repetitions with as much weight as they could lift per set (typically 70–75 % of 1RM) involving the elbow flexion exercise on a selectorized weight machine (Body Master, Rayne, LA). Rest periods between sets were timed and lasted exactly 10 s. The resistance exercise session was performed under the direct supervision of study personnel.

Venous blood sampling (visit 2, day 0 and visit 3, day 7)

Venous blood samples were obtained from the antecubital vein into 10 ml serum and plasma collection tubes using a standard vacutainer apparatus. Blood samples were allowed to stand at room temperature for 10 min and then centrifuged. The serum and plasma was removed and frozen at −80 °C for later analysis. One baseline blood sample was obtained at visit 2 and 3 samples were obtained at visit 3 (for a total of 4 blood samples). At visit 3 on day 7, the first sample was obtained immediately before ingesting the supplement, the second sample was obtained immediately after resistance exercise, and the third sample 30 min following exercise (Fig. 1).

Supplementation protocol

In a randomized, double-blind fashion participants were randomly assigned to one of four groups (n = 15 per group) involving 7 days of the oral ingestion of four capsules containing a total daily dose of either: cellulose placebo (2.52 g/day), L-citrulline (2 g/day), GSH (1 g/day), or L-citrulline (2 g/day) + GSH (200 mg/day). The total weight of the four capsules for each group was the same. Each participant ingested all four capsules containing their respective daily supplement dose each evening for six consecutive days. At Visit 3 (Day 7), participants

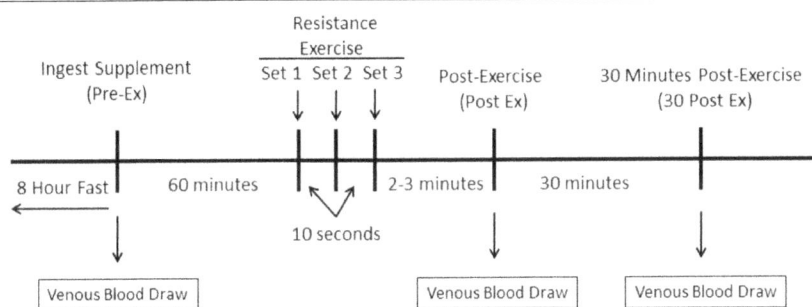

Fig. 1 An illustration of the experimental protocol for the testing session at visit 3, following seven days of L-citrulline and/or GSH supplementation

were provided the final daily dose of their respective supplement ingested one hour prior to performing the resistance exercise. Supplementation compliance was monitored by participants returning empty containers of their supplement on day 7, and also by completing a supplement compliance questionnaire.

Assessment of blood variables (L-citrulline and L-arginine)
To determine plasma L-citrulline and L-arginine concentrations, the plasma was de-proteinated by mixing equal volumes of plasma and trichloroacetic acid (TCA) (6.0 % wt/vol). The samples were vortexed and centrifuged for 15 min at 12,000 × g. Amino acids in the supernatant were analyzed with an amino acid analyzer (L-8900, Hitachi, Japan).

Assessment of plasma cGMP and nitrite
From the blood samples obtained at visit 2 (day 0) and visit 3 (day 7), using commercially-available enzyme-linked immunoabsorbent assay (ELISA) kits (Cayman Chemical, Ann Arbor, MI, USA), plasma cGMP, nitrite, and NOx were determined. Assays were analyzed in duplicate and absorbances for each variable were determined at a wavelength of 450 nm using a microplate reader (iMark, Bio-Rad, Hercules, CA). A set of standards of known concentrations for each variable utilized to construct standard curves and concentrations were determined using data reduction software (Microplate Manager, Bio-Rad, Hercules, CA).

Statistical analysis
For *in vitro* (phase 1), rodent (phase 2), and the human (phase 3) efficacy studies, results were expressed as mean ± SEM. Delta values (differences between the baseline and sequential values) were analyzed using Bonferroni's test following one-way ANOVA. For multiple comparisons to identify the statistical differences among treatments, the Bonferroni correction or Dunnett's multiple test following a comparison of the data by non-repeated ANOVA was employed. Statistical significance was considered as a

p-value ≤ 0.05. Statistical analysis was performed using Statcel software for Windows (Version 2, OMS Publishing, Inc., Saitama, Japan) and the Systat 2000 Statistical Program File (Igaku Tosho Shuppan, Tokyo, Japan).

Results

Phase 1 (*in-vitro* cell culture study)
Results demonstrated no significant differences between the control condition and cells treated with L-citrulline and GSH ($p > 0.05$) for nitrite concentration. However, cells treated with L-citrulline and GSH were significantly greater than control-treated cells ($p < 0.05$) (Fig. 2).

Phase 2 (rodent efficacy study)
For plasma NOx delta values, results demonstrated that L-citrulline + GSH was significantly greater than control and L-citrulline at one hr post-supplement infusion ($p < 0.05$) (Fig. 3).

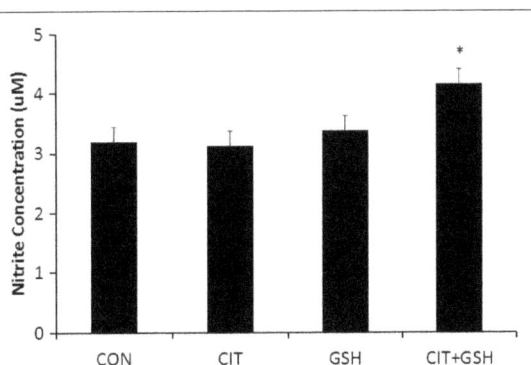

Fig. 2 From phase one, an illustration of nitrite concentration in HUVECs following supplementation with L-citrulline and/or GSH. The symbol * indicates that cells supplemented with a combination of L-citrulline (CIT) and GSH underwent significant increases in nitrite formation compared to cells supplemented with phosphate buffered saline (CON) ($p < 0.05$)

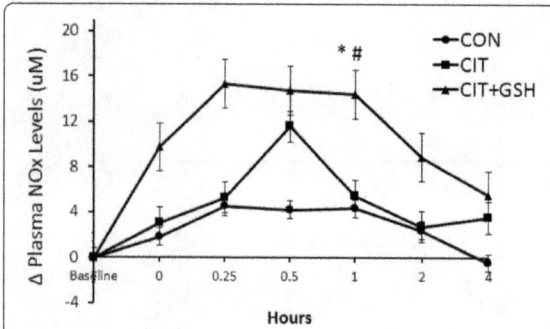

Fig. 3 From phase two, an illustration of plasma NOx levels in rats following supplementation with L-citrulline and/or GSH. The symbols * and # indicate that combined L-citrulline (CIT) and GSH-supplemented rats underwent significant increases in plasma NOx at one hr following supplement infusion compared to animals supplemented with water (CON) and CIT, respectively ($p < 0.05$)

Phase 3 (human efficacy study)
Plasma L-arginine and L-citrulline
Since no supplementation was involved at the baseline testing session, as expected, no significant differences between groups or time points ($p > 0.05$) for plasma L-citrulline and L-arginine were observed. However, at the follow-up testing session following seven 7 days of supplementation significant increases for plasma L-arginine and L-citrulline were noted. For L-arginine, no significant differences occurred between placebo and GSH at any time points ($p > 0.05$). However, at the immediate post-exercise time point L-citrulline was significantly greater than placebo and GSH, whereas L-citrulline + GSH was greater than GSH ($p < 0.05$). In addition, at 30 min post-exercise L-citrulline and L-citrulline + GSH were both significantly greater than placebo and GSH ($p < 0.05$) (Fig. 4). For plasma L-citrulline, L-citrulline and L-citrulline + GSH were both significantly greater than placebo and GSH immediately post-exercise and at 30 min post-exercise ($p < 0.05$) (Fig. 5).

Plasma cGMP, nitrite, and NOx
The delta values for the plasma levels of cGMP, nitrite, and NOx can be seen in Figs. 6, 7 and 8, respectively. For cGMP (Fig. 6), L-citrulline + GSH was elevated compared to the other three groups, but there were no significant differences between groups and time points observed ($P > 0.05$). For nitrite (Fig. 7) and NOx (Fig. 8), L-citrulline + GSH was significantly greater than placebo at 30 min post-exercise ($P < 0.05$).

Discussion
In the present study, we sought to determine the effectiveness of L-citrulline and/or GSH in increasing NO synthesis during *in vivo* conditions with rodents and humans and also in an *in vitro* condition using HUVEC.

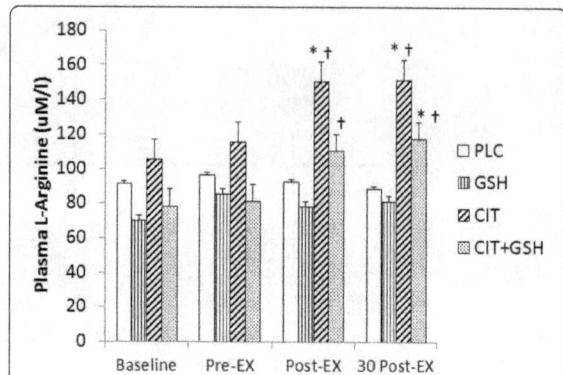

Fig. 4 From phase three, an illustration of plasma arginine levels in humans following seven days of supplementation with L-citrulline and/or GSH. Results indicated that L-citrulline (CIT) and a combination of CIT + GSH produced significant increases in plasma arginine immediately after and 30 min post-exercise compared to groups supplemented with cellulose (PLC) and GSH. The symbol * indicates a significant increase compared to PLC and the symbol † indicates a significant increase compared to GSH ($p < 0.05$)

Collectively, in phase one and three of the study we observed combining L-citrulline with GSH to be more effective at increasing the concentrations of nitrite and/or NOx than with control/placebo in HUVEC and humans, respectively. In phase two, we observed L-citrulline combined with GSH to be more effective at increasing plasma NOx.

L-citrulline is a ubiquitous amino acid in mammals [13], and in the kidneys, vascular endothelium, and other tissues can be readily converted to L-arginine thus

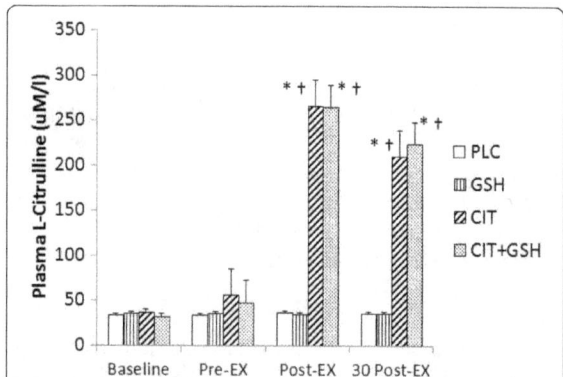

Fig. 5 From phase three, an illustration of plasma citrulline levels in humans following seven days of supplementation with L-citrulline and/or GSH. Results indicated that L-citrulline (CIT) and a combination of CIT + GSH produced significant increases in plasma CIT immediately after and 30 min post-exercise compared to groups supplemented with cellulose (PLC) and GSH. The symbol * indicates a significant increase compared to PLC and the symbol † indicates a significant increase compared to GSH ($p < 0.05$)

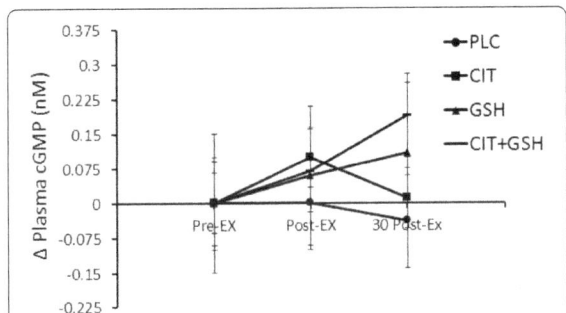

Fig. 6 From phase three, an illustration of plasma cGMP levels in humans following seven days of supplementation with L-citrulline and/or GSH. Results indicated no significant differences between any of the groups at any of the assessed time points ($p > 0.05$)

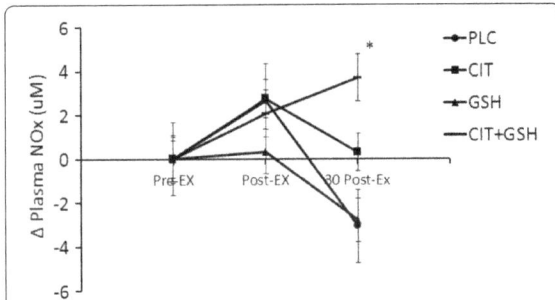

Fig. 8 From phase three, an illustration of plasma NOx levels in humans following seven days of supplementation with L-citrulline and/or GSH. The symbol * indicates that a combination of L-citrulline (CIT) and GSH produced significant increases in plasma NOx at 30 min post-exercise compared to the group supplemented with cellulose placebo (PLC) ($p < 0.05$)

raising plasma and tissue levels of L-arginine which increases NOS synthesis and subsequent NO production [14]. Additionally, L-citrulline has been indicated to be a secondary NO donor in the NOS-dependent pathway, since it can be converted to L-arginine. Nitrate and nitrite are the main substrates to produce NO via the NOS-independent pathway. These anions can be reduced *in vivo* to NO and other bioactive nitrogen oxides.

Previous studies have reported that L-citrulline could increase plasma L-arginine concentration by the L-citrulline-NO cycle [15]. Fu et al. [16] showed that pre-treatment with L-citrulline in rodents for seven days at doses of 300, 600, and 900 mg/kg increased the NO content. Since L-citrulline can be readily converted to L-arginine, it provides a recycling pathway for the conversion of L-citrulline to NO via L-arginine [14, 17]. In phase three of the present study, we observed seven days of L-citrulline supplementation, with and without GSH, to result in significant increases in the levels of plasma citrulline and arginine. Our present data support

previous results [18] showing that a 10-g oral bolus of L-citrulline significantly enhanced plasma citrulline and arginine levels compared with placebo. Therefore, our present observations indicate that L-citrulline is indeed a precursor to L-arginine formation which subsequently increases circulating levels of NOx, and that recycling of L-citrulline to L-arginine may maintain substrate concentration in favor of NO synthesis [19].

It has been shown in some mammalian cell types, that GSH and NO activity are linked [20]. Furthermore, results suggest that GSH is necessary in HUVEC for NO synthesis rather than for the NO-related effect on guanylate cyclase, because when cells were depleted of GSH, citrulline synthesis and cGMP production were inhibited in a concentration-dependent manner [21]. This may be explained based on the premise that the synthesis of NO, detected as L-citrulline production, in HUVEC and murine endothelial cells has been shown to be correlated with intracellular GSH [10]. A previous study suggested that in some cell types, the activity of NO is influenced by the endogenous antioxidant GSH [22]. It is conceivable that GSH activity may be augmented by L-citrulline as it has been shown that pre-treatment with L-citrulline in rodents for seven consecutive days lead to an elevation in the level of GSH [23].

Furthermore, in phase one of the present study, we showed that combining L-citrulline and GSH effectively increased nitrite concentration in HUVEC cells compared to control; although, both L-citrulline and GSH alone had no effect on nitrite. However, in phase two, the combined L-citrulline and GSH provided to rodents resulted in a significant increase in plasma NOx one hr following ingestion compared to control and L-citrulline. Moreover, we observed a similar response in phase three compared to phase one, where combining L-citrulline and GSH effectively increased plasma nitrite and NOx concentration in humans compared to placebo.

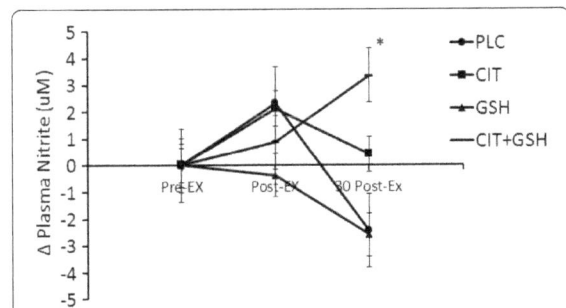

Fig. 7 From phase three, an illustration of plasma nitrite levels in humans following seven days of supplementation with L-citrulline and/or GSH. The symbol * indicates that a combination of L-citrulline (CIT) and GSH produced significant increases in plasma nitrite at 30 min post-exercise compared to the group supplemented with cellulose placebo (PLC) ($p < 0.05$)

Oral supplementation with L-arginine can increase plasma L-arginine levels; although, oral supplementation with L-citrulline, a precursor for arginine biosynthesis, has been shown to be more efficient than oral L-arginine in increasing plasma L-arginine [9], due to splanchnic catabolism of ingested L-Arginine [24]. NO synthesis is primarily dependent upon intracellular arginine availability and is affected by: 1) the transport of extracellular arginine; 2) intracellular synthesis of arginine from citrulline, which is dependent on citrulline availability; and 3) the activity of arginase [17]. Moreover, this latter point can be further supported based on the data demonstrating increased arginine availability in cultured cell model or by supplementation *in vivo* was able to overcome the effects of arginase and to enhance NO synthesis [25]. Based on results from all three phases of the present study, it is evident that L-citrulline supplementation impacted extracellular arginine concentration and the subsequent intracellular arginine synthesis based on the responses we observed in nitrite and NOx concentrations.

In phase 3 of the present study, we were also interested to determine if increased plasma arginine availability and subsequent NO synthesis due to oral L-citrulline and/or GSH supplementation was effected by resistance exercise. Interestingly, we observed increases in plasma NOx in all four groups immediately following resistance exercise, which indicates this response in plasma NOx to be particularly due to the stimulus of resistance exercise. These results are similar to our previous study where resistance exercise increased plasma NOx, independent of increased plasma arginine, due to seven days of L-arginine supplementation [5]. In the same way as NOx, plasma cGMP levels were increased by the combination of L-citrulline and GSH; however, this increase was not significantly different. Nevertheless, this suggests a possible synergistic effect from GSH that may be partially mediated by the formation of the NO-GSH complex. However, in the present study, significantly different increases in NOx occurred 30 min following resistance exercise, and only for the L-citrulline + GSH group. This suggests that a resistance exercise-related mechanism of inducing plasma NO, perhaps due to increased shear stress that triggered an up-regulation in NO-cGMP signaling, is a conceivable candidate for this response.

Consequently, there are possible physiological benefits of having high NO levels at 30 min post-exercise relative to its impact on muscle protein metabolism and possible muscle performance in response to resistance exercise training. It has been shown that NOS activity is necessary for calcium-induced activation of the Akt pathway (involved in translation initiation and thus muscle protein synthesis), and that NO is sufficient to elevate Akt activity in primary myotubes. Nitric oxide appears to influence Akt signaling though a cGMP/PI3K-dependent pathway [26], which is the primary pathway for up-regulating translation initiation and protein synthesis in skeletal muscle. Additionally, nitrite has been shown to enhance the proliferation and mTOR activity of myoblasts [27]. Similarly, NO seems to influence skeletal muscle function through effects on excitation-contraction coupling, myofibrillar function, perfusion, and metabolism. Another study showed that by using an agent to inhibit phosphodiesterase-5, that the augmentation of NO-cGMP signaling increased protein synthesis and reduced fatigue in human skeletal muscle [28]. In the present study, L-citrulline + GSH showed an improvement in cGMP activity suggesting that this outcome could likely play a role in muscle protein synthesis and muscle performance when combined with resistance training.

Our present data suggest that the oral supplementation of L-citrulline combined with GSH provides an augmenting effect on plasma NOx. Based on results from recent studies, this may be explained based on the premise that in some cell types, the activity of NO is influenced by the endogenous antioxidant, GSH [10]. Therefore, GSH may play an important role in protection against oxidative reaction of NO, thus contributing to the sustained release of NO.

Conclusions

Herein, we have presented *in vitro* and *in vivo* data demonstrating the efficacy of combining L-citrulline and GSH and the subsequent effects on NO synthesis and, collectively, we conclude that the combination of L-citrulline and GSH increases the levels of cGMP, nitrite, and NOx.

Competing interests
Masahiko Morita is an employee of KYOWA HAKKO BIO CO., LTD. The other co-authors declare no conflicts of interest.

Authors' contributions
SM served as the study coordinator and was involved in participant recruitment, testing, laboratory analyses, and assisted in manuscript preparation. TA was involved in testing and laboratory analyses. MM was involved in conducting the phase 1 and 2 portions of this study, in performing the plasma L-citrulline and L-arginine analyses in phase 3, and was involved in manuscript preparation. DSW was the principal investigator and, was responsible for securing grant funding and developing the experimental design. He was also involved in training and mentoring for laboratory analyses, provided primary oversight during the course of the study, and supervised manuscript preparation. All authors read and approved the final manuscript.

Acknowledgements
This study was supported by a research grant awarded to Baylor University from KYOWA HAKKO BIO CO., LTD. The authors would like to thank all of the individuals who participated in the study.

Author details
[1]Department of Health, Human Performance, and Recreation, Baylor University, Exercise and Biochemical Nutritional Lab, 76798 Waco, TX, USA. [2]Function Research Group, Healthcare Products Development Center, KYOWA HAKKO BIO CO., LTD., 2, Miyukigaoka, 305-0841 Tsukuba Ibaraki, Japan.

References

1. Boger R, Bode-Boger S. The clinical pharmacology of L-arginine. Annu Rev Pharmacol Toxicol. 2001;41:79–99.
2. Wu GY, Brosnan JT. Macrophages can convert citrulline into arginine. Biochem J. 1992;281:45–8.
3. Bode-Boger S, Boger R, Galland A, Tsikas D, Frolich J. L-arginine-induced vasodilation in health humans: pharmokinetic-pharmacodynamic relationship. Br J Clin Pharmacol. 1998;46:489–97.
4. Romero MJ, Yao L, Sridhar S, Bhatta A, Dou H, Ramesh G, et al. L-citrulline protects from kidney damage in type 1 diabetic mice. Front Immunol. 2013;4:480.
5. Willoughby DS, Boucher T, Reid J, Skelton G, Clark M. Effects of 7 days of arginine-alpha-ketoglutarate supplementation on blod flow, plama L-arginine, nitric oxide metabolites, and asymmetric dimethyl arginine after resistance exercise. Int J Sports Nutr Exerc Metab. 2011;21:291–9.
6. Sureda A, Pons A. Arginine and citrulline supplementation in sports and exercise: ergogenic nutrients? Med Sport Sci. 2012;59:18–28.
7. Cutrufello PT, Gadomski SJ, Zavorsky GS. The effect of l-citrulline and watermelon juice supplementation on anaerobic and aerobic exercise performance. J Sports Sci. 2014;17:1–8.
8. Wax B, Kavazis AN, Weldon K, Sperlak J. Effects of supplemental citrulline malate ingestion during repeated bouts of lower-body exercise in advanced weight lifters. J Strength Cond Res. 2015;29:786–92.
9. Schwedhelm E, Maas R, Freese R, Jung D, Lukacs Z, Jambrecine A, et al. Pharmacokinetic and pharmacodynamics properties or oral L-citrulline and L-arginine: impact on nitric oxide metabolism. Br J Clin Pharmacol. 2007;65:51–9.
10. Ghigo D, Geromin D, Franchino C, Todde R, Priotto C, Costamagna C, et al. Correlation between nitric oxide synthase activity and reduced glutathione level in human and murine endothelial cells. Amino Acids. 1996;10:277–81.
11. Hoffman H, Schmidt HH. Thiol dedepndence of nitric oxide synthase. Biochemistry. 1995;34:13443–52.
12. Mochizuki S, Toyota E, Hiramatsu O, Kajita T, Shigeto F, Takemoto M, et al. Effect of dietary control on plasma nitrate level and estimation of basal systemic nitric oxide production rate in humans. Heart Vessels. 2000;15:274–9.
13. Curis E, Nicolis I, Moinard C, Osowska S, Zerrouk N, Bénazeth S, et al. Almost all about citrulline in mammals. Amino Acids. 2005;29:177–205.
14. Schneider R, Raff U, Vornberger N, Schmidt M, Freund R, Reber M, et al. L-Arginine counteracts nitric oxide deficiency and improves the recovery phase of ischemic acute renal failure in rats. Kidney Int. 2003;64:216–25.
15. Solomonson LP, Flam BR, Pendleton LC, Goodwin BL, Eichler DC. The caveolar nitric oxide synthase/arginine regeneration system for NO production in endothelial cells. J Exp Biol. 2003;206:2083–7.
16. Fu X, Li S, Jia G, Gou L, Tian X, Sun L, et al. Protective effect of the nitric oxide pathway in L-citrulline renal ischaemia-reperfusion injury in rats. Folia Biol (Praha). 2013;59:225–32.
17. Mori M, Gotoh T. Regulation of nitric oxide production by arginine metabolic enzymes. Biochem Biophys Res Commun. 2000;275:715–9.
18. van Wijck K, Wijnands KA, Meesters DM, Boonen B, van Loon LJ, Buurman WA, et al. L-citrulline improves splanchnic perfusion and reduces gut injury during exercise. Med Sci Sports Fxerc. 2014;46:2039–46.
19. Shuttleworth CW, Conlon SB, Sanders KM. Regulation of citrulline recycling in nitric oxide-dependent neurotransmission in the murine proximal colon. Br J Pharmacol. 1997;120:707–13.
20. Walker M, Kinter M, Roberts R, Spitz D. Nitric oxide induced cytotoxicity: involvment of cellular resistance to oxidative stress and the role of glutathione in protection. Pediatr Res. 1995;37:41–9.
21. Ghigo D, Alessio P, Foco A, Bussolino F, Costamagna C, Heller R, et al. Nitric oxide synthesis is impaired in glutathione-depleted human umbilical vein endothelial cells. Am J Physiol. 1993;265:C728–32.
22. Wakulich C, Tepperman B. Role of glutathione in nitric oxide-mediated injury to rat gastric mucosal cells. Eur J Pharmacol. 1997;319:333–41.
23. Liu Y, Fu X, Gou L, Li S, Lan N, Zheng Y, et al. L-citrulline protects against glycerol-induced acute renal failure in rats. Ren Fail. 2013;35:367–73.
24. Castillo L, Chapman TE, Yu YM, Ajami A, Burke JF, Young VR. Dietary arginine uptake by the splanchnic region in adult humans. Am J Physiol. 1993;265:E532–9.
25. Oyadomari S, Gotoh T, Aoyagi K, Araki E, Shichiri M, Mori M. Coinduction of endothelial nitric oxide synthase and arginine recycling enzymes in aorta of diabetic rats. Nitric Oxide. 2001;5:252–60.
26. Drenning JA, Lira VA, Soltow QA, Canon CN, Valera LM, Brown DL, et al. Endothelial nitric oxide synthase is involved in calcium-induced Akt signaling in mouse skeletal muscle. Nitric Oxide. 2009;21:192–200.
27. Totzeck M, Schicho A, Stock P, Kelm M, Rassaf T, Hendgen-Cotta U. Nitrite circumvents canonical cGMP signaling to enhance proliferation of myocyte precursor cells. Mol Cell Biochem. 2015;401:175–83.
28. Sheffield-Moore M, Wiktorowicz JE, Soman KV, Danesi CP, Kinsky MP, Dillon EL, et al. Sildenafil increases muscle protein synthesis and reduces muscle fatigue. Clin Transl Sci. 2013;6:463–8.

## 3

The effect of turmeric (Curcumin) supplementation on cytokine and inflammatory marker responses following 2 hours of endurance cycling

Joseph N Sciberras[1*], Stuart DR Galloway[2], Anthony Fenech[3], Godfrey Grech[5], Claude Farrugia[4], Deborah Duca[4] and Janet Mifsud[3]

Abstract

Background: Endurance exercise induces IL-6 production from myocytes that is thought to impair intracellular defence mechanisms. Curcumin inhibits NF-κB and activator protein 1, responsible for cytokine transcription, in cell lines. The aim of this study was to investigate the effect of curcumin supplementation on the cytokine and stress responses following 2 h of cycling.

Methods: Eleven male recreational athletes (35.5 ± 5.7 years; W_{max} 275 ± 6 W; 87.2 ± 10.3 kg) consuming a low carbohydrate diet of 2.3 ± 0.2 g/kg/day underwent three double blind trials with curcumin supplementation, placebo supplementation, and no supplementation (control) to observe the response of serum interleukins (IL-6, IL1-RA, IL-10), cortisol, c-reactive protein (CRP), and subjective assessment of training stress. Exercise was set at 95% lactate threshold ($54 \pm 7\%$ W_{max}) to ensure that all athletes completed the trial protocol.

Results: The trial protocol elicted a rise in IL-6 and IL1-RA, but not IL-10. The supplementation regimen failed to produce statistically significant results when compared to placebo and control. IL-6 serum concentrations one hour following exercise were (Median (IQR): 2.0 (1.8-3.6) Curcumin; 4.8 (2.1-7.3) Placebo; 3.5 (1.9-7.7) Control). Differences between supplementation and placebo failed to reach statistical significance ($p = 0.18$) with the median test. Repeated measures ANOVA time-trial interaction was at $p = 0.06$ between curcumin supplementation and placebo. A positive correlation ($p = 0.02$) between absolute exercise intensity and 1 h post-exercise for IL-6 concentration was observed. Participants reported "better than usual" scores in the subjective assessment of psychological stress when supplementing with curcumin, indicating that they felt less stressed during training days ($p = 0.04$) compared to placebo even though there was no difference in RPE during any of the training days or trials.

Conclusion: The limitations of the current regimen and trial involved a number of factors including sample size, mode of exercise, intensity of exercise, and dose of curcumin. Nevertheless these results provide insight for future studies with larger samples, and multiple curcumin dosages to investigate if different curcumin regimens can lead to statistically different interleukin levels when compared to a control and placebo.

Keywords: Immunity, Interleukins, Natural polyphenols

* Correspondence: sciberras.n.joseph@gmail.com
[1]Sport Nutrition graduate from the University of Stirling, 74, San Anton Court, Pope John XXIII street, Birkirkara BKR1033, Malta
Full list of author information is available at the end of the article

Background

Research supports a role for nutritional interventions to maintain immune function in the post-exercise period [1-5] It is also widely recognized that endurance exercise stimulates an increase in circulating cytokines in the post-exercise period [6,7]. These cytokines include interleukin 1 beta (IL-1β), interleukin 6 (IL-6), interleukin 8 (IL-8), interleukin 10 (IL-10), and interleukin 1 receptor antagonist (IL1-RA). These cytokine responses following exercise do not mainly originate from circulating monocytes, but may influence secretion of other cytokines from cells which form part of the immune system [8,9]. The post-exercise rise in IL-6 is unrelated to muscle damage, but serves as a messenger from myocytes to increase hepatic glycogenolysis [10-12]. Interestingly, the release of IL-6 in the post-exercise period appears to be dependent upon carbohydrate availability [12].

IL-6 is a cell messenger which affects many cells and systems, such as lymphocytes, leads to the release of the anti-inflammatory hormone cortisol, and stimulates release of acute phase proteins and glucose from the liver [13] IL1-RA and IL-10 transcription are mediated by high IL-6 concentrations [14]. These immunomodulatory mechanisms result in a decreased amount of circulating Type 1 T-helper (Th1) cells [15]. This suggests that regular high volume exercise shifts the CD4 positive T lymphocyte profile from Th1 towards Th2. Th1 cells help neutralize intracellular infective agents like viruses and bacteria which are responsible for upper respiratory tract infections (URTI). Specific interleukins, involved in cellular immunity, are also inhibited by the increase in IL-6 [16]. Inhibition of IL-1 is mediated through IL1-RA, and IL-6 appears to blunt the effect of TNF-α, while the effects of interleukin 12 are countered by IL-10 [17]. Thus, factors that can modify the post-exercise cytokine response could assist in maintenance of immune function in athletes.

Cytokine transcription is mediated by the transcription factors NF-κB and activator protein 1 (AP-1) [18]. Activation of NF-κB is induced by several immunity mediators, cell signaling intermediates, and reactive oxygen species [19]. Curcumin found in the rhizome Curcuma longa (turmeric), is an anti-oxidant and anti-inflammatory, long used as a traditional herbal medicine [20-22]. It attenuates the activation of NF-κB and IκB kinase in cancer cell lines [23]. Researchers observed that curcumin inhibits the activity of IκB kinase and decreases the activity of NF-κB in intestinal epithelial cells [24]. Shisodia et al., reported that the activity of curcumin also affects the AP-1 pathway, and Akt signaling [25]. In a study on rats, curcumin was shown to reduce IL-6, IL-1β, and TNFα levels following eccentric exercise [26]. These authors concluded that curcumin may promote recovery following repeated strenuous activity. Curcumin has also been shown to affect

numerous physiological pathways, including inflammation, and play important roles in pathological conditions, including diabetes and arthritis, as reviewed elsewhere [27-29].

These observations with curcumin in cell and animal models, leads us to hypothesize that curcumin supplementation in humans could reduce cytokine release following exercise. An acute blunting of the cytokine response to exercise may provide a strong basis for longer term studies examining a role for curcumin on immune function and recovery during periods of strenuous exercise training. The current study, therefore, aimed to observe the effects of curcumin supplementation on interleukin and other inflammatory marker responses following two hours of cycling in a low glycogen state.

Methods

Eleven recreationally active males (regular weekly aerobic activity during the last year for at least 3 h, mean age 35.5 ± 5.7 years; mean W_{max} 275 ± 56 W; mean weight 87.2 ± 10.3 kg; mean height 1.78 ± 0.07 m) volunteered to participate in the study. All of the participants gave their written informed consent to participate in the study which was approved by the ethics committees of the University of Stirling and University of Malta. Athletes were recruited from those attending talks held at sport clubs in Malta. Participants were screened for suitability prior to the experimental trials, including a medical visit by a licensed general practitioner. None reported a history of auto-immune disorders or medical conditions which could affect the results. Moreover they were not on medication or high dose vitamin C and/or vitamin E intake. Participants reported being free from infection for at least 4 weeks prior to the trial, and were in a steady period of endurance training. The number of participants needed was calculated by sample size testing based on literature review. Power was set at 80%, $p < 0.05$, with a difference in population means of 2 pg for interleukin 6, and standard deviation of 2 pg. This gave an approximate sample size of 8–10. The sample sizes and results obtained in studies listed in the review of Fischer, 2006 [30], on interleukins and exercise were also taken as a guide.

Participants were taught how to use diabetic nutritional exchanges to comply with the pre-trial prescribed diet. Preliminary measurement of lactate threshold and maximum workload were obtained together using a Computrainer lab ergometer (Racermate, Seattle, USA) and Lactate Scout (EKF-Diagnostics, Magdeburg, Germany). The Lactate Scout was validated prior to each test using the standard solution provided by the manufacturer. Lactate was measured by skin pricking every three minutes on the computrainer® lab; following which power was increased by 30 W. This continued until volitional fatigue or until the athlete was unable to maintain a cadence of 70 rpm. This was defined as the maximum workload.

Subjects were then allocated either to the curcumin supplement or placebo in a double blind randomized cross-over fashion. Subjects performed three trials in total (supplement/placebo and control) in which they exercised for 2 h at a power output equivalent to 95% of their lactate threshold, to ensure completion of the trial task. Supplement or placebo was taken for three days prior to the trial day, and finally on arrival at the clinic for the trial. Following a one week wash-out period the trial was repeated with supplementation/placebo accordingly. An identical further trial served as a control and was held following a further week without any supplementation. The control arm of the study was scheduled after the two experimental trials in an effort to minimize data loss from curcumin and placebo trials, through athlete drop out. In addition, participants undertook a supervised one hour interval training session on a cycle ergometer in the afternoon, two days prior to each trial, in an attempt to lower muscle glycogen stores. Participants were then assigned a diet containing 2.3 ± 0.2 g/kg carbohydrate, 1.0 ± 0.2 g/kg fat, and 1.3 ± 0.2 g/kg protein. This diet was aimed at minimising carbohydrate replenishment following training two days prior to the trial. Participants returned to their habitual diet immediately after the trial. Participants were requested to refrain from strenuous physical activity for 24 h prior to trials.

Upon arrival at the laboratory for the trials a cannula was inserted in an antecubital vein. Blood samples (20 ml, 4 serum and 2 EDTA tubes) were taken just before the exercise trial, immediately after completing the two hours cycling, and one hour following the cessation of exercise (Figure 1). A pedaling cadence of 70 rpm was maintained during trials using the Computrainer® ergometer, which was calibrated as per manufacturer's instructions. Prior to all training and trial sessions participants completed a daily analysis of life demands (DALDA) questionnaire to assess stress sources (part 1) and stress symptoms (part 2) [31].

Trials, conducted at St James Highway Clinic, commenced between 1 pm and 6 pm, at least 4 h following their last meal. Heart rate was measured using a Timex®

(Middlebury, USA) telemetry strap. Temperature and humidity, measured with a calibrated thermo-hygrometer (TFA-Dostmann, Mannheim, Germany), were maintained close to 20°C and 60% RH, respectively. Rating of perceived exertion was reported after 15 min into the trial and thereafter every 30 minutes. Only water was permitted during the trial. One athlete dropped out following the second trial, and did not complete the control trial. The curcumin supplement ("Meriva®" Curcumin) and corresponding identical placebo, together with respective certificate of analysis (CoA) were donated by Indena Spa. (Milan, Italy). Meriva® curcumin was chosen because of its superior bioavailability to other curcumin products. Researchers concluded that a single dosage of 376 mg of Meriva® curcumin was eighteen times superior to a standard curcumin dose of 2 g, giving a maximum plasma concentration of 207 ng/ml four hours following supplement ingestion [32]. Dosage for the present study subjects was a single dose of 500 mg of Meriva® curcumin (5 tablets) with midday meal for three days, and then 500 mg ingested just before exercise. Samples for plasma curcumin analysis were taken at the final blood sampling time only in this study, three hours post ingestion to coincide with assessment of post-exercise interleukin response.

Plasma and serum samples obtained after centrifuging were frozen at −80°C. Plasma samples for curcumin analysis were incubated for 4 hours with helix pomatia glucuronidase (Sigma Aldrich®, Delaware, USA) in a pH 5 sodium acetate buffer. This was followed by extraction with chloroform. The organic chloroform was dried under a nitrogen stream, and reconstituted in 4 ml curcumin spiked acetonitrile. These samples were then analysed for curcumin using a Waters HPLC (Milford, USA) using a method reported in literature [33]. The method was validated for identification and linearity using curcumin standard (Sigma Aldrich, Delaware, USA). Interleukins 6, 1RA, and 10 were assayed on all serum samples using ELISA kits supplied by R&D Systems Ltd (Minneapolis, USA). Haematocrit, haemoglobin concentration, white blood cell (WBC count), neutrophil proportion, cortisol concentration, and c-reactive protein concentration were

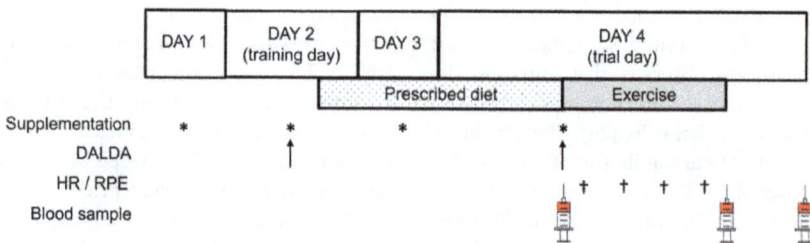

Figure 1 Trial flow chart detailing sequence of events, supplementation days, and blood sampling. DALDA – daily analysis of life demands in athletes, HR – heart rate, RPE – rating of perceived exertion.

all measured on blood taken immediately after exercise only (analyses were conducted by MLS laboratories, St James Hospital, Malta).

Repeated measures ANOVA was conducted with the values obtained for time, trial, and time x trial interactions. Any outliers in datasets were dealt with using Grubbs method [34]. Any significant within subject effects were then examined with the median test when data was not normally distributed (IL-6 conc.), otherwise student t-test was used. Ratings from the DALDA questionnaire were analysed with the wilcoxon test for paired non parametric data. Parametric results are tabulated as mean ± standard deviation, 95% confidence intervals are also given in brackets for Tables 1 and 2. Further results are graphically plotted as mean ± standard error of the mean. Median and inter-quartile range are reported when continuous data is not normally distributed. Spearman's correlation coefficient was calculated where associations were expected. The intra-assay coefficient of variation was 9.4% for IL-6; 6.4% for IL-1RA and 3.4% for the HPLC assay of curcumin.

Results

All participants undertook the trial at 95% lactate threshold. Relative to W_{max} the mean power output sustained during the 2 hour ride was 54 ± 7% of the mean maximum workload (range 39% to 63% of W_{max}). The humidity, temperature, and ergometer calibration values were all similar between trials (Table 1). Initial body mass and training volume were also not different between each trial (Table 1). None of the participants reported any adverse effect to supplementation or placebo ingestion. All participants reported adhering to their pre-trial diets on all trials. Participants completed all the trials in three weeks. Five participants started the trials with placebo and six with curcumin supplementation. HPLC analysis confirmed the presence of curcumin in plasma of all participants when taking the curcumin supplement. No curcumin was detected in plasma samples on other trials. Mean ± SD (range) curcumin concentration obtained was 79.7 ± 26.3 ng/ml (50.7 ng/ml to 125.5 ng/ml).

The reported perceived exertion increased significantly every 30 minutes during the 2 hour ride on all trials (mean (SD) RPE was: 9 ± 1; 10 ± 2; 11 ± 2 & 12 ± 2 at 15, 45, 75 and 105 minutes during exercise; p < 0.01). There were no significant differences in RPE ratings obtained during exercise between trials (11 ± 1; 11 ± 1; 11 ± 1 for curcumin, placebo and control trials, respectively). Mean (SD) heart rate during the exercise period was also not different between trials (118 ± 12; 117 ± 10; 117 ± 13 for curcumin, placebo and control trials, respectively). Whole blood analysis of the post-exercise samples revealed no differences in cortisol, c-reactive protein, haematocrit, haemoglobin, WBC, or neutrophil proportion between trials (Table 2).

Serum IL-6 data demonstrated a tendency for an interaction effect (time x trial interaction p = 0.06; F = 4.03) between curcumin and placebo trials (Figure 2). Curcumin only appeared to lower the concentration of IL-6 released one hour following exercise when compared to placebo, but this failed to reach statistical significance (p = 0.18; n = 10; 95% C.I. 1.63 ≤ x ≤ 3.81) (Figure 3). Estimation of size of effect proves difficult because one set of data is not normally distributed. Nonetheless Cohen's d is of 0.84 hinting at a possibly large effect (Figure 4). The correlation analysis revealed a significant association (p = 0.02) between IL-6 elevation and percentage W_{max} power output sustained during the exercise task (correlation coefficient rho 0.41 (df = 30)). No association was observed between attenuation of IL-6 response following exercise with the plasma concentration levels of curcumin (p = 0.92; correlation coefficient rho −0.04 (df = 9)). There was no difference between the trials for IL1-RA (time x trial interaction p = 0.85, (F = 0.44) when analysing the ANOVA for repeated measures. Correlation coefficient between percentage W_{max} power and change in IL1-RA concentration was 0.34 (df = 30), but failed to reach statistical significance (p = 0.06). There was no detectable increase in IL-10 on any of the trials.

The DALDA questionnaire (Table 3) revealed a higher number of "better than usual" results on the training day when ingesting curcumin compared to placebo and control. This was statistically significant between placebo

Table 1 Ambient conditions, ergometer calibration setting and initial body mass on the day of each trial

	Curcumin	Placebo	Control
Mean ambient humidity (% RH)	63 ± 6 (59–67)	62 ± 7 (58–66)	62 ± 6 (58–66)
Mean ambient temperature (°C)	19.9 ± 0.6 (19.5-20.3)	20.0 ± 0.4 (19.8-20.2)	20.1 ± 0.5 (19.8-20.4)
Calibration value of computrainer	2.7 ± 0.1 (2.6-2.8)	2.7 ± 0.1 (2.6-2.8)	2.8 ± 0.1 (2.7-2.9)
Body mass (kg)	86.7 ± 10.5 (80.5-92.9)	86.6 ± 10.4 (80.4-92.8)	87.5 ± 11.0 (80.7-94.3)
Training (Hours×Intensity)	11 ± 10 (5–17)	13 ± 9 (8–18)	13 ± 6 (9–17)

Habitual training load during the previous week was assessed using duration and intensity information. Training is reported in hours multiplied by intensity. Intensity was classified as low (1) medium (2) & high (3) Data are mean (± SD). Standard deviation and 95% confidence intervals are also reported following each value. No differences were noted between trials groups. Calibration value of the Computrainer is the value given to the ergometer as instructed by the manufacturer.

Table 2 Physiological parameters means (± SD) measured during trial, grouped by trial type

	Curcumin	Placebo	Control
Cortisol (nMol)	308 ± 200 (190–426)	266 ± 200 (148–384)	289 ± 228 (148–430)
C-Reactive protein (mg/l)	0.5 ± 0.3 (0.3-0.7)	0.9 ± 0.9 (0.4-1.4)	0.7 ± 0.6 (0.3-1.1)
Haematocrit (%)	43 ± 2 (42–44)	43 ± 3 (41–45)	43 ± 2 (42–43)
Haemoglobin (g/dl)	15.0 ± 0.7 (14.6-15.4)	14.0 ± 0.9 (13.5-14.5)	15.1 ± 0.8 (14.6-15.6)
WBC (10^9/L)	10.1 ± 2.7 (8.5-11.7)	9.6 ± 2.5 (8.1-11.1)	10.4 ± 2.6 (8.8-12.0)
Neutrophil (%)	61.9 ± 9.8 (56.1-67.7)	61.4 ± 9.2 (56.0-66.8)	63.5 ± 9.5 (57.6-69.4)

Confidence intervals 95% are also reported following each value.

Parameters show no significant difference between trials. These parameters were measured only at the end of exercise. Cortisol and C - reactive protein were measured to investigate any possible effects from the active compound curcumin. Haematocrit & Haemoglobin were measured to ensure that the athletes were in similar hydration status, while white blood cell and neutrophil percentage were needed to confirm that the athlete was not suffering from an infection at the time of the trial.

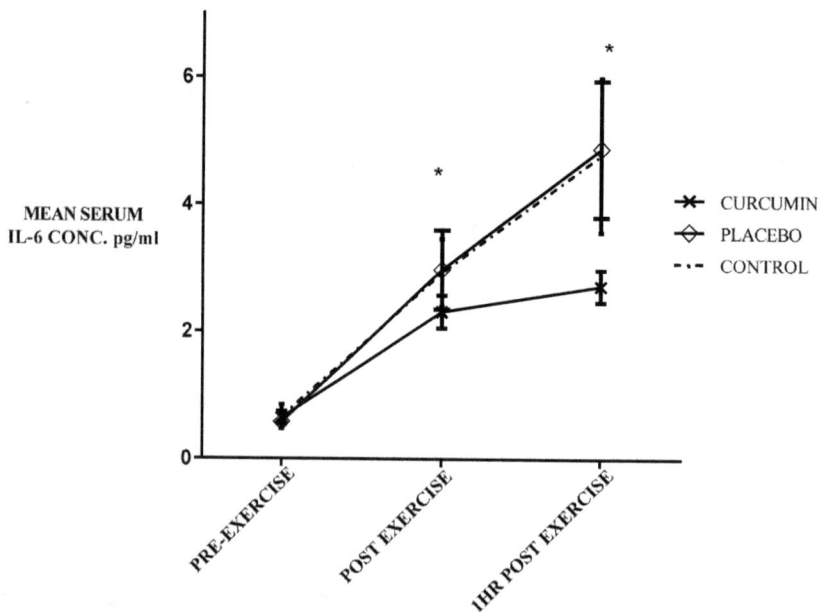

MEAN IL-6 VALUES DURING TRIALS

	CURCUMIN	PLACEBO	CONTROL
Serum IL-6 before exercise (pg/ml)	0.6±0.3 (0.4-0.8)	0.6±0.2 (±0.5-0.7)	0.7±0.6 (±0.3-1.1)
Serum IL- 6 post exercise (pg/ml)	2.3±0.8 (1.8-2.8)	3.0±2.1 (1.8-4.2)	3.0±1.7 (1.9-4.1)
Serum IL-6 1hr post exercise (pg/ml) (MEAN)	2.7±1.5 (1.8-3.6)	4.9±3.3 (2.8-7.0)	4.8±3.8 (2.4-7.2)
(MEDIAN)	2 (IQR 1.8-3.6)	4.8 (IQR 2.1-7.3)	3.5 (IQR 1.9-7.7)

Figure 2 Mean (±SEM) IL-6 concentration obtained before exercise, immediately after exercise, and one hour following exercise on each trial day. *indicates significant difference from pre-exercise on all trials. No statistical significant difference between interleukin 6 values was observed. Table shows mean cytokine levels, standard deviation, and 95% confidence intervals during trials. Median and interquartile range IQR are also shown for 1 hour post exercise.

MEAN IL1-RA VALUES DURING TRIALS

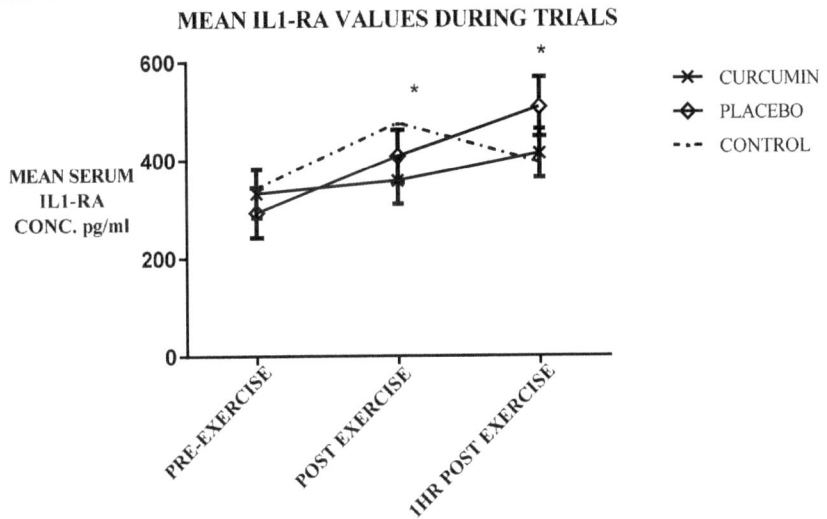

	CURCUMIN	PLACEBO	CONTROL
Serum IL1-RA before exercise (pg/ml)	332±162 (236-428)	293±170 (193-393)	343±95 (284-397)
Serum IL1-RA post exercise (pg/ml)	358±160 (263-453)	408±177 (303-513)	476±252 (327-625)
Serum IL1-RA 1hr post exercise (pg/ml)	414±158 (316-512)	508±200 (389-627)	395+131(314-476)

Figure 3 Mean (±SEM) IL1-RA concentration obtained before exercise, immediately after exercise, and one hour following exercise on each trial day. *indicates significant difference from pre-exercise. Table shows mean cytokine levels, standard deviation, and 95% confidence intervals during trials.

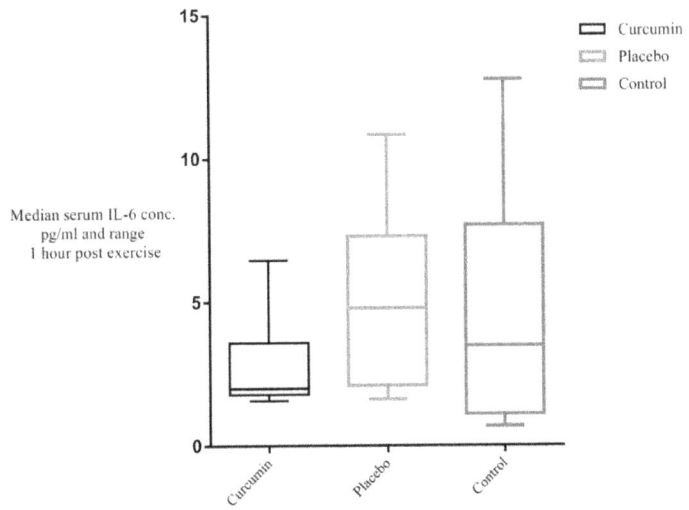

Figure 4 Median IL-6 concentration and range one hour post exercise for curcumin, placebo and control trials. Note curcumin dataset still positively skewed (towards low values) despite removing an outlier.

Table 3 DALDA (Daily Analysis of Life Demands on Athletes) questionnaire responses (median & range) for both training and trial days

	DALDA part 1 (training day) stress sources			DALDA (part 2 training day) stress symptoms		
RESPONSE	*A (Worse)*	*B (Same)*	*C (Better)*	*A (Worse)*	*B (Same)*	*C (Better)*
CURCUMIN (n = 11)	0 (0–3)	4 (4–9)	3 (0–5)[†]	1 (0–4)	21(4–25)	3 (0–19)[†]
PLACEBO (n = 11)	1 (0–5)	7 (2–9)	1 (0–6)	2 (0–7)	20 (8–25)	2 (0–15)
CONTROL (n = 10)	2 (0–3)	6 (2–9)	0 (0–7)	2 (0–9)	22 (5–25)	2 (0–18)
	DALDA part 1 (trial day) stress sources			DALDA part 2 (trial day) stress symptoms		
RESPONSE	*A (Worse)*	*B (Same)*	*C (Better)*	*A (Worse)*	*B (Same)*	*C (Better)*
CURCUMIN (n = 11)	2 (0–4)	6 (2–9)	1 (0–7)	2 (0–5)	22 (5–25)	1 (0–20)
PLACEBO (n = 11)	1 (0–5)	8 (2–9)	0 (0–6)	1 (0–6)	23 (5–25)	0 (0–18)
CONTROL (n = 10)	2 (0–3)	7 (3–9)	0 (0–6)	3 (0–8)	22 (4–25)	1 (0–19)

Data is grouped according to trial type. A – Worse than usual; B – Same as usual; C – Better than usual. [†]indicates statistical significant difference between curcumin and placebo trials, p-value in both parts between curcumin and placebo is 0.04 using Wilcoxon signed ranks.

and supplementation in both stress sources (Part 1, p = 0.04) and stress symptoms (Part 2, p = 0.04). The number of "better than usual" results obtained between curcumin and control on the training day was also higher but not statistically significant (Part 1,p = 0.06; and Part 2, p = 0.14). There were no differences in scoring on Part 1 or Part 2 of the DALDA questionnaire between treatments on the trial days.

Discussion

The current study has not revealed a statistically significant difference between the supplementation with curcumin vs. placebo or control. However these results suggest that a positive inhibitory effect of curcumin on IL-6 production/release or an enhanced uptake *in vivo could occur at* higher supplementation doses, and under different trial conditions (suggested underneath). These observations, although again not statistically significant, lend some support to the previous cell and animal model data, and suggest that further studies in humans may be warranted. The lack of statistical significance in our dataset suggests that sample size, mode of exercise, intensity of exercise, dose of curcumin, or sample collection times are interesting issues for discussion and further investigation.

Sample size estimates using the mean difference 1 hr post-exercise, and standard deviation, from the present study indicate that adequate power could be obtained with 26 participants. Given the large variance in response of IL-6 post-exercise within the current study it would be of interest to analyse responses in a similar trial on a group who may provide a more homogeneous response. The recruitment of cyclists also may have limited our ability to observe any possible effect of curcumin on post-exercise cytokine concentration, due to the absence of eccentric contractions or weight bearing impact during the exercise task. A two hour long exercise regimen was chosen because duration of exercise is

considered a better predictor of serum interleukin elevation than intensity. Running is associated with a higher rise in cytokine concentration post-exercise than observed following cycling [30], and may therefore be a mode of choice in future studies.

Despite the light exercise intensity examined in the present study a response in IL-6 and IL1-RA was still elicited, primarily because the exercise was of sufficient duration. We deliberately adopted a low carbohydrate diet in an attempt to exacerbate the cytokine response to prolonged cycling exercise [12], and this seems to have been effective. Participants whose trial was at a higher workload intensity relative to their maximum workload capacity had a greater increase in IL1-RA and IL-6 concentration one hour after exercise. This was statistically significant for IL-6, and close to statistical significance for IL1-RA. It is important to note that some studies observing higher cytokine responses employed a performance time/distance trial following a period of cycling at a submaximal steady state intensity [12]. This type of protocol would enhance the cytokine response post-exercise, and indicates that higher intensity bouts may be of most interest in future studies examining curcumin effects on cytokine response.

Although our data indicate no statistically significant effect of curcumin supplementation on IL-6 and IL1-RA response to exercise, this could be due to the curcumin dose and plasma curcumin response. Cuomo and colleagues previously indicated that serum micro-molar concentrations of curcumin would likely be necessary for pharmacological *in vivo* effects [32]. Indeed, it is possible that a significant effect on post-exercise interleukin concentrations would have been achieved with a higher plasma curcumin concentration in the present study. The curcumin concentration achieved in the present study was almost 80 ng/ml (0.22 µmoles/L). A recent paper observed an effect of curcumin on plasma oxidative stress markers following exertion in humans when plasma curcumin concentration was elevated to around 100 ng/ml [35]. Recent work [36] has demonstrated that intraperitoneal injection of curcumin counteracts muscle atrophy in rats possibly also through anti-oxidant actions. It is unclear if such effects can be demonstrated in a human model and what dose of curcumin would be required to achieve this, but translation to a human model could provide relevant outcomes for sport or clinical practice. It is, therefore, recommended that future studies quantify the plasma concentration of curcumin required to achieve significant clinically relevant outcomes and investigate any possible association with anti-oxidant activity. Furthermore, blood sampling after 2, 16, & 24 hours following exercise would have provided further data on cortisol, C-reactive protein, and interleukin 10 responses which are known to be influenced by circulating IL-6 concentration, but at a later time than the last blood sample taken in our study.

Ratings of perceived exertion significantly increased throughout the exercise period on all trials. Given the prior glycogen depleting exercise during the training day, and prescribed low carbohydrate diet, it is likely that glycogen depletion contributed towards increased ratings of exertion during the exercise period. The DALDA results indicate that participants felt better on the second day of curcumin supplementation (the training day). The number of "better than usual" responses was higher than placebo and control on the second day of supplementation. It is important to note that DALDA is a retrospective tool of psychological causes and symptoms [31], while that ratings of perceived exertion (RPE) is a prospective tool assessing the extent of exercise difficulty. The study was aimed to provide the same repeatable exercise stressor every time the trial was repeated conducted with curcumin, placebo, and control. The fact that the RPE has did not changed to the extent of its sensitivity, between experimental variables provides evidence that the study managed to reproduce similar exercise conditions in all trials. A study on patients suffering from osteoarthritis taking 1 g of curcumin supplementation for eight months showed less pain and better movement reported by patients taking the supplementation versus placebo [37]. Moreover our views are supported by a recent study on curcumin supplementation and delayed muscle onset soreness (DOMS). This study has demonstrated that, participants taking 400 mg curcumin supplementation for 2 days, report less DOMS than participants taking placebo [38]. The authors suggest that potentially acute curcumin supplementation may be of use to help participants with higher intensity training workloads.

Interestingly, researchers have recently described significant anti-inflammatory effects of curcumin, and have confirmed that curcumin acts to inhibit lipopolysaccharide stimulated NF-κB, reduce IL-6, and reduce PMA induced reactive oxygen species (ROS) production, in human neutrophils [39]. Furthermore, others [40] have noted a significant attenuation in skeletal muscle IL-6 mRNA during exercise with anti-oxidant vitamin supplementation (vitamin C and E); and lead to significantly decreased plasma IL-6 concentration. Starkie and colleagues note a significant reduction in plasma IL-6 but not in skeletal muscle IL-6 mRNA following carbohydrate intake [41]. These observations suggest that measurement of early events in cytokine production are important to monitor in future human studies, and that concurrent supplementation of carbohydrate alongside an anti-oxidant like curcumin might have a superior effect to that of carbohydrate on its own on attenuation of cytokine response following exercise. It must be noted that subjects in our study were glycogen depleted, and that further studies are needed to confirm or refute similar findings or trends in athletes who are carbohydrate replete. As such the usefulness of curcumin supplementation during competition or training needs to be studied separately.

The present study also included a control arm, intended to identify any placebo effects, especially in subjective measures and to help confirm any trends observed with curcumin supplementation. No statistical difference between placebo and control values was found for any variables and no difference was observed from control in those who commenced the study with either curcumin supplementation, or placebo supplementation. This suggests both that the washout period was sufficiently long between trials with our present protocol and that trial stress was adequately reproduced.

Conclusion

There is considerable debate concerning the impact of blunting cytokine and inflammatory marker responses to exercise on the adaptive stimulus to exercise [42], and further work is required to determine the effects of blunting cytokine and inflammatory marker responses to exercise on incidence of infection, and training adaptation in athletes. Given that the limited bioavailability of the polyphenol curcumin has been now improved with new preparations as used in the present study, it would seem prudent to direct more research towards athletic and clinical populations. In conclusion, the results from the present study did not reveal any statistical difference between intervention and placebo. However our interpretation based on the findings presented in this paper does not exclude the possibility of an attenuating effect on IL-6 by curcumin. This is supported by the results obtained in this study and corroborated by findings in other published studies. We conclude that the effect of curcumin supplementation on interleukins and other inflammatory markers needs to be further investigated with observations in a larger sample including examination of exercise mode, intensity effects, and curcumin dose effects.

Competing interests
The authors declare that they have no competing interests.

Authors' contributions
JNS designed the study including trials & analysis, collected, analysed samples & data, prepared the manuscript; SG designed the study, supervised, reviewed data, & prepared manuscript;. AF designed and supervised analysis & reviewed manuscript, GG supervised cytokine analysis, CF supervised HPLC analysis, DD designed and supervised HPLC analysis & JM supervised the study and reviewed manuscript. All authors read and approved the final manuscript.

Acknowledgements
Analysis was carried out at the department of pharmacology and therapeutics, and department of chemistry laboratories. The help of the respective laboratory officers is acknowledged. A special thanks to Dr. Bridgette Ellul, Dr. Neville Calleja, Dr. Christian Saliba, Pro-Rector Richard Muscat & Professor Roger Ellul Micallef for their support and mentorship. Many thanks to Dr. Gregory Attard & St James Highway Clinics This study was aided by a grant from the Maltese Sports Council.

Author details
[1]Sport Nutrition graduate from the University of Stirling, 74, San Anton Court, Pope John XXIII street, Birkirkara BKR1033, Malta. [2]Health and Exercise Sciences Research Group, School of Sport, University of Stirling, Stirling, Scotland. [3]Department of Clinical Pharmacology and Therapeutics, University of Malta, Msida, Malta. [4]Department of Chemistry, University of Malta, Msida, Malta. [5]Department of Pathology, University of Malta, Msida, Malta.

References
1. Nehlsen-Cannarella SL, Fagoaga OR, Nieman DC, Henson DA, Butterworth DE, Schmitt RL, et al. Carbohydrate and the cytokine response to 2.5 h of running. J Appl Physiol. 1997;82:1662–7.
2. Gleeson M, Blannin AK, Walsh NP, Bishop NC, Clark AM. Effect of low and high carbohydrate diets on the plasma glutamine and circulating leukocyte responses to exercise. Int J Sport Nutr Exerc Metab. 1998;8:49–59.
3. Mitchell JB, Pizza FX, Paquet A, Davis BJ, Forrest MB, Braun WA. Influence of carbohydrate status on immune responses before and after endurance exercise. J Appl Physiol. 1998;84:1917–25.
4. Nieman DC. Immunonutrition support for athletes [review]. Nutr Rev. 2008;66(6):310–20. DOI:10.1111/j.1753-4887.2008.00038.x.
5. Walsh NP, Gleeson M, Pyne DB, Niema D, Dhabhar FS, Shephard R, et al. Position statement part two: maintaining immune health. Exerc Immunol Rev. 2011;17:64–103.
6. Northoff H, Berg A. Immmunologic mediators as parameters of the reaction to strenuous exercise. Int J Sports Med. 1991;12(1):S9–S15.
7. Ostrowski K, Rohde T, Asp S, Schjerling P, Pedersen BK. Chemokines are elevated in plasma after strenuous exercise in humans. Eur J Appl Physiol. 2000;84(3):244–5.
8. Lancaster GL, Khan Q, Drysdale PT, Wallace F, Jeukendrup AE, Drayson MT, et al. Effect of prolonged strenuous exercise and carbohydrate ingestion on type 1 and type 2 T lymphocyte intracellular cytokine production in humans. J Appl Physiol. 2005;98:565–71. doi:10.1152/japplphysiol.00754.2004.
9. Starkie RL, Rolland J, Angus DJ, Anderson MJ, Febbraio MA. Circulating monocytes are not the source of the elevations in plasma IL-6 and TNF-α levels after prolonged running. Am J Physiol Cell Physiol. 2007;280:C769–74.
10. Ostrowski K, Rohde T, Zacho M, Asp S, Pedersen BK. Evidence that interleukin 6 is produced in human skeletal muscle during prolonged running. J Physiol. 1998;508(3):889–94.
11. Steensberg A, van Hall G, Osada T, Sacchetti M, Bengt S, Pedersen BK. Production of interleukin 6 in contracting human skeletal muscles can account for the exercise induced increase in plasma interleukin 6. J Physiol. 2000;529(1):237–42.
12. Bishop NC, Walsh NP, Haines DL, Richards DE, Gleeson M. Pre-exercise carbohydrate status and immune responses to prolonged cycling II: effect on plasma cytokine concentration. Int J Sport Nutr Exerc Metab. 2001;11:503–12.
13. Papanicolaou DA, Wilder RL, Manolagas SC, Chrousos GP. The pathophysiological roles of interleukin 6 in human disease [NIH Conference]. Ann Intern Med. 1998;128(2):128–37.
14. Steensberg A, Fischer CP, Keller C, Moller K, Pedersen BK. IL-6 enhances plasma IL1-RA, IL-10, and cortisol in humans. Am J Physiol Endocrinol Metab. 2003;285:E433–7.
15. Blannin AK. Acute exercise and the innate immune function. In: Gleeson M, editor. Immune Function in Sport and Exercise. 1st ed. Edinburgh, UK: Churchill Livingstone; 2006. p. 67–91.
16. Lakier SL. Overtraining, excessive exercise, and altered immunity, is this a T-helper-1 versus T-helper-2 lymphocyte response? Sports Med. 2003;33 (5):347–65.
17. Lancaster GL. Exercise and cytokines. In: Gleeson M, editor. Immune Function in Sport and Exercise. 2006th ed. Edinburgh, UK: Churchill Livingstone; 2006. p. 205–21.
18. Tak PP, Firestein GS. NF-κB a key role in inflammatory diseases. J Clin Investig. 2001;107(1):7–11.
19. Gloire G, Legrand-Poels S, Piette J. NF-κB activation by reactive oxygen species: fifteen years later. Biochem Pharmacol. 2006;72:1493–505. doi:10.1016/j.bcp.2006.04.011.
20. Anand P, Sherin TG, Kunnumakkara AB, Sundaram C, Harikumar KB, Sung B, et al. Biological activities of curcumin and its analogues & congeners) made by man and Mother Nature. Biochem Pharmacol. 2008;76:1590–611.
21. Pfeiffer E, Hoehle SI, Walch SG, Riess A, Solyom AM, Metzler M. Curcuminoids Form Reactive Glucuronides In Vitro. J Agric Food Chem. 2007;55:538–44.
22. Somparn P, Phisalaphong C, Nakornchai S, Unchern S, Phumala N, Morales NP. Comparative Antioxidant Activities of Curcumin and Its Demethoxy and Hydrogenated Derivatives. Biol Pharm Bull. 2007;1:74–8.
23. Bharti AC, Donato N, Singh S, Aggarwal B. Curcumin (diferuloylmethane) down-regulates the constitutive activation of nuclear factor -kB and IkBa kinase in human multiple myeloma cells, leading to suppression of proliferation and induction of apoptosis. Blood. 2003;101:1053–62. doi:10.1182/blood-2002-05-1320.
24. Jobin C, Bradham CA, Russo MP, Juma B, Narula AS, Brenner DA, et al. Curcumin blocks cytokine mediated NF-κB activation and pro-inflammatory gene expression by inhibiting inhibitory factor I-κB kinase activity. J Immunol. 1999;163:3474–83.
25. Shisodia S, Singh T, Chaturvedi MM. Modulation of transcription factors by curcumin. In: Aggarwal BB, Surh Y, Shisodia S, editors. The Molecular Targets and Therapeutic Uses of Curcumin in Health and Disease. 1st ed. New York, USA: Springer; 2007. p. 127–49.
26. Davis JM, Murph, EA, Carmichael MD, Zielinski MR, Groschwitz CM, Brown, AS, Gangemi JD, Ghaffer A, Mayer EP. Curcumin effects on inflammation and performance recovery following eccentric exercise-induced muscle damage. American Journal of Physiology - Regulatory, Integrative and Comparative Physiology 2007, 292: R2168-R2173. doi:10.1152/ajpregu.00858.2006
27. Aggarwal BB, Harikumar KB. Potential Therapeutic Effects of Curcumin, the Anti-inflammatory Agent, Against Neurodegenerative, Cardiovascular, Pulmonary, Metabolic, Autoimmune and Neoplastic Diseases. Int J Biochem Cell Biol. 2008;41(1):40–59. doi:10.1016/j.biocel.2008.06.010.
28. Kawanishi N, Kato K, Takahashi M, Mizokami T, Otsuka T, Imaizumi T, et al. Curcumin attenuates oxidative stress following downhill running-induced muscle damage. Biochem Biophys Res Commun. 2013;22:573–8.
29. Akazawa N, Choi Y, Miyakia A, Tanabe Y, Sugawara J, Ajisaka R, et al. Curcumin ingestion and exercise training improve vascular endothelial function in postmenopausal women. Nutr Res. 2012;32(10):795–9. doi:10.1016/j.nutres.2012.09.002.
30. Fischer CP. Interleukin-6 in acute exercise and training: what is the biological relevance? Exerc Immunol Rev. 2006;12:6–33.
31. Rushall BS. A tool for measuring stress tolerance in elite athletes. J Appl Sport Psychol. 1990;2:51–66.
32. Cuomo J, Appendino G, Dern AS, Schneider E, McKinnon TP, Brown MJ, et al. Comparative absorption of a standardized curcuminoid mixture and its lecithin formulation. J Nat Prod. 2011;74:664–9.
33. Hao K, Zhao XP, Liu XQ, Wang GJ. LC determination of curcumin in dog plasma for a pharmacokinetic study. Chromatographia. 2006;64(9/10):531–5.
34. Grubbs FE. Procedures for detecting outlying observations in samples. Technometrics. 1969;11(1):1–21. doi:10.1080/00401706.1969.10490657.
35. Takahashi M, Suzuki K, Kim HK, Otsuka Y, Imaizumi A, Miyashita M, Sakamoto S. Effects of curcumin supplementation on exercise-induced oxidative stress

in humans. Int J Sports Med 2013, Published online. doi:https://dx.doi.org/10.1055/s-0033-1357185

36. Vitadello M, Germinario E, Ravara B, Dalla Libera L, Danieli-Betto D, Gorsza L. Curcumin counteracts loss of force and atrophy of hindlimb unloaded rat soleus by hampering neuronal nitric oxide synthase untethering from sarcolemma. J Physiol. 2014;592:2637–52.

37. Belcaro G, Cesarone MR, Dugall M, Pellegrini L, Ledda A, Grossi MG, et al. Efficacy and safety of Meriva®, a curcumin-phoshatidylcholine complex, during extended administration in osteoarthritis patients. Altern Med Rev. 2008;15(4):337–44.

38. Drobnic F, Riera J, Appendino G, Togni S, Franceschi F, Valle X, et al. Reduction of delayed onset muscle soreness by a novel curcumin delivery system (Meriva®): a randomised, placebo-controlled trial. J Int Soc Sports Nutr. 2014;11:31. doi:10.1186/1550-2783-11-31.

39. Antoine F, Simard J, Girard D. Curcumin inhibits agent-induced human neutrophil functions in vitro and lipopolysaccharide-induced neutrophilic infiltration in vivo. Int Immunopharmacol. 2013;17:1101–7. http://dx.doi.org/10.1016/j.intimp.2013.09.024.

40. Fischer CP, Hiscock NJ, Penkowa M, Basu S, Vessby B, Kallner A, et al. Supplementation with vitamins C and E inhibits the release of interleukin 6 from contracting human skeletal muscle. J Physiol. 2004;558(2):633–45.

41. Starkie RL, Arkinstall MJ, Koukoulas I, Hawley JA, Febbraio MA. Carbohydrate ingestion attenuates the rise in plasma interleukin-6, but not skeletal muscle interleukin-6 mRNA during exercise in humans. J Physiol. 2001;533(2):585–91.

42. Peternelj T, Coombs JS. Antioxidant supplementation during exercise training: beneficial or detrimental? Sports Med. 2011;41(12):1043–69.

## 4

Safety of a dose-escalated pre-workout supplement in recreationally active females

Roxanne M Vogel[1,2], Jordan M Joy[1], Paul H Falcone[1], Matt M Mosman[1], Michael P Kim[1] and Jordan R Moon[1,3*]

Abstract

Background: Pre-workout supplements (PWS) have increased in popularity among athletic populations for their purported ergogenic benefits. Most PWS contain a "proprietary blend" of several ingredients, such as caffeine, beta-alanine, and nitrate in undisclosed dosages. Currently, little research exists on the safety and potential side effects of chronic consumption of PWS, and even less so involving female populations. Therefore, the purpose of the present study was to examine the safety of consuming a dose-escalated PWS over a 28-day period among active adult females.

Methods: 34 recreationally active, adult females (27.1 ± 5.4 years, 165.2 ± 5.7 cm, 68.2 ± 16.0 kg) participated in this study. Participants were randomly assigned to consume either 1 (G1) or 2 (G2) servings of a PWS daily or remain unsupplemented (CRL) for a period of 28 days. All were instructed to maintain their habitual dietary and exercise routines for the duration of the study. Fasting blood samples, as well as resting blood pressure and heart rate, were taken prior to and following the supplementation period. Samples were analyzed for hematological and clinical chemistry panels, including lipids.

Results: Significant ($p < 0.05$) group by time interactions were present for absolute monocytes (CRL -0.10 ± 0.10; G1 $+0.03 \pm 0.13$; G2 $+0.01 \pm 0.12 \times 10E3/uL$), MCH (CRL -0.13 ± 0.46; G1 $+0.36 \pm 0.52$; G2 -0.19 ± 0.39 pg), creatinine (CRL 0.00 ± 0.05; G1 -0.06 ± 0.13; G2 -0.14 ± 0.08 mg/dL), eGFR (CRL -0.69 ± 5.97; G1 $+6.10 \pm 15.89$; G2 $+14.63 \pm 7.11$ mL/min/1.73), and total cholesterol (CRL -2.44 ± 13.63; G1 $+14.40 \pm 27.32$; G2 -10.38 ± 15.39 mg/dL). Each of these variables remained within the accepted physiological range. No other variables had significant interactions.

Conclusion: The present study confirms the hypothesis that a PWS containing caffeine, beta-alanine, and nitrate will not cause abnormal changes in hematological markers or resting vital signs among adult females. Although there were statistically significant ($p < 0.05$) group by time interactions for absolute monocytes, MCH, creatinine, eGFR, and total cholesterol, all of the results remained well within accepted physiological ranges and were not clinically significant. In sum, it appears as though daily supplementation with up to 2 servings of the PWS under investigation, over an interval of 28 days, did not adversely affect markers of clinical safety among active adult females.

Keywords: Pre-workout, Safety, Health, Female

Background

Nutrient timing refers to the methodical, timed ingestion of carbohydrate, protein, fat and other dietary supplements either before, during, or after physical activity [1]. Supplementation during the period immediately preceding physical activity has become an increasingly popular strategy among competitive and recreational athletes alike as a means of improving performance [2]. In response to this trend, manufacturers have developed pre-workout supplements (PWS), which typically combine caffeine with any number of purported ergogenic substances, such as beta-alanine, nitrate, and amino acids. As the number of PWS available on the market grows, each containing their own "proprietary blend" of active ingredients, it must be determined which, if any, are safe for chronic consumption. This becomes particularly important as concerns have arisen over the concept of

* Correspondence: jordan@musclepharm.com
[1]MusclePharm Sports Science Institute, MusclePharm Corp., 4721 Ironton St. Building A, Denver, CO 80239, USA
[3]Department of Sports Exercise Science, United States Sports Academy, Daphne, AL, USA
Full list of author information is available at the end of the article

proprietary blends, namely the fact that the Food and Drug Administration does not monitor the amounts of ingredients used in these blends or the accuracy of product labeling by manufacturers [2].

Caffeine is one of the most commonly found ingredients in PWS. An extensive amount of scientific literature exists on the ergogenic properties of caffeine [3-5]. According to the International Society of Sports Nutrition's position stand on caffeine and performance, it is most effective when consumed in low to moderate doses, about 3–6 mg per kilogram bodyweight, 30–60 minutes prior to exercise [4]. Caffeine has been shown to improve performance in endurance events and time-trials, improve cognitive function and alertness, and delay the onset of fatigue during exhaustive exercise [3,5]. Moreover, caffeine anhydrous, which is frequently used in PWS, has been shown to have greater ergogenic effects than caffeine ingested in the form of coffee, tea, or cola [4].

Beta-alanine (BA), another common ingredient in PWS, is an amino acid which serves as a rate-limiting precursor to carnosine in skeletal muscle [6]. Carnosine's suggested mechanism of action may be to buffer hydrogen ions during exercise, thereby influencing intracellular muscle pH, and ultimately increasing work capacity [7]. In a recent review of the literature by Quesnele et al. [8], the authors concluded that although there is evidence to suggest that BA supplementation enhances athletic performance, the safety of its use remains unclear, and there is a general under-reporting of its side effects in the literature.

Despite the existing literature pertaining to individual ingredients contained in PWS and the growing number of studies that address multi-ingredient PWS specifically, we are unaware of any published reports examining the safety of PWS in a solely female population. Therefore, the purpose of the present study was to examine the safety of chronic consumption of a PWS over a 28 day period among active adult females. We hypothesized that daily PWS supplementation would not produce abnormal changes in hematological or metabolic safety markers or resting vital signs.

Methods
Experimental design
In a dose-escalated, simple randomized design, 34 subjects were randomly assigned to control (CRL, n = 16; 27.1 ± 5.9 y, 166.2 ± 4.0 cm, 65.2 ± 12.9 kg), 1 serving (G1, n = 10; 24.9 ± 3.9 y, 164.7 ± 5.8 cm, 72.4 ± 23.3 kg), or 2 serving (G2, n = 8; 29.6 ± 5.8 y, 163.8 ± 8.8 cm, 69.0 ± 11.6 kg) groups via random number generation by the investigators and asked to remain unsupplemented, or consume either 1 or 2 servings, respectively, of a pre-workout formula (Fitmiss Ignite™, MusclePharm Corp., Denver, CO) every day for 28 days. The pre-workout formula contained 1 g of carbohydrate, 23 mg of Calcium, and 5,700 mg of a proprietary blend consisting of beta-alanine, choline bitartrate, L-tyrosine, glycine, taurine, L-carnitine, beetroot extract, hawthorn berry powder, agmatine sulfate, caffeine anhydrous, and huperzine A. The supplement was analyzed by a third party (Eurofins Supplement Analysis Center, Petaluma, CA) and verified to contain all of the ingredients on the label. Subjects were instructed to consume 1–2 level scoop(s) of the supplement with 12 oz water per scoop either 30 minutes prior to exercise or at the same time of day on rest days. Compliance was monitored using supplement consumption logs, as well as by weighing supplement containers before and after the supplementation period. A total of 38 subjects were initially recruited for this study. From G1, one subject discontinued the study due to noncompliance, and from G2, three subjects discontinued due to noncompliance. The CRL group contained more total participants, as CRL group data was added from a previously conducted study which featured a design exactly identical to the present study. Participants completed the study with an average supplementation compliance of 94.6% for G1 and 100% for G2. Blood draws were taken prior to and following the supplementation period. Approval for the human subject protocol was obtained from MusclePharm Sports Science Institute's IRB, and subjects were provided with written informed consent documents prior to participation in the study.

Participants
34 recreationally active female adults (27.1 ± 5.4 years, 165 ± 5.7 cm, 68.2 ± 16.0 kg) participated in the study. Recreationally active was defined as habitually participating in moderate to vigorous physical activity on three or more days a week for a duration of thirty minutes or more. Subjects were required to be non-smokers, free of any disease or disorder which may have produced confounding effects, and have abstained from taking any other pre-workout supplements for one month prior to the beginning of the study. Exclusion criteria included having a significant history or current presence of a treated condition, such as high blood pressure (≥ 140 mmHg systolic and/or ≥ 90 mmHg diastolic), tachyarrhythmia, or heart, kidney, or liver disease, or any contraindication to physical activity. Also excluded from the study were participants whose willingness or ability to comply with the study protocol was uncertain. Eligibility was determined upon evaluation of pre-participation health history, exercise, and supplementation screening questionnaires. A caffeine usage questionnaire was given as part of the pre-participating screening process, with average self-reported caffeine consumption prior to study being 131 mg/day for G1 and 269 mg/day

for G2. Subjects were instructed to maintain their habitual dietary and exercise routines, and to not take any additional supplements during their participation in the study.

Measurements

All measurements were taken prior to and following the 28-day supplementation period in a quiet, temperature controlled private office. Upon arrival at the office, subjects were instructed to remain seated quietly for 15 minutes before resting vital signs, height, and weight were taken. Subjects then submitted a blood sample in the fasted state. All blood draws were performed in the morning to prevent diurnal variations by a trained phlebotomist via venipuncture. Samples were analyzed for comprehensive metabolic panels, complete blood counts and lipid profiles by an external laboratory (Laboratory Corporation of America, Denver, CO). Variables recorded from blood analysis consisted of white blood cell count (WBC), red blood cell count (RBC), hemoglobin, hematocrit, mean corpuscular volume (MCV), mean corpuscular hemoglobin (MCH), mean corpuscular hemoglobin concentration (MCHC), red blood cell distribution width (RDW), platelets (absolute), neutrophils (percent and absolute), lymphocytes (percent and absolute), monocytes (percent and absolute), eosinophils (percent and absolute), basophils (percent and absolute), serum glucose, blood urea nitrogen (BUN), creatinine, estimated glomerular filtration rate (eGFR), BUN:creatinine, sodium, potassium, chloride, carbon dioxide, calcium, protein, albumin, globulin, albumin:globulin, bilirubin, alkaline phosphatase, aspartate aminotransferase (AST), alanine aminotransferase (ALT), total cholesterol, triglycerides, high density lipoprotein (HDL) cholesterol, and low density lipoprotein (LDL) cholesterol. Inter-test reliability results from 12 men and women measured up to one week apart at the aforementioned laboratory resulted in no significant differences for any of the variables noted above from day-to-day ($p > 0.05$) and an average inter-test Coefficient of Variation (CV) of 6.9%.

Statistical analyses

Data was analyzed using a 3×2 repeated measures ANOVA model for all group, time, and group by time interactions. A Bonferroni post-hoc analysis was used to locate differences. Shapiro-Wilk tests were used to determine normality of the data. The Minimal Difference (MD) needed to be considered real was determined using the method previously described by Weir [9]. Data are presented as means ± standard deviation. All data were analyzed using Statistica software (Statsoft, Version 10).

Results

Significant group by time interactions were present for absolute monocytes ($p < 0.05$), wherein CRL decreased relative to G1 and G2. Absolute monocytes had a normal distribution at baseline ($p = 0.07$), yet the distribution was positively skewed ($p < 0.05$) after the supplementation period. Significant group by time interactions were observed with MCH ($p < 0.05$), with G1 increasing relative to CRL and G2. Significant group by time interactions were detected for creatinine ($p < 0.05$), with G2 decreasing relative to CRL. Significant group by time interactions were noted for eGFR ($p < 0.05$), with G2 increasing relative to control. Significant group by time interactions were also present for total cholesterol ($p < 0.05$), G1 increasing relative to CRL and G2. Total cholesterol was positively skewed at baseline ($p < 0.05$), and at post-supplementation, it became normally distributed ($p = 0.99$). MCH and eGFR were normally distributed ($p > 0.05$) at both time points, and creatinine was positively skewed ($p < 0.05$) at both time points. All variables remained within the accepted physiological range at baseline and post supplementation. No other variables had significant group by time interactions. Data are presented in Additional file 1 as means ± standard deviation. Tolerability data collected from participants reported no serious adverse events. The most common reported side effects were a tingling sensation (n = 6), itchiness (n = 2), and nausea (n = 2). Other reported side effects included dizziness, lightheadedness, dry mouth, headache, a burning sensation, and diarrhea (all n = 1). Most of these effects occurred within the first several days of supplementation and subsided over time.

Discussion

The results of the present study suggest that daily supplementation with the PWS under investigation does not appear to cause any abnormal changes in hematological and clinical chemistry/metabolic safety markers or resting vital signs in female subjects. While significant group by time interactions ($p < 0.05$) were observed for absolute monocytes, MCH, creatinine, eGFR, and total cholesterol, all group values remained well within the accepted physiological range and were not clinically significant. While remaining within range, unusual effects were observed between groups. For instance, the CRL group decreased relative to G1 and G2 for absolute monocytes, and for MCH and total cholesterol, G1 increased relative to both CRL and G2. Similar to total cholesterol, although not reaching significance ($p > 0.05$), both LDL and HDL increased in G1 but decreased in G2 over time. These findings are somewhat discrepant, since intuitively, one would think that if a lower dose increases a given parameter compared to control, then a higher dose should amplify this effect. This, however, was not the case. Such results suggest a natural variation in these clinical markers, and may not necessarily be related to supplementation. Additionally, the control group (n = 16) was larger than either of the experimental groups (G1, n = 10; G2, n = 8), so individual variations within the experimental groups had greater impact on the group mean values.

Variables that were significantly different at the group level were evaluated at the individual level to determine clinical significance. Analysis of clinical significance at the individual level was conducted using the MD statistic, which calculates the magnitude of the inter-test difference (between baseline and post-supplementation) needed to be exceeded in order for a single measurement to be considered real, as described by Weir [9]. The MD is calculated using the standard error of measurement (SEM), which is considered an absolute index of the reliability of a given test/measurement, not relative to the characteristics of the sample or population from which values were obtained. Unlike other reliability measures, such as the CV, the SEM and thus the MD, are not affected by between-subject variability [9]. If a subject's measured values exceeded the MD, the change was considered a *true* change. Clinical significance at the individual level was reached when a score that exceeded the MD crossed the upper or lower limits of the accepted physiological range for each variable. For creatinine, this occurred in three subjects, one from G1 and two from G2, wherein values decreased pre to post, bringing them within the clinical reference range. For total cholesterol, changes observed in two subjects from G1 and one from G2 exceeded the MD. Specifically, the two subjects from G1 increased over time, moving from within range to out of range, while the subject from G2 decreased pre to post, entering the accepted reference range. Also worth noting is the fact that three individuals from the CRL group experienced changes in total cholesterol values that both exceeded the MD and moved in or out of range. In this case, one subject increased over time to leave the accepted range, one started outside of the range and remained out of range, and one decreased pre to post, entering back into range. All subjects remained within 3 standard deviations of the mean and exceeded the MD. Collectively, individual analysis supports the present hypothesis and also supports the notion of intra-subject diurnal variability. Furthermore, absolute monocytes and total cholesterol were distributed differently pre to post, increasing the probability for a type 1 statistical error [10].

These findings generally agree with previous literature. Aside from the research pertaining to PWS effects on performance [11-16], only a limited number of studies have also examined the clinical safety of PWS. Kedia et al. [17] looked at the effects of a multi-ingredient PWS containing caffeine, betaine, and dendrobium extract on body composition, performance measures, and hematological markers of clinical safety in healthy, young men and women undergoing concurrent resistance training for six weeks. While the investigators did not see an improvement in objective assessments of exercise performance or body composition with supplementation, they found the PWS to be well tolerated with no significant changes in clinical laboratory safety markers at the end of six weeks.

Similarly, Shelmadine et al. [18] examined the effects of 28 days consuming a commercially available PWS, NO-Shotgun®, combined with heavy resistance exercise on body composition, muscle strength and mass, myofibrillar protein content, markers of satellite cell activation, and clinical safety markers in male subjects. They found no negative side effects or abnormal impact on clinical safety markers after 28 days of supplementation. In a follow up study of the same nature, this time with a post-workout supplement added (NO-Synthesize®), Spillane et al. [19] again found no detrimental effects on clinical safety markers following 28 days supplementation and resistance training with NO-Shotgun®.

Farney et al. [20] investigated hemodynamic and hematological effects of two supplements containing caffeine and 1,3- dimethylamylamine (a constituent of geranium) after 14 days of supplementation in men and women, and found only a significant change in blood glucose for one of the supplements (Jack3d™) over this time period. A follow up to this study conducted by Whitehead et al. [21] supplemented with the same product containing caffeine and 1,3- dimethylamylamine (Jack3d™) over a 10-week period in healthy males and also found it did not negatively impact hematological markers of health when consumed daily.

Kendall et al. [22] investigated the safety and efficacy of a PWS containing caffeine, creatine, beta-alanine, amino acids and B-vitamins in recreationally trained, college-age men over an identical period of 28 days. In that study, no adverse effects were observed for renal or hepatic clinical blood markers or resting vital signs. Researchers concluded that PWS with similar ingredients in similar doses should be safe for ingestion periods up to 28 days in healthy males. More recently, Joy et al. [23] found that supplementation with a PWS containing caffeine, nitrate, and amino acids in healthy, recreationally active men and women was apparently safe when taken within recommended dosage guidelines for 28 days.

To our knowledge, this is the first study assessing the clinical safety of a PWS in an all-female population. Female-specific recommendations for sports nutrition and supplementation is an area that warrants more attention. A review article by Volek, Forsythe, and Kraemer [24], for instance, identifies the subtle, yet important differences in exercise metabolism between male and female athletes. The authors suggest that nutritional strategies, including nutrient timing and supplement use, should be tailored to meet the sex-specific needs of female athletes. In another review article addressing gender differences in sports nutrition, Tarnopolsky [25] similarly concluded that future studies in nutrition and metabolism should examine and consider sex differences in response to supplementation and exercise. It therefore seems prudent for future research to continue to address sports nutrition supplementation in females to evaluate both safety and efficacy in this population as compared to males.

Limitations

The present study included a short duration supplementation period and small sample size. Future studies should examine the effects of supplementation for longer than 28 days among more subjects, especially given the fact that statistically significant interactions did take place over time in the present study. Again, while none of the significant variables left the accepted physiological range, the possibility that these could be the beginnings of adverse trends cannot be ruled out. This leaves long-term safety of PWS supplementation, at least greater than 28 days, still open to question.

Conclusion

This study supports the hypothesis that a PWS containing caffeine, beta-alanine, and nitrate will not cause abnormal changes in hematological or clinical chemistry/metabolic markers, or resting vital signs among recreationally active females. Although there were statistically significant (p < 0.05) group by time interactions for absolute monocytes, MCH, creatinine, eGFR, and total cholesterol, all of the results remained well within accepted physiological ranges and were not clinically significant. In sum, it appears as though daily supplementation with up to 2 servings of the PWS used in this investigation, over a period of 28 days, had no adverse impact on markers of clinical safety among active adult females.

Additional file

Additional file 1: Data collected pre and post supplementation.

Abbreviations

PWS: Pre-workout supplement(s); BA: Beta-alanine; WBC: White blood cell; RBC: Red blood cell; MCV: Mean corpuscular volume; MCH: Mean corpuscular hemoglobin; MCHC: Mean corpuscular hemoglobin concentration; RDW: Red blood cell distribution width; BUN: Blood urea nitrogen; eGFR: Estimated glomerular filtration rate; AST: Aspartate aminotransferase; ALT: Alanine aminotransferase; CV: Coefficient of variation; MD: Minimum difference; SEM: Standard error of measurement.

Competing interests

RV, JJ, PF, MM, MK and JM are employees of the funding source, MusclePharm Corporation. However, this publication should not be viewed as endorsement by the investigators, Metropolitan State University of Denver, the United States Sports Academy, or MusclePharm Corporation.

Authors' contributions

RV, JJ, and PF participated in data collection for this investigation. All authors contributed to the conception of the experimental design, drafting of the manuscript, and interpretation of data. All authors have read and approved the final manuscript.

Acknowledgements

We would like to thank all of the participants as well as MusclePharm Corporation for supplying product and funding the investigation.

Author details

[1]MusclePharm Sports Science Institute, MusclePharm Corp., 4721 Ironton St. Building A, Denver, CO 80239, USA. [2]Metropolitan State University, Denver, CO, USA. [3]Department of Sports Exercise Science, United States Sports Academy, Daphne, AL, USA.

References

1. Kerksick C, Harvey T, Stout J, Campbell B, Wilborn C, Kreider R, et al. International society of sports nutrition position stand: nutrient timing. J Int Soc Sports Nutr. 2008;5:17.
2. Eudy AE, Gordon LL, Hockaday BC, Lee DA, Lee V, Luu D, et al. Efficacy and safety of ingredients found in preworkout supplements. Am J Health Syst Pharm. 2013;70:577–88.
3. Astorino TA, Roberson DW. Efficacy of acute caffeine ingestion for short-term high-intensity exercise performance: a systematic review. J Strength Cond Res. 2010;24:257–65.
4. Goldstein ER, Ziegenfuss T, Kalman D, Kreider R, Campbell B, Wilborn C, et al. International society of sports nutrition position stand: caffeine and performance. J Int Soc Sports Nutr. 2010;7:5.
5. Graham TE. Caffeine and exercise: metabolism, endurance and performance. Sports Med. 2001;31:785–807.
6. Harris RC, Wise JA, Price KA, Kim HJ, Kim CK, Sale C. Determinants of muscle carnosine content. Amino Acids. 2012;43:5–12.
7. Derave W, Everaert I, Beeckman S, Baguet A. Muscle carnosine metabolism and beta-alanine supplementation in relation to exercise and training. Sports Med. 2010;40:247–63.
8. Quesnele JJ, Laframboise MA, Wong JJ, Kim P, Wells GD. The effects of beta-alanine supplementation on performance: a systematic review of the literature. Int J Sport Nutr Exerc Metab. 2014;24:14–27.
9. Weir JP. Quantifying test-retest reliability using the intraclass correlation coefficient and the SEM. J Strength Cond Res. 2005;19:231–40.
10. Delaney HD, Vargha A. The effect of nonnormality on student's two-sample t test. In: The education resources information center. U.S. Department of Education. 2000. http://eric.ed.gov/?q=ED443850&id=ED443850. Accessed 20 November 2014.
11. Fukuda DH, Smith AE, Kendall KL, Stout JR. The possible combinatory effects of acute consumption of caffeine, creatine, and amino acids on the improvement of anaerobic running performance in humans. Nutr Res. 2010;30:607–14.
12. Hoffman JR, Kang J, Ratamess NA, Hoffman MW, Tranchina CP, Faigenbaum AD. Examination of a pre-exercise, high energy supplement on exercise performance. J Int Soc Sports Nutr. 2009;6:2.
13. Lowery RP, Joy JM, Dudeck JE, Oliveira de Souza E, McCleary SA, Wells S, et al. Effects of 8 weeks of Xpand(R) 2X pre workout supplementation on skeletal muscle hypertrophy, lean body mass, and strength in resistance trained males. J Int Soc Sports Nutr. 2013;10:44.
14. Outlaw JJ, Wilborn CD, Smith-Ryan AE, Hayward SE, Urbina SL, Taylor LW, et al. Acute effects of a commercially-available pre-workout supplement on markers of training: a double-blind study. J Int Soc Sports Nutr. 2014;11:40.
15. Smith AE, Fukuda DH, Kendall KL, Stout JR. The effects of a pre-workout supplement containing caffeine, creatine, and amino acids during three weeks of high-intensity exercise on aerobic and anaerobic performance. J Int Soc Sports Nutr. 2010;7:10.
16. Spradley BD, Crowley KR, Tai CY, Kendall KL, Fukuda DH, Esposito EN, et al. Ingesting a pre-workout supplement containing caffeine, B-vitamins, amino

acids, creatine, and beta-alanine before exercise delays fatigue while improving reaction time and muscular endurance. Nutr Metab (Lond). 2012;9:28.

17. Kedia AW, Hofheins JE, Habowski SM, Ferrando AA, Gothard MD, Lopez HL. Effects of a pre-workout supplement on lean mass, muscular performance, subjective workout experience and biomarkers of safety. Int J Med Sci. 2014;11:116–26.

18. Shelmadine B, Cooke M, Buford T, Hudson G, Redd L, Leutholtz B, et al. Effects of 28 days of resistance exercise and consuming a commercially available pre-workout supplement, NO-Shotgun(R), on body composition, muscle strength and mass, markers of satellite cell activation, and clinical safety markers in males. J Int Soc Sports Nutr. 2009;6:16.

19. Spillane M, Schwarz N, Leddy S, Correa T, Minter M, Longoria V, et al. Effects of 28 days of resistance exercise while consuming commercially available pre- and post-workout supplements, NO-Shotgun(R) and NO-Synthesize(R) on body composition, muscle strength and mass, markers of protein synthesis, and clinical safety markers in males. Nutr Metab (Lond). 2011;8:78.

20. Farney TM, McCarthy CG, Canale RE, Allman Jr RJ, Bloomer RJ. Hemodynamic and hematologic profile of healthy adults ingesting dietary supplements containing 1,3-dimethylamlamine and caffeine. Nutr Metab Insights. 2012;5:1–12.

21. Whitehead PN, Schilling BK, Farney TM, Bloomer RJ. Impact of a dietary supplement containing 1,3-dimethylamylamine on blood pressure and bloodborne markers of health: a 10-week intervention study. Nutr Metab Insights. 2012;5:33–9.

22. Kendall KL, Moon JR, Fairman CM, Spradley BD, Tai C-Y, Falcone PH, et al. Ingesting a preworkout supplement containing caffeine, creatine, beta-alanine, amino acids, and B vitamins for 28 days is both safe and efficacious in recreationally active men. Nutr Res. 2014;34:442–9.

23. Joy JM, Mosman MM, Falcone PH, Tai C-Y, Carson LR, Kimber D, et al. Safety of 28 days consumption of a pre-workout supplement. J Int Soc Sports Nutr. 2014;11 Suppl 1:30.

24. Volek JS, Forsythe CE, Kraemer WJ. Nutritional aspects of women strength athletes. Br J Sports Med. 2006;40:742–8.

25. Tarnopolsky MA. Gender differences in metabolism; nutrition and supplements. J Sci Med Sport. 2000;3:287–98.

## 5

The risks of self-made diets: the case of an amateur bodybuilder

Lucio Della Guardia[*], Maurizio Cavallaro and Hellas Cena

Abstract

Background: Following DIY (do it yourself) diets as well as consuming supplements exceeding by far the recommended daily intake levels, is common among athletes; these dietary habits often lead to an overconsumption of some macro and/or micronutrients, exposing athletes to potential health risks.

The aim of this study is to document the development of possible adverse effects in a 33 year-old amateur bodybuilder who consumed for 16 years a DIY high protein diet associated to nutrient supplementation. Body composition, biochemical measures and anamnestic findings were evaluated.

We present this case to put on alert about the possible risks of such behavior repeated over time, focusing on the adverse gastrointestinal effects. We discuss the energy and nutrient composition of his DIY diet as well as the use of supplements.

Conclusion: This study provides preliminary data of the potential risks of a long-term DIY dietary supplementation and a high protein diet. In this case, permanent abdominal discomfort was evidenced in an amateur body builder with an intake exceeding tolerable upper limit for vitamin A, selenium and zinc, according to our national and updated recommendations.

As many amateur athletes usually adopt self-made diets and supplementation, it would be advisable for them to be supervised in order to prevent health risks due to a long-term DIY diet and over-supplementation.

Keywords: Supplementation, Vitamin and micronutrients overdose, Gastrointestinal, High-protein diet, Bodybuilding, DIY diets

Background

Nutritional supplements are commonly used by elite and amateur athletes. Supplements are often considered necessary to maintain strength as well as to enhance endurance performance and to improve the ability to train longer [1].

It is estimated that up to 90 percent of all the athletes globally use supplements to some extent [2] mainly because these substances are freely available to purchase. In particular, amateur athletes frequently follow their own prescriptions despite the recommendations regarding the risks connected with prolonged and excessive intake of specific nutrients [3-5]. Indeed, although various nutrients are required for normal growth, maintenance and repair of tissues, it has been demonstrated that the excess of nutrient intake may cause adverse effects on organs and metabolism [3-5].

Furthermore, there is a substantial risk of supplements contamination with prohibited substances such as stimulants or hormone-like compounds [6,7].

Whether a scheduled supplementation of some and specific macronutrient compounds could enhance muscle adaptation to training [8], no precise reason, even among athletes, seems to justify a massive intake of some nutrients, especially vitamins and minerals, if the dietary regimen provides for a sufficient variety of foods [9]. Therefore, many efforts have been performed to identify macro and micronutrient intake ranges of safety.

The purpose of this study is to document the development of possible adverse effects in an amateur bodybuilder on a long term DIY high protein diet associated to nutrient supplementation.

* Correspondence: lucio.dellaguardia@unimi.it
Department of Public Health, Experimental and Forensic Medicine, Unit of Human Nutrition, University of Pavia, via Bassi 21, 27100 Pavia, Italy

Case presentation

According to the international dietary guidelines [10] and the dietary reference intakes (IOR)[a] [11] a balanced diet should respect some paradigms regarding the macro and micronutrient intake. In detail, the guidelines specify that carbohydrate (CHO), lipids and protein intake should represent specific percentages of the total energy intake (CHO 55%, lipids less than 30% and protein around 15%) [11,12]. Although, as far as protein intake is concerned, the daily-recommended amount should be related to the body weight (0.9 g of protein/kg/day) [11,12].

In case of trained athletes, the protein intake can be increased to 1.2-1.7 g/kg/day, in order to satisfy the augmented muscle turnover depending on the type and amount of sport activity [9].

Fiber intake is recommended in a quantity of 20–30 g/day in order to maintain a correct gastrointestinal activity and mucosal tropism.

Moreover, recommendations of daily vitamins and minerals intakes have been provided in order to satisfy the body metabolic request and to avoid toxicity [12].

Amateur athletes often go on do-it-yourself (DIY) diets that differ somewhat from the above recommendations and may lead to health hazards.

We discuss the development of possible adverse effects in a 33 year-old amateur bodybuilder on a long term DIY high protein diet associated to micronutrient supplementation, referred to our department by his personal trainer after reporting deep weakness and recurrent episodes of diarrhea in the previous 6 months.

The patient was a warehouse worker. He used to follow a DIY diet along with a multivitamin and mineral supplementation.

Symptoms

The patient complained of feeling fatigue and tiredness, interfering with his work activity as well as with his training and performance. The anamnestic interview did not record any insomnia episodes or other sleep disturbances. The sleep period was around the 6 hours per night. Moreover, the patient described a strong gastrointestinal discomfort such as post-prandial fullness, nausea and dyspepsia; the main symptoms reported by the patient were frequent episodes of diarrhea that occurred around 3 times per day, minutes to hours after the ingestion of food, followed by moderate-to-intense low abdominal pain. Diarrhea and the gastrointestinal distress reported had occurred approximately for 6 months before the patient underwent our medical examination.

Anthropometric and nutritional evaluation

We conducted a complete nutritional evaluation. The medical inspection included: physical examination, blood tests recording, anthropometric measurements, nutritional and medical history collection, body composition analysis by bioelectrical-impedance (BIA-101 model; Akern srl, Florence, Italy) and resting energy expenditure by indirect calorimetry (Vmax Spectra 29n; Sensormedics, Yorba Linda, California, US). The last two tests were conducted under standard conditions: the patient was dressed in light clothing and the average room temperature was around 21°C; the patient had been advised to fast for 12 hours, abstain from alcohol consumption and refrain from any physical activity in the 24 hours before the measurements.

Heart rate and blood pressure were in the normal range (61 bpm and 125/80 mmHg); no signs of respiratory, skin or mucosal alterations were reported. Notably, the patient felt pain in epigastrium and in the right iliac fossa during abdominal palpation.

Height (m 1.86) and weight (86.3 kg) of the subject were measured and recorded in nearest 0.1 and 1 cm, respectively. BMI (24.9 kg/m^2) was then calculated dividing the weight (kg) by the height in square meters (m^2).

Body composition by bioelectrical-impedance analysis, revealed a moderate-to-high percentage of metabolically active mass (body cellular mass 48.5%, body fat-free mass 79.9%, body fat mass 20.1%, phase angle 6.8°)[b].

Anthropometric, body composition and blood pressure characteristics are reported in Table 1.

Indirect calorimetry measured a respiratory quotient of 0.9 and a resting energy expenditure (REE) of 1554 kcal/day, equivalent to the 79% of the estimated value according to Harris-Benedict equation [13]. This disparity was probably due both to the complete suspension of rigorous training (for a 6 months period) than to the self-induced food restriction in the effort to try to manage the gastrointestinal discomfort. The prolonged training suspension period was likely to lead to a muscle mass loss and relative increase of fat mass [14]. Besides, the low resting energy expenditure observed is likely to reflect the body-self adjustment secondary to the scarce physical activity performed as well as the spontaneously decreased energy daily intake [12,15].

Table 1 Patient's characteristics

Variable	Value
Height (m)	1.86
Weight (kg)	86.3
BMI (kg/m^2)	24.9
WC (cm)	89
SBP/DBP (mmHg)	120/80
Arm circumference (cm)	33
Fat mass kg (%)	17.3 (20.1)
Fat-free mass kg (%)	69 (79.9)
Body cellular mass kg (%)	33.5 (48.5)
Extracellular water kg (%)	19.1 (38.5)

Unfortunately, not in possession of the body composition data prior the 6-month suspension of training, we are not able to comment in more detail the above-reported findings.

Laboratory analysis

All measured biochemical parameters (blood count as well as serum electrolytes, total protein, hepatic markers, ferritin, creatinine, C-reactive protein, pancreatic enzymes and insulin) were within the reference values. The patient also underwent a cardiological assessment (electrocardiography and echocardiography) that did not show any alteration. The fecal fat test identified a slight fat malabsorption. Markers of celiac disease, Helicobacter Pylori antibodies and parasite exam were all negative. The total IgE value resulted within the range . The allergen-specific IgE assay showed no positivity for the food allergens tested. The H_2 breath test showed lactose intolerance. Basal biochemical data are shown in Table 2.

The oral glucose tolerance test revealed impaired glucose tolerance (glycaemia: 153 mg/dl after 2 hours). The esophagogastroduodenoscopy performed did not display any remarkable anatomic alteration.

Dietary data

The diet history collected by trained nutrition professionals included a detailed interview about usual pattern of eating, a food list asking for amount and frequency usually eaten, and a 7-day dietary record.

The major strength of the diet history method is its assessment of meal patterns and details of food intake rather than intakes for a short period of time. We used this approach since our patient had been following a specific DIY eating pattern and this method is a tool able to ascertain the usual eating patterns for an extended period of time, including type, frequency and amount of foods consumed [16].

Portion sizes were estimated through a validated colour food photography atlas for quantifying the portion size eaten [17].

Supplement use, frequency and dosage were investigated. According to the 7-day food diary compiled by the patient and the 24-h recall performed, the patient's daily energy intake, at the time of the medical examination, was approximately 2160 kcal/day (Table 3). Furthermore, the vitamin and mineral supplementation, he reported he had never stopped, exceeded by far the micro nutrients intake recommended by the Italian Official Reccomendations (IOR) [11] (Table 4).

Data about the remote dietary history were collected. The DIY dietary scheme, handed out by the subject, was then analyzed for energy, macro and micronutrient content and compared to the dietary intakes recommended by the IOR [11] using a software with BDA food composition tables [18] as database.

The results showed that the patient usual dietary intake for up to 6 months before was very high in protein and poor in fiber; protein daily intake, mainly from

Table 2 Patient's biochemical data

Metabolite	Value
Urea nitrogenum (mg/dl)	47
Creatinine (mg/dl)	0.92
Total protein (g)	8.0
Fasting glucose (mg/dl)	69
TSH (UI/l)	1.17
Ca^{2+} (mg/dl)	10.1
Na^+/K^+ (mEq/l)	139/3.8
Helicobacter Pilory IgG	Negative
Anti-gliadine IgA-IgG	Negative
H_2 breath test	Positive
Fecal occult blood test	Negative
Basal insulin (mUI/l)	14
Fecal simple sugars (g/l)	1.8
Fecal fats (g/dl)	2.2
Total IgE (UI/ml)	110

Table 3 Dietary intake at the time of the medical examination (7-day food diary assessment)

Component	Quantity	% of TE	IOR§
Energy (kcal)	2160	-	-
Total protein (g)	106.9	19.7	-
Total fats (g)	46.1	19.2	20-35%
Saturated fats (g)	9.1	3.8	<10%
MUFA (g)	24.8	10.3	10-15%
PUFA (g)	9.4	3.9	5-10%
Total carbohydrates (g)	352	61.1	45-60%
Starch (g)	297	51.5	45-53%
Simple sugars (g)	55	9.5	<15%
Dietary fiber (g)	16	-	12.6-16.7*
Iron (mg)	15	-	10
Cholesterol (mg)	212	-	0-300
Vitamin A (RE) (µg)	174	-	700
Niacin (mg)	35	-	18
Selenium (µg)	25	-	55
Zinc (mg)	14	-	12

% of TE: percentage of total energy intake.
IOR: Italian official recommendations reference values.
§IOR reference values are reported as % of TE for macronutrient and as daily total amount for micronutrient and fiber.
*g/1000 kcal of energy intake.

Table 4 Reference values and content of vitamins and minerals per tablet of supplement (1 tablet/day)

Vitamin	IOR (per day)	UL (per day)	MPL*	TC
Vitamin A (µg)	700**	3000	1200	6000
Vitamin D (µg)	15	100	25	10
Vitamin E (mg)	13	300	60	66.7
Vitamin K (µg)	140	-	105	-
Vitamin C (mg)	105	-	1000	150
Thiamin (mg)	1.2	-	25	25
Riboflavin (mg)	1,6	-	25	25
Niacin (mg)	18	900§	36	100
Vitamin B6 (mg)	1,3	25	9,5	25
Folic acid (µg)	400	1000	400	800
Vitamin B12 (µg)	2,4	-	33	100
Biotin (µg)	-	-	0.450	300
Minerals				
Calcium (mg)	1000	2500	1200	25
Magnesium (mg)	240	250	450	7.2
Iron (mg)	10	-	30	10
Zinc (mg)	12	25	12.5	15
Copper (mg)	0.9	5	2	2
Manganese (mg)	2.7	-	10	5
Selenium (µg)	55	300	83	200

IOR: Italian official recommendations.
MPL: maximum permitted level in supplements (per unit of dosage).
TC: content per table of supplement.
UL: tolerable upper levels of intake.
*Maximum daily dosage of supplement allowed according to Italian Ministry of Health.
§Vitamin A is reported as Retinol Activity Equivalents.

Table 5 Composition of the DIY dietary scheme followed during the last 16 years * (except for the last 6 months)

Component	Quantity	% of TE	IOR§
Energy (kcal)	2967	-	-
Total protein (g)	199	26.8	-
Total fats (g)	74	22.5	20-35%
Saturated fats (g)	17	5.2	<10%
MUFA (g)	44	13.6	10-15%
PUFA (g)	8	2.4	5-10%
Total carbohydrates (g)	401	50.7	45-60%
Starch (g)	316	39.9	45-53%
Simple sugars (g)	85	10.7	<15%
Dietary fiber (g)	19	-	12.6-16.7**
Iron (mg)	20	-	10
Cholesterol (mg)	493	-	0-300
Vitamin A (RE) (µg)	1087	-	700
Niacin (mg)	71	-	18
Selenium (µg)	88	-	55
Zinc (mg)	19	-	12

% of TE: percentage of total energy intake.
IOR: Italian official recommendations reference values.
§IOR reference values are reported as % of TE for macronutrient and as daily total amount for micronutrient and fiber.
*Milk-protein supplementation is not reported in the list.
**g/1000 kcal of energy intake.

animal-sources, was around 2.3 g/kg/day (Table 5). Moreover, in the same period, the patient used to train about 5 times a week, also supplementing his diet with milk-derived protein drinks (30 g of whey protein/day, right after each training session), along with multivitamin and mineral supplementation. According to the data collected, the patient's mean daily energy intake was about 3000 kcal/day (Table 5). The usual daily water intake was up to 5 liters per day. The patient has not been consuming coffee, tea, fructose or sweeteners of any type.

He reported to have followed the same dietary pattern for 16 years with no adverse effects.

Six months before our medical nutrition evaluation, the patient switched to a lactose-free diet, suspending the milk-derived protein supplements as well, since he stated he had developed lactose intolerance symptomatology.

At the time of the medical examination, the patient had not yet resumed workouts, suspended 6 months before, due to persistent tiredness, gastrointestinal discomfort and mood deflection.

Dietary therapy

We estimated the daily energy expenditure multiplying REE measured by indirect calorimetry to physical activity level (PAL = 1.65)[c] [19] and therefore developed a physiological dietary plan meeting the actual energy, macro and micronutrient requirements (Table 6). The dietary plan was aimed primarily to establish a correct energy intake in order to counteract the feeling of weakness and to correct inappropriate eating habits. It was also paid particular attention to those nutrients possibly implicated in the development of gastrointestinal distress (simple sugars, fats, fiber). In addition, in order to rebalance the intestinal microflora and improve the enteric trophism reducing diarrhea and GI discomfort we prescribed a multiple strain probiotic with a mixture of prebiotics and antioxidants vitamins especially useful in intestinal dysbiosis and inflammations [20,21]. To this was added a EPA /DHA and Vitamin E supplement (300 mg/200 mg and 1.8 mg per tablet) for 2 weeks to further reduce the gastrointestinal inflammation [11,15].

Finally we encouraged the patient to suspend the multivitamin and mineral supplementation and to restrain from taking protein supplements.

The follow-up visit conducted 1 month later reported a slight improvement of the gastric post-prandial discomfort and the diarrhea episodes frequency reduction.

Table 6 Dietary composition of the nutritional therapy prescribed

Component	Quantity	% of TE	IOR[§]
Energy (kcal)	2601	-	-
Total protein (g)	122	18.8	-
Total fats (g)	71	24.5	25-35%
Saturated fats (g)	13	4.5	<10%
MUFA (g)	44	15.2	10-15%
PUFA (g)	11	3.8	5-10%
Total carbohydrates (g)	393	56.6	45-60%
Starch (g)	343	49.4	45-53%
Simple sugars (g)	50	7.2	<15%
Dietary fiber (g)	29	-	12.6-16.7*
Iron (mg)	19	-	10
Cholesterol (mg)	207	-	0-300
Vitamin A (RE) (μg)	835	-	700
Niacin (mg)	27	-	18
Selenium (μg)	35	-	55
Zinc (mg)	14	-	12

% of TE: percentage of total energy.
IOR: Italian official recommendations reference values.
[§]IOR reference values are reported as % of TE for macronutrient and as daily total amount for micronutrient and fiber.
*g/1000 kcal of energy intake.

The improvement of gastrointestinal symptoms allowed the patient to increase the daily energy intake as assessed by the 24 h recall method.

Discussion

A resistance athlete's diet needs to be different in macronutrient and in micronutrient composition compared to a normally active subject's diet. For a resistance athlete it should be considered a higher daily protein requirement in order to satisfy the muscle accretion needs as well as the muscle protein synthesis increase [8,9]. Protein intake should be increased to 1.2-1.7 g/kg/day, enough to ensure the increased muscle needs [9]. Besides proteins, CHO intake and remarkably its timing, seems to be important for the muscle accretion and weight lift performance of these athletes. The reference range is 8–10 g/kg/day of CHO [8,22].

Although exercise leads to an oxidative stress increase and loss of some minerals, there are no evidences justifying the massive intake of vitamin-mineral supplements, especially among amateur athletes [9,22]. Even considering the hypothetical augmented needs of a bodybuilder, in our case-report, the daily intake of some nutrients was far higher than advisable. According to the data we obtained from the dietary scheme he handed us out and the nutritional anamnesis we collected, the patient's dietary pattern differs somewhat from the official

guidelines [10]: quite higher in protein, vitamins and minerals intake than recommended [11,12]. The diet history collected showed a 16-year period of large dietary protein intake (approximately around the 2.5 g/kg/day, also considering the extra protein supplementation) mostly from animal sources. It is conceivable that the long period of unsupervised supplementation and self-made diet consumption may have led to the development of adverse effects. It is not uncommon that the large fortified food consumption, associated with supplements, may lead to an excessive intake of vitamins and minerals that come close to or exceed the Tolerable Upper Intake Level (UL).

Indeed, many of the side effects exerted by the supplements are related to the gastrointestinal tract [3].

The patient reported the continuative and habitual intake of milk-derived protein supplements. Although the metabolic side effects of a high protein diet is not completely clarified, it is possible that the prolonged high protein load may have induced a slight bowel mucosal dysfunction; some bacterial protein-derived metabolites such as ammonia and short-chain fatty acids are likely to interfere with the colonic epithelium metabolism and physiology [23]; ammonia at millimolar concentrations in the bowel lumen has been shown to exert deleterious effects on the colonic epithelium [24] and to alter short-chain fatty acids oxidation in isolated colonocytes [25]. Interestingly, recent research has reported [26] that feeding mice with a very high protein diet causes the development of peculiar alterations in the enterocytes metabolism, such as t the mucosa thinning and an overall impairment in water absorption.

In our case, we noticed that more than five components listed in the supplement nutritional label, exceeded the IOR as well as the Maximum Permitted Level in supplements (MPL) in Italy [27]. Therefore, given that the patient has been exposed to a high level of micronutrients intake, consuming many fortified foods apart from supplements, it seems reasonable that the overall excessive micronutrient intake may partially explain the reported symptomatology.

In particular Vitamin A, Niacin, Zinc and Selenium overdose intake will be discussed.

Vitamin A is an essential component for human growth, gene expression and immune system. Vitamin A includes a family of fat-soluble molecules such as retinol and pro-vitamins A carotenoids (mainly β-carotene). The RDA for men is around the 900 μg/day of retinol activity equivalents (RE) while the UL for adults is set at 3000 μg/day of preformed vitamin [11,28]. Notably, the recent IOR for men is 700 μg of RE/day [11,3]. Excessive prolonged intake of vitamin A (months or years) may produce toxicity with symptoms such as nausea, vomiting and diarrhea [4]. The patient's daily intake of Vitamin A as a supplement (β-carotene and retinyl palmitate, in 1 tablet of supplement) was 6000 µg of RE. The whole dietary daily intake (dietary + supplementation) had been around the 7080 µg of RE for several years.

Niacin, as a precursor of nicotinamide, plays its biological role in many reactions connected to the energy production. In the form of nicotinic acid it is employed to treat different types of dyslipidemia and to lower overall risk of developing atherosclerosis [29,30]. Its recommended intake in adult males is be around the 18 mg/day and should not exceed 30–35 mg/day (which corresponds to 900 mg/day of nicotinamide and 10 mg/day of nicotinic acid) [11,31]. In our case report, the overall niacin daily intake (mean dietary intake plus supplement) was around the 170 mg/day. Although the common side effects reported by niacin overconsumption are usually related to skin flushing (niacin intake from 30 to 1000 mg/day) and hepatotoxicity as shown in several studies [5,31], niacin "overdose" might also be related to gastrointestinal discomfort, as already reported for doses > 2000 mg with subsequent episodes of severe diarrhea and/or transaminase increase [31]. The development or exacerbation of peptic ulcer as well as nausea and vomiting have been described by several authors, in cases of very high doses of niacin intake during anti-atherosclerotic therapy [5,31].

Zinc is another nutrient presumably involved in the development or exacerbation of abdominal discomfort. The mechanism of damage could be related to a direct corrosive action of the metal on the mucosal wall, after reacting with the gastric secretion [32]. The recommended zinc intake should be in the range of 8–13 mg/day, without exceeding 25 mg/day [11,30]. Higher zinc intake might promote nausea, abdominal cramping, vomiting, and diarrhea [32-34]. In our case, this micronutrient intake (dietary intake plus supplementation) was about 34 mg/day. High doses of zinc sulfate, as those employed in the treatment of Wilson's disease, have been associated to the development of some gastrointestinal disorders such as dyspepsia, vomiting, nausea and loss of appetite [35].

Selenium is an important co-factor for several biological molecules and enzymes playing an important role in redox reactions and hormone production. The currently recommended safety range intake for male adults is less than the 400 µg/day, while the IOR UL is set at 300 µg/day [11,36]. The patient's overall intake was about 288 µg/day. A higher intake is likely to lead to the toxic effects on the endocrine function as well as on the gastrointestinal tract [37]. In 2008, a poorly manufactured multivitamin was responsible for more than 200 cases of selenium poisoning with symptoms including diarrhea, fatigue, hair loss, and joint pain [38].

Moreover, the development of gastrointestinal adverse effect could also be interpreted considering the possible presence of contaminating compounds within the supplements. Many supplements have been found to be adulterated with pharmaceuticals or pharmaceutical analogues, including stimulants, anabolic steroids, antidepressants, psychotropic substances [39,40]. Stimulants and doping compounds [7,41], as well as new analogue of amphetamine, have been found in widespread sport supplements [7]. Also the above-mentioned selenium contamination of multivitamin supplement was considered a case of supplementation poisoning [38]. Other studies pointed out the presence, frequently, of compounds with 17β-estradiol-like activity or GHPR-2 in these supplements, which may interfere with some key points of the hormonal metabolism [11,42]. The presence of such hidden substances may determine the development of side effects that go beyond simple constituents of the supplement-in-itself, especially when the supplementation is carried out with more than a single supplement and consumed every day for years.

The fecal test (mucus, blood, erythrocytes, leucocytes) and all the biochemical parameters connected with a possible IBD (Hb, leucocytes, RCP) resulted in the normal range. The external medical inspection also led to rule out an IBD in existence. The gastroscopy performed and the negative result of celiac antibodies confuted any diagnostic suspect of celiac disease. No history of inhaled or food allergy was recorded. The value of the total IgE was in a normal range. The specific IgE test performed on different food allergens showed no positivity. The last findings led us to rule out the presence of food allergies. Although the patient resulted lactose intolerant, we excluded that it could be connected with the symptoms suffered because since he developed the lactose intolerance he self-suspended any milk and milk-derived food consumption as well as supplementation with milk derived proteins, without achieving any amelioration of the gastrointestinal distress. The low amount of simple sugars introduced (Tables 3 and 5) as well as the result from fecal analysis led us to rule out any possibility of osmotic diarrhea. After excluding this common causes of abdominal distress and diarrhea, we infer that the gastrointestinal symptoms reported by this patient of ours such as osmotic diarrhea, abdominal cramping and/or nausea might be linked to the poor quality of his dietary pattern and in particular to the massive intake of protein and micronutrients, secondary to suboptimal diet and supplementation [22-26,29-42]. Although we believe that our patient's clinical situation did not completely match for the established criteria of diagnosis of irritable bowel syndrome (IBS), we cannot completely rule it out. The low mood, the low visceral pain threshold and the symptomatology reported lead to suppose the presence of an IBS as well. Actually, given that the IBS is a nosological status with a complex and not well-defined pathogenesis, we are likely to believe that the IBS could have been triggered or possibly enhanced by the patient's suboptimal diet. The glucose intolerance detected still remains an unsolved question. The basal insulin and HOMA index were in a normal range. The fasting glucose level was even slightly lower than recommended. To partially explain the findings we supposed that the GI distress and the patent's whole clinical situation were likely to determine an increase in stress hormone levels (adrenaline, cortisol). As these hormones play a diabetogenic effect, we can assume that the detected glucose intolerance may be thus explained.

The main limitation of this study is related to the short period of follow-up carried out (the results are related to 1 month therapy) due to the poor compliance of the patient to the new dietary scheme and recommendations. We are likely to believe that the low mood and the vicious circle induced by the GI discomfort, the low training level and the partial disappearance of the symptoms played an important role in the dropout. Furthermore, the patient did not willingly accept the indication to the micronutrient supplementation suspension, which he considered necessary to cover his metabolic needs. The follow-up brevity and the patient's scarce compliance to the therapy did not allow us to obtain any further data to confirm or disprove our diagnostic hypothesis. Another limit regards the lack of any data about his physical condition or muscular strength in order to prove the basal performance and the improvement after our nutritional intervention. Similarly, we were unable to report any training log, which would have been helpful to better understand the clinical situation. Finally, the lack of epidemiological and human studies useful to confirm our hypothesis or contradict it, the absence of significant similar reports in literature, the atypical clinical presentation and the differential diagnosis make our hypothesis speculative and the case difficult to interpret but worthy of being reported.

Conclusion

The present study highlights the risk of adverse effects in prolonged suboptimal macro and micronutrient supplementation in a subject involved in non-competitive sport.

As showed in this case, the common practice of adopting "self-made" nutritional regimes among amateur athletes may lead to an unusual gastrointestinal symptomatology. Moreover, future chronic complications cannot be completely ruled out. Although many amateur bodybuilders believe that "more is better" underestimate the importance of diet and overestimate the effects of supplements, unaware of "over supplementation" side effects.

In order to prevent severe and chronic health effects, nutritionists and trainers should advise the athletes about the possible risks of self-made diets that provide for extra supplementation, especially when carried out for long time.

Consent

Written informed consent was obtained from the patient for publication of this Case Report. A copy of the written consent is available for review by the Editor-in-Chief of this journal.

Endnotes

[a]The considered IOR are referred to adult males aged between 30–59 y-old.
[b]Body fat mass and fat-free mass were estimated by BODYGRAM software (AKERN, Florence, Italy).
[c]The 1.65 value of PAL has been chosen considering a light level of physical activity in accordance to the WHO/FAO/UNU guidelines.

Abbreviations
IOR: Italian official recommendations; DIY: Do it yourself; BIA: Bioelectrical-impedance; MPL: Maximum permitted in supplements; RE: Retinol activity equivalents; UL: Tolerable upper intake level; TC: content per tablet of supplement.

Competing interests
The authors declare that they have not received any funding, or salary from an organization that may in any way gain or lose financially from the publication of this manuscript.
The authors declare that they do not hold any stock or shares in an organization that may in any way gain or lose financially from the publication of this manuscript.
The authors declare that they do not hold or are currently applying for any patents relating to the content of the manuscript.
The authors declare that they do not have any other financial competing interest.

Authors' contributions
LDG carried out all the medical examinations, designed the study and drafted the manuscript. MC participated in the design of the study and in the manuscript drafting. HC conceived of the study and participated in its design and coordination. All authors read and approved the final manuscript.

Authors' information
LDG: MD. Resident at the School of Human Nutrition, University of Milano, Italy. Internship at the Department of Public Health, Experimental and Forensic Medicine, Unit of Human Nutrition, University of Pavia, Italy.
MC: PhD. Resident at the School of Human Nutrition, University of Milano, Italy. Internship at the Department of Public Health, Experimental and Forensic Medicine, Unit of Human Nutrition, University of Pavia, Italy.
HC: MD, PhD. Professor of Dietetics and Clinical Nutrition, Head of the Clinical Nutrition Laboratory, Department of Public Health, Experimental and Forensic Medicine University of Pavia, Italy.

References
1. Petrotti A, Naughton DP, Pearce G, Bailey R, Bloodworth A, McNamee M. Nutritional supplement use by elite young UK athletes: fallacies of advice regarding efficacy. J Int Soc Sports Nutr. 2008;15:5–22.
2. Giannopoulou I, Noutsos K, Apostolidis N, Bayios I, Nassis GP. Performance level affects the dietary supplement intake of both individual and team sports athletes. J Sports Sci Med. 2013;12(1):190–6. 2013.
3. Walter P. Towards ensuring the safety of vitamins and minerals. Toxicol Lett. 2001;120:83–7.
4. Allen LH, Haskell M. Estimating the potential for vitamin a toxicity in women and young children. J Nutr. 2002;132(9 Suppl):2907S–19.
5. Mosher LR. Nicotinic acid side effects and toxicity: a review. Am J Psychiatry. 1970;126:1290–6.

6. Cohen PA, Travis JC, Venhuis BJ. A methamphetamine analog (N,α-diethyl-phenylethylamine) identified in a mainstream dietary supplement. Drug Test Anal. 2013;6(7-8):805–7.

7. Plotan M, Elliott CT, Frizzell C, Connolly L. Estrogenic endocrine disruptors present in sports supplements. A risk assessment for human health. Food Chem. 2014;159:157–65.

8. Kerksick C, Harvey T, Stout J, Campbell B, Wilborn C, Kreider R, et al. International society of sports nutrition position stand: nutrient timing. J IntSoc Sports Nutr. 2008;5:17.

9. American Dietetic Association; Dietitians of Canada; American College of Sports Medicine, Rodriguez NR, Di Marco NM, Langley S. American college of sports medicine position stand. Nutrition and athletic performance. Med Sci Sports Exerc. 2009;41(3):709–31.

10. Food based dietary guidelines in the WHO European Region. Nutrition and Food Security Program WHO Regional Office for Europe, 2003. Copenhagen Denmark, Volume id: E79832, 10-35. http://www.euro.who.int/__data/assets/pdf_file/0017/150083/E79832.pdf.

11. Società Italiana di nutrizione clinica. LARN, Livelli Di Assunzione di Riferimento di Nutrienti ed energia per la popolazione Italiana, IV Revisione. Coordinamento editoriale SINU-INRAN. Milano: SICS; 2014.

12. Margie Lee G. The nutrition and their metabolsim. In: Mahan LK, Eschott-Stump S, editors. Krause's food and nutrition therapy. Philadelphia: Saunders, Elsevier; 2008. p. 43–109.

13. Harris JA, Benedict FG. A biometric study of basal metabolism in man. Proc Natl Acad Sci U S A. 1918;4(12):370–3.

14. Campbell EL, Seynnes OR, Bottinelli R, McPhee JS, Atherton PJ, Jones DA, et al. Skeletal muscle adaptations to physical inactivity and subsequent retraining in young men. Biogerontology. 2013;14(3):247–59.

15. Calder PC. Polyunsaturated fatty acids, inflammatory processes and inflammatory bowel diseases. Mol Nutr Food Res. 2008;52(8):885–97.

16. Thompson FE, Subar AF. Dietary assessment methodology. In: Coulston AM, Boushey CJ, Ferruzzi MG, editors. Nutrition in the prevention and treatment of disease. 3rd ed. Oxford: Elsevier; 2013. p. 5–29.

17. Turconi G, Guarcello M, Berzolari FG, Carolei A, Bazzano R, Roggi C. An evaluation of a colour food photography atlas as a tool for quantifying food portion size in epidemiological dietary surveys. Eur J Clin Nutr. 2005;59(8):923–31.

18. Banca dati di composizione alimenti per studi epidemiologici in Italia. Istituto Europeo di Oncologia. http://www.bda-ieo.it/. Accessed on 18 Jan 2015.

19. FAO/WHO/UNU. Food and Agriculture Organization/World Health Organization/United Nation University. Human energy requirements. Report of a joint FAO/WHO/UNU Expert Consultation Rome. FAO Food and nutrition technical report series No 1, 2004.

20. Sarowska J, Choroszy-Król I, Regulska-Ilow B, Frej-Mądrzak M, Jama-Kmiecik A. The therapeutic effect of probiotic bacteria on gastrointestinal diseases. Adv Clin Exp Med. 2013;22(5):759–66.

21. Cappello C, Tremolaterra F, Pascariello A, Ciacci C, Iovino P. A randomised clinical trial (RCT) of a symbiotic mixture in patients with irritable bowel syndrome (IBS): effects on symptoms, colonic transit and quality of life. Int J Colorectal Dis. 2013;28(3):349–58.

22. McArdle WD, Katch FI, Katch VL. Sport and exercise nutrition. 3rd ed. Philadephia: Lippincott Williams & Wilkins; 2008.

23. Blachier F, Mariotti F, Huneau JF, Tome D. Effects of amino acid-derived luminal metabolites on the colonic epithelium and physiopatho-logical consequences. Amino Acids. 2007;33:547–62.

24. Lin HC, Visek WJ. Colon mucosal cell damage by ammonia in rats. J Nutr. 1991;121:887–93.

25. Cremin Jr JD, Fitch MD, Fleming SE. Glucose alleviates ammonia-induced inhibition of short-chain fatty acid metabolism in rat colonic epithelial cells. Am J Physiol Gastrointest Liver Physiol. 2003;285:G105–14.

26. Andriamihaja M, Davila AM, Eklou-Lawson M, Petit N, Delpal S, Allek F, et al. Colon luminal content and epithelial cell morphology are markedly modified in rats fed with a high-protein diet. Am J Physiol Gastrointest Liver Physiol. 2010;299:G1030–7.

27. Italian Ministry of Health. http://www.salute.gov.it/imgs/c_17_paginearee_1268_listafile_itemname_5_file.pdf. Accessed on 15 Oct 2014.

28. Institute of Medicine: Dietary Reference Intakes for Vitamin A, Vitamin K, Arsenic, Boron, Chromium, Copper, Iodine, Iron, Manganese, Molybdenum, Nickel, Silicon, Vanadium, and Zinc. Panel on Micronutrients, Subcommittees on Upper Reference Levels of Nutrients and of Interpretation and Use of Dietary Reference Intakes, and the Standing Committee on the Scientific Evaluation of Dietary Reference Intakes: National Academy Press. Washington; 2001.

29. Lavigne PM, Karas RH. The current state of niacin in cardiovascular disease prevention: a systematic review and meta-regression. J Am CollCardiol. 2013;61(4):440–6.

30. Guyton JR, Goldberg AC, Kreisberg RA, Sprecher DL, Superko HR, O'Connor CM. Effectiveness of once-nightly dosing of extended- release niacin alone and in combination for hypercholesterolemia. Am J Cardiol. 1998;82:737–43.

31. Guyton JR, Bays HE. Safety considerations with niacin therapy. Am J Cardiol. 2007;99(suppl):22C–31.

32. Bothwell DN, Mair EA, Cable BB. Chronic ingestion of a zinc-based penny. Pediatrics. 2003;111(3):689–91.

33. Maret W, Sandstead HH. Zinc requirements and the risks and benefits of zinc supplementation. J Trace Elem in Med Biol. 2006;20(1):3–18.

34. World Health Organization. Environmental Health Criteria 221: Zinc. Geneva: World Health Organization; 2001. p. 123–253.

35. Wiernicka A, Jańczyk W, Dądalski M, Avsar Y, Soch P, Schmidt H. Gastrointestinal side effects in children with Wilson's disease treated with zinc sulphate. World J Gastroenterol. 2013;19(27):4356–62.

36. Yang G, Zhou R. Further observations on the human maximum safe dietary selenium intake in a seleniferous area of China. J Trace Elem Electrolytes Health Dis. 1994;8(3–4):159–65.

37. Vinceti M, Wei ET, Malagoli C, Bergomi M, Vivoli G. Adverse health effects of selenium in humans. Rev Environ Health. 2001;16(4):233–51.

38. Mac Farquhar JK, Broussard DL, Melstrom P, Hutchinson R, Wolkin A, Martin C, et al. Acute selenium toxicity associated with a dietary supplement. Arch Intern Med. 2010;170(3):256–61.

39. Cohen PA. Hazards of hindsight — monitoring the safety of nutritional supplements. N Engl J Med. 2014;370:1277–80.

40. Food and Drug Administration: Tainted supplements CDER. Silver Spring, MD. http://www.accessdata.fda.gov/scripts/sda/sdNavigation.cfm?sd=tainted_supplements_cder&displayAll=false&page=6. Accessed on 5 Oct 2014.

41. Geyer H, Parr MK, Koehler K, Mareck U, Schänzer W, Thevis M. Nutritional supplements cross-contaminated and faked with doping substances. J Mass Spectrom. 2008;43(7):892–902.

42. Thomas A, Kohler M, Mester J, Geyer H, Schänzer W, Petrou M, et al. Identification of the growth-hormone-releasing peptide-2 (GHRP-2) in a nutritional supplement. Drug Test Anal. 2010;2(3):144–8.

## 6

The effect of a decaffeinated green tea extract formula on fat oxidation, body composition and exercise performance

Justin D Roberts[1,2*], Michael G Roberts[2†], Michael D Tarpey[2†], Jack C Weekes[2†] and Clare H Thomas[2†]

Abstract

Background: The cardio-metabolic and antioxidant health benefits of caffeinated green tea (GT) relate to its catechin polyphenol content. Less is known about decaffeinated extracts, particularly in combination with exercise. The aim of this study was therefore to determine whether a decaffeinated green tea extract (dGTE) positively influenced fat oxidation, body composition and exercise performance in recreationally active participants.

Methods: Fourteen, recreationally active males participated in a double-blind, placebo-controlled, parallel design intervention (mean ± SE; age = 21.4 ± 0.3 yrs; weight = 76.37 ± 1.73 kg; body fat = 16.84 ± 0.97%, peak oxygen consumption [$\dot{V}O_{2peak}$] = 3.00 ± 0.10 L·min^{-1}). Participants were randomly assigned capsulated dGTE (571 mg·d^{-1}; n = 7) or placebo (PL; n = 7) for 4 weeks. Following body composition and resting cardiovascular measures, participants cycled for 1 hour at 50% $\dot{V}O_{2peak}$, followed by a 40 minute performance trial at week 0, 2 and 4. Fat and carbohydrate oxidation was assessed via indirect calorimetry. Pre-post exercise blood samples were collected for determination of total fatty acids (TFA). Distance covered (km) and average power output (W) were assessed as exercise performance criteria.

Results: Total fat oxidation rates increased by 24.9% from 0.241 ± 0.025 to 0.301 ± 0.009 g·min^{-1} with dGTE (P = 0.05; ηp^2 = 0.45) by week 4, whereas substrate utilisation was unaltered with PL. Body fat significantly decreased with dGTE by 1.63 ± 0.16% in contrast to PL over the intervention period (P < 0.001; ηp^2 = 0.84). No significant changes for FFA or blood pressure between groups were observed. dGTE resulted in a 10.9% improvement in performance distance covered from 20.23 ± 0.54 km to 22.43 ± 0.40 km by week 4 (P < 0.001; ηp^2 = 0.85).

Conclusions: A 4 week dGTE intervention favourably enhanced substrate utilisation and subsequent performance indices, but did not alter TFA concentrations in comparison to PL. The results support the use of catechin polyphenols from dGTE in combination with exercise training in recreationally active volunteers.

Keywords: Green tea, Body composition, Fat oxidation, Exercise performance

Introduction

The health benefits of polyphenols found in green tea (GT), the unfermented leaves of the tea plant, *Camellia sinensis*, have been extensively investigated in the last fifteen years [1-7]. Studies have demonstrated antioxidant [8,9] and chemoprotective properties [4], as well as improvements in cardio-metabolic health from various

GT strategies (including reduced circulating cholesterol and triglyerides [10], increased thermogenesis and whole body fat oxidation [1,3,11], reduced blood pressure [7,12,13] and improved body mass index ratios [5,14-17]). These health benefits, in part, relate to the bioactive catechin polyphenol content of GT, of which (−)-epigallocatechin-3-gallate (EGCG) can account for between 50–80% of the total catechin content [18].

GT catechins have been proposed to influence metabolic and thermogenic activities in the short term, via inhibition of catechol-o-methyl transferase (COMT) leading to enhanced catecholamine, cAMP and lipolytic activity

* Correspondence: justin.roberts@anglia.ac.uk

†Equal contributors

[1]Department of Life Sciences, Anglia Ruskin University, East Road, Cambridge, UK

[2]School of Life & Medical Sciences, University of Hertfordshire, College Lane, Hatfield, Hertfordshire, UK

[17,19,20], although this has been disputed [20]. GT catechins, particularly EGCG, may also activate endothelial nitric oxide synthase, leading to mild reductions in blood pressure [13,21].

In the longer term, GT catechins may influence specific signalling molecules, including PGC1α, leading to gene expression of fat metabolism enzymes [20]. Whilst such mechanisms are currently under debate, strategies to enhance fat oxidation, body composition and cardiovascular efficiency in conjunction with physical activity are of pertinence to the general population. Additionally the indirect sparing of glycogen stores may support improved exercise tolerance and/or performance.

Research investigating GT extracts (GTE) and exercise have produced conflicting results. Modest EGCG dosage in the short term (270 mg·d^{-1} EGCG for 6 days [22], and 68 mg·d^{-1} EGCG for 3 weeks [23,24]) did not alter metabolic or performance variables in healthy or endurance trained volunteers. However, the inclusion of 100.5 mg·d^{-1} EGCG over a 10 week training period enhanced whole-body metabolic efficiency elsewhere [11]. One confounding factor though is the use of caffeinated GTE in these studies. When decaffeinated GTE (dGTE) has been employed, 366 mg EGCG was found to acutely increase fat oxidation by 17% [3]. Conversely, higher dosage dGTE (624 ± 3 mg·d^{-1} EGCG for 28 days) did not significantly affect fat oxidation in healthy, male volunteers [25].

We were therefore invited to undertake an independent assessment of the cardio-metabolic and performance effects of a dGTE formula (571 mg·d^{-1} GTE providing 400 mg·d^{-1} EGCG) over a 4 week period in comparison to placebo in healthy, male volunteers. It was hypothesised that moderate dose dGTE would significantly improve fat oxidation and performance, supporting longer term mechanisms linking GTE catechins to enhanced metabolic enzyme gene expression.

Materials and methods

Participants

Fourteen healthy, male participants volunteered following power calculation assessment (G*Power3, Dusseldorf [26]; using α = 0.05; 1-β = 0.95; based on observed data [3,22-24] and 2 groups). Participants were required to be recreationally active non-smokers, and have no known sensitivities to tea products or be regular green tea consumers. Prior to study inclusion, all participants provided written informed consent and satisfactorily completed a general health screen. The study was approved by the University of Hertfordshire Life and Medical Sciences Ethics Committee. Participant characteristics are displayed in Table 1.

Procedures

Preliminary testing

All testing took place in the Human Physiology Laboratory, University of Hertfordshire. Participants were instructed to refrain from consuming caffeinated products for 48 hours prior to initial testing, and not be consuming other supplementation.

Peak oxygen consumption ($\dot{V}O_{2peak}$) was assessed at least one week prior to experimental trials using a standard incremental step protocol increasing by 30 W each 3 minutes until volitional exhaustion as previously reported [27]. Tests were performed on a Monark Ergomedic 874E stationary bike (Monark Exercise AB, Varberg, Sweden) using a Metalyser 3B automated gas-analyser (Cortex Biophysik, Leipzig, Germany). On a separate occasion, subjects undertook a familiarisation trial to confirm exercise intensity at 50% $\dot{V}O_{2peak}$. This intensity was selected based on pilot work in which average fat oxidation rates during sustained submaximal exercise were statistically greater at 50% $\dot{V}O_{2peak}$ compared to both 40 and 60% $\dot{V}O_{2peak}$.

Treatments

Participants were randomly assigned to an experimental or placebo group, and provided with either capsulated dGTE (571 mg·d^{-1} dGTE, delivering 70% or 400 mg·d^{-1} EGCG (equivalent to 6–7 cups of green tea per day), Changsha Active Ingredients Group Inc., Changsha, China*), or placebo (700 mg·d^{-1} corn flour). All participants received capsules on a weekly basis to monitor compliance, with instructions to consume one capsule daily before breakfast with 250 ml water. *Analysis of the main active ingredient (EGCG) was undertaken prior to and independently of the main study by Changsha Active Ingredients Group Inc., using high performance liquid chromatography. The certificate of analysis provided by the supplying company demonstrated that the product contained 91.21% total catechins, from which 70.74% was EGCG. The product did not appear to be assessed for other catechins, so it is likely that the remaining percentage comprised other catechins (GCG, EGC, GC, EC, ECG, etc.).

Experimental design and intervention

A randomised, double blind, placebo controlled parallel design was employed over a 4 week intervention. Participants completed three laboratory trials at week 0, 2 and 4 under controlled conditions following an overnight fast. Upon arrival, nude body mass (Seca 780, Hamburg, Germany), height (Seca 200 stadiometer, Hamburg, Germany) and body composition [28] (Tanita Body Segmental Analyser 418-BC, Tokyo, Japan) were assessed.

Participants were then fitted with a Polar FS2c telemetric monitor (Polar Electro Ltd., Kempele, Finland) and

Table 1 Baseline characteristics and resting measurements across the intervention

Variable	PL (n = 7)			dGTE (n = 7)		
Age (years)	21.4 ± 0.6			21.4 ± 0.3		
Height (m)	1.77 ± 0.03			1.78 ± 0.01		
$\dot{V}O_{2peak}$ (L·min^{-1})	3.13 ± 0.18			2.87 ± 0.08		
	Baseline	Week 2	Week 4	Baseline	Week 2	Week 4
Weight (kg)	75.46 ± 2.91	75.11 ± 2.94*	74.81 ± 2.88*	77.29 ± 2.05	76.96 ± 2.03*	76.69 ± 1.95* [B]
Bodyfat (%)	16.63 ± 1.58	16.34 ± 1.69	15.97 ± 1.69*#	17.06 ± 1.24	16.23 ± 1.39*	15.43 ± 1.33*# [A,B]
HR (bpm)	61.00 ± 2.70	62.14 ± 1.81	61.00 ± 1.83	62.00 ± 1.25	62.43 ± 2.01	62.57 ± 1.92
SBP (mm Hg)	129.29 ± 1.73	125.71 ± 3.64	127.00 ± 2.44	130.00 ± 1.18	126.57 ± 2.14	126.86 ± 3.64
DBP (mm Hg)	67.57 ± 4.35	66.14 ± 1.72	69.71 ± 2.37	69.57 ± 2.40	65.71 ± 2.55	67.71 ± 2.11

Table 1 shows the key participant characteristics for each group, including absolute changes for weight, body fat, heart rate and blood pressure over the intervention. Data are presented as mean ± SE. PL, Placebo; dGTE, decaffeinated green tea extract; $\dot{V}O_{2peak}$, peak oxygen uptake; HR, heart rate; SBP, systolic blood pressure; DBP, diastolic blood pressure. [A]denotes significant overall group x time interaction effect ($P = 0.002$). [B]denotes significant overall time interaction effect only ($P < 0.001$). *denotes significant difference ($P \leq 0.05$) to baseline only within group. #denotes significant difference to week 2 within group only ($P < 0.046$).

seated for 5 minutes prior to resting heart rate and blood pressure readings (Omron MX3 plus, Kyoto, Japan). A venous wholeblood sample was then collected into duplicate 4 ml K$_3$EDTA Vacutainers (Greiner Bio-One GmbH, Kremsmunster, Austria) by a qualified phlebotomist. Samples were centrifuged for 10 minutes at 2000 rpm, with aliquotted plasma immediately frozen at −80°C for later assessment of TFA.

Exercise trials

Exercise trials comprised a submaximal assessment and performance stage. During the submaximal assessment, participants exercised for one hour at 50% $\dot{V}O_{2peak}$ on a Monark Ergomedic 874E cycle ergometer. Gas exchange data was recorded continuously throughout exercise using a Metalyser 3B gas analyser, with average data taken over the final 45 minutes of submaximal exercise. Rating of perceived exertion (RPE) [29] and heart rate were recorded every 20 minutes.

Rates of total carbohydrate oxidation (CHO$_{TOT}$), total fat oxidation (FAT$_{TOT}$) (g·min^{-1}) and energy expenditure (EE) (kJ·min^{-1}) were calculated from $\dot{V}O_2$ and $\dot{V}CO_2$ (L·min^{-1}) using stoichiometric equations [30], with protein oxidation assumed negligible, as follows:

$$CHO_{TOT} = 4.210 \cdot (\dot{V}CO_2) - 2.962 \cdot (\dot{V}O_2) \quad (1)$$

$$FAT_{TOT} = 1.695 \cdot (\dot{V}O_2) - 1.701 \cdot (\dot{V}CO_2) \quad (2)$$

$$EE = [(0.550 \cdot \dot{V}CO_2) - (4.471 \cdot \dot{V}O_2)] \cdot 4.2 \quad (3)$$

Upon completion, seated blood pressure and post exercise venous sampling was repeated as previously described. Following this, participants were instructed to undertake a 40 minute self-paced performance trial using a Computrainer erogometer system (RaceMate

Inc., Seattle, USA). Distance covered (km) and power output (W) were recorded each 10 minutes, with only time elapsed visible to the subjects. Verbal encouragement was provided each 10 minutes. At the end of the exercise trial, subjects recovered for 5 minutes at 50 W.

Dietary intake and exercise activity

All participants recorded a 3 day dietary recall preceding each exercise trial to assess for habitual dietary compliance. Dietary analyses were undertaken using Dietplan 6.50 (Forestfield Software Ltd, West Sussex, United Kingdom), with no differences reported between groups for macronutrients and/or energy intake. Additionally, participants were requested to consume similar meals the day before the exercise trials at regular time intervals to provide increased control of oxidation variables. This was based on pilot work assessment of fat oxidation stability at 50% $\dot{V}O_{2peak}$ (assessed by calculating the amount of time (minutes) throughout the exercise that was spent within ±0.02 g·min^{-1} of the average fat oxidation rate, expressed as a percentage for each individual), which was greater when the 24 hour pre exercise period was controlled for dietary intake (68.22 ± 5.70%) compared to when only the evening meal preceding the testing session was controlled (60.78 ± 8.42%).

The standardised menu was based on typical foods consumed by participants at breakfast, lunch and dinner, and provided similar caloric intake to habitual dietary records (values as calorie totals and per kilogram mean bodyweight: energy intake: 2484.70 kcal·d^{-1} (32.68 kcal·kg^{-1}·d^{-1}); carbohydrate: 1127.7 kcal·d^{-1} (14.83 kcal·kg^{-1}·d^{-1}); fat: 565.4 kcal·d^{-1} (7.43 kcal·kg^{-1}·d^{-1}) and protein: 791.96 kcal·d^{-1} (10.42 kcal·kg^{-1}·d^{-1}). Throughout the intervention period, participants were instructed to minimise consumption of polyphenol rich foods. Participants were additionally required to cycle for one hour at 50% $\dot{V}O_{2peak}$ three times per week as part of a regulated exercise programme. All participants provided training diaries to monitor compliance.

Blood analyses

All blood analyses for TFA were independently undertaken by ABS Laboratories (Biopark, Welwyn Garden City, Hertfordshire) employing previously validated methods [31]. TFA concentrations were based on assessment of palmitic, palmitoleic, stearic, oleic and linoleic acids. Briefly, 100 µl plasma aliquots were spiked with internal standard (heptadecanoic acid), with free fatty acids being extracted using the 'Dole Extraction Solvent' (isopropanol/heptane/sulphuric acid (1 M) (40:10:1)). After drying under nitrogen, the extracts were resuspended using 200 µL of dichoromethane and the FFAs derivatised using diethylamine and Deoxo-Fluor. The diethylamide derivatives were then extracted into heptane. The heptane was then removed using nitrogen in a dry-block at 70°C. The dried extracts were reconstituted into 100 µL of heptane and quantified by gas chromatography using a mass spectrometer as the detector in the selected ion monitoring (SIM) mode.

Statistical analyses

Statistical analyses were performed using SPSS (v19, Chicago, USA). Baseline variables were assessed using an independent samples t-test. A mixed design repeated measures analysis of variance (ANOVA) was employed to assess treatment and time interactions. Where pertinent, a one way ANOVA with Bonferroni post hoc adjustments was utilised to assess within treatment effects. An alpha level of ≤ 0.05 was employed for statistical significance. Data are reported as means ± SE.

Results

Baseline characteristics and resting measures

Intervention groups were matched for age, height, weight, body fat and $\dot{V}O_{2peak}$ at baseline (Table 1). A significant interaction effect for bodyweight was found across time only (F = 16.98, $P < 0.001$). Net bodyweight reduction was similar between groups across the intervention (0.64 ± 0.17 kg for PL; F = 12.33, $P = 0.001$; $\eta p^2 = 0.67$), and 0.60 ± 0.21 kg for dGTE; F = 6.27, $P = 0.014$; $\eta p^2 = 0.51$ within group). There was a significant group x time interaction for percentage body fat (F = 7.81, $P = 0.002$), with an overall reduction of 1.63 ± 0.16% with dGTE ($P < 0.001$; $\eta p^2 = 0.84$ within group) compared to 0.66 ± 0.15% for PL ($P = 0.002$; $\eta p^2 = 0.66$ within group). No significant effects were reported for resting heart rate or blood pressure.

Submaximal exercise measures

Weekly contribution of substrate to total energy expenditure (EE) for PL and dGTE are reported in Figures 1 and 2 respectively. No significant differences were reported for EE either between or within groups over time ($P > 0.05$), demonstrating consistency of the submaximal exercise trials.

A significant overall group x time interaction for FAT_{TOT} was observed (F = 3.39, $P = 0.05$). FAT_{TOT} during exercise remained similar for PL across the intervention period (week 0 = 0.277 ± 0.038 g·min^{-1}; week 2 = 0.274 ± 0.031 g·min^{-1}; week 4 = 0.279 ± 0.030 g·min^{-1}, $P > 0.05$) despite a non-significant increase in percentage contribution to total EE (week 0 = 34.61 ± 3.72%; week 2 = 35.23 ± 2.99%; week 4 = 35.53 ± 2.53%, $P > 0.05$).

FAT_{TOT} for dGTE increased from 0.241 ± 0.025 g·min^{-1} at week 0 to 0.256 ± 0.023 g·min^{-1} at week 2, and to 0.301 ± 0.009 g·min^{-1} by week 4 (F = 4.10, $P = 0.05$; $\eta p^2 = 0.45$). This represented a 24.9% or 0.060 ± 0.027 g·min^{-1} increase in FAT_{TOT} with dGTE. Correspondingly, percentage contribution of total fat to exercise EE increased with dGTE from 32.61 ± 3.53% at week 0 to 34.71 ± 2.57% at week 2, and to 41.45 ± 1.31% at week 4 (F = 4.28, $P = 0.045$; $\eta p^2 = 0.46$).

A significant time interaction was observed only for CHO_{TOT} (F = 4.28, $P = 0.028$). CHO_{TOT} reduced with dGTE from 1.203 ± 0.078 g·min^{-1} at week 0, to 1.144 ± 0.044 g·min^{-1} at week 2, and finally to 1.025 ± 0.048 g·min^{-1} by week 4, representing a reduction of 14.8% or 0.178 ± 0.069 g·min^{-1} (F = 4.02, $P = 0.05$; $\eta p^2 = 0.45$).

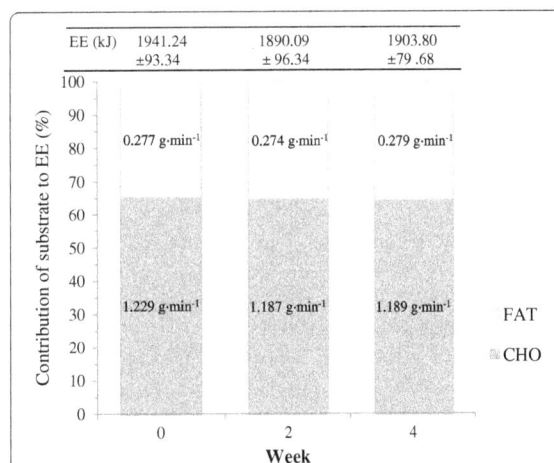

Figure 1 Weekly contribution of substrate to total energy expenditure (EE) for the PL group. Figure 1 shows the contribution of both fat and carbohydrate (based on oxidation rates) to energy expenditure during submaximal exercise for the placebo condition. Data are presented as mean ± SE. PL, Placebo; FAT, average fat oxidation rates; CHO, average carbohydrate oxidation rates. No significant differences were found with ANOVA ($P > 0.05$).

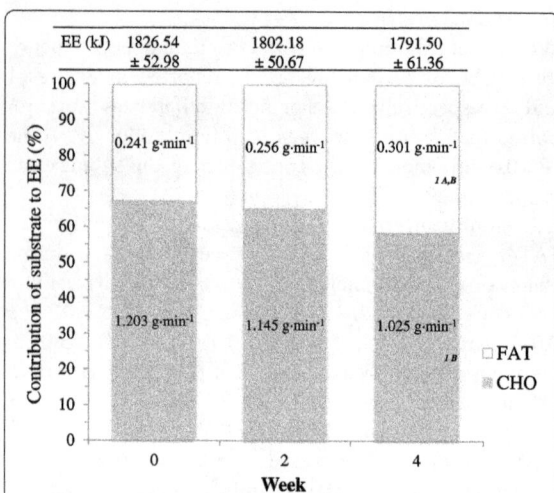

Figure 2 Weekly contribution of substrate to total energy expenditure (EE) for the dGTE group. Figure 2 shows the contribution of both fat and carbohydrate (based on oxidation rates) to energy expenditure during submaximal exercise for the dGTE condition. Data are presented as mean ± SE. dGTE, decaffeinated green tea extract; FAT, average fat oxidation rates; CHO, average carbohydrate oxidation rates. [A]denotes significant overall group × time interaction effect compared with PL (Figure 1; $P = 0.05$). [B]denotes significant overall time interaction effect in conjunction with PL (Figure 1; $P \leq 0.03$). [1] denotes significant interaction over time within GTE only ($P \leq 0.05$).

Correspondingly, percentage contribution of total CHO to exercise EE also reduced with dGTE from 67.39 ± 3.53% at week 0 to 65.28 ± 2.57% at week 2, and to 58.55 ± 1.31% at week 4 (F = 4.28, $P = 0.045$; $\eta p^2 = 0.46$). CHO_{TOT} and contribution of CHO to EE were largely unaffected with PL ($P > 0.05$).

Despite an improvement in FAT_{TOT} for dGTE, no significant differences were observed for TFA concentrations either within or between groups pre-post intervention (Figure 3, $P > 0.05$). It was however noted that TFA concentrations were elevated pre-exercise by week 4 with PL (249.3 ± 46.2 $\mu M \cdot L^{-1}$ at week 0 to 315.4 ± 98.1 $\mu M \cdot L^{-1}$ at week 4, a 26.5% increase, $P > 0.05$) and dGTE (227.9 ± 37.6 $\mu M \cdot L^{-1}$ at week 0 to 289.7 ± 54.8 $\mu M \cdot L^{-1}$ at week 4, a 27.1% increase, $P > 0.05$), with lack of significance most likely explained by individual variance.

It was also noted that whereas TFA concentrations reduced by 18.8% post exercise in the PL group from 616.5 ± 114.8 $\mu M \cdot L^{-1}$ at week 0 to 500.3 ± 141.8 $\mu M \cdot L^{-1}$ at week 4; post exercise TFA concentrations were maintained with dGTE (509.3 ± 90.0 $\mu M \cdot L^{-1}$ at week 0 to 514.3 ± 71.1 $\mu M \cdot L^{-1}$ at week 4), although no significant differences were reported within or between groups ($P > 0.05$). No significant differences were reported for any of the individual fatty acids measured.

Submaximal oxygen uptake values were not different across time either within or between groups (Table 2)

demonstrating compliance to the set intensity ($P > 0.05$). No significant interaction effects were found for expired carbon dioxide, despite a modest reduction in $\dot{V}CO_2$ during submaximal exercise with dGTE from 1.31 ± 0.05 $L \cdot min^{-1}$ at week 0, to 1.25 ± 0.05 $L \cdot min^{-1}$ at week 4 ($P > 0.05$). However, in conjunction with improved FAT_{TOT}, a significant overall group × time interaction was observed for the respiratory exchange ratio (RER; F = 3.30, $P = 0.05$), with values reducing from 0.90 ± 0.01 at week 0 to 0.87 ± 0.01 at week 4 (F = 4.36, $P = 0.044$; $\eta p^2 = 0.47$, within group) supporting reduced reliance on CHO with dGTE. No such modifications for RER were observed with PL ($P > 0.05$).

Although submaximal exercise heart rate reduced by 6.24 ± 3.85 $b \cdot min^{-1}$ (4.8% by week 4) in the PL group, significance across time was only found with dGTE where submaximal exercise heart rate reduced by 8.8% from 124.95 ± 3.69 $b \cdot min^{-1}$ at week 0 to 113.90 ± 4.03 $b \cdot min^{-1}$ at week 4 (F = 4.07, $P = 0.045$; $\eta p^2 = 0.40$). A significant overall group × time interaction was also found for RPE (F = 3.43, $P = 0.05$), with subjects perceiving exercise to be progressively easier with dGTE by week 4 (10.0 ± 0.6 relative effort rating) compared to week 0 (11.9 ± 0.4; $P = 0.015$; $\eta p^2 = 0.58$). No differences were reported for systolic or diastolic blood pressure immediately post exercise over time for either group ($P > 0.05$).

Performance measures

A significant overall group × time interaction was found for distance covered (F = 9.84, $P = 0.001$; Figure 4). The use of dGTE resulted in a progressive increase in distance covered from 20.23 ± 0.54 km at week 0, to 21.77 ± 0.49 km at week 2 and finally 22.43 ± 0.40 km by week 4, representing a 10.9% significant increase in performance (F = 28.66, $P < 0.001$; $\eta p^2 = 0.85$). A similar interaction effect was also observed for PL (F = 7.94, $P = 0.009$; $\eta p^2 = 0.61$) with distance covered significantly improving by week 2 (21.75 ± 0.40 km) compared to week 0 (20.79 ± 0.30 km; $P = 0.002$) only.

In a similar manner, a significant overall group × time interaction was found for average power output (F = 14.43, $P < 0.001$; Figure 4). Average power output increased with dGTE (F = 40.01, $P < 0.001$; $\eta p^2 = 0.89$) by 17.9% or 29.02 ± 5.53 W from week 0 (162.06 ± 10.08 W) to week 2 (191.08 ± 10.85 W; $P = 0.01$); and by 22.7% (or 36.85 ± 3.20 W) from week 0 to week 4 (198.91 ± 8.61 W; $P < 0.001$), but was not significantly different between week 2 and 4 ($P > 0.05$). No significant differences across time for average power output were observed for PL ($P > 0.05$).

Discussion

The use of a 4 week dGTE strategy significantly enhanced FAT_{TOT} by 24.9% or 0.060 ± 0.027 $g \cdot min^{-1}$ compared to

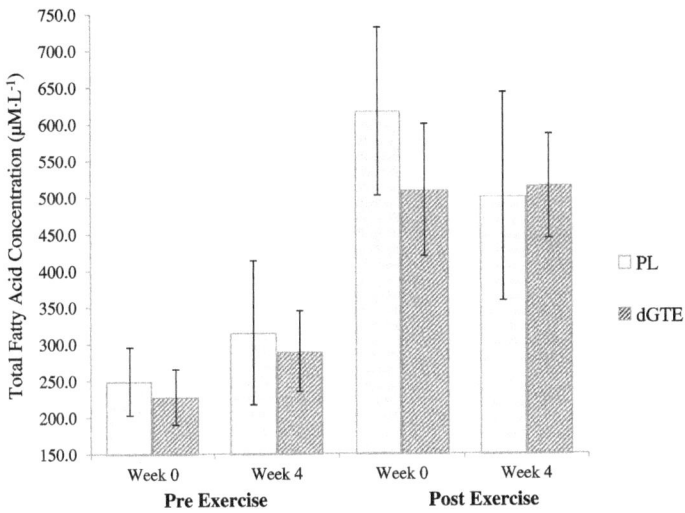

Figure 3 Total fatty acid concentrations pre and post exercise. Figure 3 shows the absolute total fatty acid concentrations at rest and post exercise for both treatment conditions at week 0 and week 4. Data are presented as mean ± SE. PL, Placebo; dGTE, decaffeinated green tea extract. No significant differences were found with ANOVA ($P > 0.05$).

PL supporting the hypothesis set. The increased contribution of total fat to EE with dGTE supports the proposal that EGCG positively influences substrate utilisation, particularly in combination with exercise training. The use of a capsulated dGTE formula in the present study potentially offers a more practical means to regularly consume a sufficient daily dosage to elicit such effects (compared to consumption of ~6-7 cups of green tea per day, especially considering the notable variability of catechin content in commercial green teas).

Improvements in FAT_{TOT} have been demonstrated elsewhere [1,11,32], with current values comparable to those reported when employing an acute dGTE strategy with similar EGCG content [3]. Conversely, higher dose

dGTE over a 28 day period did not enhance substrate metabolism in healthy, male volunteers [25] in contrast to these findings. However, in this latter study, the higher FAT_{TOT} are more typical of endurance trained athletes. It has been inferred that the combined effect of exercise training and GTE may be more relevant for untrained individuals who 'respond' to GTE intervention [25]. Participants in this study were recreationally active. It is therefore plausible that adaptations in exercise metabolism with dGTE are more pronounced with less trained individuals, as opposed to physically active or endurance trained volunteers assessed elsewhere [23-25].

Improved FAT_{TOT}, and reduced reliance on CHO_{TOT} during exercise are of clinical and performance relevance.

Table 2 Assessment of oxygen uptake, mean heart rate, perceived exertion and blood pressure related to submaximal exercise

Variable	PL (n = 7)			dGTE (n = 7)		
	Week 0	Week 2	Week 4	Week 0	Week 2	Week 4
$\dot{V}O_2$ (L·min^{-1})	1.55 ± 0.08	1.51 ± 0.08	1.52 ± 0.06	1.46 ± 0.04	1.44 ± 0.04	1.44 ± 0.05
$\dot{V}CO_2$ (L·min^{-1})	1.38 ± 0.06	1.35 ± 0.06	1.35 ± 0.05	1.31 ± 0.05	1.29 ± 0.03	1.25 ± 0.05
RER	0.89 ± 0.01	0.89 ± 0.01	0.89 ± 0.01	0.90 ± 0.01	0.89 ± 0.01	0.87 ± 0.01 [1, A,B]
HR (b·min^{-1})	127.8 ± 5.5	122.7 ± 4.4	121.5 ± 3.8	124.9 ± 3.7	117.0 ± 2.5	113.9 ± 4.0 [1, B]
RPE (6–20)	11.1 ± 0.8	11.7 ± 0.6	11.6 ± 0.3	11.9 ± 0.4	11.2 ± 0.4	10.0 ± 0.6* [A]
SBP (mm Hg)	132.7 ± 2.9	127.4 ± 3.0	127.7 ± 2.9	132.3 ± 2.4	127.6 ± 1.8	126.3 ± 2.9
DBP (mm Hg)	80.1 ± 3.3	74.7 ± 1.9	73.0 ± 2.0	74.4 ± 1.8	76.6 ± 5.1	70.1 ± 3.5

Table 2 demonstrates the influence of the dGTE on cardio-respiratory measures during submaximal steady state exercise across the intervention. Data are presented as mean ± SE. PL, Placebo; dGTE, decaffeinated green tea extract; $\dot{V}O_2$, submaximal oxygen uptake; $\dot{V}CO_2$, submaximal expired carbon dioxide; RER, respiratory exchange ratio; HR, heart rate; RPE, rating of perceived exertion; SBP, systolic blood pressure; DBP, diastolic blood pressure. [A]denotes significant overall group x time interaction effect ($P \le 0.05$). [B]denotes significant overall time interaction effect only ($P \le 0.02$). [1]denotes significant within group time interaction effect only ($P \le 0.045$). *denotes significant difference within group to baseline ($P = 0.015$).

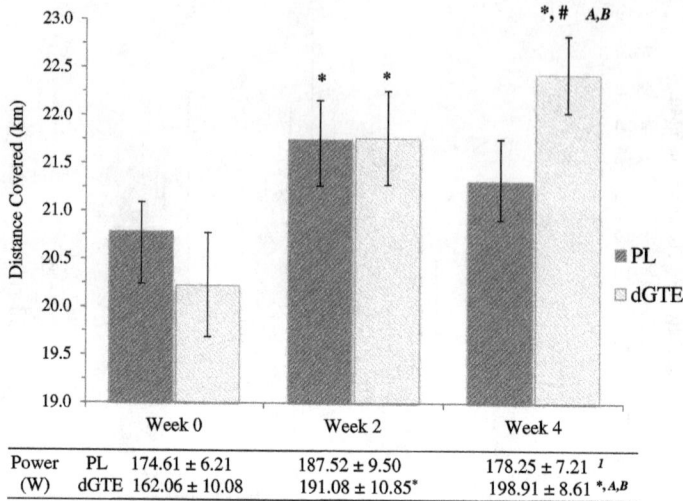

Power (W)		Week 0	Week 2	Week 4
	PL	174.61 ± 6.21	187.52 ± 9.50	178.25 ± 7.21 [1]
	dGTE	162.06 ± 10.08	$191.08 \pm 10.85^{*}$	198.91 ± 8.61 [*,A,B]

Figure 4 Distance covered and average power output during the performance trial. Figure 4 shows the distance covered and average power output elicited during the 40 minute performance trial for both treatment conditions at week 0, 2 and 4 of the intervention. Data are presented as mean ± SE. PL, Placebo; dGTE, decaffeinated green tea extract. [A]denotes significant overall group × time interaction effect ($P \leq 0.001$). [B]denotes significant overall time interaction effect ($P < 0.001$). [1]denotes significant within group time interaction effect only ($P = 0.039$). [*]denotes significant difference ($P \leq 0.02$) to baseline only within group. [#]denotes significant difference to week 2 within group only ($P = 0.03$).

Although resting and post exercise TFAs were not significantly different between groups, the increase in FAT_{TOT} with dGTE supports the contention that the inhibition of COMT may not be a dominant mechanism.

Independently of antioxidant protective mechanisms, it has been proposed that EGCG positively modulates cell signalling via PGC1α [20], sirtuin 1 (SIRT1) and mitogen activated protein kinase (MAPK) pathways [33,34]. In the longer term (>4 weeks), it is feasible that EGCG at moderate dose facilitates up-regulation of gene expression leading to enhanced FAT_{TOT} with exercise.

Although bodyweight reductions were similar between groups, the use of dGTE combined with regulated exercise significantly reduced body fat compared to PL. These findings are similar to those reported elsewhere [10,32,35], particularly when either higher dose GTE or low dose caffeine has been employed. Alterations in body composition, coupled with increased FAT_{TOT} infer that catechin polyphenols favourably modulate cellular metabolism, possibly via a calorie restriction mimetic (CRM) action [36]. This contention is further supported via studies demonstrating enhanced glucose tolerance, insulin sensitivity and adiponectin levels with EGCG [3,37].

In the current study, resting and submaximal exercise heart rate and blood pressure decreased over the intervention period in both groups. However, results were only significant over time with dGTE for exercising heart rate and perceived exertion, possibly relating to substrate utilisation efficiency and improved exercise economy. Additionally, whilst the results could also indicate an acute training stimulus, non-significant reductions in SBP found were comparable to those observed elsewhere [10,13,37]. It is therefore suggested that any mild hypotensive effects are likely due to the short-term influence of regular aerobic activity on nitric oxide pathways than dGTE impacting on endothelial production of nitric oxide synthase.

There has been much interest in the use of GTE to enhance physical performance. In animal studies, time to exhaustion has been shown to improve with GTE by 8-24%, with corresponding evidence of increased ß-oxidation and fatty acid translocase/CD36 mRNA expression [38]. When relatively low GTE/EGCG doses have been employed in humans, improvements in time trial or performance measures have not been observed [22,24]. However, the inclusion of matched caffeine placebo or pre-exercise feeding may explain these findings. Conversely, with higher dose GTE strategies, improvements in maximal oxygen uptake and time trial performance have been observed [39,40].

To the authors' knowledge, this is the first study to demonstrate a significant impact of dGTE on subsequent exercise performance. Performance indices improved by 10.9% for distance covered, and 22.7% for average power output with dGTE. This is unlikely to be fully explained via a training effect as improvements with PL were only observed at week 2 of the trial. Reduced reliance on CHO_{TOT} may have contributed to improved performance following submaximal exercise.

Future research investigating specific effects of EGCC from dGTE on exercise tolerance, performance and recovery is warranted, particularly in light of metabolomic advances [41]. High dose GTE has been demonstrated to reduce muscle soreness following strenuous exercise [42], potentially via signalling interactions leading to reduced post exercise inflammatory cascades [43]. Results in the current study may have been augmented due to utilisation of a low polyphenol diet. Further research combining dietary polyphenols with dGTE is warranted.

Conclusions

In conclusion, dGTE in conjunction with exercise training reduced relative FAT_{TOT} and body composition in recreationally active, male volunteers. Improved metabolic efficiency during submaximal exercise may potentiate improved metabolic economy and hence adherence to longer term training programmes. Combined with the observed impact of dGTE on subsequent performance indices, this supports the contention that EGCG use may modulate cellular signalling pathways leading to more efficient substrate use, resulting in improved exercise output.

Abbreviations

CHO: Carbohydrate; CHO_{TOT}: Total carbohydrate oxidation rate (measured in $g \cdot min^{-1}$); COMT: Catechol-o-methyl transferase; dGTE: Decaffeinated green tea extract; EE: Energy expenditure (measured in $kJ \cdot min^{-1}$); EGCG: (–)-Epigallocatechin-3-gallate; FAT_{TOT}: Total fat oxidation rate (measured in $g \cdot min^{-1}$); GT: Green tea; PL: Placebo formula used in the study; RER: Respiratory exchange ratio the ratio from dividing expired carbon dioxide with oxygen uptake; RPE: Rating of perceived exertion; TFA: Total fatty acids; $\dot{V}O_2$: Volume of oxygen uptake (measured in $L \cdot min^{-1}$); $\dot{V}O_{2peak}$: Peak oxygen uptake (measured in $L \cdot min^{-1}$); $\dot{V}CO_2$: Volume of expired carbon dioxide (measured in $L \cdot min^{-1}$).

Competing interests

Research funding and product supply to support this study was received from High 5 Ltd. All data was collected, analysed and reported by the investigatory team fully independently of the company. The authors declare that they have no competing interest.

Authors' contributions

All authors were involved in the study. JDR was the principal researcher, involved with liaison with the company, project organisation, statistical analysis and manuscript generation; MGR was co-supervisor involved with project co-ordination, quality control and technical accuracy in preparation of the manuscript; MDT was involved with confirmation of statistical analyses, and manuscript editing; JCW and CHT were involved with participant recruitment, pilot data collection, experimental interventions, data analysis and manuscript editing. All authors read and approved the final manuscript.

Acknowledgements

The authors wish to acknowledge High5 Ltd. for providing the support and funding to undertake this study. dGTE was supplied by High 5 Ltd. independently of the investigatory team. The authors also wish to acknowledge the support and external collaboration with ABS Laboratories, Biopark, Welwyn Garden City, for independent assessment of blood samples.

References

1. Dulloo AG, Duret C, Rohrer D, Girardier L, Mensi N, Fathi M, et al. Efficacy of a green tea extract rich in catechin polyphenols and caffeine in increasing 24-h energy expenditure and fat oxidation in humans. Am J Clin Nutr. 1999;70:1040–50.
2. Ryu OH, Lee J, Lee KW, Kim HY, Seo JA, Kim SG, et al. Effects of green tea consumption on inflammation, insulin resistance and pulse wave velocity in type 2 diabetes patients. Diabetes Res Clin Pract. 2006;71:356–8.
3. Venables MC, Hulston CJ, Cox HR, Jeukendrup AE. Green tea extract ingestion, fat oxidation, and glucose tolerance in healthy humans. Am J Clin Nutr. 2008;87:778–84.
4. Mukhtar H, Ahmad N. Tea polyphenols: prevention of cancer and optimizing health. Am J Clin Nutr. 2000;71(6):1698S–702.
5. Maki KC, Reeves MS, Farmer M, Yasunaga K, Matsuo N, Katsuragi Y, et al. Green tea catechin consumption enhances exercise-induced abdominal fat loss in overweight and obese adults. J Nutr. 2009;139(2):264–70.
6. Moore RJ, Jackson KG, Minihane AM. Green tea (Camellia Sinensis) catechins and vascular function. Br J Nutr. 2009;102(12):1790–802.
7. Nantz MP, Rowe CA, Bukowski JF, Percival SS. Standardised capsule of Camellia sinensis lowers cardiovascular risk factors in a randomized, double-blind, placebo-controlled study. Nutr. 2009;25(2):147–54.
8. Valcic S, Burr JA, Timmermann BN, Liebler TC. Antioxidant chemistry of green tea catechins. New oxidation products of (–)-epigallocatechin gallate and (–)-epigallocatechin from their reactions with peroxyl radicals. Chem Res Toxicol. 2000;13(9):801–10.
9. Henning SM, Niu Y, Lee NH, Thames GD, Minutti RR, Wang H, et al. Bioavailability and antioxidant activity of tea flavanols after consumption of green tea, black tea, or a green tea extract supplement. Am J Clin Nutr. 2004;80:1558–64.
10. Nagao T, Hase T, Tokimitsu I. A green tea extract high in catechins reduces body fat and cardiovascular risks in humans. Obesity. 2007;15(6):1473–83.
11. Ichinose T, Nomura S, Someya Y, Akimoto S, Tachiyashiki K, Imaizumi K. Endurance training supplemented with green tea extract on substrate metabolism during exercise in humans. Scand J Med Sci Sports. 2011;21:598–605.
12. Galleano M, Pechanova O, Fraga CG. Hypertension, nitric oxide, and dietary plant polyphenols. Curr Pharm Biotech. 2010;11(8):837–48.
13. Brown AL, Lane J, Coverly J, Stocks J, Jackson S, Stephen A, et al. Effects of dietary supplementation with the green tea polyphenol epigallocatechin-3-gallate on insulin resistance and associated metabolic risk factors: a randomised control trial. Br J Nutr. 2009;101(6):886–94.
14. Rains TM, Agarwal S, Maki KC. Antiobesity effects of green tea catechins: a mechanistic review. J Nutr Biochem. 2011;22(1):1–7.
15. Phung OJ, Baker WL, Matthews LJ, Lanosa M, Thorne A, Coleman CI. Effect of green tea catechins with or without caffeine on anthropometric measures: a systematic review and meta-analysis. Am J Clin Nutr. 2010;91(1):73–81.
16. Hursel R, Viechtbauer W, Westerterp-Plantenga MS. The effects of green tea on weight loss and weight maintenance: A meta-analysis. Int J Obes. 2009;33(9):956–61.
17. Hursel R, Westerterp-Plantenga MS. Thermogenic ingredients and body weight regulation. Int J Obes. 2010;34(4):659–69.
18. Feng WY. Metabolism of green tea catechins: An overview. Curr Drug Metab. 2006;7(7):755–809.
19. Chen C, Wang CY, Lambert JD, Ali N, Welsh WJ, Yang CS. Inhibition of human liver catechol-O-methyltransferase by tea catechins and their metabolites: structure-activity relationship and molecular-modelling studies. Biochem Pharma. 2005;69(10):1523–31.
20. Hodgson AB, Randell RK, Jeukendrup AE. The effect of green tea extract on fat oxidation at rest and during exercise: Evidence of efficacy and proposed mechanisms. Adv Nutr. 2013;4:129–40.
21. Reiter CEN, Kim JA, Kwon MJ. Green tea polyphenol epigallocatechin gallate reduces endothelin-1 expression and secretion in vascular endothelial cells: Roles for AMP activated protein kinase, Akt and FOXO1. Endocrinol. 2009;151(1):103–14.
22. Dean S, Braakhuis A, Paton C. The effects of EGCG on fat oxidation and endurance performance in male cyclists. Int J Sport Nutr Exerc Metab. 2009;20(6):624–44.
23. Eichenberger P, Colombani PC, Mettler S. Effects of a 3-week consumption of green tea extracts on whole-body metabolism during cycling exercise in endurance-trained men. Int J Vitam Nutr Res. 2009;79(1):24–33.

24. Eichenberger P, Mettler S, Arnold M, Colombani PC. No effects of three-week consumption of a green tea extract on time trial performance in endurance trained men. Int J Vitam Nutr Res. 2010;80(1):54–64.

25. Randell RK, Hodgson AB, Lotito SB, Jacobs DM, Rowson M, Mela DJ. Variable duration of decaffeinated green tea extract ingestion on exercise metabolism. Med Sci Sports Exerc. 2014;46(6):1185–93.

26. Faul F, Erdfelder E, Lang A-G, Buchner A. G*power 3: a flexible statistical power analysis program for the social, behavioral, and biomedical sciences. Behav Res Meth. 2007;39(2):175–91.

27. Roberts JD, Tarpey MD, Kass LS, Tarpey RJ, Roberts MG. Assessing a commercially available sports drink on exogenous carbohydrate oxidation, fluid delivery and sustained exercise performance. J Int Soc Sports Nutr. 2014;11(8):1–14.

28. Kao M-F, Lu H-K, Jang T-R, Yang W-C, Chen C-H, Chen Y-Y, et al. Comparison of different measurement equations for body composition estimation in male athletes. Int J Sport Exerc Sci. 2010;3(1):11–6.

29. Borg G. Ratings of perceived exertion and heart rates during short term cycle exercise and their use in a new strength test. Int J Sports Med. 1982;3(3):153–8.

30. Jeukendrup AE, Wallis GA. Measurement of substrate oxidation during exercise by means of gas exchange measurements. Int J Sports Med. 2005;26(1):S28–37.

31. Kangani CO, Kelley DE, DeLany JP. New method for GC/FID and GC-C-IRMS analysis of plasma free fatty acid concentration and isotopic enrichment. J Chromatogr B Analyt Technol Biomed Life Sci. 2008;873(1):95–101.

32. Westerterp-Plantenga MS, Lejeune MPGM, Kovacs EMR. Body weight loss and weight maintenance in relation to habitual caffeine intake and green tea supplementation. Obes Res. 2005;13:1195–204.

33. Ayissi VBO, Ebrahimi A, Schluesenner H. Epigenetic effects of natural polyphenols: a focus on SIRT1-mediated mechanisms. Mol Nutr Food Res. 2014;58:22–32.

34. Kim H-S, Quon MJ, Kim J-A. New insights into the mechanisms of polyphenols beyond antioxidant properties: lessons from the green tea polyphenol, epigallocatechin 3-gallate. Redox Biol. 2014;2:187–95.

35. Wang H, Wen Y, Du Y, Yan X, Guo H, Rycroft JA, et al. Effects of catechin enriched green tea on body composition. Obesity. 2010;18:773–9.

36. Madeo F, Pietrocola F, Eisenberg T, Kroemer G. Calorie restriction mimetics: towards a molecular definition. Nat Rev: Drug Disc. 2014;13(10):727–40.

37. Potenza MA, Marasciulo FL, Tarquinio M, Tiravanti E, Colantuono G, Federici A, et al. EGCG, a green tea polyphenol, improves endothelial function and insulin sensitivity, reduces blood pressure, and protects against myocardial I/R injury in SHR. Am J Physiol Endocrinol Metab. 2007;292:E1378–87.

38. Murase T, Haramizu S, Shimotoyodome A, Tokimitsu I, Hase T. Green tea improves running endurance in mice by stimulating lipid utilization during exercise. Am J Physiol Reg Integr Comp Physiol. 2006;290(6):R1550–6.

39. MacRae HSH, Mefferd KM. Dietary antioxidant supplementation combined with quercetin improves cycling time trial performance. Int J Sport Nutr Exer Metab. 2006;16(4):405–19.

40. Richards JC, Lonac MC, Johnson TK, Schweder MM, Bell C. Epigallocatechin-3-gallate increases maximal oxygen consumption in adult humans. Med Sci Sports Exerc. 2010;42(4):739–44.

41. Nieman DC, Gillitt ND, Knab AM, Shanely RA, Pappan KL, Jin F, et al. Influence of a polyphenol-enriched protein powder on exercise-induced inflammation and oxidative stress in athletes: a randomized trial using a metabolomics approach. Plos One. 2013;8(8):1–11.

42. Moradpourian MR, Ashkavand Z, Venkatesh C, Vishwanath BS. Effect of different doses of green tea on oxidative stress and muscle soreness in downhill treadmill running. Asian J Pharm Clin Res. 2014;7(2):192–3.

43. Cunha CA, Lira FS, Neto JCR, Pimentel GD, Souza GIH, da Silva CMG, et al. Green tea extract supplementation induces the lipolytic pathway, attenuates obesity, and reduces low-grade inflammation in mice fed a high-fat diet. Mediators Inflamm. 2013;2013:1–8.

## 7

A review on effects of conjugated linoleic fatty acid (CLA) upon body composition and energetic metabolism

Tatiana Ederich Lehnen[1,4], Marcondes Ramos da Silva[2], Augusto Camacho[1,2], Aline Marcadenti[2,3] and Alexandre Machado Lehnen[1,2*]

Abstract

Conjugated linoleic acid (CLA) is highly found in fats from ruminants and it appears to favorably modify the body composition and cardiometabolic risk factors. The capacity of CLA to reduce the body fat levels as well as its benefic actions on glycemic profile, atherosclerosis and cancer has already been proved in experimental models. Furthermore, CLA supplementation may modulate the immune function, help re-synthetize of glycogen and potentiate the bone mineralization. CLA supplementation also could increase the lipolysis and reduce the accumulation of fatty acids on the adipose tissue; the putative mechanisms involved may be its action in reducing the lipase lipoprotein activity and to increase the carnitine-palmitoil-transferase-1 (CAT-1) activity, its interaction with PPARγ, and to raise the expression of UCP-1. Although studies made in human have shown some benefits of CLA supplementation as the weight loss, the results are still discordant. Moreover, some have shown adverse effects, such as negative effects on glucose metabolism and lipid profile. The purpose of this article is to review the available data regarding the benefits of CLA on the energetic metabolism and body composition, emphasizing action mechanisms.

Introduction

Although many research studies are inconclusive about functional foods, their benefits to health have often been discussed, calling the attention of the scientific community [1–3]. Thus, several studies were performed claiming that functional foods are essential for health and have helped reduce the risk of developing various chronic diseases [4–6]. This functional property concerns the metabolic or physiological role played by the nutrient or non-nutrient in growth, development, maturity and other normal functions of the human organism. However, studies on nutraceutics (foods with a medicinal function) lack further explanation, especially regarding the associated protective effects. The doses indicated generate doubts that these effects will be achieved, and also regarding the possible adverse effects of their long term use [1–3].

Several classes of substance which are naturally present in foods or produced by food technology have functional properties. One of these substances is conjugated linoleic acid (CLA) - a fatty acid which presents a linoleic acid isomer (C18:2, n-6) and has been considered an antiobesity agent, and can be useful in the weight reduction process [7]. Although the initial results were found only in an animal model [8, 9], more recent research on humans suggests that CLA would act to reduce adiposity through modulating properties in the lipid metabolism [10, 11]. However, doubts remain as to the action mechanisms of CLA in adipocytes, leading to the reduction of body fat and, especially, the safety of supplementation of this compound.

Therefore, the purpose of this review is to describe the effect of CLA supplementation on body composition, particularly on the reduction of adiposity, focusing on possible action mechanisms.

* Correspondence: amlehnen@gmail.com
[1]Faculdade Sogipa de Educação Física, Porto Alegre, Brazil
[2]Instituto de Cardiologia/Fundação Universitária de Cardiologia (IC/FUC), Porto Alegre, Brazil
Full list of author information is available at the end of the article

Conjugated linoleic acid

Conjugated linoleic acid (CLA) is a term that describes a group of fatty acids with 18 atoms of carbon, and the geometric isomers consist of linoleic acid [12]. This is a common name given to a group of position isomers with two double bonds separated by a methylene group [7, 13]. This conjugation of the double bond is generally in positions 9 and 11 or 10 and 12, and may be a *cis* or *trans* configuration (Fig. 1).

CLA is produced naturally in the digestive tract of ruminants such as cattle, goats, sheep, buffalo, and to a lesser degree in pigs, chickens and turkeys, and the synthesis occur due to fermentative bacteria, *Butyrivibrio Fibrisolvens*, which isomerize the linoleic acid in CLA or by synthesis via α9-desaturase of 11-*trans* octadecanoic acid [14]. The fat in beef contains about 1.7 to 10.8 mg CLA/g of fat with 9-*cis* and 11-*trans* isomers. It is also found in dairy products (milks and derivatives) [6].

CLA can be obtained by means of enzyme α9-desaturase which promotes the desaturation of the 11-*trans* octadecanoic acid. Several different isomers of CLA such as 11-*trans* and 9-*cis* are the best known because they are found in food [7, 12]. It is also possible to obtain CLA in an industrial form, through the partial hydrogenation of linoleic acid or by thermal treatments, aiming to produce a compound with maximum biological activity and with a defined chemical composition [10].

CLA has a major role in the lipid metabolism, especially as regards the oxidative cellular system, which explains many physiological properties of fatty acids. Their

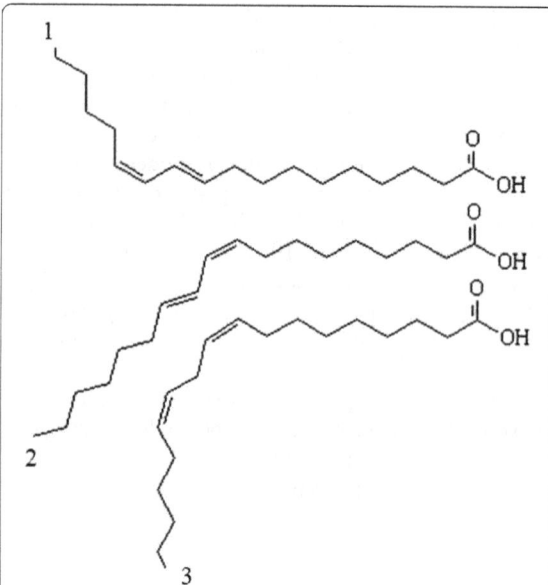

Fig. 1 Isomer structure. (1) represents CLA 10-trans and 12-cis; (2) indicate CLA 9-cis and 11-trans; (3) C18:2 9-cis and 12-cis

action on the lipid metabolism is associated with the inhibition of the entry of glucose into the adipocytes, and may lead to changes in the insulin metabolism and cause situations of hyperinsulinemia, as well as the increase of inflammatory markers [15, 16].

There are many investigations to evaluate the influences of CLA on the energetic metabolism, promoting significant changes in the lipid metabolism and in body composition [9–11, 17–20]. As a result, some effects can be cited such as: reduction of body fat, improved insulin resistance, antithrombogenic and anticarcinogenic effects, reduction of atherosclerosis, improved lipid profile, modulation of the immune system and stimulation of bone mineralization, and also reduced blood glucose. The most studied CLA supplementation effect is its capacity to alter the body composition, promoting an increase in lean mass and reduction of the fatty mass.

Putative mechanisms of action

The possible action mechanisms which show that CLA can alter the body composition involve metabolic changes that favor the reduction of the lipogenesis and the potentiation of lipolysis, accompanied by the oxidation of fatty acid in the skeletal muscle, due to increased carnitine palmitoil-transferase-1 activity and action, or possibly because of adipocyte differentiation inhibition [7]. Therefore, researchers have evaluated the action of CLA supplementation on the lipid and hormone profile, and the activity of the enzymes involved in the oxidation process [21].

Studies have demonstrated that isomers 10-*trans* and 12-*cis*, differently from the 9-*cis* 11-*trans* of CLA, increase lipolysis significantly in the human adipocytes, and also have the function of diminishing the synthesis of fatty acids [15]. This would explain, in part, the possible action mechanisms of CLA on the body composition. Although various studies were *in vitro*, the metabolic hypotheses to explain the body fat reducing action of CLA began based on control of the expression of genes involved in the differentiation of pre-adipocytes into mature adipocytes, in other words, the expression of these genes would result in reducing lipogenesis [22, 23].

In turn, the peroxisome proliferator-activated receptors (PPARs) are nuclear transcription factors that play a central role in the storage and catabolism of fatty acids (FA). They are part of a class of nuclear receptors that belong to the family of the nuclear receptor of the steroid, retinoid and thyroid receptors. Three isoforms of the nuclear receptor have already been identified, PPARα, PPARβ and PPARγ. PPARα and β are involved in the lipid metabolism (especially the proteins related to FA oxidation) and glucose, and PPARγ is involved in adipocyte differentiation [24, 25].

Figure 2 shows the activation mechanism and re-quires the release of the co-repressor complex (histone deacetylase activity) by a binder, and the recruitment of the co-activator complex (acetyltransferase activity). The activated PPAR:RxR complex binds to the elements that are responsive to peroxisome proliferators (PPRE), producing changes in the chromatin structure, giving rise to a transcriptionally competent structure. Hence, it seems that the CLA interacts with the Co-activator complex PPAR increasing the gene transcription related to the differentiation of adipocytes, lipolysis (β-oxidation), mitochondrial biogenesis and insulin sensitivity, and col-lectively, it is related to the weight loss effect [24].

The effects of CLA in lipid and glucose metabolism on body composition are mediated by the activation or in-hibition of the PPARs, especially PPARγ. The inhibition of PPARγ by CLA (isomer 10-*trans*, 12-*cis*) leads to the reduction of body fat by modulation of the gene expres-sion in the sense that it inhibits cell differentiation and alters the activity of proteins involved in lipogenesis and in lipolysis [26]. Evidence suggests that the activation of PPARγ can diminish the progression of atherosclerosis and increase sensitivity to insulin, and may be a poten-tial therapeutic target for the treatment of various dis-eases, including diabetes mellitus type 2 (DM2) and dyslipidemia.

In adipocytes, PPARγ regulates the expression of genes involved in the lipid metabolism, including acyl CoA-synthetase and lipoprotein lipase (LPL). The expression of the transport protein of fatty acids involved in the up-take of lipids by the adipocytes is also controlled by PPARγ [25].

The reduction of body fat occurs not due to the reduc-tion in the number of adipocytes but rather by the re-duction of their size. Considering that the size of the adipose cells is directly elated to the triglyceride content inside the cells, its reduction results in a smaller cell size. The increased β-oxidation of mitochondrial fatty acids induced by CLA may be responsible for the

reduction of triacylglycerol synthesis, not depositing them in the adipocyte, but reducing their size [8].

The fatty acid is transported into the mitochondria by the carnitine-palmitoil-transferase (CPT) complex. Three enzymatic components are involved: CPT-1, CPT-2 and carnitine acylcarnitine translocase (CATC) [27]. The fatty acids are activated by the acyl-CoA synthetase enzyme forming an activated complex (fatty acyl-CoA), with the carnitine-palmitoil-transferase (CPT-1) enzyme. This com-plex penetrates the mitochondrial membrane and reaches the intermembrane space. Acyl-CoA is regenerated with the release of carnitine in the CPT-2 reaction. Once it reaches the mitochondrial matrix, the long chain fatty acid (LCFA) is oxidized to generate adenosine triphosphate (ATP) through the β-oxidation of the fatty acids [27]. CLA supplementation would increase the concentration and ac-tivity of CPT-1. Thus, collectively, the increased lipolysis, the reduction of lipase lipoprotein activity and increased carnitine-palmitoil-transferase-1 (CAT-1) activity lead to the reduction of the accumulation of fatty acids in the adi-pose and muscle tissues. These action mechanisms are those most discussed by the researchers [8]. Inside the mitochondria the fatty acids are oxidized by β–oxidation reactions and Cycle of Krebs (CK), releasing the H^+ and e- which are carried ($NADH^{+2}$ and $FADH_2$) to the respiratory chain (1). The gradient of H^+ and e- between the inter-membrane space and the matrix determines its return passing by the ATP synthase protein (2) with a synthesis of ATP (coupled reaction) or by the uncoupling protein (3) producing heat.

However, the rationale that CLA stimulates lipolysis only by increasing CPT-1 is valid (and limited) for situa-tions in which β-oxidation (capacity to generate ATP through the successive break down of fatty acid carbon) is more efficient than the transport of the fatty acyl-CoA complex to the mitochondrial matrix. In this way it is possible and logical to say that CLA supplementation (in-creasing CPT-1 concentration and activation) would only have a potential effect on physically active individuals,

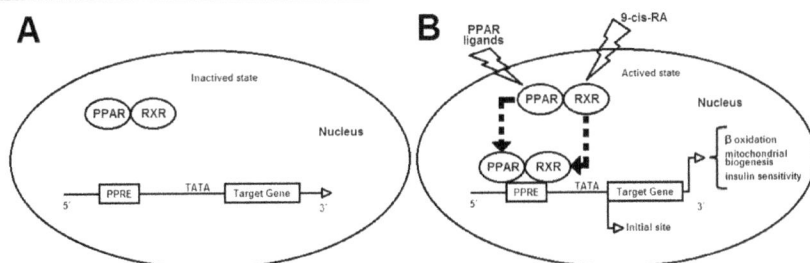

Fig. 2 Mechanism for transcriptional activation by PPAR. Panel **a** shows the inactivated state, without gene transcriptional of any target genes. Panel **b** shows the activation of PPAR by PPAR ligands and RXR by 9-cis-RA (9-cis-retinoic acid), thereby stimulating target genes transcription by binding to specific DNA sequence (peroxisome proliferators – PPRE) leading to increased β-oxidation, mitochondrial biogenesis and insulin sensitivity

particularly for those whose β-oxidation is more efficient than the transport of fatty acid itself to the mitochondrial matrix.

On the other hand, weight loss with CLA supplementation could be explained by its association with the uncoupling protein of the respiratory chain (UCP), potentiating the β-oxidation capacity [28]. The respiratory chain or electron transport chain is formed by a series of transport compounds located in the inner membrane of the mitochondria. The last of these of these compounds is called cytochrome-oxidase, the only one that presents all necessary conditions to deliver electrons directly to the O_2. However, not all of the energy contained in the electrons will be contained in the ATP, since part of it evolves as heat to maintain the spontaneity of the successive transfers. As the electrons flow through the respiratory chain, they lose their free energy. Part of this energy can be picked up and stored to produce ATP from ADP and inorganic phosphate. The rest of the free energy, which is not taken up for ATP re-synthesis, is released in the form of heat, increasing UCP activity [29, 30].

UCPs are proteins found in the inner mitochondrial membrane that allow proton flow from the intermembrane space to the mitochondrial matrix. However, the return of protons to the mitochondrial matrix does not lead to energy storage in the form of ATP thereby releasing heat. UCP-1, also known as thermogenin, often speeds up the proton return to the mitochondrial matrix so that energy from Krebs cycle, originated from the oxidation of energetic substrates (including lipids), is lost in the form of heat (which can lead to weight loss if this UCP is stimulated) [31].

UCPs can be subdivided into UCP-1, UCP-2 and UCP-3. They differ in their distribution among tissues and possible function. UCP1 is exclusively expressed in brown adipose tissue; UCP3 is expressed in muscle and a number of other tissues; and UCP2 is expressed in a variety of tissues including white adipose tissue (WAT) and is the most highly expressed UCP [32]. These proteins can exert a thermogenic effect and are capable of depleting the proton gradient, but their functions are not yet completely clear [13, 26, 31].

UCP-1 is responsible for lipid oxidation and heat production in brown adipose tissue (abundant in hibernating animals). Human adults have higher levels of white adipose tissue and have UCP-2 and UCP-3, which appears to be related to heat generation. Other UCPs (UCP-4, for instance) are also being investigated [31]. The administration of thyroid hormones leads to respiratory chain uncoupling, which might be explained by an increase in UCPs [33]. Moreover, lipolysis resulting from fasting appears to stimulate UCPs, and the interaction of fatty acids with PPAR seems to increase the expression of UCPs [34].

Supplementation with a CLA mixture or 10,12 CLA in rodents has been shown to induce UCP2 transcription in WAT [32, 35, 36], but whether it plays a role in energy dissipation is unclear. It would appear that CLA interacts with PPARγ, increases CTP-1 and expression of UCP-1 resulting in greater capacity for lipolysis and fat mass weight reduction [28].

Evidences from experimental animal

According to Gaze et al. [37], the effect of CLA is not the same in all animal models. Rats supplemented with 0.5 % of CLA, for instance, presented a small, but fast (7 days) reduction of adipose tissue, compared to mice [37].

Botelho [8] evaluated the effects of supplementation with CLA on the body composition of healthy Wistar rats supplemented for 3 weeks with CLA at the concentrations of 1 %, 2 % and 4 % on the daily consumption of the diet + control group (2 % linoleic acid). At the end of the period, the groups that were supplemented at a concentration of 2 % and 4 % with CLA presented a greater body fat reduction compared to the control group [8].

Other researchers evaluated coconut oil, maize oil and CLA. In this study 28 rats were allocated to 4 different diets: supplementation with coconut oil, coconut oil and CLA, maize oil and maize oil and CLA. After 28 days, total cholesterol, HDL−c and triglycerides were evaluated. It was found that the triglycerides diminished in the diet supplemented with coconut oil and CLA, and HDL-c diminished with the maize oil diet. The total cholesterol concentrations were lowest in the rats on the coconut oil and CLA diet, but not in the diet with maize oil and CLA. This study suggests that the CLA might diminish adiposity and improve the lipid profile under some conditions [9].

Evidences from human studies

In recent years, CLA supplementation has also been used in sports, aiming to reduce body fat and possibly improve performance [38]. Furthermore, other supposed benefits include improved lipid profile [39] and/or anti-inflammatory effects [40] that can reduce oxidative stress [41] and ameliorate insulin signaling [42], among others. Collectively, these mechanisms improve body composition and energetic metabolism. Table 1 shows 16 randomized clinical trials (RCT) using CLA as intervention (last 5 years, Pubmed database) on putative benefits. It is possible to see that 9 RCTs, from a total of 16, showed no benefit on aspects related to CLA supplementation. In addition, the studies shown in Table 1, other evidence from human studies are shown below.

Few studies have evaluated changes in body composition with the use of CLA alone or in combination with physical exercise in humans. Blankson et al. [10] showed

Table 1 Randomized clinical trials using CLA as intervention on putative benefits

Author	Sampling	Study design	Intervention	Results
BACHMAIR et al., 2015 [55]	Forty-three healthy adults at low to moderate risk of cardiovascular disease	Double-blind, placebo controlled study	Sample received 4 g/day of CLA80:20 or placebo for two weeks	No clear evidence was found for inhibition or activation of platelet function as well as inflammation by CLA80:20 in a low to moderate cardiovascular risk group.
JENKINS et al., 2014a [56]	Thirty-four untrained to moderately trained men	Double-blind, placebo controlled study	Randomly assigned to either a CLA (Clarinol A-80; $n = 18$) or placebo (PLA; sunflower oil; $n = 16$) group Prior to and following 6 weeks of aerobic training (50 % VO$_2$peak for 30 min, twice per week) and supplementation (5.63 g of total CLA isomers [of which 2.67 g was 9-cis, 11-trans and 2.67 g was 10-trans, 12-cis] or 7.35 g high oleic sunflower oil per day)	Serum triacylglycerol concentrations were lower (p < 0.05) in the CLA than the PLA group. For VO$_2$peak and glucose, there were group x time interactions (p < 0.05). However, post-hoc statistical tests did not reveal any differences between the CLA and PLA groups.
JENKINS et al., 2014b [57]	Thirty-four untrained to moderately trained men	Double-blind, placebo controlled study	Randomly assigned to either a CLA (Clarinol A-80; $n = 17$) or placebo (PLA; sunflower oil; $n = 16$) group. Before and after 6 weeks of aerobic training (50 % VO$_2$peak for 30 min, twice per week) and supplementation (8 ml CLA or PLA per day), each subject completed an incremental cycle ergometer test, maximal number of sit-ups in 1 min, and the standing long jump	There were no differences between the CLA and PLA groups for the analysis of covariance-adjusted post-test mean values for physical working capacity, sit-ups, or standing long jump. The physical working capacity increased from pre- to post-training in the CLA (p = 0.003) and PLA (p = 0.003) groups. There were no differences from pre- to post-training for sit-ups and standing long jump in either the CLA or PLA groups. There was no effect of CLA on physical working capacity, maximum number of sit-ups or standing long jump.
ARYAEIAN et al., 2014 [58]	Seventy eight adults with active rheumatoid arthritis	Double-blind clinical trial	Four groups receiving one of the following daily supplement for 3 months; group C: 2.5 g CLAs, group E: 400 mg Vitamin E, group CE: CLAs plus Vitamin E, group P: Placebo. Cytokines, matrix metalloproteinase (MMP-3) and citrullinated antibody (CCP-A)	Co-supplementation CLAs and Vitamin E may be effective in the level of inflammatory markers in rheumatoid arthritis patients.
EFTEKHARI et al., 2014 [59]	Ninety atherosclerotic patients	clinical randomized trial	Patients were classified into 3 groups receiving 3 g/d CLA or 1 920 mg/d ω3 or placebo for 2 months.	Although CLA did not appear to have a significant effect on triglycerides, ω3 supplementation significantly reduced triglycerides level. Consumption of CLA and ω3 supplementation did not significantly affect HDL cholesterol, LDL cholesterol, and total cholesterol.
MOHAMMADZADEH et al., 2013 [60]	Thirty four volunteers patients with rectal cancer	Randomized, double-blind, placebo-controlled pilot	CLA group ($n = 16$), receiving 3 g CLA/d, and placebo group ($n = 18$) receiving placebo capsules (sunflower oil) for 6 weeks	CLA supplementation improved inflammatory factors, MMP-2, and MMP-9 as biomarkers of angiogenesis and tumor invasion. It seems that CLA may provide new complementary treatment by reducing tumor invasion and resistance to cancer treatment in patients with rectal cancer.

Table 1 Randomized clinical trials using CLA as intervention on putative benefits (Continued)

Reference	Study design	Participants	Intervention	Results
PENETO et al., 2013 [61]	Double-blind clinical trial	Twenty nine healthy adult volunteers (nineteen women and ten men, aged twenty two to thirty six years)	CLA depletion was achieved through an 8-week period of restricted dairy fat intake (depletion phase; CLA intake was 5.2 ± 5.8 mg/day), followed by an 8-week period in which individuals consumed 20 g/day of butter naturally enriched with 9-cis, 11-trans CLA (repletion phase; CLA intake of 1020 ± 167 mg/day)	The intake of a 9-cis, 11-trans CLA-enriched butter by normal-weight subjects induces beneficial changes in immune modulators associated with sub-clinical inflammation in overweight individuals.
CARVALHO et al., 2013 [62]	Randomized clinical trial, placebo-controlled	Fourteen women diagnosed with metabolic syndrome	Participants received strawberry jam enriched or not with microencapsulated CLA (3 g/day) as a mixture of 38.57 % 9-cis, 11-trans, and 39.76 % 10-trans, 12-cis CLA isomers associated with a hypocaloric diet for 90 days	There were no significant effects of CLA on the lipid profile or blood pressure. Mean plasma insulin concentrations were significantly lower in women supplemented with CLA, did not alter the waist circumference, but there was a reduction in body fat mass detected after 30 days, and had a reduced waist circumference
BULUT et al., 2013 [63]	Randomized double blind experiment	Eighteen sedentary male volunteers	Volunteers were randomly divided into CLA and placebo supplementation groups; both groups underwent daily supplementation of either 3 g CLA or 3 g placebo for 30 days and performed exercise on a bicycle ergometer 3 times per week	CLA is not more effective than exercise alone.
LÓPEZ PLAZA, et al., 2013 [64]	A prospective, placebo-controlled, randomised double-blind, parallel clinical trial	Thirty eight volunteers (29w, 9 m)	Volunteers consumed 200 ml/day of skimmed milk with 3 g of CLAs or 3 g olive oil (placebo).	The consumption of skimmed milk enriched with 3 g of a 1:1 mixture of 9-cis, 11-trans and 10-trans, 12-cis for 24 weeks led to a decrease in body weight and total fat mass in healthy, overweight subjects who maintained habitual diets and exercise patterns. No adverse effects were observed
ENGBERIN et al. 2012 [65]	Double-blind, placebo controlled study	Sixty-one healthy volunteers	The diets were identical except for 7 % of energy (18.9 g in a diet of 10 MJ/day) that was provided either by oleic acid, by industrial trans fatty acids or by 9-cis, 11-trans CLA.	The effect of the CLA diet compared with the oleic acid diet was 0.11 mm Hg (95 % confidence interval: −1.27, 1.49) systolic and −0.45 mm Hg (−1.63, 0.73) diastolic. Short-term high intakes of 9-cis, 11-trans CLA do not affect blood pressure in healthy volunteers.
JOSEPH et al., 2011 [66]	Double-blinded, 3-phase crossover trial	Twenty seven volunteers with overweight, borderline hypercholesterolemic,	Participants consumed under supervision in random order 3.5 g/d of safflower oil (control), a 50:50 mixture of 10-trans, 12-cis, and 9-cis, 11-trans CLA:Clarinol G-80, and 9-cis, 11-trans isomer CLA	Compared with the control treatment, the CLA treatments did not affect changes in body weight, body composition, or blood lipids. In addition, CLA did not affect the β-oxidation rate of fatty acids or induce significant alterations in the safety markers tested.

Table 1 Randomized clinical trials using CLA as intervention on putative benefits *(Continued)*

MICHISHITA et al., 2010 [67]	Forty-one healthy subjects	Single-centre, randomized, double-blind, placebo-controlled trial	Subjects were randomized to receive either placebo or one of three test supplements: amino acid mixture 0.76 g/day; amino acid mixture 1.52 g/day; or amino acid mixture 1.52 g/day coadministered with conjugated linoleic acid 1.6 g/day and exercises for a period of 12 weeks	The results suggest that ingestion of these supplements might enhance the fat-burning effects of exercise.
WANDERS et al., 2010 [68]	Sixty-one healthy women and men	Double-blind, placebo controlled study	It was provided either by oleic acid, by industrial trans fatty acids or by a mixture of 80 % 9-*cis*, 11-*trans* and 20 % 10-*trans*, 12-*cis* CLA.	High intakes of an 80:20 mixture of 9-*cis*, 11-*trans*, and 10-*trans*, 12-*cis* CLA raise the total to HDL cholesterol ratio in healthy volunteers. The effect of CLA may be somewhat less than that of industrial trans fatty acids.
SLUIJS et al., 2010 [69]	Four hundred and one	Double-blind, randomized, placebo-controlled and parallel-group trial	Subjects receive either 4 g CLA/d (2.5 g 9-*cis*, 11-*trans* CLA/d and 0.6 g 10-*trans*, 12-*cis* CLA/d) or placebo supplements for 6 months	There was no effect of 9-*cis*, 11-*trans* CLA supplementation on blood pressure, body composition, insulin resistance, or concentrations of lipid, glucose, and C-reactive protein.
SYVERTSEN et al., 2007 [70]	One hundred and eighteen volunteers	Randomized, double-blind, placebo-controlled trial	Supplementation with either placebo (olive oil) or CLA (Clarinol) for 6 months	CLA does not affect glucose metabolism or insulin sensitivity in a population of overweight or obese volunteers.

that CLA may reduce the percentage of fat in humans over a 12-months period, besides increasing the lean mass and not presenting any additional effect at doses above 3.4 g of CLA per day. However since physical training was performed at the same time as the CLA was used, and the levels of exercise were different among the groups, it was not possible to evaluate whether the effect of the body changes was due to the use of CLA, exercise, or the combination of both.

Gaullier et al. [11] performed a 24-month randomized, double-blind placebo–controlled study, during which 6 capsules of gel were administered daily, totaling 4.5 g of CLA. The authors observed that the CLA supplementation for this period in overweight adults is well tolerated, and CLA reduces body fat in overweight humans and can help maintain the initial fat and weight losses over the long term [11].

As to gender, Santos-Zago et al. [20] showed the effect of body fat reduction on healthy, eutrophic women who consumed 3 kg of CLA per day, during 64 days. The results, however, were not significant, since CLA consumption during this period did not alter the women's body composition [20]. On the other hand, individuals with overweight and obesity, who consumed the amount of 3.4 g of CLA per day for 12 weeks reduced their body fat, as previously shown [10].

The responses to the different CLA isomers do not appear to present differences, although it was found that the 10-*trans*, 12-*cis* isomer increased the concentration of triglycerides and LDL cholesterol in a greater proportion in healthy men compared to the 9-*cis*, 11-*trans* isomer [21]. In a review study, obese men diagnosed with metabolic syndrome used CLA for 4 weeks. The final result was a reduction of the abdominal circumference, however other anthropometric measures did not undergo a relevant change [37].

A randomized, double blind, placebo-controlled study looked at the effects of CLA supplementation on body composition and weight loss for 12 weeks, in individuals with obesity or grade I obesity in the Chinese population. Bioelectric impedance was the method used to evaluate body composition changes during the study. Individuals randomly received 1.7 g of 9-*cis*, 11-*trans* and 10-*trans*, 12-*cis* of CLA ($n = 30$) or placebo ($n = 33$) in 200 ml of sterilized milk twice a day. As a result it was found that the group supplemented with CLA presented a reduction of obesity and/or overweight besides other benefits, without evidence of adverse effects [18].

Kim et al. [43] tested the supplementation of CLA 2.4 g/day CLA mixture (36.9 % of 9-*cis*, 11-*trans* and 37.9 % of 10-*trans*, 12-*cis*) as an antioxidant agent in healthy overweight/obese Korean individuals. Eight weeks of conjugated linoleic acid supplementation has no effect on antioxidant status (plasma total radical-trapping antioxidant potential, lipid peroxidation, lipid-soluble antioxidant vitamin concentration, erythrocyte antioxidant enzyme – superoxide dismutase, catalase, glutathione peroxidase), and leukocyte DNA damage between the CLA, compared to placebo group.

Thirty-seven recreationally-trained women (mean BMI = 25.1 ± 3.4) were randomized for three dietary interventions: 1) a control diet (without changing their usual dietary habits); 2) a high-protein, low-calorie diet supplemented with protein gels (22 g of protein per serving), encapsulated thermogenic (Burn®), multivitamin (Balance®), and CLA (Tone®); and 3) a high-protein diet with isocaloric placebo supplements. After three weeks, women in the supplementation group had their body weight and percentage of body fat (assessed by DEXA and skinfolds) significantly decreased when compared to placebo or control diets. Despite these positive results, it is noteworthy the fact that CLA was used concomitant to other nutritional supplements, and it is thus difficult to assess its effect individually on body adiposity [44].

In another study, 101 moderately obese subjects who lost >8 % of their baseline body weight in a previous study were subsequently assigned to a 1-year double-blind CLA (3.4 g/day) or placebo (olive oil) supplementation regime in combination with a modest hypocaloric diet. The authors found no significant difference in body weight or body fat regain (assessed by DEXA) between the treatments; however, there was a significant increase in the number of leukocytes with CLA supplementation [45].

Individuals with type 2 diabetes mellitus (T2DM) using metformin (30 females and 26 males) were allocated to an eight-week randomized trial and stratified by sex, age and BMI into one of three groups: 1) 3 g CLA/day (3 × 1 g capsules; a 50:50 isomer blend of 9-*cis*, 11-*trans* and 10-*trans*, 12-*cis* CLA) plus 100 IU/day of vitamin E; 2) 3 g CLA/day plus vitamin E placebo; 3) or CLA placebo (soy bean oil) plus vitamin E placebo. By the end of the study there were no significant differences regarding body weight, body composition, glycemic index and inflammatory profile among the three groups; however, there was a trend toward an increase in malondialdehyde levels (a marker of oxidative stress) and decrease in apoB100 (linked to HDL-cholesterol levels) among those receiving CLA [46].

Thirty-five obese postmenopausal women with T2DM were also randomized to receive safflower oil (8 g/day) or CLA (6.4 g CLA isomers/day) in a 36-week randomized crossover trial (two 16-week diet periods separated by a 4-week washout period). DEXA analysis was used for the assessment of body composition. Supplementation with CLA reduced BMI and total adipose mass without changing lean mass; in contrast, safflower oil reduced trunk adipose mass, increased lean mass and significantly lowered fasting glucose. It is suggested that both oils have different effects on body composition in obese women with T2DM who are not also on a weight-loss diet or exercise plan [47].

Finally, a meta-analysis that included 7 clinical assays in the final analysis for the purpose of evaluating the use of CLA during a long time did not show significant results to support changes in the body composition when using CLA for a longer period [48].

Recommended dose

Most of the studies were a mixture of the two predominant isomers, 9-*cis*, 11-*trans* and 10-*trans*, 12-*cis*, in equal proportions. The daily doses of CLA varied from 3 to 6 g/day, according to several studies and these doses appear safe [49]. Although some studies indicate that doses above 3.4 g/day would not have any additional effect, they suggest that there is a very great variation compared to the results due to different doses, type of isomer, and evaluation of the body composition, which makes it difficult to compare different studies [10, 18].

Adverse effects

Despite the positive effects of CLA supplementation on some health-related parameters, there are a few reports of possible adverse effects, mainly in rats and due to the 10-*trans* and 12-*cis* isomer. In the animal models procarcinogenic effects and of increased production of prostaglandins attributed to CLA 10-*trans* and 12-*cis* have been identified [50].

Other negative effect may be due to the increase in the lipid oxidation products (isoprostanes), besides the diminished leptin and greater probability of developing insulin resistance [51]. Studies also show undesirable effects in human beings as increased levels of triglycerides and LDL-cholesterol and reduction of the HDL levels, suggesting a negative alteration in the serum lipids profile [52]. Obese individuals also presented negative alterations in the glucose metabolism with insulin resistance in some studies [53, 54].

Conclusions

Despite studies on CLA supplementation for the purpose of investigating changes in body composition and other benefits, both in animals and in humans, they are very discordant. The capacity of CLA to alter the body composition positively by reducing the fat mass was proved in experimental models, and, in some studies on human beings. In fact, few studies have evaluated the use of CLA alone or in combination with physical exercise in humans, regarding changes in body composition. Therefore, the clinical evidence appears to be insufficient and not unanimous regarding the effects on body fat

reduction and major side effects have already been described.

In this sense, the consumption of foods naturally enriched with CLA (and not from supplementation) during lifetime would be an alternative to reduce increased adiposity. Besides, it could reduce de risk of other diseases associated with obesity, since they would ensure the beneficial effects on body composition and would not add effects that are adverse to health.

Competing interests
The authors declare that they have no competing interests (financial and non-financial).

Authors' contributions
Each author has made a valuable contribution to the preparation of this manuscript: TEL was involved in conception and design of the paper, as well as drafting and editing the final document for publication. MRC and AC were equally involved in the collection of articles involving CLA, as well as drafting and editing the final document for publication. AM was involved in reviewing all parts of the final document for publication, in particular on nutritional issues. AML was involved in conception and design of the study, articles analysis, as well as writing, drafting and editing the final document for publication. All authors read and approved the final manuscript.

Author details
[1]Faculdade Sogipa de Educação Física, Porto Alegre, Brazil. [2]Instituto de Cardiologia/Fundação Universitária de Cardiologia (IC/FUC), Porto Alegre, Brazil. [3]Universidade Federal de Ciências da Saúde de Porto Alegre (UFCSPA), Porto Alegre, Brazil. [4]Instituto de Cardiologia do Rio Grande do Sul, Av. Princesa Isabel, 395 Santana, 90620-001 Porto Alegre, RS, Brazil.

References
1. Hasler CM. Functional foods: benefits, concerns and challenges-a position paper from the american council on science and health. J Nutr. 2002;132:3772–81.
2. Hite AH, Bernstein LH. Functional foods: needs, claims, and benefits. Nutrition. 2012;28:338–9.
3. Williamson C. Functional foods: what are the benefits? Br J Community Nurs. 2009;14:230–6.
4. Chen S, Osaki N, Shimotoyodome A. Green tea catechins enhance norepinephrine-induced lipolysis via a protein kinase A-dependent pathway in adipocytes. Biochem Biophys Res Commun. 2015. Epub ahead of print.
5. Roberfroid MB. Concepts and strategy of functional food science: the European perspective. Am J Clin Nutr. 2000;71:1660S–4S.
6. Oliveira RL, Ladeira MM, Barbosa MAAF, Assunção DMP, Matsushita M, Santos GT, et al. Linoleic conjugated acid and fatty acids profile in the muscle and fat layer of water buffalo steers fed different fat sources. Braz J Vet Anim Sci. 2008;60:169–78.
7. Churruca I, Fernandez-Quintela A, Portillo MP. Conjugated linoleic acid isomers: differences in metabolism and biological effects. Biofactors. 2009;35:105–11.
8. Botelho AP, Santos-Zago LF, Reis SMPM, Oliveira AC. Conjugated linoleic acid suplementation decreased the body fat in Wistar rats. Braz J Nutr. 2005;18(4):561-565.
9. Kloss R, Linscheid J, Johnson A, Lawson B, Edwards K, Linder T, et al. Effects of conjugated linoleic acid supplementation on blood lipids and adiposity of rats fed diets rich saturated versus unsaturated fat. Pharmacol Res. 2005;51(6):503–7.
10. Blankson H, Stakkestad JA, Fagertun H, Thom E, Wadstein J, Gudmundsen O. Conjugated linoleic acid reduces body fat mass in overweight and obese humans. J Nutr. 2000;130:2943–8.
11. Gaullier JM, Halse J, Hoye K, Kristiansen K, Fafertun H, Vik H, et al. Supplementation with conjugated linoleic acid for 24 months is well

tolerated by and reduces body fat mass in healthy, overweight humans. J Nutr. 2005;135:778–84.

12. Campbell B, Kreider R. Conjugated linoleic acids. Curr Sports Med Rep. 2008;7:237–41.

13. Ryder JW, Portocarrero CP, Song XM, Cui L, Yu M, Combatsiaris T, et al. Isomer-specific antidiabetic properties of conjugated linoleic acid. Improved glucose tolerance, skeletal muscle insulin action, and UCP-2 gene expression. Diabetes. 2001;50:1149–57.

14. Kishino S, Ogawa J, Omura Y, Matsumura K, Shimizu S. Conjugated linoleic acid production from linoleic acid by lactic acid bacteria. J Am Oil Chem Soc. 2002;70:159–63.

15. Martins SV, Madeira A, Lopes PA, Pires VM, Alfaia CM, Prates JA, et al. Adipocyte membrane glycerol permeability is involved in the anti-adipogenic effect of conjugated linoleic acid. Biochem Biophys Res Commun. 2015;458:356–61.

16. Poirier H, Shapiro JS, Kim RJ, Lazar MA. Nutritional supplementation with trans-10, cis-12-conjugated linoleic acid induces inflammation of white adipose tissue. Diabetes. 2006;55:1634–41.

17. Whigham LD, Watras AC, Schoeller DA. Efficacy of conjugated linoleic acid for reducing fat mass: a meta-analysis in humans. Am J Clin Nutr. 2007;85:1203–11.

18. Chen SC, Lin YH, Huang HP, Hsu WL, Houng JY, Huang CK. Effect of conjugated linoleic acid supplementation on weight loss and body fat composition in a Chinese population. Nutrition. 2012;28:559–65.

19. Kamphuis MMJW, Lejeune MPGM, Saris WHM, Westerterp-Plantenga MS. The effect of conjugated linoleic acid supplementation after weight loss on body weight regain, body composition, and resting metabolic rate in overweight subjects. Int J Obes. 2003;27:840–7.

20. Santos-Zago LF, Botelho AP, Oliveira AC. Effects of conjugated linoleic acid on animal metabolism: advances in research and perspectives for the future: [review]. Braz J Nutr. 2008;21(2):195-221.

21. McGowan MM, Eisenberg BL, Lewis LD, Froehlich HM, Wells WA, Eastman A, et al. A proof of principle clinical trial to determine whether conjugated linoleic acid modulates the lipogenic pathway in human breast cancer tissue. Breast Cancer Res Treat. 2013;138:175–83.

22. Reardon M, Gobern S, Martinez K, Shen W, Reid T, McIntosh M. Oleic acid attenuates trans-10, cis-12 conjugated linoleic acid-mediated inflammatory gene expression in human adipocytes. Lipids. 2012;47:1043–51.

23. Vaughan RA, Garcia-Smith R, Bisoffi M, Conn CA, Trujillo KA. Conjugated linoleic acid or omega 3 fatty acids increase mitochondrial biosynthesis and metabolism in skeletal muscle cells. Lipids Health Dis. 2012;11:142.

24. Abduljabbar R, Al-Kaabi MM, Negm OH, Jerjees D, Muftah AA, Mukherjee A, et al. Prognostic and biological significance of peroxisome proliferator-activated receptor-gamma in luminal breast cancer. Breast Cancer Res Treat. 2015;150:511–22.

25. Tavares V, Hirata MH, Hirata RDC. Peroxisome proliferator-activated receptor gamma (PPARgamma): molecular study in glucose homeostasis, lipid metabolism and therapeutic approach. Arch Endocrinol Metabol. 2007;51:526–33.

26. Boschini RP, Garcia Júnior JR. UCP2 and UCP3 genic expression: regulation by food restriction, fasting and physical exercise. Braz J Nutr. 2005;18:753–64.

27. Yamashita AS, Lira FS, Lima WP, Carnevali LC, Gonçalves DC, Tavares FL, et al. Influence of aerobic physical training in the motochondrial transport of long chain fatty acids in the skeletal muscle: role of the carnitine palmitoil transferase. Brazilian journal of sports medicine. 2008;14(2):150-154.

28. Peters JM, Park Y, Gonzalez FJ, Pariza MW. Influence of conjugated linoleic acid on body composition and target gene expression in peroxisome proliferator-activated receptor α-null mice. Biochim Biophys Acta. 2001;1533(3):233–42.

29. Toda C, Diano S. Mitochondrial UCP2 in the central regulation of metabolism. Best Pract Res Clin Endocrinol Metab. 2014;28(5):757–64.

30. Sugimoto S, Nakajima H, Kodo K, Mori J, Matsuo K, Kosaka K, et al. Miglitol increases energy expenditure by upregulating uncoupling protein 1 of brown adipose tissue and reduces obesity in dietary-induced obese mice. Nutr Metab (Lond). 2014;11(1):14.

31. Busiello RA, Savarese S, Lombardi A. Mitochondrial uncoupling proteins and energy metabolism. Front Physiol. 2015;6:36.

32. Kennedy A, Martinez K, Schmidt S, Mandrup S, LaPoint K, McIntosh M. Antiobesity mechanisms of action of conjugated linoleic acid. J Nutr Biochem. 2010;21(3):171–9.

33. Ribeiro MO, Bianco SD, Kaneshige M, Schultz JJ, Cheng SY, Bianco AC, et al. Expression of uncoupling protein 1 in mouse brown adipose tissue is thyroid hormone receptor-beta isoform specific and required for adaptive thermogenesis. Endocrinology. 2010;151(1):432–40.

34. Aubert J, Champigny O, Saint-Marc P, Negrel R, Collins S, Ricquier D, et al. Up-regulation of UCP-2 gene expression by PPAR agonists in preadipose and adipose cells. Biochem Biophys Res Commun. 1997;238:606–11.

35. Takahashi Y, Kushiro M, Shinohara K, Ide T. Dietary conjugated linoleic acid reduces body fat mass and affects gene expression of proteins regulating energy metabolism in mice. Comp Biochem Physiol B Biochem Mol Biol. 2002;133(3):395–404.

36. Nagao K, Wang YM, Inoue N, Han SY, Buang Y, Noda T, et al. The 10trans, 12cis isomer of conjugated linoleic acid promotes energy metabolism in OLETF rats. Nutrition. 2003;19(7–8):652–56.

37. Gaze BS, Nanci DP, Oliveira VAJ, Clemente M. Effect of the supplementation of conjugated linoleic acid (CLA) and the loss of weight in animals and human beings. Revista Brasileira de Obesidade, Nutrição e Emagrecimento. 2007;1:48-55.

38. Barone R, Macaluso F, Catanese P, Marino Gammazza A, Rizzuto L, Marozzi P, et al. Endurance exercise and conjugated linoleic acid (CLA) supplementation up-regulate CYP17A1 and stimulate testosterone biosynthesis. PLoS One. 2013;8:e79686.

39. Agueda M, Zulet MA, Martínez JA. Effect of conjugated linoleic acid (CLA) on human lipid profile. Arch Latinoam Nutr. 2009;59(3):245–52.

40. Viladomiu M, Hontecillas R, Bassaganya-Riera J. Modulation of inflammation and immunity by dietary conjugated linoleic acid. Eur J Pharmacol. 2015;2999(15):459–8.

41. Eftekhari MH, Aliasghari F, Babaei-Beigi MA, Hasanzadeh J. Effect of conjugated linoleic acid and omega-3 fatty acid supplementation on inflammatory and oxidative stress markers in atherosclerotic patients. ARYA Atheroscler. 2013;9(6):311–8.

42. Evans JL, Maddux BA, Goldfine ID. The molecular basis for oxidative stress-induced insulin resistance. Antioxid Redox Signal. 2005;7(7–8):1040–52.

43. Kim J, Paik HD, Shin MJ, Park E. Eight weeks of conjugated linoleic acid supplementation has no effect on antioxidant status in healthy overweight/obese Korean individuals. Eur J Nutr. 2012;51:135–41.

44. Falcone PH, Tai CY, Carson LR, Joy JM, Mosman MM, Vogel RM, et al. Subcutaneous and segmental fat loss with and without supportive supplements in conjunction with a low-calorie high protein diet in healthy women. PLoS One. 2015;10:e0123854.

45. Larsen TM, Toubro S, Gudmundsen O, Astrup A. Conjugated linoleic acid supplementation for 1 y does not prevent weight or body fat regain. Am J Clin Nutr. 2006;83(3):606–12.

46. Shadman Z, Taleban FA, Saadat N, Hedayati M. Effect of conjugated linoleic acid and vitamin E on glycemic control, body composition, and inflammatory markers in overweight type2 diabetics. J Diabetes Metab Disord. 2013;12:42.

47. Norris LE, Collene AL, Asp ML, Hsu JC, Liu LF, Richardson JR, et al. Comparison of dietary conjugated linoleic acid with safflower oil on body composition in obese postmenopausal women with type 2 diabetes mellitus. Am J Clin Nutr. 2009;90:468–76.

48. Onakpoya IJ, Posadzki PP, Watson LK, Davies LA, Ernst E. The efficacy of long-term conjugated linoleic acid (CLA) supplementation on body composition in overweight and obese individuals: a systematic review and meta-analysis of randomized clinical trials. Eur J Nutr. 2012;51:127–34.

49. Iwata T, Kamegai T, Yamauchi-Sato Y, Ogawa A, Kasai M, Aoyama T, et al. Safety of dietary conjugated linoleic acid (CLA) in a 12-weeks trial in healthy overweight Japanese male volunteers. J Oleo Sci. 2007;56:517–25.

50. Wendel AA, Purushotham A, Liu LF, Belury MA. Conjugated linoleic acid fails to worsen insulin resistance but induces hepatic steatosis in the presence of leptin in ob/ob mice. J Lipid Res. 2008;49:98–106.

51. Cooper MH, Miller JR, Mitchell PL, Currie DL, McLeod RS. Conjugated linoleic acid isomers have no effect on atherosclerosis and adverse effects on lipoprotein and liver lipid metabolism in apoE−/− mice fed a high-cholesterol diet. Atherosclerosis. 2008;200:294–302.

52. Funck LG, Barrera-Arellano D, Block JM. Conjugated linoleic acid (CLA) and its relationship with cardiovascular disease and associated risk factors. Arch Latinoam Nutr. 2006;56:123–34.

53. Kennedy A, Martinez K, Chung S, LaPoint K, Hopkins R, Schmidt SF, et al. Inflammation and insulin resistance induced by trans-10, cis-12 conjugated linoleic acid depend on intracellular calcium levels in primary cultures of human adipocytes. J Lipid Res. 2010;51:1906–17.

54. Kennedy A, Overman A, Lapoint K, Hopkins R, West T, Chuang CC, et al. Conjugated linoleic acid-mediated inflammation and insulin resistance in human adipocytes are attenuated by resveratrol. J Lipid Res. 2009;50(2):225–32.

55. Bachmair EM, Wood SG, Keizer HG, Horgan GW, Ford I, de Roos B. Supplementation with a 9c,11 t-rich conjugated linoleic acid blend shows no clear inhibitory effects on platelet function in healthy subjects at low and moderate cardiovascular risk: a randomized controlled trial. Mol Nutr Food Res. 2015;59:741–50.

56. Jenkins ND, Buckner SL, Baker RB, Bergstrom HC, Cochrane KC, Weir JP, et al. Effects of 6 weeks of aerobic exercise combined with conjugated linoleic acid on the physical working capacity at fatigue threshold. J Strength Cond Res. 2014;28:2127–35.

57. Jenkins ND, Buckner SL, Cochrane KC, Bergstrom HC, Goldsmith JA, Weir JP, et al. CLA supplementation and aerobic exercise lower blood triacylglycerol, but have no effect on peak oxygen uptake or cardiorespiratory fatigue thresholds. Lipids. 2014;49:871–80.

58. Aryaeian N, Djalali M, Shahram F, Djazayery A, Eshragian MR. Effect of conjugated linoleic Acid, vitamin E, alone or combined on immunity and inflammatory parameters in adults with active rheumatoid arthritis: a randomized controlled trial. Int J Prev Med. 2014;5:1567–77.

59. Eftekhari MH, Aliasghari F, Beigi MA, Hasanzadeh J. The effect of conjugated linoleic acids and omega-3 fatty acids supplementation on lipid profile in atherosclerosis. Adv Biomed Res. 2014;9:3–15.

60. Mohammadzadeh M, Faramarzi E, Mahdavi R, Nasirimotlagh B, Asghari JM. Effect of conjugated linoleic acid supplementation on inflammatory factors and matrix metalloproteinase enzymes in rectal cancer patients undergoing chemoradiotherapy. Integr Cancer Ther. 2013;12:496–502.

61. Penedo LA, Nunes JC, Gama MA, Leite PE, Quirico-Santos TF, Torres AG. Intake of butter naturally enriched with cis9, trans11 conjugated linoleic acid reduces systemic inflammatory mediators in healthy young adults. J Nutr Biochem. 2013;24:2144–51.

62. Carvalho RF, Uehara SK, Rosa G. Microencapsulated conjugated linoleic acid associated with hypocaloric diet reduces body fat in sedentary women with metabolic syndrome. Vasc Health Risk Manag. 2012;8:661–7.

63. Bulut S, Bodur E, Colak R, Turnagol H. Effects of conjugated linoleic acid supplementation and exercise on post-heparin lipoprotein lipase, butyrylcholinesterase, blood lipid profile and glucose metabolism in young men. Chem Biol Interact. 2013;203:323–9.

64. López-Plaza B, Bermejo LM, Koester Weber T, Parra P, Serra F, Hernández M, et al. Effects of milk supplementation with conjugated linoleic acid on weight control and body composition in healthy overweight people. Nutr Hosp. 2013;28:2090–8.

65. Engberink MF, Geleijnse JM, Wanders AJ, Brouwer IA. The effect of conjugated linoleic acid, a natural trans fat from milk and meat, on human blood pressure: results from a randomized crossover feeding study. J Hum Hypertens. 2012;26:127–32.

66. Joseph SV, Jacques H, Plourde M, Mitchell PL, McLeod RS, Jones PJ. Conjugated linoleic acid supplementation for 8 weeks does not affect body composition, lipid profile, or safety biomarkers in overweight, hyperlipidemic men. J Nutr. 2011;141:1286–91.

67. Michishita T, Kobayashi S, Katsuya T, Ogihara T, Kawabuchi K. Evaluation of the antiobesity effects of an amino acid mixture and conjugated linoleic acid on exercising healthy overweight humans: a randomized, double-blind, placebo-controlled trial. J Int Med Res. 2010;38:844–59.

68. Wanders AJ, Brouwer IA, Siebelink E, Katan MB. Effect of a high intake of conjugated linoleic acid on lipoprotein levels in healthy human subjects. PLoS One. 2010;5:e9000.

69. Sluijs I, Plantinga Y, de Roos B, Mennen LI, Bots ML. Dietary supplementation with cis-9, trans-11 conjugated linoleic acid and aortic stiffness in overweight and obese adults. Am J Clin Nutr. 2010;91:175–83.

70. Syvertsen C, Halse J, Høivik HO, Gaullier JM, Nurminiemi M, Kristiansen K, et al. The effect of 6 months supplementation with conjugated linoleic acid on insulin resistance in overweight and obese. Int J Obes (Lond). 2007;31:1148–54.

## 8

Ergogenic effects of caffeine and sodium bicarbonate supplementation on intermittent exercise performance preceded by intense arm cranking exercise

Matthaus Marriott[1], Peter Krustrup[1,2] and Magni Mohr[3,4*]

Abstract

Background: Caffeine and sodium bicarbonate ingestion have been suggested to improve high-intensity intermittent exercise, but it is unclear if these ergogenic substances affect performance under provoked metabolic acidification. To study the effects of caffeine and sodium bicarbonate on intense intermittent exercise performance and metabolic markers under exercise-induced acidification, intense arm-cranking exercise was performed prior to intense intermittent running after intake of placebo, caffeine and sodium bicarbonate.

Methods: Male team-sports athletes (n = 12) ingested sodium bicarbonate ($NaHCO_3$; 0.4 $g.kg^{-1}$ b.w.), caffeine (CAF; 6 $mg.kg^{-1}$ b.w.) or placebo (PLA) on three different occasions. Thereafter, participants engaged in intense arm exercise prior to the Yo-Yo intermittent recovery test level-2 (Yo-Yo IR2). Heart rate, blood lactate and glucose as well as rating of perceived exertion (RPE) were determined during the protocol.

Results: CAF and $NaHCO_3$ elicited a 14 and 23% improvement ($P < 0.05$), respectively, in Yo-Yo IR2 performance, post arm exercise compared to PLA. The $NaHCO_3$ trial displayed higher [blood lactate] ($P < 0.05$) compared to CAF and PLA (10.5 ± 1.9 vs. 8.8 ± 1.7 and 7.7 ± 2.0 $mmol.L^{-1}$, respectively) after the Yo-Yo IR2. At exhaustion CAF demonstrated higher ($P < 0.05$) [blood glucose] compared to PLA and $NaHCO_3$ (5.5 ± 0.7 vs. 4.2 ± 0.9 vs. 4.1 ± 0.9 $mmol.L^{-1}$, respectively). RPE was lower ($P < 0.05$) during the Yo-Yo IR2 test in the $NaHCO_3$ trial in comparison to CAF and PLA, while no difference in heart rate was observed between trials.

Conclusions: Caffeine and sodium bicarbonate administration improved Yo-Yo IR2 performance and lowered perceived exertion after intense arm cranking exercise, with greater overall effects of sodium bicarbonate intake.

Keywords: Yo-Yo IR2 test performance, Fatigue, Blood lactate, Rating of perceived exertion, Team sport athletes

Introduction

Fatigue during high-intensity intermittent exercise is complex and multifaceted. Early speculation regarding the aetiology of fatigue commends that high rate of lactic acid production and a concomitant fall in blood and muscle pH [1], which may have multiple indirect and direct impairing effects on centrally and peripherally mediated fatigue-resistance. Caffeine and sodium bicarbonate

($NaHCO_3$) are two supplements frequently consumed to elicit ergogenic effects on high-intensity exercise performance [2].

Effects of caffeine on intense intermittent exercise performance have for example been studied by Stuart et al. [3] demonstrating improved repeated sprint performance during a simulated rugby game trial. Moreover, team-sport athletes improved both total work and mean power output during an intermittent cycle sprint protocol [4] and Yo-Yo IR2 performance by 16% after caffeine intake [5]. However, Glaister et al. [6] showed that although the fastest sprint time in a repeated sprint test was observed with caffeine intake, the magnitude of

* Correspondence: magnim@setur.fo
[3]Faculty of Natural and Health Sciences, University of the Faroe Islands, Jónas Broncks gøta 25. 3rd floor, Tórshavn, Faroe Islands
[4]Center of Health and Human Performance, Department of Food and Nutrition, and Sport Science, University of Gothenburg, Gothenburg, Sweden
Full list of author information is available at the end of the article

fatigue in the caffeine condition appeared to be greater compared to a placebo trial. Furthermore, no ergogenic effect has been found on sprint performance during the Loughborough intermittent shuttle test [7]. Thus, the effects of caffeine intake on intense intermittent exercise protocols are equivocal.

$NaHCO_3$ ingested 90–150 min prior exercise has been used as an ergogenic aid for athletic events highly dependent on anaerobic glycolysis, since the ergogenic potential that $NaHCO_3$ might elicit is suggested to depend upon the demands of the activity being sufficient to induce performance inhibiting levels of metabolic acidosis [8]. $NaHCO_3$ ingestion has been reported to improve competitive and laboratory-based protocols lasting 1–7 min including swimming, middle distance running, rowing and repeated sprinting [9]. In addition, improvement in performance during a repeated sprint protocol is reported [10]. However, other studies are less affirmative and demonstrating no performance enhancing effects on high-intensity intermittent cycling [11]. Further discrepancies have been illustrated by Cameron et al. [12] whereby no benefits were observed during a high-intensity rugby-specific training session followed by a repeated-sprint test. The absence of effects within the aforementioned studies is potentially due to insufficient metabolic taxation.

The Yo-Yo Intermittent Recovery test level 2 (Yo-Yo IR2) consists of 20-m shuttle runs at progressive running speed and has a high anaerobic energy turnover [13]. Thus, in order to examine the effect of caffeine and $NaHCO_3$ intake on high-intensity intermittent exercise the Yo-Yo IR2 test can be utilized. Moreover, engaging in intense arm exercise prior to repeated high-intensity running elevates the levels of leg muscle and blood [lactate] and [H^+] [14], as well as increasing the accumulation rate in muscle interstitial [K^+] resulting in decreased knee extensor exercise performance [15]. Therefore, intense upper-body exercise prior to running exercise can be applied to induce pre-exercise muscle acidosis and high metabolic disturbance without exercising the legs.

Thus, the aim of the present study was therefore to compare the effects of caffeine and $NaHCO_3$ supplementation 70–90 min prior to exercise, respectively, on Yo-Yo IR2 performance and physiological response to intense intermittent exercise with prior metabolic acidosis induced by intense arm cranking exercise.

Methods
Participants
Twelve healthy male participants involved in sub-elite team-sports (age: 20.8 ± 1.4 (±SD) yrs.; height: 183 ± 7 cm; body mass: 78.9 ± 5.4 kg) volunteered to participate in this study. Participants gave their written informed consent to participate prior to the experimental procedures and the study conforms the ethical guidelines of the Declaration of Helsinki. The study was approved by the University of Exeter Ethics Committee.

Design
The participants reported to the laboratory on five separate occasions with at least four days between visits. On the initial visit to the laboratory the participants were familiarised to the arm exercise protocol conducted on an upper body arm cranking ergometer (Lode BV, Angio, Netherlands) to determine individual specific power outputs as previously described [15]. On the second occasion participants performed a baseline, control (CON) Yo-Yo IR2 that they were familiarized to prior to the study [13]. The CON-trial was performed without any supplementation or prior arm-exercise. Participants were then assigned in a single-blind, randomized, crossover design to receive placebo (PLA; plain flour), caffeine (CAF) or sodium bicarbonate ($NaHCO_3$) supplementation.

Experimental procedure
On each experimental visit, participants were asked to report to the laboratory 100 min prior to the initiation of the Yo-Yo IR2 in a fully hydrated state and ≥2 h postprandial. The tests were carried out at the same time of the day (±1 h). The participants were not permitted to consumed alcohol 24 h prior to testing or to take any other form of dietary supplements for the duration of the study and to avoid strenuous exercise 24 h preceding each experimental trial. In addition the participants were asked to avoid food items containing caffeine prior to the experimental days. Moreover, the food intake was noted the day prior to the first test trial and replicated prior to the remaining trials. Upon arrival to the laboratory participants were fitted with a heart rate (HR) monitor (Polar Electro, Kempele, Finland) and a baseline fingertip capillary blood sample was obtained. Participants were then given either CAF or PLA (blinded) or $NaHCO_3$ to orally ingest under the supervision of the researchers. 70 min before the start of the Yo-Yo IR2 either CAF or PLA was taken orally in gelatine capsule (6 mg.kg^{-1} body mass; 474 ± 31 mg; see Mohr et al. [5]). $NaHCO_3$ was ingested orally in 21–25 gelatine capsules (0.4 g.kg^{-1} body mass; 31.6 ± 1.6 g) and supplementation began 90 min prior to the start of the Yo-Yo IR2 with 7 ml.kg^{-1} of water drank ad libitum over a 30 min period as described by Carr et al. [9]. The respective $NaHCO_3$ intake protocol has in a pilot study been demonstrated to markedly raise the blood HCO_3^- concentration (data not shown).

The arm exercise protocol lasted for 17 min, during which the participants maintained a constant cadence (80 ± 5 RPM) at individualised power outputs (157.6 ±

7.4 W). The protocol, adapted from others [14,15] consisting of 4×1-min and 1×1.5-min exercise periods separated by 0.5-min recovery, followed by 4.5 min of recovery and a final 1-min exercise period. Immediately after completion of the arm exercise, a blood sample was taken. The Yo-Yo IR2 began 4 min after the completion of the arm exercise protocol corresponding to 70 min post CAF and PLA intake and 90 min after the NaHCO₃ ingestion. The Yo-Yo IR2 test was completed on a wooden surface and consists of repeated two 20-m runs at a progressively increased speed controlled by audio bleeps from a CD player [13]. The test-leader controlling the Yo-Yo IR2 test was blinded in relation to drug-treatment.

Fingertip capillary 300 μL blood samples were collected in heparin-fluoride coated Microvette CB 300 tubes (Sarstedt Ltd, UK) which were immediately stored on ice and subsequently analysed to determine blood [lactate] and [glucose] after the protocol [5] using a YSI 2500 Lactate Analyser (YSI, Yellow Springs, US) having a test-retest coefficient of variance of <2%. Blood samples were obtained: prior to supplementation on arrival to the laboratory, immediately after arm exercise, immediately after Yo-Yo IR2 exhaustion, 1, 3 and 5 min post exhaustion. Heart rate was determined during the entire protocol while rating of perceived exertion (RPE) values using the Borg scale [16] were recorded during the Yo-Yo IR2 at 160, 280, 440, 600 m and at exhaustion.

Statistical analyses

Differences between baseline Yo-Yo IR2 performance and PLA Yo-Yo IR2 after arm exercise were analysed using a paired-samples t-test. A one-way repeated measures ANOVA was used to determine the influence of supplementation on the performance in the Yo-Yo IR2 after intense arm exercise. Where analyses revealed a significant main effect, the origin of this effect was determined by Bonferroni adjusted post hoc paired t-tests. Differences in plasma [glucose], [lactate], HR and RPE between the three conditions (PLA, CAF and NaHCO₃) were analysed using multiple separate two-way repeated measures ANOVAs (supplement x time). Significant main effects were further analysed by Bonferroni adjusted post hoc paired t-tests. All repeated measures data was checked for the assumption of sphericity using Mauchly's test. All data were analysed using the statistical software package SPSS (version 20). Statistical significance was accepted at $P < 0.05$. Results are presented as means ± SD.

Results

Performance

Yo-Yo IR2 performance was reduced ($P < 0.05$) by 41% when the test was preceded by an intense intermittent arm cranking (CON: 696 ± 185 m vs. PLA: 413 ± 121 m; $P < 0.01$, Figure 1A). However, after CAF and NaHCO₃ supplementation Yo-Yo IR2 performance was 14 and 23% higher ($P < 0.05$) compared to PLA (480 ± 113 and 540 ± 138 m, respectively), with a greater ($P < 0.05$) improvement in NaHCO₃ than CAF (Figure 1B).

Blood metabolites

Baseline blood [Lactate] was similar (0.9 ± 0.3, 1.0 ± 0.5 and 0.9 ± 0.6 mmol.L⁻¹; $P > 0.05$) for PLA, CAF and NaHCO₃, respectively, but increased ($P < 0.01$) post arm crank (7.3 ± 1.8, 7.4 ± 1.5 and 8.3 ± 1.8 mmol.L⁻¹, respectively, Figure 2A) with no significant differences between the three trials, although there was a trend ($P = 0.09$) for higher blood [lactate] for the NaHCO₃ trial. Blood [lactate] did not change ($P > 0.05$) during Yo-Yo IR2 for PLA at exhaustion (7.7 ± 2.0 mmol.L⁻¹), but rose ($P < 0.05$) for both CAF and NaHCO₃ (8.8 ± 1.7 vs. 10.5 ± 1.9 mmol.L⁻¹, respectively, Figure 2A). Between group comparisons revealed that blood [lactate] values were similar between PLA and CAF, but higher ($P < 0.01$) for the NaHCO₃ trial compared to PLA and CAF trials at exhaustion (Figure 2A). At 1 min post exhaustion PLA blood [lactate] rose (9.4 ± 1.8 mmol.L⁻¹; $P < 0.05$) compared to exhaustion whereas CAF and NaHCO3 remained unchanged ($P > 0.05$) and blood [lactate] in the NaCHO₃ trial still remained higher (11.6 ± 1.7 mmol.L⁻¹; $P < 0.01$) when compared to PLA and CAF. At 3 min post Yo-Yo IR2 [lactate] was not different between groups (8.1 ± 1.9, 8.5 ± 2.2 and 8.8 ± 1.7 mmol.L⁻¹; $P > 0.05$) PLA, CAF and NaHCO₃, respectively. At 5 min into recovery Yo-Yo IR2 blood [lactate] was reduced in the PLA trial when compared to CAF and NaHCO₃ (7.2 ± 2.2 vs. 8.5 ± 2.3 and 9.1 ± 1.9 mmol.L⁻¹; $P < 0.05$, respectively) whereas CAF and NaCHO₃ were similar at this time point ($P > 0.05$).

Baseline blood [glucose] was not significantly different between trials (4.5 ± 0.5 vs. 4.2 ± 0.4 vs. 4.4 ± 0.9 mmol.L⁻¹; $P > 0.05$, Figure 2B) for PLA, CAF and NaHCO₃, respectively. For all trials at Yo-Yo IR2 exhaustion there was no difference ($P > 0.05$) in blood [glucose] within and between the supplements (3.9 ± 0.9 vs. 4.5 ± 1.1 vs. 4.2 ± 0.8 mmol.L⁻¹, respectively, Figure 2B). In the PLA and NaHCO₃ trials blood [glucose] rose ($P < 0.05$) between exhaustion and 1 min post Yo-Yo IR2 (4.9 ± 0.9 and 4.9 ± 0.7 mmol.L⁻¹). In the CAF trial blood [glucose] rose by 30% at the end of the protocol (Figure 2B), compared to the PLA ($P < 0.05$). However, no differences ($P > 0.05$) were in [glucose] between PLA and NaHCO₃ at any protocol time points (Figure 2B). Between group comparisons revealed that at 5 min post Yo-Yo IR2 blood [glucose] in the CAF trial was greater ($P < 0.05$) compared to the PLA and NaHCO₃ (5.5 ± 0.7 vs. 4.2 ± 0.9 and 4.1 ± 0.9 mmol.L⁻¹, respectively).

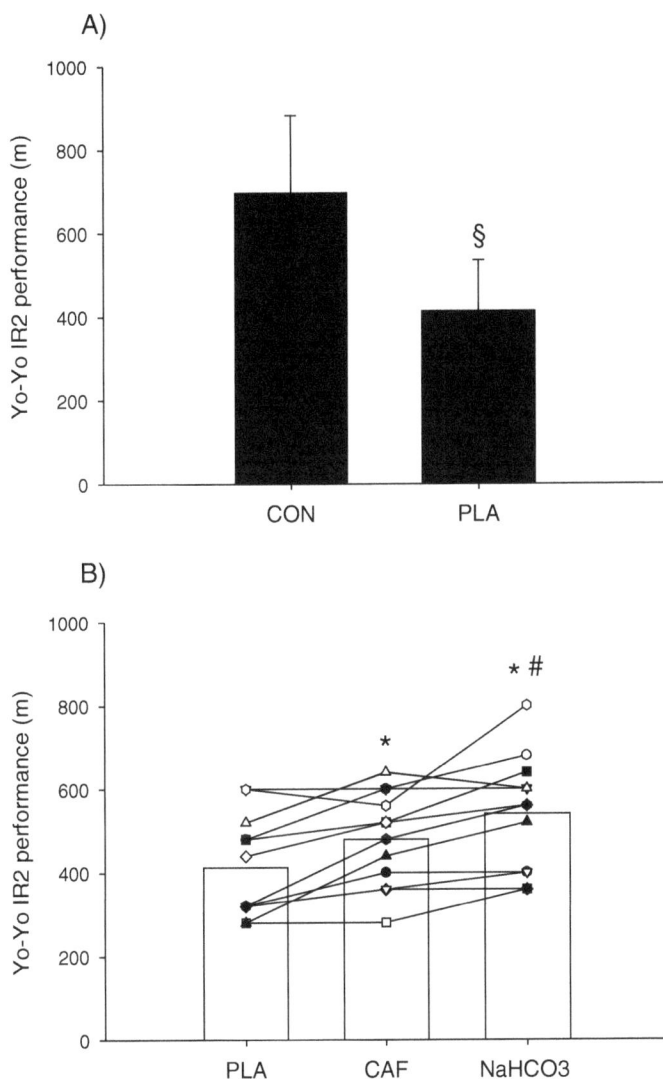

Figure 1 Yo-Yo Intermittent Recovery level 2 test (Yo-Yo IR2) performance in control (CON) and placebo (PLA) trials (A) and individual Yo-Yo IR2 performance during PLA and after caffeine (CAF) and sodium bicarbonate (NaHCO₃) supplementation (B) (n = 12). §: Denotes a significant difference from CON. *Denotes a significant difference from PLA. # Denotes a significant difference from CAF. Significance level P < 0.05.

Rating of perceived exertion and heart rate loading

Between group comparisons revealed that RPE was reduced ($P < 0.05$) in the NaHCO₃ trials at both 160 m and 280 m (160 m: 15.3 ± 2.3 and 15.0 ± 1.6 vs. 13.1 ± 2.0), (280 m: 17.8 ± 1.2 and 17.3 ± 1.8 vs. 15.8 ± 1.5) for PLA, CAF and NaHCO₃, respectively (Figure 3). No differences ($P > 0.05$) were observed at Yo-Yo IR2 exhaustion (19.3 ± 1.0, 19.3 ± 0.9 and 19.3 ± 0.7 in PLA, CAF and NaHCO₃, respectively, Figure 3). Arm exercise caused a rise ($P < 0.01$) in heart rate during all trials (179 ± 7, 178 ± 8 and 177 ± 9 bts.min^{-1}) for PLA, CAF and NaHCO₃, respectively. At Yo-Yo IR2 exhaustion a

further rise ($P < 0.05$) in heart rate for CAF and NaHCO₃ was observed (187 ± 7 and 186 ± 7 bts.min^{-1}, respectively). Comparisons between trials revealed that there was no difference between PLA, CAF and NaHCO₃ at any time points during the testing protocol.

Discussion

The principle findings of the present study were that Yo-Yo IR2 performance after intense arm cranking exercise was markedly reduced compared to a control trial, while both caffeine and NaHCO₃ intake improved fatigue resistance during the Yo-Yo IR2 test. NaHCO₃

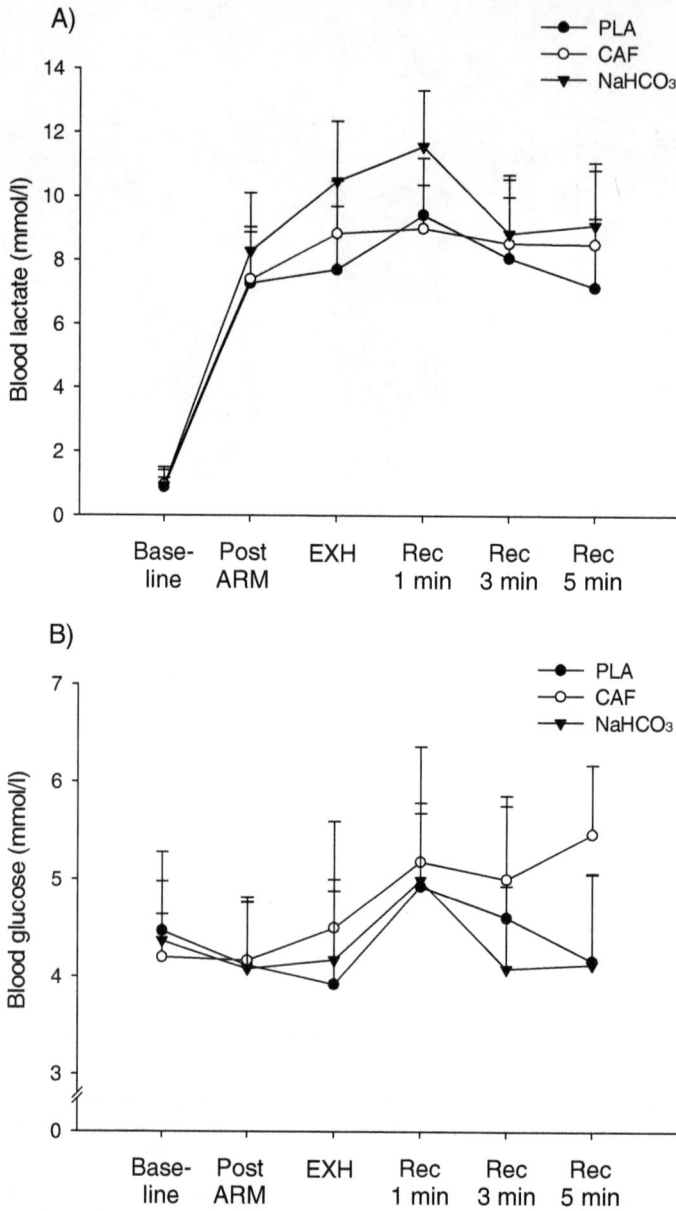

Figure 2 Capillary blood lactate (A) and glucose (B) concentrations before, during and after the Yo-Yo IR2 test protocol (n = 12) in the placebo (PLA), caffeine (CAF) and sodium bicarbonate (NaHCO₃) trials.

intake elicited a further ergogenic effect on Yo-Yo IR2 performance when performed after intense arm cranking exercise compared to that of caffeine. The present study is the first to report performance effects of caffeine and NaHCO₃ intake using high-intensity intermittent running exercise preceded by intense arm cranking exercise and to demonstrate additional performance and perceptual benefits of NaHCO₃ beyond that of caffeine.

The reduction in high-intensity running performance when performed after intense arm cranking exercise is consistent with previous research studying isolated muscle performance [14,15]. In the present study, Yo-Yo IR2 performance was reduced by 41% when preceded by arm exercise, which is of a similar magnitude as the performance decrements of 35% and ~48%, respectively, observed during intense exhaustive one-legged knee extensor exercise performed after intense arm cranking

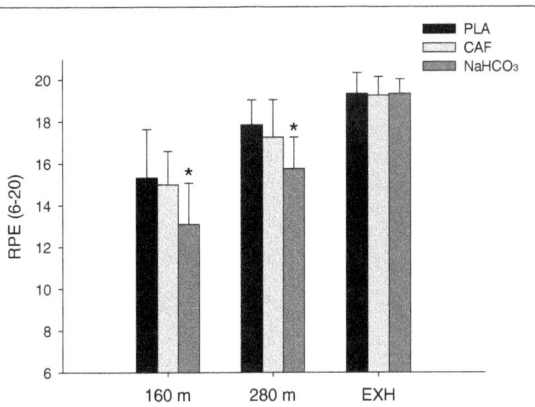

Figure 3 Rating of Perceived Exertion (RPE) at 160 and 280 m during the Yo-Yo IR2 test, as well as at exhaustion in PLA, CAF and NaHCO₃. *Denotes a significant difference from PLA. Significance level P < 0.05.

[14,15]. These two studies also showed that the arm exercise resulted in metabolic acidosis with arterial blood lactate being elevated by ~11-fold resting levels, as well as higher leg muscle lactate and H^+ concentrations [14] and elevated accumulation rate of leg muscle interstitial $[K^+]$ [15]. In the present study capillary blood lactate was elevated ~8-fold after the arm cranking protocol, confirming that the metabolic environment was markedly altered prior to the Yo-Yo IR2 test compared to baseline conditions.

Yo-Yo IR2 performance was improved by 23% after NaHCO₃ supplementation, which is supported by others [9,10]. Indeed performance enhancement in the final sprints of a repeated sprint test after NaHCO₃ intake has been reported [10], indicating an ergogenic effect of NaHCO₃ on fatigue resistance during high intensity exercise conditions performed under metabolic stress. However, some studies applying intense exercise protocols report no beneficial effect of NaHCO₃ supplementation (for review see Carr et al. [9]). In the present study intense arm cranking markedly elevated blood lactate, confirming findings of an increased leg muscle lactate and H^+ concentration following the same arm protocol [14]. Part of the longer exercise time level in the NaHCO₃-trial may be explained by an elevated NaHCO₃ induced buffer capacity in the blood, which will increase the muscle-to-blood H^+ and lactate gradient. Since the monocarboxylate transporters (MCT) are gradient dependent [17], this will increase the removal of H^+ and lactate ions from the leg muscles before and during the Yo-Yo IR2 test. This may reduce the degree of intramuscular acidification and corresponding fatigue development [1]. The higher blood lactate levels were observed in the NaHCO₃-trial, may also partly be a direct consequence of the greater fatigue resistance,

and thereby higher glycolytic contribution and concomitant muscle lactate production compared to the caffeine and placebo trials. A limitation with the present study is that blood was not drawn during the Yo-Yo IR2 test, which have been done on other comparable studies [5,13], so we are unable to compare the three intervention trial at fixed time points due to the different exercise times.

The intake of NaHCO₃ may also affect the activity of sarcolemmal ion transporters. For example elevated extracellular Na^+ concentration may stimulate the Na^+/H^+ exchangers [18] and thereby increase the efflux of hydrogen ions from the exercising muscles and attenuate intramuscular acidification. In a study by Street et al. [19] muscle interstitial pH decreased gradually during graded exercise comparable to the Yo-Yo IR2 test. However, in a follow-up study sodium citrate was ingested prior to intense exercise, which on one hand elevated plasma HCO_3^- and lowered the accumulation of muscle interstitial H^+ [18]. Finally, the accumulation rate of interstitial K^+ was significantly reduced, which was suggested to relate to less opening probability of the K_{ATP} channels, which tend to open during intracellular acidification [20]. In addition, the elevated systemic Na^+ may directly stimulate the activity in the Na^+-K^+ ATPase [1,18]. Thus, the intake of NaHCO₃ may have elevated fatigue resistance by inducing maintenance of a more optimum intracellular pH [21] and/ or by enhancing Na^+/K^+ pump activity and potentially $Na^+/K^+/2Cl^-$ co-transporter activity, contributing to lower muscle interstitial $[K^+]$ preserving sarcolemma excitability, allowing enhanced high intensity repeated muscular performance [1].

RPE was lower in NaHCO₃-trial during the Yo-Yo IR2 test, which may suggest that centrally mediated mechanisms were affected. The participants experienced less exertion during the Yo-Yo IR2 in the NaHCO₃-trial, and that although distance covered before exhaustion was increased the RPE values remained the same as the caffeine and placebo trials at the point of fatigue. Thus, a greater distance could be covered yet reporting an equal level of perceived fatigue at exhaustion. Peripheral changes may cause modulation of neural strategies via group III and IV muscle afferents which are widely distributed through the muscle and are responsive to chemical stimuli such as altered H^+ and K^+ [22]. Different mechanisms have been proposed by which such peripheral inputs might lead to modulation of motor neuron firing rates and muscle function including facilitation or inhibition of spinal reflexes, pre-synaptic inhibition of the group Ia afferents thus reducing inhibitory input into the motoneurons, and altered supraspinal drive [22]. Thus, part of the improved performance after NaHCO₃ treatment may relate to less negative feedback from the muscle and thereby less effect on the descending drive to the motoneurons [22,23].

In the present study caffeine increased Yo-Yo IR2 performance by 14% compared to the placebo-trial, which is in line with other findings [3,4]. Caffeine has multiple physiological effects that may promote fatigue resistance during intense exercise, such as elevating the catecholamine levels [24] and reducing muscle interstitial K^+ accumulation [5]. Peak blood glucose concentrations were higher in the caffeine-trial than placebo, which is in accordance with findings by others [5], indicating an elevated catecholamine response, which may facilitate the Na^+-K^+ ATPase activity [25]. The arm protocol has been shown to increase the accumulation of interstitial potassium during leg exercise [15], and caffeine may reduce this effect by increasing the pump activity in the Na^+-K^+ APTase directly or via an elevated catecholamine response [5,25]. Finally caffeine may have an effect on central mechanisms associated with fatigue [23,26], however, the RPE rating were not different between the caffeine and placebo trials in the present study. Caffeine is well-known to affect the central nervous system response mediated via antagonism of adenosine receptors, which dampens pain perception and attenuates fatigue [27]. However, during high-intensity intermittent exercise caffeine-induced effects on RPE appear to be negated [6], which is supported by this study.

Intriguingly, there were no differences in HR between the trials, suggesting that the aerobic demands were similar, yet participant's perception of fatigue was attenuated during the NaHCO$_3$-trial, indicating that NaHCO$_3$ in contrast to caffeine might impact upon central fatigue as well as peripheral fatigue.

The possibility of a 'high-responders' and 'low-responders' phenomena for both caffeine and NaHCO$_3$ has been previously reported [27-29]. This effect was apparent in the present study, whereby three subjects and one subject, respectively, after caffeine and NaHCO$_3$ intake, showed no improvement compared to PLA. Moreover five of the subjects reported experiencing some form of gastrointestinal discomfort after sodium bicarbonate intake; however this was apparently not detrimental to exercise performance.

Conclusions
The present study demonstrates that high-intensity intermittent exercise performance is impaired when preceded by intense arm exercise. However, fatigue resistance can be markedly improved by caffeine and NaHCO$_3$ administration 70–90 min prior to exercise. Moreover, for the first time NaHCO$_3$ has been shown to elicit an improvement above that of caffeine in a sport-specific high-intensity intermittent test with concomitant reductions in RPE and higher blood lactate levels.

This study suggests that caffeine and NaHCO$_3$ might be effective ergogenic aids for intermittent high-intensity exercise performance in sub-elite team sport athletes.

Competing interests
The authors declare that they have no competing interests.

Authors' contributions
MM and MM participated in the design of the study, and carried out the data collection in cooperation with PK. MM, PK and MM performed the data treatment including statistical analyses. MM and MM drafted the manuscript with help from PK. All authors read and approved the manuscript.

Acknowledgement
The authors would like to thank the athletes for committed participation. Moreover, we thank Dr. Nikolai Nordsborg, Dr. Sarah R. Jackman and Giorgios Ermidis for excellent technical assistance. The authors have no conflict of interest in relation to the study.

Author details
[1]Sport and Health Sciences, College of Life and Environmental Sciences, St. Luke's Campus, University of Exeter, Exeter, UK. [2]Department of Nutrition, Exercise and Sports, Section of Human Physiology, Copenhagen Centre for Team Sport and Health, University of Copenhagen, Copenhagen, Denmark. [3]Faculty of Natural and Health Sciences, University of the Faroe Islands, Jónas Broncks gøta 25. 3rd floor, Tórshavn, Faroe Islands. [4]Center of Health and Human Performance, Department of Food and Nutrition, and Sport Science, University of Gothenburg, Gothenburg, Sweden.

References
1. Fitts R. Cellular mechanism of muscle fatigue. Physiol Rev. 1994;74:49–94.
2. Kilding AE, Overton C, Gleave J. Effects of caffeine, sodium bicarbonate, and their combined ingestion on high-intensity cycling performance. Int J Sport Nutr Exerc Metab. 2012;22:175–83.
3. Stuart GR, Hopkins WG, Cook C, Cairns SP. Multiple effects of caffeine on simulated high-intensity team-sport performance. Med Sci Sports Exerc. 2005;37:1998–2005.
4. Schneiker KT, Bishop D, Dawson B, Hackett LP. Effects of caffeine on prolonged intermittent-sprint ability in team-sport athletes. Med Sci Sports Exerc. 2006;38:578–85.
5. Mohr M, Nielsen JJ, Bangsbo J. Caffeine intake improves intense intermittent exercise performance and reduces muscle interstitial potassium accumulation. J Appl Physiol. 2011;111:1372–9.
6. Glaister M, Howatson G, Abraham CS, Lockey RA, Goodwin JE, Foley P, et al. Caffeine supplementation and multiple sprint running performance. Med Sci Sports Exerc. 2008;40:1835–40.
7. Foskett A, Ali A, Gant N. Caffeine enhances cognitive function and skill performance during simulated soccer activity. Int J Sport Nutr Exerc Metab. 2009;19:410–23.
8. McNaughton LR, Siegler J, Midgley A. Ergogenic effects of sodium bicarbonate. Curr Sports Med Rep. 2008;7:230–6.
9. Carr AJ, Slater GJ, Gore CJ, Dawson B, Burke LM. Effect of sodium bicarbonate on [HCO$_3$-], pH, and gastrointestinal symptoms. Int J Sport Nutr Exerc Metab. 2011;21:189–94.
10. Bishop D, Edge J, Davis C, Goodman C. Induced metabolic alkalosis affects muscle metabolism and repeated-sprint ability. Med Sci Sports Exerc. 2004;36:807–13.
11. Bishop D, Claudis B. Effects of induced metabolic alkalosis on prolonged intermittent-sprint performance. Med Sci Sports Exerc. 2005;37:759–67.
12. Cameron SL, McLay-Cooke RT, Brown RC, Gray AR, Fairbairn KA. Increased blood pH but not performance with sodium bicarbonate supplementation in elite rugby union players. Int J Sport Nutr Exerc Metab. 2010;20:307–21.
13. Krustrup P, Mohr M, Nybo L, Nielsen JJ, Jensen JM, Bangsbo J. The Yo-Yo IR2 test: physiological response, reliability, and application to elite soccer. Med Sci Sports Exerc. 2006;38:1666–73.
14. Bangsbo J, Madsen K, Kiens B, Richter EA. Effect of muscle acidity on muscle metabolism and fatigue during intense exercise in man. J Physiol. 1996;495:587–96.

Ergogenic effects of caffeine and sodium bicarbonate supplementation on intermittent...

75

15. Nordsborg N, Mohr M, Pedersen LD, Nielsen JJ, Langberg H, Bangsbo J. Muscle interstitial potassium kinetics during intense exhaustive exercise: effect of previous arm exercise. Am J Physiol Regul Integr Comp Physiol. 2003;285:143–8.

16. Borg G. Borg's perceived exertion and pain scales. IL, USA: Champaign; 1998.

17. Juel C, Klarskov C, Nielsen JJ, Krustrup P, Mohr M, Bangsbo J. Effect of high-intensity intermittent training on lactate and H+ release from human skeletal muscle. Am J Physiol Endocrinol Metab. 2004;286:e245–51.

18. Street D, Nielsen JJ, Bangsbo J, Juel C. Metabolic alkalosis reduces exercise-induced acidosis and potassium accumulation in human skeletal muscle interstitium. J Physiol. 2005;566:481–9.

19. Street D, Bangsbo J, Juel C. Interstitial pH in human skeletal muscle during and after dynamic graded exercise. J Physiol. 2001;537:993–8.

20. Davis NW, Standen NB, Stanfield PR. ATP-dependent potassium channels of muscle cells: their properties, regulation, and possible functions. J Bioenerg Biomembr. 1991;23:509–35.

21. Raymer GH, Marsh GD, Kowalchuk JM, Thompson RT. Metabolic effects of induced alkalosis during progressive forearm exercise to fatigue. J Appl Physiol. 2004;96:2050–6.

22. Gandevia SC. Spinal and supraspinal factors in human muscle fatigue. Physiol Rev. 2001;81:1725–89.

23. Nybo L, Secher NH. Cerebral perturbations provoked by prolonged exercise. Prog Neurobiol. 2004;72:223–61.

24. Greer F, McLean C, Graham TE. Caffeine, performance, and metabolism during repeated Wingate exercise tests. J Appl Physiol. 1998;85:1502–8.

25. Clausen T. Na+-K+ pump regulation and skeletal muscle contractility. Physiol Rev. 2003;83:1269–324.

26. Del Coso J, Muñoz-Fernández VE, Muñoz G, Fernández-Elías VE, Ortega JF, Hamouti N, et al. Effects of a caffeine containing energy drink on simulated soccer performance. PLoS One. 2012;7:e31380.

27. Davis JK, Green JM. Caffeine and anaerobic performance: ergogenic value and mechanisms of action. Sports Med. 2009;39:813–32.

28. Wu CL, Shih MC, Yang CC, Huang MH, Chang CK. Sodium bicarbonate supplementation prevents skilled tennis performance decline after a simulated match. J Int Soc Sports Nutr. 2010;7:33–41.

29. Siegler JC, Marshall PW, Bray J, Towlson C, et al. Sodium bicarbonate supplementation and ingestion timing: does it matter? J Strength Cond Res. 2012;26:1953–8.

## 9

The effects of whey protein with or without carbohydrates on resistance training adaptations

Juha J. Hulmi[*], Mia Laakso, Antti A. Mero, Keijo Häkkinen, Juha P. Ahtiainen and Heikki Peltonen

Abstract

Background: Nutrition intake in the context of a resistance training (RT) bout may affect body composition and muscle strength. However, the individual and combined effects of whey protein and carbohydrates on long-term resistance training adaptations are poorly understood.

Methods: A four-week preparatory RT period was conducted in previously untrained males to standardize the training background of the subjects. Thereafter, the subjects were randomized into three groups: 30 g of whey proteins ($n = 22$), isocaloric carbohydrates (maltodextrin, $n = 21$), or protein + carbohydrates ($n = 25$). Within these groups, the subjects were further randomized into two whole-body 12-week RT regimens aiming either for muscle hypertrophy and maximal strength or muscle strength, hypertrophy and power. The post-exercise drink was always ingested immediately after the exercise bout, 2–3 times per week depending on the training period. Body composition (by DXA), quadriceps femoris muscle cross-sectional area (by panoramic ultrasound), maximal strength (by dynamic and isometric leg press) and serum lipids as basic markers of cardiovascular health, were analysed before and after the intervention.

Results: Twelve-week RT led to increased fat-free mass, muscle size and strength independent of post-exercise nutrient intake ($P < 0.05$). However, the whey protein group reduced more total and abdominal area fat when compared to the carbohydrate group independent of the type of RT ($P < 0.05$). Thus, a larger relative increase (per kg bodyweight) in fat-free mass was observed in the protein vs. carbohydrate group ($P < 0.05$) without significant differences to the combined group. No systematic effects of the interventions were found for serum lipids. The RT type did not have an effect on the adaptations in response to different supplementation paradigms.

Conclusions: Post-exercise supplementation with whey proteins when compared to carbohydrates or combination of proteins and carbohydrates did not have a major effect on muscle size or strength when ingested two to three times a week. However, whey proteins may increase abdominal fat loss and relative fat-free mass adaptations in response to resistance training when compared to fast-acting carbohydrates.

Keywords: Hypertrophy, Resistance training, Nutrition, Skeletal muscle, Supplement

* Correspondence: juha.hulmi@jyu.fi
Department of Biology of Physical Activity, Neuromuscular Research Center, University of Jyväskylä, Rautpohjankatu 8, P.O. Box 35FI-40014 Jyväskylä, Finland

Background

Adequate size and function of skeletal muscle are of paramount importance for health [1–3]. Conversely, excessive fat, especially in the abdominal area, is linked to increased risk of premature death [4] and comorbidities such as negatively altered blood lipid profile [5]. Therefore, it is important to identify lifestyle choices that enhance muscle size and function while concurrently decreasing fat mass, especially in the areas harmful for health.

Resistance training (RT) is the most effective strategy to enhance muscle strength and size, and it may also provide many other health benefits such as enhanced cardiovascular and bone health and functional capacity in daily activities [6, 7]. Of nutritional choices, protein ingestion in the context of a RT bout can enhance skeletal muscle hypertrophy and strength [8, 9]. However, the importance of timing of the protein intake has been questioned lately [10], and possible beneficial effects of post-workout protein nutrition on skeletal muscle has been suggested to be affected by exercise volume, intensity and frequency and the total protein intake of the subjects [9, 11].

Dairy whey proteins seem to promote a reduction of body fat in addition to other potential health benefits [12–14]. In contrast, added sugar, at least in excessive amounts, is linked to increased risk for morbidities and early death [15]. A recent study suggests positive effects of whey proteins on abdominal fat [16], but the effects of whey proteins when compared to carbohydrates in connection with RT are less well known.

Acute protein synthesis and breakdown studies suggest that carbohydrates alone or combination of protein and carbohydrates does not further improve muscle protein balance versus protein alone after single resistance exercise bout when protein alone is sufficient, i.e. at least 20–25 grams [17–19]. However, acute measures after a single exercise bout may not always reflect long-term adaptations to RT [20].Therefore, also long term studies are needed. Bird et al. [21] investigated the effects of added carbohydrates to a small amount of essential amino acid ingestion during resistance exercise bout on RT adaptations. It was found that the combination may be slightly more effective on muscular adaptations than either essential amino acids or carbohydrates alone. This reflects the results of a protein balance study [22] in which added carbohydrates to a small amount of essential amino acids was found to increase protein balance acutely after a resistance exercise bout.

The aim of this randomized, controlled and double-blinded trial was to examine the effects of different post-exercise supplementation regimens on RT adaptation. More specifically, the purpose of this study was to examine the effects of protein and carbohydrate supplementation on body composition and strength as well as blood lipid profile. We hypothesized that proteins alone, along with the combination of proteins and carbohydrates would facilitate a greater increases in muscle size, lean mass and muscle strength with positive effects of whey proteins also on abdominal fat mass and blood lipid profile when compared to isocaloric carbohydrates. The effects of nutritional supplementations were hypothesized to occur independent of the type of RT.

Methods

Subjects

A total of 86 healthy, recreationally active men without previous systematic RT background, recruited by newspaper, email list and university web page advertisements, commenced the study. Smokers and those with chronic diseases or prescribed medications, abnormal resting electrocardiography patterns and those training habitually ≥ 2 endurance exercise sessions per week were excluded from the study. The subjects were not allowed to ingest any nutritional supplements during the study other than what were provided, except basic vitamins and minerals.

After comprehensive verbal and written explanations of the study, all subjects gave their written informed consent to participate. The study was conducted according to the Declaration of Helsinki, and ethical approval for the study procedures were granted by the Ethical Committee at the University of Jyväskylä and by the Ethical Committee of the Central Hospital, Jyväskylä.

Study design

The first phase of the study was a four-week long preparatory RT period, during which subjects were familiarized to RT. This RT period was conducted to standardize training status, to minimize the effects of stressors related to unaccustomed exercise, and to overcome strong neural and learning adaptations known to occur within the first few weeks of RT [23]. In this preparatory RT period, subjects were exercising whole-body workouts two times per week. The subjects used on average nine exercises in one workout, 2–3 sets of every exercise, and 10–15 repetition in every set. Recovery time between the sets lasted two minutes. Training loads were 50–80 % of one repetition maximum (1 RM) increasing throughout the preparatory phase. Bilateral leg press, bilateral knee extension, and bilateral knee flexion exercises were performed during each RT session. The preparatory RT period also included exercises for the other main muscle groups of the body, conducted once a week using machines: chest and shoulders, upper back, trunk extensors and flexors, and upper arms rotated during 2 weekly exercises. Table 1 and 2 lists the main details of the preparatory RT period.

Table 1 An overview of the RT program: the first block was a preparatory phase after which supplementations started and within those the subjects were separated into 2 different training regimens. Training bout consisted always of four main exercises trained with the spesific regimen of using either MS, HS or PS as a focus. Five accessory exercises were trained in a HS manner

	Weeks	Training sessions per week	Main aim of training legs BP and LPD	Aim for other accessory exercises	Exercises per session
Prep. period	1–4	2	100 %	ME	ME	9
SHP-group	5–8	2 to 3	75 %	MS	HS	9
			25 %	PS	HS	9
	9–12	2 to 3	25 %	MS	HS	9
			75 %	PS	HS	9
	13–16	2	12.5 %	MS	HS	9
			87.5 %	PS	HS	9
HS-group	5–8	2 to 3	100 %	HS	HS	9
	9–12	2 to 3	75 %	HS	HS	9
	13–16	2	25 %	HS	HS	9
			75 %	MS	HS	9

ME muscle endurance, *SHP* Strength-hypertrophy-power training, *HS* Hypertrophy-strength training, *MS* maximal strength, *PS* power & strength, *UFC* until concentric failure, *RM* repetition maximum, *2 to 3* every second week twice per week / thrice per week, *BP* bench press, *LPD* lat pull down

Before randomization further into different intervention groups, eight subjects declined to continue with the study during the preparatory RT period. This resulted in 78 subjects (age 34.4 ± 1.3 years, height 1.80 ± 0.08 m, weight 83.6 ± 1.4 kg) who started the actual RT program with different supplementary nutrition. These were randomized into three groups: whey protein ($n = 25$), carbohydrates (CHO, $n = 25$) or whey protein + carbohydrates ($n = 28$). The variation in the responses to body composition and strength was hypothesized to be larger in the combination group than in the protein or carbohydrate groups, so the n size was slightly larger in that group at the start. Within these groups, the subjects were further divided into two different RT regimens: 1) training aiming especially for muscle hypertrophy and strength (HS) and 2) training aiming especially for muscle strength, hypertrophy and power (SHP) for 12 weeks. Subjects were advised to continue their normal recreational physical activities such as low-intensity walking, skiing, cycling and swimming during the study.

Resistance training protocols

Whole-body RT that started after the preparatory RT period was undertaken 2–3 times per week, depending on the phase of the training program, for a total of 28 training sessions. Table 1 and 2 lists the main details of the RT period. The training techniques were carefully supervised and the training was controlled throughout the whole RT period. The individual loads were determined by the strength tests (repetitions to failure: 2–6RM) for all main exercise during the first week of each 4-week training block using the Brzycki

Table 2 Typical exercise bout performed 2–3 x week contained exercises for legs, whereas exercises for other muscle groups rotated and thus were trained on average once per week

Exercises in every session:	In HS session:			In MS session:			In PS session:		
	Rest								
Leg press	3–4 × 8–12 or UCF	75–85 % of 1RM	1'	3–5 × 4–6 or UCF	86–95 % of 1RM	3'	3–5 × 3–6	50–80 % of 1RM	3'
Knee flexion	3–4 × 8–12 or UCF	75–85 % of 1RM	1'	3–5 × 4–6 or UCF	86–90 % of 1RM	3'	3–5 × 3–6	50–80 % of 1RM	3'
Knee extension	2–3 × 10–15 or UCF	75–85 % of 1RM	1'	3–5 × 4–6 or UCF	86–90 % of 1RM	3'	3–5 × 3–6	50–80 % of 1RM	3'
Accessory exercises rotated between session I and II:									
Bench press / LPD	3–4 × 10–15 or UCF	70–85 % of 1RM	1'	3–5 × 4–6 or UCF	86–95 % of 1RM	3'	3–5 × 3–8	50–80 % of 1RM	3'
Other exercises	2–4 × 8–15 or UCF	70–85 % of 1RM	1'	2–4 × 8–15	70–85 % of 1RM	2'	2–4 × 8–15	70–85 % of 1RM	2'

Exercises in every 2nd session

Session I: main exercise: bench press. Other exercises: shoulder press, elbow extensors, upper-back/rear deltoideus, hip abductors and adductors.

Session II: main exercise: lat pulldown. Other exercises horizontal row, elbow flexors, torso rotators, abdominals, back extensions.

ME muscle endurance, *SHP* Strength-hypertrophy-power training, *HS* Hypertrophy-strength training, *MS* maximal strength, *PS* power & strength, *UCF* until concentric failure, *RM* repetition maximum, *2 to 3* every second week twice per week / thrice per week, *LPD* lat pull down

formula [24]. The loads were then adjusted through-out the training in each training block. The sets were conducted to a last possible repetition that could be performed with good technique or until concentric failure. The exception to this were the power-strength (PS) sets that were conducted with maximal concentric speed and, thus, not close to concentric failure. The sets, repetitions and loads fluctuated throughout each training block in a modern manner using aspects from block and non-linear periodization [25, 26]. This is important as training variety is crucial for stimulating further development in muscle strength after the first few weeks of training [26]. However, a general long-term plan was to increase absolute and relative (%-1RM) loads in a progressive manner with a short peaking period at the end of each training block before the outcome measurements.

The following exercises were used in each training session: bilateral leg press, knee extension, and knee flexion. The training program also included exercises for the other main muscle groups of the body: chest and shoulders, upper back, trunk extensors and flexors, and upper arms conducted every second training session. Hypertrophy-focused strength (HS) training contained mainly sets of 8–12 repetitions with 75–85 % loads of 1 RM. Maximal strength (MS) training in both RT regimens consisted of neural enhancing RT with lower repetitions per set (typically 4–6) and higher intensity (86–95 % 1 RM), but also more traditional hypertrophy sets to increase muscle size. PS training consisted of sets with lower loads of 1 RM (50–80 % 1 RM) performed with maximal concentric speed.

To shortly describe the RT program, the 12-week periodized RT was divided further into three different blocks. Every block consisted of four weeks of RT. In the first block, SHP group had 25 % power-strength (PS) and 75 % maximal-strength (MS) training sessions, in the second 75 % PS and 25 % MS training sessions and in the last 87.5 % PS and 12.5 % MS training sessions.

By contrast, in HS training groups, the first block consisted of 100 % HS sessions, in the second block 75 % HS and 25 % MS training sessions and in the last block 25 % HS and 75 % MS of the total training sessions per block. This type of RT program has been used in previous studies in our lab [27], and it is in line with the American College of Sports Medicine (ACSM) position stand [28] recommendations of progression models in RT.

Thus, in short, the main difference between these two training regimens (SHP vs. HS) was that in SHP power-strength sets replaced part of the hypertrophy-focused sets, especially at the end of the training program and therefore the volume of sets aiming for maximal hypertrophy was higher in HS than in SHP.

Nutritional supplementation during resistance training
During the 12-week RT intervention, pre-sweetened post-workout supplements were mixed in 0.5 L water and consumed immediately following every training bout in a double blind fashion. One group received protein, one group carbohydrate, and one group protein plus carbohydrate. Protein and carbohydrates were provided by Northforce (Kuusamon Juusto Oy, Kuusamo, Finland). Protein group received 37.5 grams of whey concentrate (30 g of whey proteins, 5 g of lactose < 1 g of fat) and carbohydrate group received 34.5 grams of maltodextrin being thus isocaloric to whey protein. In contrast, protein plus carbohydrate group received 37.5 grams of whey concentrate (30 g of whey proteins) and 34.5 grams of maltodextrin. The supplements were mixed with non-caloric sugar-free drinks (FUN Light provided by Orkla Foods Finland, Turku, Finland) depending on the week and subject's preference (either strawberry, forest fruit, pomegranate-strawberry, apple-pear or raspberry-lemon). The subjects were advised to eat normal recommended mixed meal based on the Finnish Nutrition Recommendations 2014 (see below) 1–2 hours after the exercise bout.

Daily nutrient intake
Subjects kept 4-day food diaries during the second block of the 12-week RT period. Dietary intake was recorded over three weekdays and one weekend day. The researchers gave subjects both verbal and written nutritional recommendations based on the Finnish Nutrition Recommendations 2014. As a rule, these follow the recommendations for the Nordic countries in Europe published in Autumn 2013 (NNR2012) and are very close to USDA and HHS dietary guidelines (2010) for normal healthy adults. The subjects were instructed on how to report nutritional intake in the diaries. Nutrients provided by the supplements were included in the analysis. The food diaries were analyzed by nutrient analysis software (Nutri-Flow; Flow-team Oy, Oulu, Finland).

Body composition
Body composition was estimated by Dual-energy X-ray absorptiometry (DXA, Lunar Prodigy Advance, GE Medical Systems – Lunar, Madison WI USA) before the preparatory RT period, before the supplementations started and after the experimental RT. DXA measurements were conducted following a 12-hour overnight fast and 24-h absence of alcohol and strenuous exercise. Subjects were tested on their back in a supine position on the DXA table with their arms at their sides and feet together with minimal clothing (i.e., a pair of shorts). Legs were secured by non-elastic straps at the knee and ankles, and the arms were aligned along the trunk with the palms facing the

thighs. All metal objects were removed from the subject before the scan. Analyses (using enCORE 2005, version 9.30 and Advance 12.30) provided total, lean (including muscle) and fat masses. The same investigator conducted all the analyses. Automatically generated regions of the legs were manually adjusted by the same investigator to include the hamstrings and gluteal muscles. Thus, legs were separated from the trunk by a horizontal line right above the iliac crest providing lean and fat mass for legs and upper body separately. In fat-free mass (FFM) excluding bones, the present study focuses on total and leg mass as also the other measurements (muscle CSA and muscle strengths) in the current study are from the legs. The results are presented as absolute measures and as normalized to total body mass. The trunk region includes the neck, chest, abdominal and pelvic areas except the gluteal area that was included into legs. The android region is the area between the ribs and the pelvis within the trunk region (the upper part of the trunk). This area correlates with visceral fat measures [29] and is highly associated with metabolic abnormalities [30] and, thus, was selected for the present investigation. These customized range of interests were then copied to the DXA scans obtained at weeks 0 and 12 to assure that analyses were conducted from the same areas at all measurement times. In a previous study in our laboratory an intraclass correlation coefficient (ICC) for the body composition measures were 0.786–0.975 [31].

Muscle cross-sectional area

Cross-sectional area (CSA) of the knee extensor muscles at the mid-thigh (vastus lateralis, rectus femoris, and vastus intermedius) were measured by the extended field of view mode using a B-mode axial plane ultrasound (model SSD-2000, Aloka, Tokyo, Japan) with a 10-MHz linear-array probe. A customized convex-shaped probe support coated with water-soluble transmission gel was used to assure a perpendicular measurement and to constantly distribute pressure on the tissue. The measurements were conducted twice: before the supplementations started and after the experimental RT. The transducer was moved manually from lateral to medial along a marked line on the skin. Panoramic cross sectional images were conducted at 50 % of the femur length (lateral aspect of the distal diaphysis to the greater trochanter), and CSA was analysed manually using ImageJ software (version 1.44p; National Institutes of Health, Bethesda, MD). Each leg extensor muscle CSA was analysed three times. The two closest values for each muscle were averaged, summed for total knee extensor CSA, and this value was used for statistical analyses. The method has been shown to be very reliable and valid against magnetic resonance imaging (MRI) to detect RT-induced change in muscle

size in our laboratory, e.g. ICC > 0.9 and high limits of agreement by Bland Altman method [32].

Maximal strength testing

Maximal strength was measured before the 4-week preparatory RT period, after the preparatory RT period and thus before the supplementation started, and after the 12-week experimental RT period. In addition, the subjects came to the laboratory once before the study began to learn the techniques in the strength test devices. Isometric strength was already then performed maximally to investigate the reliability of the testing between this preliminary session and the actual pre-test session in these subjects. The analysis of reliability revealed an ICC of 0.945 for isometric strength measurement.

In the actual measurements, the subjects were carefully familiarized with the test procedures and had several warm-up contractions on all devices. A David 210 horizontal leg press device (David Health Solutions Ltd, Finland) was used to measure maximal bilateral dynamic concentric strength of the leg extensors (hip and knee extensors). In the actual test, the subjects had as many trials as required to determine 1 RM. Between the trials, subjects were allowed to rest for one minute in the first light weights and thereafter two minutes when the maximal weights were approached. The device was set up so that the knee angle in the initial flexed position was on average 60° and a successful trial was accepted when the knees were fully extended (approximately 180°). The greatest load that the subject could lift to full knee extension was accepted as 1RM.

In addition, a horizontal leg press extension dynamometer (Department of Biology of Physical Activity, University of Jyväskylä, Jyväskylä, Finland) was used to determine maximal isometric bilateral leg press force (maximal voluntary contraction, MVC). Subjects were seated with a hip and knee angle of 110° and 107°, respectively, and were instructed to produce maximal force on verbal command and to maintain the force plateaued for 3–4 s. In total, 3 maximal trials with one minute rest were performed. At least three trials separated by a rest period of 1 minute or more when needed were conducted, and up to two additional trials were performed if the maximum force during the last trial was greater by 5 % compared with that during the previous attempt. The trial with the highest maximal force measured was used for statistical analysis.

Venous blood sampling and analysis

Venous blood samples were collected before the preparatory RT period and every four weeks thereafter. Venous blood samples were drawn after 12 h of fasting to obtain concentrations of total cholesterol, LDL, HDL and triglycerides. Subjects were asked to rest for at least 8 h during the preceding night and were required to refrain from strenuous physical activity for at least 48 h. Blood samples were taken from the antecubital vein into serum tubes (Venosafe; Terumo Medical Co., Leuven, Hanau, Belgium) using standard laboratory procedures. Blood samples were stored in room temperature for 10 min, after which they were centrifuged at 3500 rpm for 10 minutes (Megafure 1.0 R Heraeus; DJB Lab Care, Germany) and the serum obtained was immediately analyzed by spectrophotometry (Konelab 20XTi; Thermo Fisher Scientific, Vantaa, Finland). LDL concentration was estimated using the Friedewald [33] equation: LDL = total cholesterol - HDL - (triglycerides/2.2).

Statistical analysis

All data are expressed as means ± SE, except where designated. The data were analysed by a repeated measures General Linear Model ANOVA and using time and nutrition as factors with training type as a covariate when appropriate. Possible training-type x nutrition x time interactions were analysed using a 3-factor repeated measures General Linear Model ANOVA. Any violations of the assumptions of sphericity were explored and, if needed, corrected with a Greenhouse-Geisser (if estimated epsilon (ε) is < 0.75) or Huynh-Feldt estimator (if estimated epsilon (ε) is ≥ 0.75). The differences in the changes from pre to post measurements between different supplement groups were analysed using univariate ANOVA and training type (HS or SP) as a covariate. Bonferroni post hoc tests were performed to localize differences between and within the treatments and/or time-points. For the data that was not normally distributed, a non-parametric Wilcoxon signed rank test was used. SPSS version 13.0 for Windows was used for statistical analyses (SPSS, Inc., Chicago, IL). The level of significance was set at $P < 0.05$.

Results

There were no differences among the groups in the rate of noncompliance or drop-outs (carbohydrates, $n = 4$, protein, $n = 3$, protein + carbohydrates, $n = 3$). Baseline physical characteristics of the subjects ($n = 68$) who completed the different supplemental and training programs are presented in Table 3.

Preparatory RT period

The 4-week preparatory RT period was used to standardize the training background of the subjects. This short RT period increased FFM (total and in legs) ($P < 0.001$) (Fig. 1). Total body, trunk, android ($P < 0.001$, Fig. 2) and leg fat masses (not shown, $P < 0.05$), all decreased. Muscle strength (1 RM and MVC) increased ($P < 0.001$) (Fig. 3). Of serum lipids, total

cholesterol decreased after the preparatory RT period ($P = 0.001$) (Table 4). There were no differences between the groups later randomized into different supplement groups.

Training type

After the preparatory RT period, the subjects within all three supplementation groups trained with either the hypertrophic-strength (HS) or strength-hypertrophy-power (SHP) focused program for 12 weeks. Muscle strength and size increased and fat mass decreased in both training groups ($P < 0.05$). The comparison between the training types per se is not the focus of the present study concentrating on the three groups of supplemental nutrition. There were no nutrition x training-type x time interaction effects on any variables investigated ($P > 0.05$). This means that the type of RT did not have an effect on the nutrition responses. Therefore in the following figures and results, the two different training types are shown as pooled. However, to minimize even the small possible effects of the training type, the statistics were always conducted with the training type (HS or SHP) as a covariate.

Daily nutrient intake

All three groups reported to consume approximately 20 E% proteins and 40 E% carbohydrates, which was slightly high for protein and low for carbohydrates (10–20 % of proteins and 45–60 % of carbohydrates). Although the protein group tended to have lower energy intake ($P = 0.1$), the dietary intake did not differ significantly between the groups when expressed relative to body weight (Table 3).

Body composition

Fat-free mass

Significant increases following RT for all three supplemental groups were seen for total FFM ($P < 0.001$) and leg FFM ($P = 0.001$) (Fig. 1). There were no differences in the changes between the different supplemental groups for the absolute FFM changes. However, the protein group increased relative FFM (per kg bodyweight) more than the carbohydrate group ($P < 0.05$) (Fig. 1d).

Fat mass

Total fat mass (FM) ($P = 0.001$) (Fig. 2) and leg FM ($P = 0.002$) (not shown) decreased following RT. Leg FM decreased similarly in all nutrition groups (no nutrition x time interaction: $P = 0.302$). However, total FM showed a nutrition x time interaction effect ($P = 0.032$). This was seen as a decrease following RT in the protein ($P = 0.001$) and protein + carbohydrate ($P = 0.02$) groups, but not in the carbohydrate alone group ($P = 0.98$) (Fig. 2). This change in total FM ($P =$

Table 3 Characteristics of subjects after the habituation before the actual 12 -week RT interventions started and average daily dietary intakes from four-day diary during the second four-week training block

	CHO ($n = 21$)	Protein ($n = 22$)	Protein + CHO ($n = 25$)	All ($n = 68$)
Age (y)	36.4 ± 4.2	31.4 ± 1.4	36.2 ± 1.2	34.7 ± 1.4
Height (m)	1.79 ± 0.02	1.81 ± 0.02	1.80 ± 0.02	1.80 ± 0.01
Weight (kg)	81.4 ± 2.5	83.8 ± 2.4	85.1 ± 2.3	83.6 ± 1.4
Energy (kJ/kg/day)	146.5 ± 8.4	124.0 ± 10.3	122.5 ± 8.9	129.4 ± 5.5
Protein (g/kg)	1.7 ± 0.1	1.5 ± 0.1	1.4 ± 0.1	1.5 ± 0.1
Protein (%)	20.0 ± 0.6	21.2 ± 1.1	20.2 ± 1.1	20.5 ± 0.6
Fat (g/kg)	1.4 ± 0.1	1.1 ± 0.1	1.1 ± 0.1	1.2 ± 0.1
CHO (g/kg)	3.5 ± 0.3	3.0 ± 0.3	3.0 ± 0.3	3.2 ± 0.2
HS (n)	10	13	14	37
SP (n)	11	9	11	31

Data are means ± SE. There were no significant differences between the groups. FFM = fat-free mass, CHO = carbohydrates. HS = hypertrophic-strength training and SP = strength-and power training. The nutrition results also include the supplement that was ingested for 1 or 2 days during the four day diary recording.

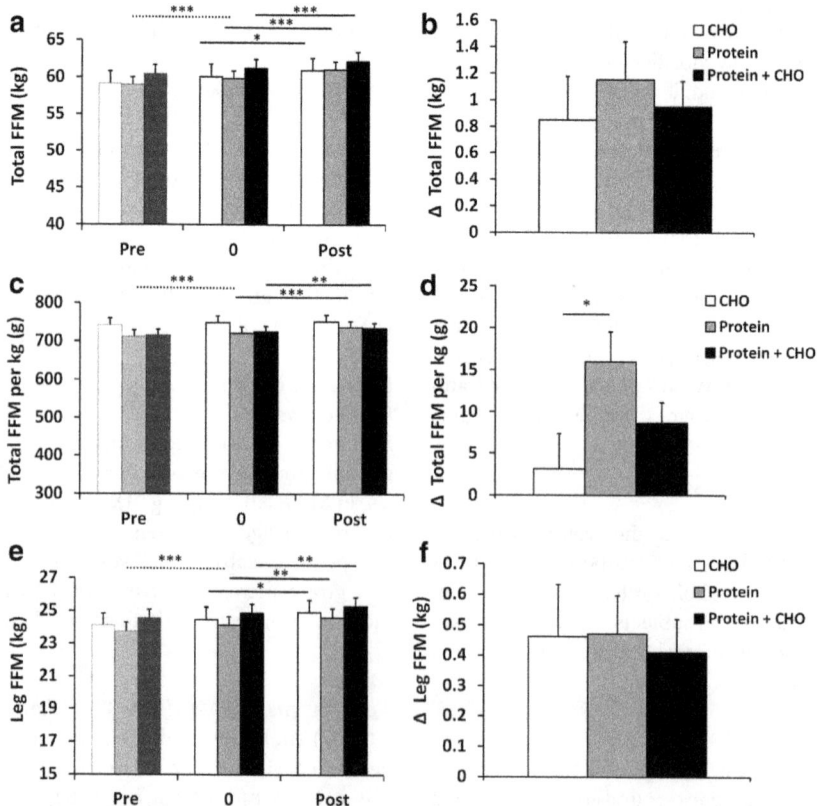

Fig. 1 a Total fat-free mass (FFM), (**b**) total FFM changes, (**c**) relative FFM (total FFM divided by the body weight), (**d**) relative FFM changes, (**e**) leg FFM, and (**f**) leg FFM changes. The changes are from the beginning of supplementation (week 0) to the end of the training period (week 12) in carbohydrate (CHO), protein, and protein and carbohydrate groups. * $p < 0.05$, ** $p < 0.01$, *** $p < 0.001$ depict significant differences. During the preparatory RT period the difference to the week 0 is analyzed as one group and depicted using dashed line as no supplementation was provided before the week 0

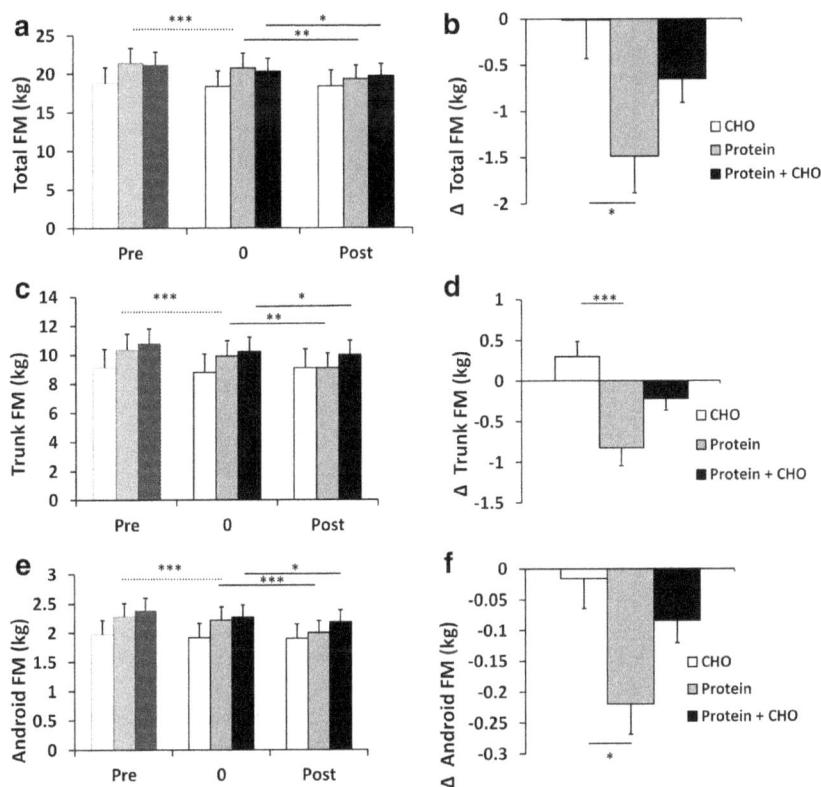

Fig. 2 Total fat mass (**a**), total fat mass changes (**b**), trunk fat mass (**c**), trunk fat mass changes (**d**), android fat mass (**e**), android fat mass changes (**f**) in carbohydrate (CHO), protein, and protein and carbohydrate groups. * ($p < 0.05$), ** ($p < 0.01$), *** ($p < 0.001$) depict significant differences within each treatment (**a, c, e**) or between the treatments (**b, d, f**).

0.03) was also larger in the protein group compared with the carbohydrate group without differences in the leg FM ($P = 0.427$).

Trunk FM was unchanged following RT ($P = 0.07$) whereas android FM decreased due to RT ($P < 0.001$) (Fig. 2). A nutrition x time interaction was detected for trunk FM ($P = 0.001$) and for android FM ($P = 0.011$). Both trunk ($P = 0.001$ and $P = 0.001$) and android ($P < 0.001$ and $P = 0.02$) FM decreased following RT in the protein and protein + carbohydrate groups, respectively (Fig. 2). A post hoc test showed that these changes in trunk and android FM were larger in the protein group compared to the carbohydrate group ($P < 0.001$ and $P = 0.01$), respectively (Fig. 2).

Muscle size
The CSA of leg extensor muscles increased following RT ($P < 0.001$) without nutrition x time effects ($P = 0.715$) (Fig. 4). Thus, CSA increased in all supplemental groups ($P < 0.001$).

Maximal strength
Significant increases following RT were seen for 1 RM ($P < 0.001$) and for isometric strength ($P < 0.001$) of leg and hip extensor muscles (Fig. 3). No nutrition x time interaction effects were observed for 1 RM strength ($P = 0.360$) and for isometric strength ($P = 0.129$).

Blood lipid profile
Serum lipids were measured every 4 weeks. Total cholesterol ($P = 0.753$), HDL ($P = 0.162$), LDL ($P = 0.110$) or triglycerides ($P = 0.433$) did not show significant overall RT effect from the beginning of the training, i.e. 16 weeks of training (Table 4). No nutrition x time interaction effects were observed for total cholesterol ($P = 0.126$), HDL ($P = 0.953$), LDL ($P = 0.476$) and for triglycerides ($P = 0.752$).

Discussion
The purpose of this study was to investigate the effects of postexercise protein and carbohydrate supplementation alone or in combination on RT adaptations. Significant increases following RT were observed for

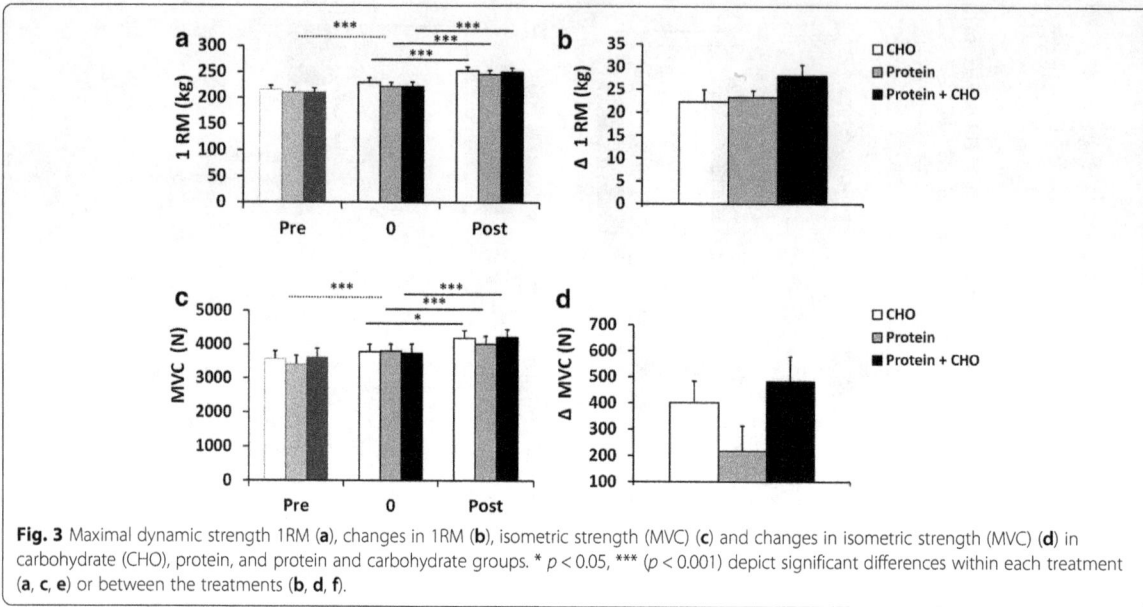

Fig. 3 Maximal dynamic strength 1RM (**a**), changes in 1RM (**b**), isometric strength (MVC) (**c**) and changes in isometric strength (MVC) (**d**) in carbohydrate (CHO), protein, and protein and carbohydrate groups. * $p < 0.05$, *** ($p < 0.001$) depict significant differences within each treatment (**a**, **c**, **e**) or between the treatments (**b**, **d**, **f**).

quadriceps muscle cross-sectional area (~9 %), total body FFM (~2 %) and muscle strength (~10-11 %) with only marginal effects of the supplemental nutrition. However, postexercise whey protein intake reduced total (~6 % vs. 0 %) and abdominal (~8 % vs. 0 %) fat when compared to carbohydrates (fast acting glucose polymers) supplementation, respectively. This led to an increased relative FFM change in the protein (~2.5 %) when compared to the carbohydrate group (~0.5 %), independent of the type of RT. These results

Table 4 Blood lipids

	CHO (n = 21)	Protein (n = 22)	Protein + CHO (n = 25)	All (n = 68)
S-Chol Pre				5.00 ± 0.12**
S-Chol 0	4.70 ± 0.21	4.61 ± 0.19	4.98 ± 0.20	4.77 ± 0.18
S-Chol 12	5.02 ± 0.22	4.52 ± 0.17	5.07 ± 0.24	4.87 ± 0.13
S-HDL Pre				1.45 ± 0.05
S-HDL 0	1.46 ± 0.08	1.46 ± 0.08	1.48 ± 0.07	1.47 ± 0.04
S-HDL 12	1.39 ± 0.10	1.33 ± 0.07	1.37 ± 0.07	1.36 ± 0.05
S-LDL Pre				3.12 ± 0.10
S-LDL 0	2.98 ± 0.18	2.87 ± 0.19	3.24 ± 0.18	3.04 ± 0.11
S-LDL 12	2.89 ± 0.21	2.65 ± 0.14	3.09 ± 0.20	2.88 ± 0.11
S-Trig. Pre				1.20 ± 0.09
S-Trig. 0	1.08 ± 0.16	1.05 ± 0.08	1.12 ± 0.11	1.09 ± 0.07
S-Trig. 12	1.40 ± 0.21**	1.20 ± 0.11*	1.30 ± 0.15	1.30 ± 0.09**

Data are mean ± SE (mmol/L). *Trig* triglycerides / triacylglyerols. * ($p < 0.05$), ** ($p < 0.01$), *** ($p < 0.001$) depict significant differences from the representative 0-time-point. Note that even though from weeks 0 to 12 there was an increasing trend in all the groups, resistance training from Pre to week 12 (16 weeks in total) did not have significant effect on blood triglycerides

were not accompanied by changes in serum lipid profile.

Adequate size and function of skeletal muscle [1–3] and rather low fat mass in the abdominal areas are of paramount importance for health [4]. The only significant effect of the supplements observed in the present study on lean or muscular tissue was the larger relative gains of FFM in the protein group when compared to the carbohydrate group. This was driven by the significantly larger decrease in fat mass and non-significantly higher increase in FFM by the protein group. Therefore, more positive body composition changes may be achieved with post-exercise ingestion of whey proteins when compared to isocaloric carbohydrates. Previous studies have shown that protein ingestion can enhance skeletal muscle hypertrophy and strength in response to chronic RT [8, 9]. Whey contains high quality proteins [34] which have increased muscle CSA adaptation to RT even in subjects ingesting 1.4–1.5 g/kg body weight of protein in their daily nutrition [27]. However, not all studies have found positive effects of protein ingestion and the importance of timing of the protein intake and the post-exercise intake of protein *per se* has been questioned lately [10]. Indeed, the possible beneficial effects of the post-workout protein nutrition may be affected by at least the volume, intensity and frequency of training and of the nutritional state of the subjects [9, 11]. In the present study, however, the type of training did not have major influence on the effects of the supplements. Previously, Farup et al. [35] observed improved muscle size gains by whey protein when compared to carbohydrates independent of training type (eccentric vs. concentric

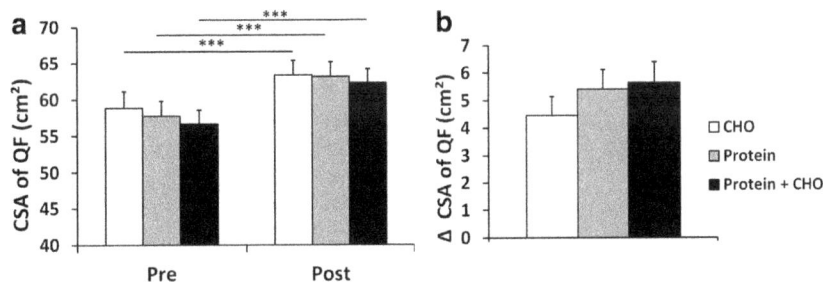

Fig. 4 Cross sectional area (CSA) of leg extensor muscles (quadriceps femoris, QF) excluding (vastus medialis muscle) (**a**) and absolute changes in CSA (**b**) in carbohydrate (CHO), protein, and protein and carbohydrate groups. *** ($p < 0.001$) depict significant differences within each treatment (**a**, **c**, **e**).

RT). More studies are needed to investigate the effects of nutrition in different types of resistance training modalities in the future studies.

No effects of supplementation were observed on muscle strength. The reason for a lack of change may be due to small differences in muscle size and also the fact that increased muscle strength during the first months of RT is achieved through not just increased muscle size, but especially through neural adaptations [23] that may be less responsive to nutrition. This may have occurred, even though we had a 4-week preparatory RT period to accommodate the influence of neural adaptations on muscle strength as has been suggested [9, 36]. Thus, neural and possibly other confounding factors and high individual variation on muscle strength adaptation [37] may be the reason why the effects of postexercise nutrient supplementation have been less consistent for muscle strength adaptation than for muscle hypertrophy [9].

In addition to protein vs. carbohydrate comparison, an important aim of the study was to investigate the effects of adding carbohydrates to the postexercise drink. Acute protein synthesis and breakdown studies suggest that the addition of carbohydrates does not further improve muscle protein balance versus sufficient ingestion of protein alone acutely after a single resistance exercise bout [17–19]. The present study also supports this evidence showing that adding carbohydrates to a protein drink did not enhance muscular adaptation to RT. Previously, Bird et al. [21] investigated the effects of added carbohydrates to a small amount of essential amino acid (total 6 g) ingestion divided into small doses ingested between each set of resistance exercise bout. They reported that the combination may be slightly more effective on muscular adaptations than the choices alone. This supports a protein balance study also using small amount (~6 g) of essential amino acids [22]. Clearly, more long-term training studies are needed to investigate this phenomenon.

Long-term RT can provide benefits to body composition such as improved muscle mass and decreased fat

mass [6], which were also observed in the present study. In addition to RT, many studies support replacing dietary carbohydrates or fats with dietary protein for favorable changes on decreasing fat mass [38, 39]. However, the effect of whey protein supplementation during RT on fat mass are conflicting [40]. Volek et al. [41] demonstrated that whey protein supplementation did not promote fat loss more than carbohydrate supplementation during RT. However, Cribb et al. [42] reported that fat mass decreased in a group consuming whey proteins during 10 weeks of RT. Moreover, a study by Arciero et al. [16], although lacking a placebo group, suggests that whey alone and whey protein combined with RT reduces total fat, abdominal fat and visceral fat mass. This is consistent with the results of the present study, where total, trunk and android fat of the whey protein group reduced when compared to the carbohydrate group. Interestingly, unlike the total and trunk area fat, however, the leg fat mass that decreased after RT, was not affected by the supplemental nutrition. Recently, Antonio et al. [43] investigated the effects of a very high protein ingestion (on average 3.4 g/kg per day) during 8 weeks of RT. Whey or beef protein powder was provided for the subjects to supplement their normal meals so that they achieve this high level of protein ingestion. The adaptations where compared to a group with rather high protein ingestion (2.3 g/kg per day). The result was that the very high protein group lost an average of 1.6 kg of fat mass when compared to only 0.3 kg in the high protein group. These studies combined suggest that supplementary whey protein ingestion can decrease fat mass during RT when ingested in the context of a resistance exercise workout or throughout the day.

The present study did not have a RT only group so we can only speculate whether the supplementary carbohydrate ingestion blocked the effects of RT on fat mass loss or whether whey proteins potentiated or maintained the fat mass loss of RT in the present study. Nevertheless, whey protein may have either decreased energy intake and/or increased energy expenditure when compared to the carbohydrate group in the subjects with a written and verbal recommendations to follow the Nordic recommendations published in Autumn 2013 (NNR2012). Indeed, although not significant, total energy intake tended to be lower in the whey protein group compared to the carbohydrate group ($P = 0.1$). The known effect of dairy proteins on satiety and decreased energy intake [13, 44] may, in part, explain why the whey protein group showed decreased fat mass when compared to carbohydrates. In addition to a rather short 12-week length of the study, this slightly lower macronutrient intake and not higher total protein intake may also explain why in the absolute terms the whey group did not increase muscle size and strength more that carbohydrates alone, only relative FFM [11]. Another potential reason that there was no observed increase in FFM or muscle CSA compared to carbohydrates alone was that the subjects only took supplements after workouts, i.e. 2–3 times per week. In addition to energy intake, whey proteins have been reported to increase postexercise resting energy expenditure (REE) when compared to carbohydrates [45] or non-energy placebo [46], up to 24 hours [45]. Whey proteins have been also shown to increase fat oxidation [47] and lipolysis [48] when compared to carbohydrates and also markers of lipolysis directly in visceral fat pad at least in rodents [49]. Therefore, it is speculated that both energy intake and expenditure were affected in the whey protein group contributing to the ~1 kg larger decrease in total and 0.2 kg of abdominal / android fat mass when compared to the carbohydrate group. The beneficial effects of whey proteins on abdominal fat were not, however, associated with altered blood lipid profile. Previously, dairy whey proteins have been shown to have various health benefits [12–14] in contrast to excessive amounts of added sugar [15]. Future studies should investigate in humans whether a form of whey proteins (e.g. intact vs. hydrolyzed) also may have an effect on body fat and muscle masses and their regulation as may be suggested based on recent rodent studies [49, 50].

Interestingly, the replacement of carbohydrates by whey protein did offer benefits to fat mass decrease, but when whey was added to carbohydrates, the result was in between the carbohydrate and whey group. Indeed, a meta-analysis [40] suggests that whey when consumed as a replacement, not as a supplement, may decrease fat mass. It is possible that in a study with *ad libitum* diet, such as the present one, whey protein ingestion alone may offer benefits for the athlete if he/she wants to decrease fat mass. However, it can be speculated that if the main goal is to increase muscle and body mass, one has to be careful to potentially eat more when ingesting these high satiating, REE-inducing proteins, otherwise the energy intake may be too low for optimal adaptations and recovery, at least in some individuals.

The major strengths of the present study were the relatively large number of subjects, two different types of RT and perhaps especially, a preparatory RT period at the start. Most of the training and nutrition studies are conducted in previously untrained subjects, which is problematic as the stressors related to unaccustomed exercise may potentially confound interpretation of the true effects of different types of training or even nutrition and the neural effects can be overriding the effects of muscle mass [23]. We believe that this strategy should be used more in the future studies as well.

A limitation of our study is that we only had one time point for the dietary diaries. By having a dietary diary also before the study period we could have directly assessed the effects of different supplemental groups on changes in daily dietary intake. We were also not able to get diaries from the last weeks of the study due to the already very demanding study for the subjects. Due to a careful randomization and such a large n-size, we find, however, it very improbable that there would have been consistent differences between the groups by a chance alone. Furthermore, DXA measures the total fat of the entire region of interest and thus both visceral and subcutaneous. However, the upper abdominal android region measure of DXA well correlates between visceral fat measured by computed tomography (CT) scan (R = 0.78) [29] and the response of trunk/abdominal and visceral fat masses to RT and protein nutrition have been shown to very closely mimic each other [16]. Furthermore, android area in DXA includes liver, pancreas and lower part of the heart, and fat accumulation in these areas is associated with metabolic abnormalities, even more closely than the accumulation of visceral fat [30].

Conclusions
This first long-term study supports the acute protein balance studies showing that adding carbohydrates to postexercise protein ingestion may not have large effect on the RT adaptations. Whey proteins, however, increased abdominal fat loss and relative fat-free mass adaptations in response to resistance training when compared to fast-acting carbohydrates. Therefore, if the main goal is to maximize fat loss responses to RT especially from abdominal area without compromising increases in muscle hypertrophy, whey protein instead of carbohydrates can be recommended for the postexercise nutrition.

Abbreviations
REE: Resting energy expenditure; 1 RM: One repetition maximum; ANOVA: Analysis of variance; CHO: Carbohydrates; CSA: Cross-sectional area; DXA: Dual-energy X-ray absorptiometry; FFM: Fat-free mass; FM: Fat mass; HDL: High-density lipoprotein; HS: Hypertrophy and strength; ICC: Intraclass correlation coefficient; LDL: Low-density lipoprotein; MS: Maximal-strength; MVC: Maximal voluntary contraction; PS: Power-strength; QF: Quadriceps femoris; RT: Resistance training; SHP: Strength, power and hypertrophy.

Competing interests
The authors declare that they have no competing interests in relation to the present study.

Authors' contribution
ML carried out the experiments and analysis with the help from JJH, HP, students and laboratory technicians. JJH drafted the manuscript with the help of ML. HP and JJH designed the study with help from ML, JPA, AAM and KH. All authors read and approved the final manuscript.

Acknowledgements
This work was supported by Tekes-National Technology Agency of Finland with University of Jyväskylä (Decision No. 70007/13).
The authors thank Pirkko Puttonen, Henna Syväoja, Risto Puurtinen, Aila Ollikainen, Johanna Stenholm and many students for their help in the data collection and analysis and in supervising the RT bouts. We also thank Joonas Järvinen form Northforce Ltd and Olli Kiviniemi from Orkla Foods Finland Ltd for providing us the proteins/carbohydrates and sugar-free drinks, respectively, and the subjects who made this project possible.

References

1. Zhou X, Wang JL, Lu J, Song Y, Kwak KS, Jiao Q, et al. Reversal of cancer cachexia and muscle wasting by ActRIIB antagonism leads to prolonged survival. Cell. 2010;142:531–43.
2. Wolfe RR. The underappreciated role of muscle in health and disease. Am J Clin Nutr. 2006;84:475–82.
3. Cooper R, Kuh D, Hardy R, Mortality Review Group, FALCon and HALCyon Study Teams. Objectively measured physical capability levels and mortality: systematic review and meta-analysis. BMJ. 2010;341:c4467.
4. Pischon T, Boeing H, Hoffmann K, Bergmann M, Schulze MB, Overvad K, et al. General and abdominal adiposity and risk of death in Europe. N Engl J Med. 2008;359:2105–20.
5. Despres JP, Lemieux I. Abdominal obesity and metabolic syndrome. Nature. 2006;444:881–7.
6. Westcott WL. Resistance training is medicine: effects of strength training on health. Curr Sports Med Rep. 2012;11:209–16.
7. Mekary RA, Grontved A, Despres JP, De Moura LP, Asgarzadeh M, Willett WC, et al. Weight training, aerobic physical activities, and long-term waist circumference change in men. Obesity (Silver Spring). 2015;23:461–7.
8. Cermak NM, Res PT, de Groot LC, Saris WH, van Loon LJ. Protein supplementation augments the adaptive response of skeletal muscle to resistance-type exercise training: a meta-analysis. Am J Clin Nutr. 2012;96:1454–64.
9. Pasiakos SM, McLellan TM, Lieberman HR. The effects of protein supplements on muscle mass, strength, and aerobic and anaerobic power in healthy adults: a systematic review. Sports Med. 2015;45:111–31.
10. Schoenfeld BJ, Aragon AA, Krieger JW. The effect of protein timing on muscle strength and hypertrophy: a meta-analysis. J Int Soc Sports Nutr. 2013;10:53-2783-10-53.
11. Bosse JD, Dixon BM. Dietary protein to maximize resistance training: a review and examination of protein spread and change theories. J Int Soc Sports Nutr. 2012;9:42-2783-9-42.
12. Sousa GT, Lira FS, Rosa JC, de Oliveira EP, Oyama LM, Santos RV, et al. Dietary whey protein lessens several risk factors for metabolic diseases: a review. Lipids Health Dis. 2012;11:67-511X-11-67.
13. Bendtsen LQ, Lorenzen JK, Bendsen NT, Rasmussen C, Astrup A. Effect of dairy proteins on appetite, energy expenditure, body weight, and composition: a review of the evidence from controlled clinical trials. Adv Nutr. 2013;4:418–38.
14. Pal S, Radavelli-Bagatini S. The effects of whey protein on cardiometabolic risk factors. Obes Rev. 2013;14:324–43.
15. Yang Q, Zhang Z, Gregg EW, Flanders WD, Merritt R, Hu FB. Added sugar intake and cardiovascular diseases mortality among US adults. JAMA Intern Med. 2014;174:516–24.
16. Arciero PJ, Baur D, Connelly S, Ormsbee MJ. Timed-daily ingestion of whey protein and exercise training reduces visceral adipose tissue mass and improves insulin resistance: the PRISE study. J Appl Physiol (1985). 2014;117:1–10.
17. Koopman R, Beelen M, Stellingwerff T, Pennings B, Saris WH, Kies AK, et al. Coingestion of carbohydrate with protein does not further augment postexercise muscle protein synthesis. Am J Physiol Endocrinol Metab. 2007; 293:E833–42.
18. Staples AW, Burd NA, West DW, Currie KD, Atherton PJ, Moore DR, et al. Carbohydrate does not augment exercise-induced protein accretion versus protein alone. Med Sci Sports Exerc. 2011;43:1154–61.
19. Gorissen SH, Burd NA, Hamer HM, Gijsen AP, Groen BB, van Loon LJ. Carbohydrate coingestion delays dietary protein digestion and absorption but does not modulate postprandial muscle protein accretion. J Clin Endocrinol Metab. 2014;99:2250–8.
20. Mitchell CJ, Churchward-Venne TA, Parise G, Bellamy L, Baker SK, Smith K, et al. Acute post-exercise myofibrillar protein synthesis is not correlated with resistance training-induced muscle hypertrophy in young men. PLoS ONE. 2014;9:e89431.
21. Bird SP, Tarpenning KM, Marino FE. Independent and combined effects of liquid carbohydrate/essential amino acid ingestion on hormonal and muscular adaptations following resistance training in untrained men. Eur J Appl Physiol. 2006;97:225–38.
22. Miller SL, Tipton KD, Chinkes DL, Wolf SE, Wolfe RR. Independent and combined effects of amino acids and glucose after resistance exercise. Med Sci Sports Exerc. 2003;35:449–55.
23. Folland JP, Williams AG. The adaptations to strength training : morphological and neurological contributions to increased strength. Sports Med. 2007;37:145–68.
24. Brzycki M. Strength testing - predicting a one-rep max from reps-to-fatigue. J Phys Educ Recreation Dance. 1993;64:88.
25. Bartolomei S, Hoffman JR, Merni F, Stout JR. A comparison of traditional and block periodized strength training programs in trained athletes. J Strength Cond Res. 2014;28:990–7.
26. Harries SK, Lubans DR, Callister R. Systematic review and meta-analysis of linear and undulating periodized resistance training programs on muscular strength. J Strength Cond Res. 2015;29:1113–25.
27. Hulmi JJ, Kovanen V, Selanne H, Kraemer WJ, Häkkinen K, Mero AA. Acute and long-term effects of resistance exercise with or without protein ingestion on muscle hypertrophy and gene expression. Amino Acids. 2009;37:297–308.
28. American College of Sports Medicine. American College of Sports Medicine position stand. Progression models in resistance training for healthy adults. Med Sci Sports Exerc. 2009;41:687–708.
29. Hill AM, LaForgia J, Coates AM, Buckley JD, Howe PR. Estimating abdominal adipose tissue with DXA and anthropometry. Obesity (Silver Spring). 2007;15:504–10.
30. Kang SM, Yoon JW, Ahn HY, Kim SY, Lee KH, Shin H, et al. Android fat depot is more closely associated with metabolic syndrome than abdominal visceral fat in elderly people. PLoS ONE. 2011;6:e27694.
31. Schumann M, Kuusmaa M, Newton RU, Sirparanta AI, Syvaoja H, Hakkinen A, et al. Fitness and lean mass increases during combined training independent of loading order. Med Sci Sports Exerc. 2014;46:1758–68.
32. Ahtiainen JP, Hoffren M, Hulmi JJ, Pietikäinen M, Mero AA, Avela J, et al. Panoramic ultrasonography is a valid method to measure changes in skeletal muscle cross-sectional area. Eur J Appl Physiol. 2010;108:273–9.
33. Friedewald WT, Levy RI, Fredrickson DS. Estimation of the concentration of low-density lipoprotein cholesterol in plasma, without use of the preparative ultracentrifuge. Clin Chem. 1972;18:499–502.
34. Hulmi JJ, Lockwood CM, Stout JR. Effect of protein/essential amino acids and resistance training on skeletal muscle hypertrophy: A case for whey protein. Nutr Metab (Lond). 2010;7:51-7075-7-51.
35. Farup J, Rahbek SK, Vendelbo MH, Matzon A, Hindhede J, Bejder A, et al. Whey protein hydrolysate augments tendon and muscle hypertrophy independent of resistance exercise contraction mode. Scand J Med Sci Sports. 2014;24:788–98.
36. Erskine RM, Fletcher G, Hanson B, Folland JP. Whey protein does not enhance the adaptations to elbow flexor resistance training. Med Sci Sports Exerc. 2012;44:1791–800.
37. Hubal MJ, Gordish-Dressman H, Thompson PD, Price TB, Hoffman EP, Angelopoulos TJ, et al. Variability in muscle size and strength gain after unilateral resistance training. Med Sci Sports Exerc. 2005;37:964–72.
38. Bosse JD, Dixon BM. Dietary protein in weight management: a review proposing protein spread and change theories. Nutr Metab (Lond). 2012;9: 81-7075-9-81.

39. Evans EM, Mojtahedi MC, Thorpe MP, Valentine RJ, Kris-Etherton PM, Layman DK. Effects of protein intake and gender on body composition changes: a randomized clinical weight loss trial. Nutr Metab (Lond). 2012;9: 55-7075-9-55.
40. Miller PE, Alexander DD, Perez V. Effects of whey protein and resistance exercise on body composition: a meta-analysis of randomized controlled trials. J Am Coll Nutr. 2014;33:163–75.
41. Volek JS, Volk BM, Gomez AL, Kunces LJ, Kupchak BR, Freidenreich DJ, et al. Whey protein supplementation during resistance training augments lean body mass. J Am Coll Nutr. 2013;32:122–35.
42. Cribb PJ, Williams AD, Carey MF, Hayes A. The effect of whey isolate and resistance training on strength, body composition, and plasma glutamine. Int J Sport Nutr Exerc Metab. 2006;16:494–509.
43. Antonio J, Ellerbroek A, Silver T, Orris S, Scheiner M, Gonzalez A, et al. A high protein diet (3.4 g/kg/d) combined with a heavy resistance training program improves body composition in healthy trained men and women–a follow-up investigation. J Int Soc Sports Nutr. 2015;12:39.
44. Pesta DH, Samuel VT. A high-protein diet for reducing body fat: mechanisms and possible caveats. Nutr Metab (Lond). 2014;11:53.
45. Hackney KJ, Bruenger AJ, Lemmer JT. Timing protein intake increases energy expenditure 24 h after resistance training. Med Sci Sports Exerc. 2010;42:998–1003.
46. Hulmi JJ, Volek JS, Selanne H, Mero AA. Protein ingestion prior to strength exercise affects blood hormones and metabolism. Med Sci Sports Exerc. 2005;37:1990–7.
47. Acheson KJ, Blondel-Lubrano A, Oguey-Araymon S, Beaumont M, Emady-Azar S, Ammon-Zufferey C, et al. Protein choices targeting thermogenesis and metabolism. Am J Clin Nutr. 2011;93:525–34.
48. Hector AJ, Marcotte GR, Churchward-Venne TA, Murphy CH, Breen L, von Allmen M, et al. Whey protein supplementation preserves postprandial myofibrillar protein synthesis during short-term energy restriction in overweight and obese adults. J Nutr. 2015;145:246–52.
49. Mobley CB, Fox CD, Ferguson BS, Pascoe CA, Healy JC, McAdam JS, et al. Effects of protein type and composition on postprandial markers of skeletal muscle anabolism, adipose tissue lipolysis, and hypothalamic gene expression. J Int Soc Sports Nutr. 2015;12:14-015-0076-9. eCollection 2015.
50. Roberts MD, Cruthirds CL, Lockwood CM, Pappan K, Childs TE, Company JM, et al. Comparing serum responses to acute feedings of an extensively hydrolyzed whey protein concentrate versus a native whey protein concentrate in rats: a metabolomics approach. Appl Physiol Nutr Metab. 2014;39:158–67.

## 10

Glutathione supplementation suppresses muscle fatigue induced by prolonged exercise via improved aerobic metabolism

Wataru Aoi[1*], Yumi Ogaya[1], Maki Takami[1], Toru Konishi[2], Yusuke Sauchi[2], Eun Young Park[3], Sayori Wada[1], Kenji Sato[4] and Akane Higashi[1]

Abstract

Backgrounds: Glutathione is an endogenous redox couple in animal cells and plays important roles in antioxidant defense and detoxification, although it is unknown if oral glutathione supplementation affects exercise-induced physiological changes. The present study investigated the effect of glutathione intake on exercise-induced muscle metabolism and fatigue in mice and humans.

Methods: ICR mice were divided into 4 groups: sedentary control, sedentary supplemented with glutathione (2.0%, 5 µL/g body weight), exercise control, and exercise supplemented with glutathione. After 2 weeks, the exercise groups ran on a treadmill at 25 m/min for 30 min. Immediately post-exercise, intermuscular pH was measured, and hind limb muscle and blood samples were collected to measure biochemical parameters. In a double-blind, cross-over study, 8 healthy men (35.9 ± 2.0 y) were administered either glutathione (1 g/d) or placebo for 2 weeks. Then, they exercised on a cycle ergometer at 40% maximal heart rate for 60 min. Psychological state and blood biochemical parameters were examined after exercise.

Results: In the mouse experiment, post-exercise plasma non-esterified fatty acids were significantly lower in the exercise supplemented with glutathione group (820 ± 44 mEq/L) compared with the exercise control group (1152 ± 61 mEq/L). Intermuscular pH decreased with exercise (7.17 ± 0.01); however, this reduction was prevented by glutathione supplementation (7.23 ± 0.02). The peroxisome proliferator-activated receptor-γ coactivator-1α protein and mitochondrial DNA levels were significantly higher in the sedentary supplemented with glutathione group compared with the sedentary control group (25% and 53% higher, respectively). In the human study, the elevation of blood lactate was suppressed by glutathione intake (placebo, 3.4 ± 1.1 mM; glutathione, 2.9 ± 0.6 mM). Fatigue-related psychological factors were significantly decreased in the glutathione trial compared with the placebo trial.

Conclusions: These results suggest that glutathione supplementation improved lipid metabolism and acidification in skeletal muscles during exercise, leading to less muscle fatigue.

Keywords: Glutathione, Dkeletal muscle, Lipid metabolism, Running exercise, PGC-1α

* Correspondence: waoi@kpu.ac.jp
[1]Laboratory of Health Science, Graduate School of Life and Environmental Sciences, Kyoto Prefectural University, 1-5 Hangi-cho Shimogamo, Sakyo-ku, Kyoto 606-8522, Japan
Full list of author information is available at the end of the article

Background

Glutathione, a tripeptide consisting of glutamate, cysteine, and glycine, is synthesized primarily in the hepatic cells. It is stored in an oxidized or reduced form at high concentrations in the majority of cells. Glutathione is reported to be involved in the regulation of various physiological functions, in particular, antioxidation and detoxification functions [1,2]. Reduced glutathione is easily oxidized by reactive oxygen species and subsequently reduced again by glutathione reductase, and the redox balance of glutathione has been used as a marker of antioxidant status in various conditions. Physical exercise decreases the reduced form and increases the oxidized form of glutathione [3,4]. In addition, prolonged exercise decreases total plasma and tissue glutathione content over time [5,6], which suggests that glutathione may be associated with aerobic energy metabolism and maintenance of muscle contraction.

Energy and nutrient metabolism in skeletal muscle plays an important role in muscular fatigue. In particular, the energy source can affect muscle performance. For example, a carbohydrate-based energy source results in decreased muscular pH owing to increased lactic acid production, which leads to impaired muscle contraction. However, when the energy expended during exercise is derived from lipids, a large amount of energy can be continuously supplied via aerobic metabolism. Therefore, increased lipid utilization in the mitochondria of skeletal muscle cells is associated with continued muscle contraction, and the number and activity of mitochondria influence the utilization of fatty acids in muscle cells.

Over the past decade, peroxisome proliferator-activated receptor-γ coactivator-1α (PGC-1α) has been demonstrated as a key transcriptional co-activator, providing a mechanistic insight into nuclear regulatory pathways in the biogenesis of mitochondria in skeletal muscle [7-9]. Its contents are changed by differing levels of physical activity, metabolic disorders, and aging, which are all associated with metabolic capacity [9-11]. Moreover, it interacts with nuclear receptors and transcription factors to activate the transcription of lipid metabolic genes, and its activity is responsive to aerobic metabolic events [9,10].

Recently, Kovacs-Nolan et al. [12] demonstrated, in in vitro and ex vivo intestinal absorption model, that intact glutathione can be transported across human intestinal epithelial cells. In addition, we reported that the plasma glutathione concentration is transiently elevated after oral glutathione supplementation [13], which suggests that exogenous glutathione can be absorbed into the body and act as an important glutathione supply. Therefore, we hypothesized that glutathione supplementation may contribute to aerobic metabolism during

exercise as a result of activated mitochondria via PGC-1α in skeletal muscle. The purpose of this study was to examine the effects of glutathione supplementation on muscle fatigue in exercise as a result of improved muscular aerobic metabolism.

Methods

Animal experimental design

This study complied with the guidelines of the Japanese Council on Animal Care and was approved by the Committee for Animal Research at Kyoto Prefectural University of Medicine (No. 23–77). ICR mice (7-week-old; Shimizu Laboratory Supplies, Kyoto, Japan) were acclimatized for 1 week in an air-conditioned ($22 \pm 2°C$) room on a 12-h light/dark cycle (lights on from 7:30 to 19:30). Mice were divided into 4 groups containing 8 animals each: sedentary control, sedentary supplemented with glutathione, exercise control, and exercise supplemented with glutathione. Glutathione was purified and crystalized after separation from the fermented food-grade yeast Candida utilis which approved by the U.S. food and drug administration (FDA), and used for experiments.

A glutathione solution (2% w/w) was provided 1 time per d (5 µL/g body weight) for 2 weeks. Saline was provided to control mice in the same volume. After 2 weeks of treatment, the exercise groups ran on a treadmill; after an initial 5-min warm up, the running speed was gradually increased to 25 m/min, which was maintained for 30 min. Immediately following the exercise, intermuscular pH was measured under anesthesia; then the hind limb muscles and blood were collected. The control mice underwent the same measurements. Blood glucose was measured (GluTest; Arkray, Inc., Kyoto, Japan), following which the blood samples were centrifuged at 3,500 rpm for 15 min at 4°C to collect plasma. Plasma nonesterified fatty acid (NEFA) was measured using a NEFA-C assay kit (WAKO, Osaka, Japan).

pH measurements in animals

pH levels in the interstitial fluid of exercised muscle tissue were measured under anesthesia using a glass microelectrode that was inserted into the interstitium between the gastrocnemius and tibialis anterior muscles.

Western blotting

Protein was extracted from muscle tissues obtained from sedentary groups using a lysis buffer (Sigma, St. Louise, MO) containing protease inhibitor. Equal amounts of protein in the lysates were separated by 10% sodium dodecyl sulfate-polyacrylamide gel electrophoresis, and proteins were then transferred onto nitrocellulose membrane. The blots were incubated with primary antibodies against PGC-1α (Chemicon International, Temecula, CA) and

AMP-activated protein kinase (AMPK) (Cell Signaling Technology, Beverly, MA), and the reaction products were visualized using a horseradish peroxidase-conjugated secondary antibody (Invitrogen, Carlsbad, CA) and enhanced chemiluminescence (Chemi-Lumi One Super, Nakarai Tesque, Kyoto, Japan) (Additional file 1: Figure S1). Band densities were measured using ImageQuant LAS4000 (GE Healthcare, Buckinghamshire, UK).

Mitochondrial DNA
To determine the mitochondrial DNA (mtDNA), polymerase chain reaction (PCR) analysis was performed using DNA obtained from muscle tissues. Total DNA was extracted using the extraction reagent (DNA zol® BD Reagent, Invitrogen) following homogenization. The relative copy numbers of mitochondrial to nuclear DNA were determined by real-time PCR with primers specific to cytochrome c oxidase subunit II (COX II) (mitochondrial) 5′-ATCCCAGGCCGACTAAATCA (forward) and 5′-TT TCAGAGCATTGGCCATAGAA (reverse) and β-actin (nuclear) genes 5′-TATCCACCTTCCAGCAGATGT (forward) and 5′-AGCTCAGTAACAGTCCGCCTA (reverse).

Human experimental design
Eight healthy men (age, 35.9 ± 2.0 y; height, 172.6 ± 1.9 cm; body weight, 70.6 ± 3.2 kg; BMI, 23.8 ± 1.2 kg/m^2) were recruited to participate in a double-blind, cross-over study, which was complied with the principles outlined in the Helsinki Declaration and approved by the ethics committee of Kyoto Prefectural University (No. 46). All of the subjects provided written, informed consent. The subjects did not have a current or prior chronic disease or a history of smoking, and they were not currently using any medications. The subjects were also not habituated to a regular exercise regimen.

A single-bout exercise experiment was performed following 2 weeks of glutathione (1 g/d) or placebo supplementation in capsule form. The subjects were asked to fast, except for water, from 22:00 the night prior to the experiment. On the experiment day, all subjects consumed the same breakfast (200 g of steamed rice) 90 min before the exercise session to normalize the effects of a pre-exercise meal. All participants performed a single bout of steady-state cycling exercise at 40% maximum heart rate for 60 min. Heart rate and the rating of perceived exertion (RPE; Borg scale) were monitored every 10 min during exercise. Blood samples were collected from the antecubital vein before and after exercise, and blood glucose and lactate were measured using simple measuring instruments (Lactate Pro, GluTest; Arkray, Kyoto, Japan). Data obtained from seven subjects was analyzed for glucose and lactate due to failure of blood collection during exercise for one subject. Psychological state was assessed after blood collection using the

Profile of Mood State test, of which we were interested in 2 mood factors (fatigue–inertia and vigor–activity). In addition, the degree of relaxation was examined using a visual analogue scale (VAS). A 4-week washout period separated the conditions, and all of the subjects completed both testing conditions.

Measurement of plasma glutathione
Plasma glutathione concentration was measured according to our previously reported protocol [13]. Briefly, collected plasma was mixed with ethanol and then centrifuged. The supernatant was dried and added to 5% trichloroacetic acid (TCA) containing 2% 2-mercaptoethanol to reduce the oxidized form of glutathione, and the mixture was used as the deprotenized plasma fraction. The ethanol precipitate of the plasma was mixed with the 5% (final concentration) TCA and 2% 2-mercaptoethanol. After centrifugation, the supernatant was used as the protein-bound plasma fraction. The concentrations of both fractions were determined by precolumn derivation with 6-aminoquinolyl-N-hydroxy succinimidyl carbamate and liquid chromatography-tandem mass spectrometry (LC-MS/MS).

Statistical analysis
All data are reported as mean ± SE. Differences between groups or time course comparisons were evaluated using 2-way ANOVA. When significant interactions were detected, *post hoc* multiple comparisons were conducted using the Bonferroni method. Differences between the control and glutathione groups in the animal study were determined using Student's t-tests. Differences between the placebo and glutathione trials in the human study were tested using Wilcoxon signed-rank tests. $P < 0.05$ was considered statistically significant.

Results
Body weight and blood parameters in animals
Body weight was similar in all of the groups (sedentary control, 41.4 ± 0.9 g; sedentary supplemented with glutathione, 39.8 ± 0.9 g; exercise control 41.3 ± 0.8 g; exercise supplemented with glutathione, 40.2 ± 0.7 g). There were no significant differences in blood glucose levels between the control and glutathione groups in both sedentary and exercise conditions (degree of freedom (df) = 31, F = 0.039) (Figure 1A). In contrast, plasma NEFA after exercise was significantly lower with supplementation of glutathione compared with the control group (df = 31, F = 5.90, p < 0.01) (Figure 1B).

Intermuscular pH in animals
The interstitial pH levels in muscle were significantly reduced by exercise (df = 31, F = 4.36, p < 0.001; Figure 1C). However, the pH following exercise of the glutathione

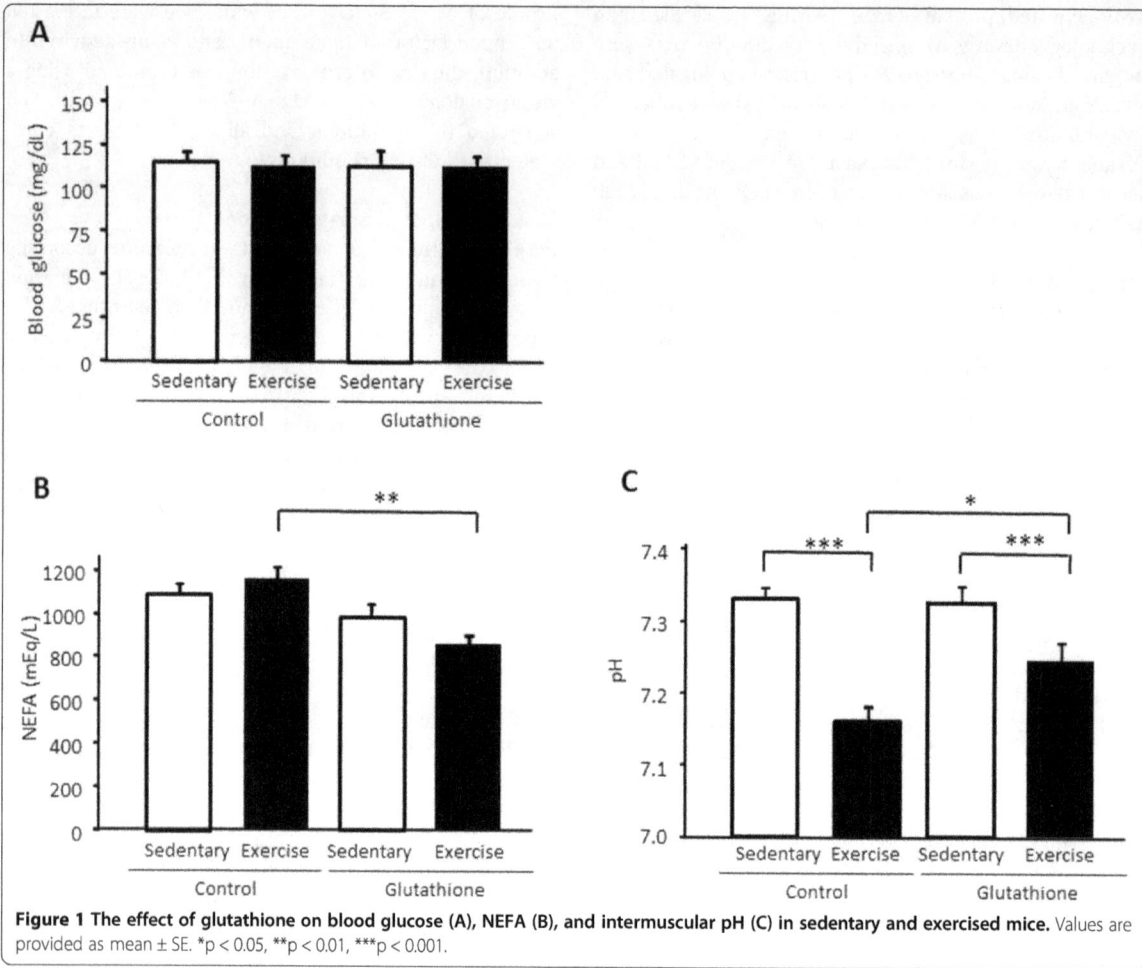

Figure 1 The effect of glutathione on blood glucose (A), NEFA (B), and intermuscular pH (C) in sedentary and exercised mice. Values are provided as mean ± SE. *p < 0.05, **p < 0.01, ***p < 0.001.

group was significantly higher than that of the control group (p < 0.05).

PGC-1α, AMPK, and mitochondrial DNA in mouse muscle
PGC-1α was significantly higher with glutathione intake (df = 14, t = −1.88, p < 0.05; Figure 2A). In addition, AMPK, an upstream protein of PGC-1α, was also significantly higher in the sedentary treated with glutathione group than in the sedentary control group (df = 13, t = −2.76, p < 0.05; Figure 2B). In addition, mtDNA was significantly higher with glutathione supplementation (df = 14, t = −1.98, p < 0.05; Figure 2C).

Blood biochemical parameters in humans
There was a significant decrease in the blood glucose concentrations at 30 and 60 min after exercise compared with pre-exercise in both the placebo and glutathione trials (df = 41, F = 23.9, p < 0.01) (Figure 3A); however, there was no difference between the trials. There was a significant increase in blood lactate concentrations at

30 min after exercise compared with pre-exercise in the placebo trial (df = 41, F = 3.90, p < 0.05) but not in the glutathione trial (Figure 3B). The free form of glutathione in plasma was not changed by either exercise or glutathione intake. In contrast, protein-bound plasma glutathione was significantly reduced by exercise in the placebo trial (p < 0.05) although the reduction was moderated in the glutathione-supplemented group (Figure 4).

Heart rate and psychological parameters in humans
There was a trend for lower heart rates during exercise at 40 and 60 min in the glutathione trial compared with the placebo trial (Z = −1.47, p = 0.071 and Z = −1.26, p = 0.104, respectively) (Figure 5). There was also a trend for a lower RPE at 50 min (Z = −1.44, p = 0.075) and a significant decrease at 60 min (Z = −1.78, p < 0.05) in the glutathione trial compared with the placebo trial.

The Profile of Mood State vigor–activity factor after exercise was significantly higher following exercise in the glutathione trial compared with the placebo trial

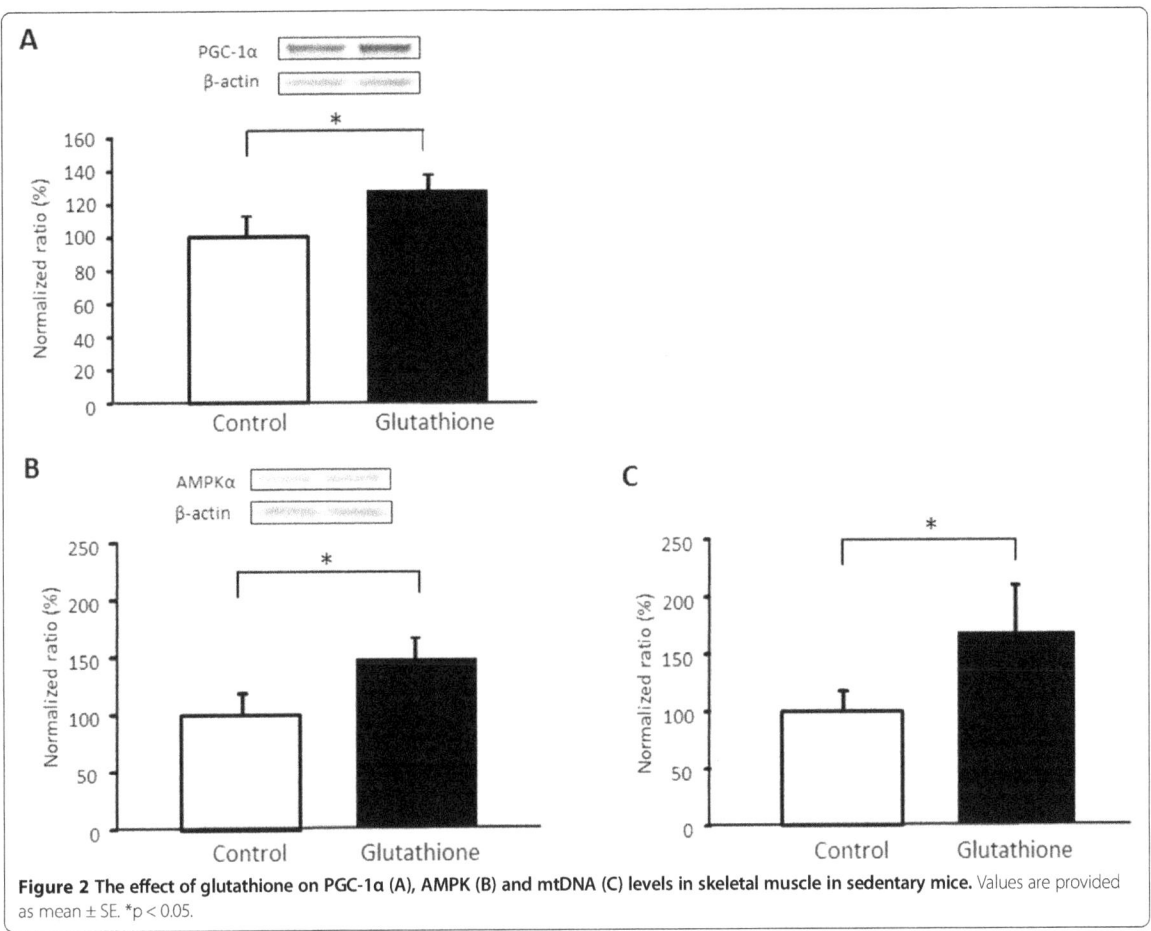

Figure 2 The effect of glutathione on PGC-1α (A), AMPK (B) and mtDNA (C) levels in skeletal muscle in sedentary mice. Values are provided as mean ± SE. *p < 0.05.

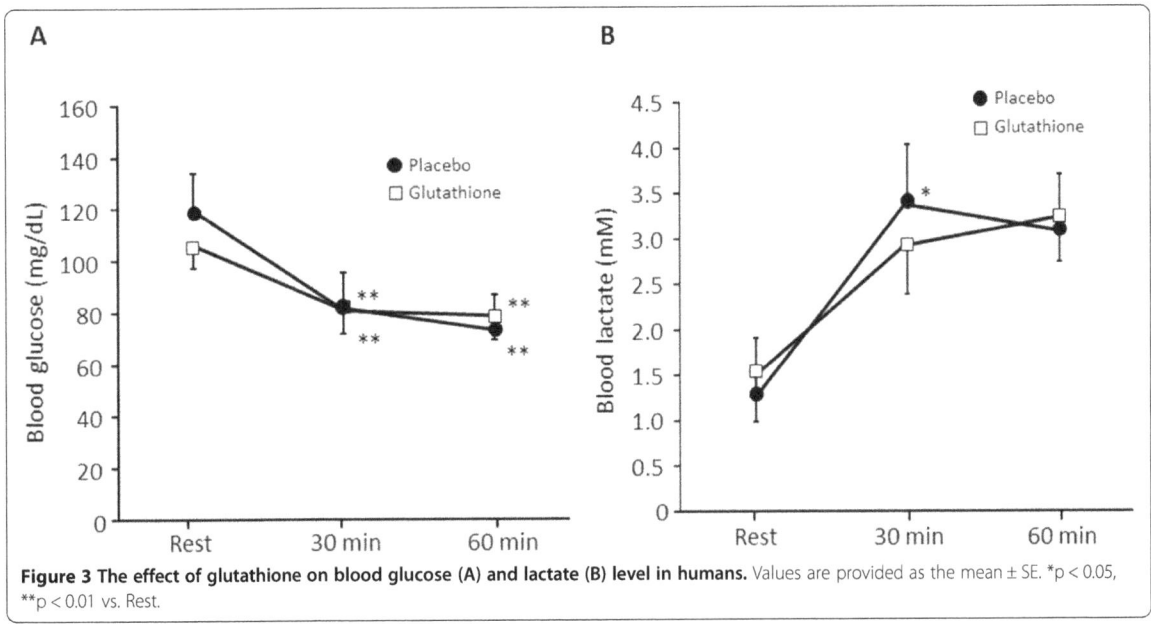

Figure 3 The effect of glutathione on blood glucose (A) and lactate (B) level in humans. Values are provided as the mean ± SE. *p < 0.05, **p < 0.01 vs. Rest.

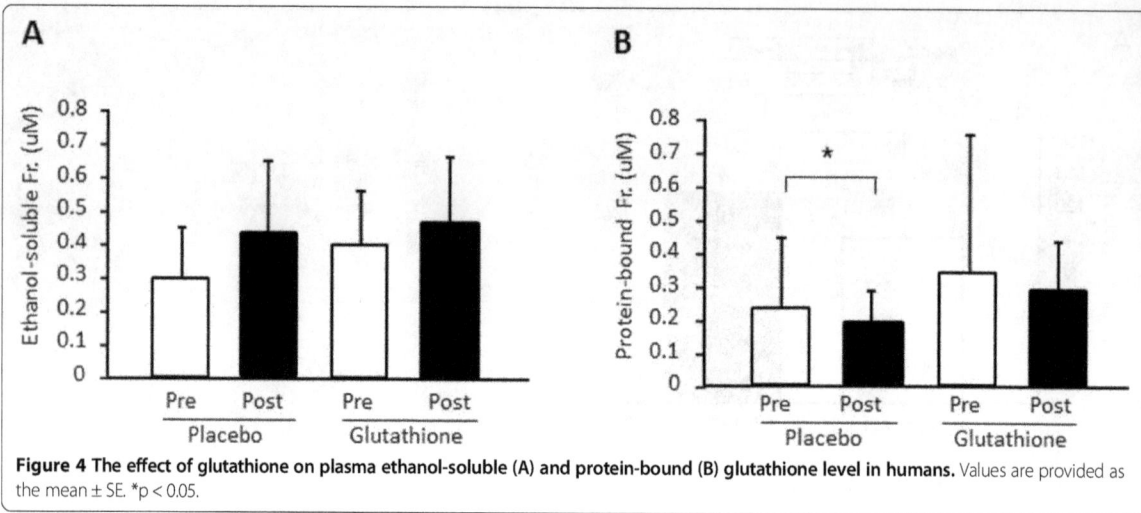

Figure 4 The effect of glutathione on plasma ethanol-soluble (A) and protein-bound (B) glutathione level in humans. Values are provided as the mean ± SE. *$p < 0.05$.

($Z = -2.11$, $p < 0.05$) (Table 1). In contrast, the fatigue–inertia factor was significantly lower in the glutathione trial compared with the placebo trial ($Z = -1.82$, $p < 0.05$), while marked difference was not found in the VAS scores between trials ($Z = -0.98$, $p = 0.163$).

Discussion

In the present study, glutathione supplementation resulted in higher levels of PGC-1α and mtDNA biogenesis in mouse skeletal muscle and prevented the exercise-induced reduction in intermuscular pH in mice. Moreover, in humans, glutathione supplementation suppressed fatigue-related parameters during and after exercise. While it has been well documented that glutathione plays a central role in the antioxidant network in animal cells and redox balance can act as a marker of antioxidant status in various pathological and physiological conditions

including exercise [3,4,14,15], the role of exogenous glutathione on phenotypic changes relating to physical exercise has not been explored. To the best of our knowledge, the present study is the first to demonstrate that glutathione supplementation improves aerobic metabolism in skeletal muscle, leading to reduced exercise-induced muscle fatigue.

During muscle contraction, lactic acid, a major source of protons, is rapidly produced by increased glycolytic metabolism, lowering the pH and inhibiting muscle contraction [16]. The protons generated from cytosolic lactic acid are immediately buffered in the cell or exported to the interstitial fluid and further transported to the blood. The buffering capacity is relatively high in the cytosol and blood, whereas this capacity is low in interstitial fluid where the presence of buffering factors, such as proteins, is limited [17,18]. Therefore, the pH of the

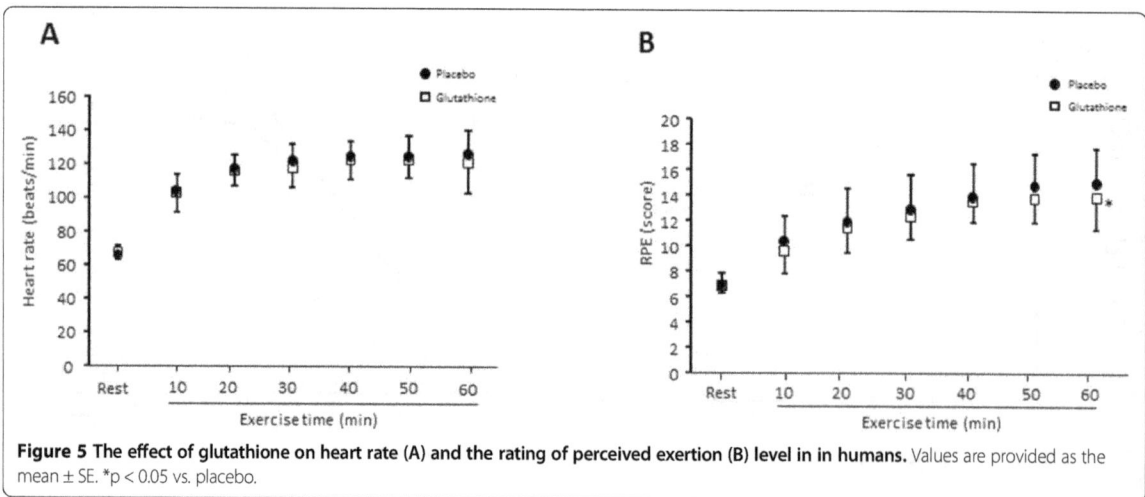

Figure 5 The effect of glutathione on heart rate (A) and the rating of perceived exertion (B) level in in humans. Values are provided as the mean ± SE. *$p < 0.05$ vs. placebo.

Table 1 Psychological examination after exercise

	Placebo	Glutathione
POMS test		
Vigor-activity	54.5 ± 2.8	58.8 ± 3.2*
Fatigue-inertia	51.0 ± 2.8	45.1 ± 2.7*
VAS	6.0 ± 0.7	4.7 ± 0.8

Values are provided as mean ± SE. *$p < 0.05$ vs. placebo.
POMS, Profile of Mood State; VAS, visual analogue scale.

interstitial fluid in muscle tissues can drastically change in response to muscle contraction and can also be a marker of acid–base conditions in muscle tissue. In contrast, the majority of lactate anions are released into the circulation or immediately metabolized as an energy substrate through aerobic metabolism [19-21]; therefore, their levels are not suitable as a marker. The results of both the animal and human studies indicate that glutathione supplementation inhibited the decrease in intermuscular pH after exercise; in the human study, this was demonstrated by the differences in blood lactate concentrations following exercise between the placebo and glutathione trials. These results may also explain the differences observed between the trials in RPE and subjective fatigue during and after exercise; in particular, an improvement in muscular acidosis results in less fatigue.

Circulating NEFA concentrations are regulated by a balance between catabolic processes in adipose tissue and fatty acid substrate utilization by the skeletal muscle. Circulating catecholamines such as adrenalin and noradrenalin are increased in response to exercise and stimulate lipolysis of triglycerides in adipose tissue [22], which causes an elevation of circulating fatty acids. In contrast, muscle contraction increases uptake of fatty acids from the circulation into muscle cells [23], which leads to a decrease in circulating fatty acids. Therefore, we suggest that the reduction of NEFA observed in the glutathione-supplemented mice was due to an increase in muscle utilization rather than a release from adipose tissue. Because energy consumed in muscle during exercise is mainly supplied by carbohydrates and lipids, glutathione-induced lipid utilization can decrease energy obtained from carbohydrates, which may lead to a decrease in lactate/proton production. Collectively, this indicates that glutathione improves metabolic acidosis through the activation of lipid metabolism, which leads to suppression of exercise-induced fatigue.

PGC-1α is a central member of a family of transcriptional co-activators involved in aerobic metabolism. Activation of PGC-1α alters the metabolic phenotype through interactions with nuclear respiratory factor and peroxisome proliferator-activated receptor-α [8-10], which leads to increased mitochondrial biogenesis and activity. It has

been reported that PGC-1α activation causes significant improvements in athletic performance [24,25], prevention and treatment of muscle weakness in the elderly, obesity, and other metabolic diseases such as mitochondrial myopathies and diabetes [10,11,26]. Here, we detected an increase in PGC-1α with 2 weeks of glutathione intake, along with an increase in mtDNA content, indicating the activation of mitochondrial biogenesis. Therefore, the observed elevation of PGC-1α by glutathione intake strongly suggests an acceleration in lipid metabolism. In addition, the increase of mitochondria content could also lead to a decrease of lactate generation by accelerating aerobic metabolism of glucose, which would prevent muscle acidosis during exercise even further.

The regulatory mechanism for glutathione-induced increases in PGC-1α is unclear. One explanation is the elevation of AMPK, which is an upstream factor of PGC-1α regulation [27,28]. Recently, it has been argued that oral intake of other antioxidants, including vitamin C and E, do not elevate PGC-1α in the skeletal muscle of mice and humans [29,30]; thus, this may be a specific action of glutathione as a signal factor, but not its antioxidant properties. We found that 2 weeks of glutathione supplementation did not affect plasma glutathione concentration in the basal state. However, glutathione is transported across the intestines with in its intact form [12], and its plasma concentration, along with the glutathione-derived dipeptides γ-glutamyl-cysteine and cysteinyl-glycine, is markedly elevated during the 60–120-min period after oral administration, as shown in our previous report [13]. Therefore, the transient elevation of glutathione or the derived dipeptides following supplementation over 2 weeks may indicate stimulation of specific signaling factors that lead to elevated AMPK and PGC-1α. Alternatively, glutathione content in muscle tissues may also increase with supplementation, leading to the up-regulation of these factors. Further studies are needed to determine the specific mechanism(s) by which glutathione affects muscle aerobic metabolism. In addition, we also observed that reduction of the protein-bound glutathione concentration in plasma after exercise was suppressed following glutathione supplementation, which may also be related to the regulation of energy metabolism or fatigue. Future studies should also aim to identify the bound protein in plasma and examine the mechanism of protein binding or release from the protein and its source.

Conclusions

The present results demonstrated that 2 weeks of glutathione supplementation decreased plasma fatty acids and suppressed the exercise-induced reduction in intermuscular pH. Glutathione supplementation also resulted in elevated concentrations of PGC-1α and mitochondria in skeletal muscle. These observations suggest that glutathione induces aerobic metabolism and improves an acidic environment in skeletal muscle during exercise by elevating PGC-1α, which would prevent exercise-induced fatigue.

Additional file

Additional file 1: Figure S1. Images of western blotting for PGC-1α, AMPK, and β-actin in control (C) and glutathione (G) groups.

Abbreviations

AMPK: AMP-activated protein kinase; COX II: Cytochrome c oxidase subunit II; mtDNA: Mitochondrial DNA; NEFA: Nonesterified fatty acid; PCR: Polymerase chain reaction; PGC-1α: Peroxisome proliferator-activated receptor-γ coactivator-1α; RPE: Rating of perceived exertion; VAS: visual analogue scale.

Competing interests

This study was supported in part by a research fund from the KOHJIN Life Sciences Company, Ltd.

Authors' contributions

WA, YO, MT, YS, and AH conceived and designed the experiments. WA, YO, MT, EYP, SW, and KS performed research. TK, YS, EYP, and KS contributed reagents/materials/analysis tools. WA wrote the paper. All authors read and approved the final manuscript.

Acknowledgements

We would like to express our appreciation to the Kyoto Integrated Science & Technology Bio-Analysis Center for the use of their LC-MS/MS.

Author details

[1]Laboratory of Health Science, Graduate School of Life and Environmental Sciences, Kyoto Prefectural University, 1-5 Hangi-cho Shimogamo, Sakyo-ku, Kyoto 606-8522, Japan. [2]KOHJIN Life Sciences Company, Ltd., Tokyo, Japan. [3]Laboratory of Food Science, Graduate School of Life and Environmental Sciences, Kyoto Prefectural University, Kyoto, Japan. [4]Division of Applied Biosciences, Graduate School of Agriculture, Kyoto University, Kyoto, Japan.

References

1. Meister A. Glutathione-ascorbic acid antioxidant system in animals. J Biol Chem. 1994;269:9397–400.
2. Tedeschi M, Bohm S, Di Re F, Oriana S, Spatti GB, Tognella S, et al. Glutathione and detoxification. Cancer Treat Rev. 1990;17:203–8.
3. Gambelunghe C, Rossi R, Micheletti A, Mariucci G, Rufini S. Physical exercise intensity can be related to plasma glutathione levels. J Physiol Biochem. 2001;57:9–14.
4. Ji LL, Fu R. Responses of glutathione system and antioxidant enzymes to exhaustive exercise and hydroperoxide. J Appl Physiol (1985). 1992;72:549–54.
5. Pyke S, Lew H, Quintanilha A. Severe depletion in liver glutathione during physical exercise. Biochem Biophys Res Commun. 1986;139:926–31.
6. Lew H, Pyke S, Quintanilha A. Changes in the glutathione status of plasma, liver and muscle following exhaustive exercise in rats. FEBS Lett. 1985;185:262–6.
7. Wu Z, Puigserver P, Andersson U, Zhang C, Adelmant G, Mootha V, et al. Mechanisms controlling mitochondrial biogenesis and respiration through the thermogenic coactivator PGC-1. Cell. 1999;98:115–24.
8. Olesen J, Kiilerich K, Pilegaard H. PGC-1-alpha-mediated adaptations in skeletal muscle. Pflugers Arch. 2010;460:153–62.
9. Finck BN, Kelly DP. PGC-1 coactivators: inducible regulators of energy metabolism in health and disease. J Clin Invest. 2006;116:615–22.
10. Patti ME, Butte AJ, Crunkhorn S, Cusi K, Berria R, Kashyap S, et al. Coordinated reduction of genes of oxidative metabolism in humans with insulin resistance and diabetes: Potential role of PGC1 and NRF1. Proc Natl Acad Sci USA. 2003;100:8466–71.
11. Wenz T, Rossi SG, Rotundo RL, Spiegelman BM, Moraes CT. Increased muscle PGC-1alpha expression protects from sarcopenia and metabolic disease during aging. Proc Natl Acad Sci USA. 2009;106:20405–10.
12. Kovacs-Nolan J, Rupa P, Matsui T, Tanaka M, Konishi T, et al. In vitro and ex vivo uptake of GSH across the intestinal epithelium, and fate of oral GSH after in vivo supplementation. J Agric Food Chem. in press
13. Park EY, Shimura N, Konishi T, Sauchi Y, Wada S, Aoi W, et al. Increase in the protein-bound form of glutathione in human blood after oral administration of glutathione. J Agric Food Chem. 2014;62:6183–9.
14. Johnson WM, Wilson-Delfosse AL, Mieyal JJ. Dysregulation of glutathione homeostasis in neurodegenerative diseases. Nutrients. 2012;4:1399–13440.
15. Franco R, Schoneveld OJ, Pappa A, Panayiotidis MI. The central role of glutathione in the pathophysiology of human diseases. Arch Physiol Biochem. 2007;113:234–58.
16. Mainwood GW, Renaud JM. The effect of acid–base balance on fatigue of skeletal muscle. Can J Physiol Pharmacol. 1985;63:403–16.
17. Fogh-Andersen N, Altura BM, Altura BT, Siggaard-Andersen O. Composition of interstitial fluid. Clin Chem. 1995;41:1522–5.
18. Aukland K, Fadnes HO. Protein concentration of interstitial fluid collected from rat skin by a wick method. Acta Physiol Scand. 1973;88:350–8.
19. Brooks GA. The lactate shuttle during exercise and recovery. Med Sci Sports Exerc. 1986;18:360–8.
20. Bangsbo J, Aagaard T, Olsen M, Kiens B, Turcotte LP, Richter EA. Lactate and H+ uptake in inactive muscles during intense exercise in man. J Physiol. 1995;488:219–29.
21. Juel C, Halestrap AP. Lactate transport in skeletal muscle - role and regulation of the monocarboxylate transporter. J Physiol. 1999;517:633–42.
22. Wahrenberg H, Bolinder J, Arner P. Adrenergic regulation of lipolysis in human fat cells during exercise. Eur J Clin Invest. 1991;21:534–41.
23. Sahlin K, Harris RC. Control of lipid oxidation during exercise: role of energy state and mitochondrial factors. Acta Physiol (Oxf). 2008;194:283–91.
24. Calvo JA, Daniels TG, Wang X, Paul A, Lin J, Spiegelman BM, et al. Muscle-specific expression of PPAR-gamma coactivator-1alpha improves exercise performance and increases peak oxygen uptake. J Appl Physiol (1985). 2008;104:1304–12.
25. Tadaishi M, Miura S, Kai Y, Kano Y, Oishi Y, Ezaki O. Skeletal muscle-specific expression of PGC-1α-b, an exercise-responsive isoform, increases exercise capacity and peak oxygen uptake. PLoS One. 2011;6:e28290.
26. Zechner C, Lai L, Zechner JF, Geng T, Yan Z, Rumsey JW, et al. Total skeletal muscle PGC-1 deficiency uncouples mitochondrial derangements from fiber type determination and insulin sensitivity. Cell Metab. 2010;12:633–42.
27. Lee WJ, Kim M, Park HS, Kim HS, Jeon MJ, Oh KS, et al. AMPK activation increases fatty acid oxidation in skeletal muscle by activating PPARalpha and PGC-1. Biochem Biophys Res Commun. 2006;340:291–5.
28. Terada S, Goto M, Kato M, Kawanaka K, Shimokawa T, Tabata I. Effects of low-intensity prolonged exercise on PGC-1 mRNA expression in rat epitrochlearis muscle. Biochem Biophys Res Commun. 2002;296:350–4.
29. Ristow M, Zarse K, Oberbach A, Klöting N, Birringer M, Kiehntopf M, et al. Antioxidants prevent health-promoting effects of physical exercise in humans. Proc Natl Acad Sci USA. 2009;106:8665–70.
30. Gomez-Cabrera MC, Domenech E, Romagnoli M, Arduini A, Borras C, Pallardo FV, et al. Oral administration of vitamin C decreases muscle mitochondrial biogenesis and hampers training-induced adaptations in endurance performance. Am J Clin Nutr. 2008;87:142–9.

## 11

Acute and chronic safety and efficacy of dose dependent creatine nitrate supplementation and exercise performance

Elfego Galvan[1], Dillon K. Walker[2], Sunday Y. Simbo[2], Ryan Dalton[1], Kyle Levers[1], Abigail O'Connor[1], Chelsea Goodenough[1], Nicholas D. Barringer[3], Mike Greenwood[1], Christopher Rasmussen[1], Stephen B. Smith[4], Steven E. Riechman[5], James D. Fluckey[6], Peter S. Murano[7], Conrad P. Earnest[8] and Richard B. Kreider[1*]

Abstract

Background: Creatine monohydrate (CrM) and nitrate are popular supplements for improving exercise performance; yet have not been investigated in combination. We performed two studies to determine the safety and exercise performance-characteristics of creatine nitrate (CrN) supplementation.

Methods: Study 1 participants ($N = 13$) ingested 1.5 g CrN (CrN-Low), 3 g CrN (CrN-High), 5 g CrM or a placebo in a randomized, crossover study (7d washout) to determine supplement safety (hepatorenal and muscle enzymes, heart rate, blood pressure and side effects) measured at time-0 (unsupplemented), 30-min, and then hourly for 5-h post-ingestion. Study 2 participants ($N = 48$) received the same CrN treatments vs. 3 g CrM in a randomized, double-blind, 28d trial inclusive of a 7-d interim testing period and loading sequence (4 servings/d). Day-7 and d-28 measured Tendo™ bench press performance, Wingate testing and a 6x6-s bicycle ergometer sprint. Data were analyzed using a GLM and results are reported as mean ± SD or mean change ± 95 % CI.

Results: In both studies we observed several significant, yet stochastic changes in blood markers that were not indicative of potential harm or consistent for any treatment group. Equally, all treatment groups reported a similar number of minimal side effects. In Study 2, there was a significant increase in plasma nitrates for both CrN groups by d-7, subsequently abating by d-28. Muscle creatine increased significantly by d-7 in the CrM and CrN-High groups, but then decreased by d-28 for CrN-High. By d-28, there were significant increases in bench press lifting volume (kg) for all groups (PLA, 126.6, 95 % CI 26.3, 226.8; CrM, 194.1, 95 % CI 89.0, 299.2; CrN-Low, 118.3, 95 % CI 26.1, 210.5; CrN-High, 267.2, 95 % CI 175.0, 359.4, kg). Only the CrN-High group was significantly greater than PLA ($p < 0.05$). Similar findings were observed for bench press peak power (PLA, 59.0, 95 % CI 4.5, 113.4; CrM, 68.6, 95 % CI 11.4, 125.8; CrN-Low, 40.9, 95 % CI −9.2, 91.0; CrN-High, 60.9, 95 % CI 10.8, 111.1, W) and average power.

Conclusions: Creatine nitrate delivered at 3 g was well-tolerated, demonstrated similar performance benefits to 3 g CrM, in addition, within the confines of this study, there were no safety concerns.

Keywords: Creatine, Nitrate, Creatine nitrate, Nutrition, Supplementation, Exercise performance

* Correspondence: rkreider@hlkn.tamu.edu
[1]Department of Health and Kinesiology, Exercise and Sport Nutrition Laboratory, Texas A&M University, College Station, TX 77843-4243, USA
Full list of author information is available at the end of the article

Background

Numerous nutrition supplements have been investigated to determine their ergogenic benefits related to exercise performance. Two supplements that are currently popular in the marketplace are creatine and nitrate. Creatine has been extensively researched and has been the subject of numerous reviews and position statements attesting to its efficacy and safety in sport and in health [5, 7, 8]. It has been well established that supplementation with creatine can increase strength performance and improve overall body anthropometry via a reduction in percent body fat and increased fat-free mass [5]. Recently, dietary nitrate ingestion has gained in popularity as a means of improving endurance performance.

Inorganic nitrate (NO_3^-) is an ion exhibiting limited synthesis in the body, therefore usually obtained from the diet via green leafy vegetables, while nitrites (NO_2^-) are also found in food as processing additives, but to a much lesser degree [13]. The ingestion of nitrate have demonstrated its importance to health in that nitrate and nitrite can be reduced to nitric oxide, which has shown to have numerous physiologic effects in exercise and health [16, 17, 19]. While extensive reviews are available elsewhere, nitrate ingestion has been shown to reduce the oxygen cost of exercise and improve exercise tolerance [22, 24]. For example, Larsen et al., reported a reduction in maximal oxygen consumption; yet a trend for improvement in time-to-exhaustion accompanying the ingestion of sodium nitrate intake at 0.1 mmol/kg/day for three days [22]. In a similar study by the same group, investigators reported a significant reduction in oxygen consumption and improvement in gross efficiency at sub-maximal workloads using the same ingestion schema [24]. Bescos et al., (2011) investigated the impact of sodium nitrate in highly trained cyclist and triathletes and found that the consumption of 10 mg/kg prior to a cycle ergometer test reduced VO_{2peak} without influencing time to exhaustion or maximal power output [3]. Further research has elaborated on these findings, showing a reduction in the amplitude of the VO_2 slow component; hence an improvement in muscle efficiency associated with nitrate ingestion [2, 18].

Despite the number of studies associated with endurance performance, a dearth of literature exists examining nitrate supplementation on strength performance; and no studies that we are aware of have examined the role of creatine and nitrate in combination. However, the two nutrients have the potential to work synergistically. The primary aim of our current study was to examine the effects of creatine nitrate (CrN) in a two-phase, dose dependent study administering CrN at 1.5 g (CrN-Low) and 3 g (CrN-High). Study 1 of our trial examined the acute ingestion of the respective treatments for five hours following ingestion. Study 2 of our trial examined

each respective treatment for 28 days. Each CrN condition was compared to a placebo (PLA) and creatine monohydrate (CrM) treatment condition. We hypothesized that CrN would increase exercise performance and related performance indices (e.g., peak power, mean power, total work, etc.) in a dose dependent manner and be equal in effectiveness to CrM. We further hypothesized that CrN ingestion would not adversely affect hepatorenal function or hemodynamics indices following acute and chronic ingestion.

Methods

The current report represents studies examining the [1] acute and [2] chronic supplementation of a CrN formula. Study 1 was an acute phase study with participants ingesting each respective supplement one time in a randomized, double blind, crossover manner. Study 2 was a 28-d study using different participants receiving treatments in a randomized, double blind manner. Figure 1 presents a CONSORT schematic for Study 1 (Fig. 1a) and Study 2 (Fig. 1b). Each study was performed at the Exercise & Sport Nutrition Laboratory (ESNL) at Texas A&M University after obtaining ethical approval from the university's ethics committee and signed informed consent from each participant. Herein we describe our overall procedures for each study followed by a detailed methodology for each test used within the studies (see below, Testing Methodology).

STUDY ONE: acute supplementation
Participants

Thirteen healthy and recreationally active men (age: 22 ± 5 y, height: 177.8 ± 7.4 cm, weight: 84.1 ± 18.9 kg) were recruited to participate in Study 1. Inclusion criteria required that each participant have at least 6 mo. of resistance training immediately prior to entering the study inclusive of performing bench press and leg press or squats. Participants were excluded if they had a history of treatment for metabolic disease, hypertension, thyroid disease, arrhythmias, cardiovascular disease; currently using any prescription medication, or had ingested creatine within 6 wk of the intervention. Further exclusion criteria also included women; a history of smoking; and excessive alcohol consumption (>12 drinks/wk).

Familiarization session

Each participant initiated Study 1 by participating in a familiarization session and was assessed for standard anthropological measurements including height, weight, blood pressure, and heart rate. Participants also completed a general health screening form that was reviewed by a registered nurse. Prior to baseline testing, each participant completed a dietary record to include three weekdays and one weekend day.

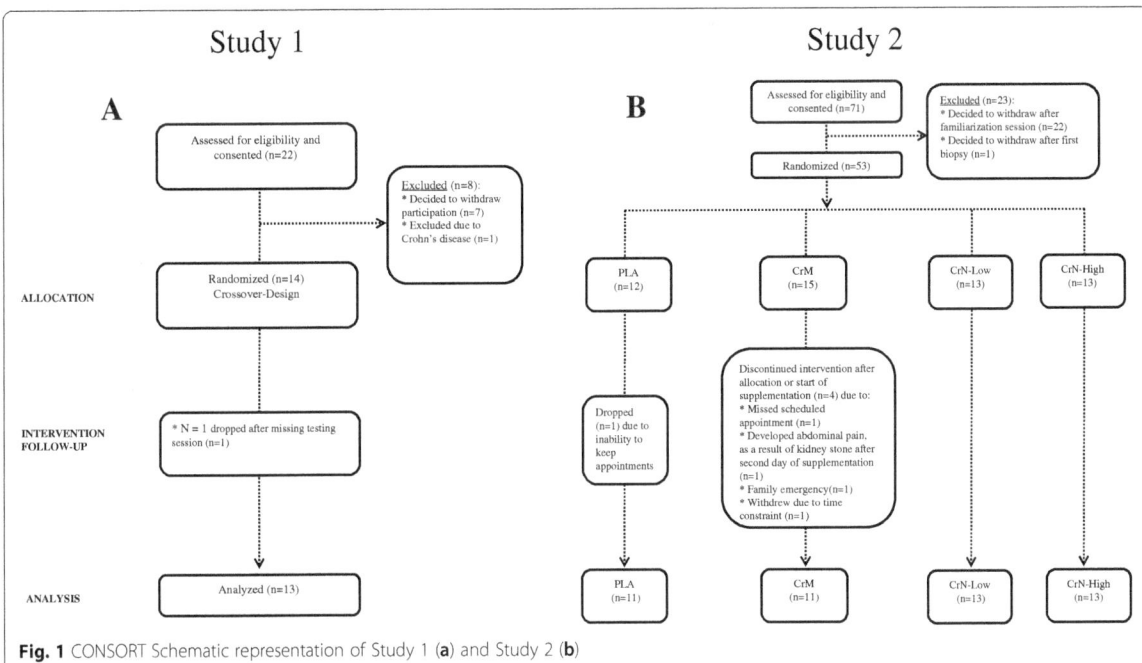

Fig. 1 CONSORT Schematic representation of Study 1 (**a**) and Study 2 (**b**)

Testing procedures

Participants were instructed to refrain from drinking alcohol, exercise, and non-steroidal anti-inflammatory drugs (NSAIDs) for 48 h before testing. Testing was initiated by obtaining participant weight, body composition measure (DXA), resting blood pressure (BP), and resting heart rate (HR). Participants were then fitted with an indwelling catheter for collection of a 20 mL blood sample at time-0 prior to supplement ingestion.

Supplementation and assessment protocol

Upon completion of the pre-supplementation procedures, each participant was randomized in a counterbalanced manner to ingest their respective supplements providing 6.5 g total ingredients per dose. Treatments consisted of a [1] placebo (PLA: 6.5 g dextrose), [2] creatine monohydrate (CrM, 5 g creatine monohydrate, 1.5 g dextrose), [3] CrN-Low (1.5 g creatine nitrate, 5 g dextrose) or [4] CrN-High (3 g creatine nitrate, 3.5 g dextrose). All supplements were provided by Nutrabolt (Bryan, TX). Following the ingestion of each respective supplement, participants were placed into a semi-recumbent position where HR and BP were measured and blood was drawn in regular time increments of 30 min and then 1–5 h on the hour. All blood samples were analyzed for standard blood chemistries to assess hepatorenal and muscle enzyme function, as well as glucose, and blood lipids. A complete blood count with platelet differential was measured in addition to determining plasma nitrate and nitrite levels. All treatment

assessments were separated by at least a 7-d washout period.

STUDY TWO: chronic supplementation
Participants

Forty-eight, healthy and recreationally active males volunteered to participate in Study 2 (age: 21 ± 3 y, height: 176.8 ± 5.8 cm, weight: 77.4 ± 20.9 kg). Baseline testing followed a similar pattern to Study 1. Participants also were asked to follow a standardized resistance-training program 2 wk before their baseline testing session (d-0) that was continued throughout the supplementation period. Participants were further requested not to change their dietary intake throughout the investigation.

Familiarization testing

During the familiarization period, testing procedures were initiated by explaining measurements for body composition measurements, blood collection, biopsies, and exercise testing. Participants also completed a 1-repetition maximum (1RM) bench press test and a practice anaerobic sprint test on a cycle ergometer. The strength test and anaerobic capacity procedures are explained in greater detail below. Strength tests were performed using a standardized isotonic lifting protocol on an Olympic bench press [21]. Participants then were scheduled to return to the laboratory and were requested to start a standardized resistance-training program 2 wk before their baseline laboratory visit. After the baseline testing session (d-0) for Study 2 participants were assigned randomly to one of the four treatment groups, providing 5.5 g total ingredients per dose. In Study 2, participants were assigned randomly to [1] PLA (5 g dextrose, 0.5 g flavoring), [2] CrM (3 g CrM, 0.5 g flavoring, 2 g dextrose), [3] CrN-Low (1.5 g CrN, 0.5 g flavoring, 3.5 g dextrose), and [4] CrN-High (3 g CrN, 0.5 g flavoring, 2 g dextrose). Exercise testing occurred on baseline (d-0) and d-28.

Testing procedures

Participants arrived at the laboratory on the day before baseline testing, at baseline (d-0), d-7, d-27, and d-28 for a total of five laboratory visits. Percutaneous muscle biopsies from the *vastus lateralis* occurred on the day before baseline testing, d-7, and d-27 using a modified Bergstrom needle biopsy technique following standard procedures and subsequently examined for creatine concentrations [10]. Participants were requested to fast for 12 h and refrain from exercise, alcohol, and NSAIDs consumption for 48 h prior to baseline, d-7, and d-28 testing. Participants turned in their food records upon arrival to the lab at baseline, d-7, and d-28. Participants were weighed and body composition was determined via a DXA scan. Total body water was measured via bioelectrical impedance analysis (BIA). A fasted blood sample was collected after determining body composition. On d-7, participants completed the testing session with a muscle biopsy. At baseline and d-28, after the blood sample collection, participants continued with the exercise tests, which consisted of a bench press test and an anaerobic sprint test. Following their respective treatment assignment, participants were requested to ingest four doses of their respective supplements per day (at approximately 0800, 1200, 1600, and 2000 h.) for the first 7-d. Thereafter, participants ingested supplements one time per day for the remainder of the study (d 8–28). Nutrabolt (Bryan, TX) provided all of the supplements for this study.

A side effect questionnaire was completed weekly for the duration of the study. The questionnaires were completed to determine how well participants tolerated supplementation; how well participants followed the supplementation protocol; and if participants experienced any symptoms as a result of the supplement. Supplement logs and verbal confirmation were used to monitor compliance to the supplementation protocol. After completing the first performance testing session at baseline, participants were given their required supplements and written directions on how to properly ingest the supplements during the supplementation period. Participants also engaged in a standardized, 4 d/wk, split routine, encompassing upper and lower body workouts

for a total of 6 wk. Training logs were completed and maintained by each participant to detail each training session workload. A training partner or fitness instructor monitored the training sessions to verify each session was completed.

Testing methodology
Anaerobic capacity

After completion of the third bench press set, participants rested for ~5 min before starting the anaerobic sprint test on a Lode Excalibur Sport 925900 cycle ergometer (Lode BV, Groningen, The Netherlands). The anaerobic sprint test consisted of a 3-min warm-up comprised of pedaling at 60 – 70 rpm against a resistance of 50 W for the first minute, 75 W for the second minute, and 100 W for the third minute. The test consisted of six sprints, lasting 6-sec each, interspersed with a 30-sec rest between each repetition. Participants were then allowed to rest for 3 min before initiating a Wingate test. Participants practiced the anaerobic sprint test during the familiarization session. They were given detailed instructions and verbal encouragement to pedal as fast as possible, at an 'all out' pace at each sprint during the anaerobic sprint test.

During the six, 6-sec sprints and the Wingate test (30-sec sprint), each participant pedaled, all out, against a standard workload of 7.5 J/kg/rev on the Lode ergometer. To initiate the test, we instructed each individual to pedal as fast as possible, at an 'all out' pace prior to application of the workload and then sprint as fast as possible (all out) for the duration of each sprint. Test-to-test variability in performing repeated Wingate anaerobic capacity tests in our lab have yielded correlation coefficients of $r = 0.98 \pm 15 \%$ for mean power. Following each test, we recorded the seat height, pedal position, and handlebar height to use for each testing session.

Anthropometry

Standardized anthropological testing included assessments for body mass and height on a calibrated scale (Cardinal Detecto Scale Model 8430, Webb City, MO) and body composition via DXA (excluding cranium; Hologic Inc., Waltham, MA). Test/retest reliability studies performed on male athletes with DXA yielded mean deviation for total bone miner content and total fat-free/soft tissue mass of 0.31-0.45 %, with a mean intra-class correlation of 0.985 [1].

Blood collection procedures

Participants provided a (8 h) fasted blood sample via venipuncture, using intravenous (IV) catheterization (BD Insyte Autoguard, Bection, Dickinson and Company, Franklin Lakes, NJ) from the antecubital vein in the forearm according to standard phlebotomy procedures.

Approximately 20 mL of whole blood was collected at each time point (i.e., 0 [unsupplemented], 0.5, 1, 2, 3, 4, 5 h) in three, pre-chilled, 10-mL (18 mg K_2 ethylene-diaminetera-acetic acid) tubes (BD Hemogard, Franklin Lakes, New Jersey). The 10-mL EDTA tubes were pre-chilled on ice and immediately placed back on ice after each blood sampling period. Two collection tubes were centrifuged at 3000 x g for 10 min at 4 °C within 3 min of collection. Plasma was extracted and stored at −80 °C for later analysis. The third collection tube was stored at 4 °C for approximately 5 h and analyzed for a complete blood count with platelet differential.

Blood chemistry

All blood samples were analyzed for standard blood chemistries inclusive of alkaline phosphatase (ALP), aspartate transaminase (AST), alanine transaminase (ALT), creatinine, blood urea nitrogen (BUN), creatine kinase (CK), lactate dehydrogenase (LDH), glucose, and blood lipids (total cholesterol, high density lipoprotein [HDL], low density lipoprotein [LDL], triglycerides [TG] using a Cobas® c 111 (Roche Diagnostics, Basel, Switzerland).

The Cobas® automated clinical chemistry analyzer was calibrated according to manufacturer guidelines. This analyzer has been known to be valid and reliable in previously published reports [15]. The internal quality control for the Cobas c 111 was performed using two levels of control fluids purchased from the manufacturer to calibrate acceptable SD and coefficients of variation (C_V) values for all aforementioned assays. Samples were re-run if the observed values were outside control values and/or clinical norms according to standard procedures. Participants were also given questionnaires at each time point of the study to assess how well participants tolerated supplementation, how well participants followed the supplementation protocol, and if participants experienced any symptoms as a result of the supplementation.

A complete blood count with platelet differential (hemoglobin, hematocrit, red blood cell counts, MCV, MCH, MCHC, RDW, white blood cell counts, lymphocytes, granulocytes, and mid-range absolute count (MID) was measured using a Abbott Cell Dyn 1800 (Abbott Laboratories, Abbott Park, IL, USA) automated hematology analyzer. The internal quality control for Abbott Cell Dyn 1800 was performed using three levels of control fluids purchased from manufacturer to calibrate acceptable SD and C_V values for all whole blood cell parameters. Calorimetric assay kits were used to measure plasma creatine (Sigma-Aldrich, St. Louis, MO) and plasma nitrate (Cayman Chemical, Ann Arbor, MI) concentrations. These assays yielded mean C_V value for

plasma nitrate (±3.21 %) and plasma creatine (±6.66 %) with a test/retest correlation of $r = 0.98$ and $r = 0.99$ for plasma nitrate and creatine, respectively.

Food frequency

A registered dietitian collected all food logs and analyzed the results using dietary analysis software (ESHA Food Processor Version 8.6, Salem, OR). Participants were asked to record all food and beverage consumption for three days and one weekend day prior to each testing session during Study 1 and prior to baseline, d-7, and d-28 during Study 2.

Muscle biopsies

During the study, we collected and analyzed muscle biopsy samples to assay for creatine concentration. All samples were collected while the participant was in the supine position, where the region around the biopsy site was shaved and sterilized with 3 povidone-iodine swab sticks (Professional Disposables International, Inc., Orangeburg, NY). Lidocaine HCl (1 %) was injected underneath the skin, followed by an injection through the fascia and to the epidermis using a 10 mL syringe to anesthetize the biopsy region. After approximately 5 – 10 min a small incision of about 0.5 cm was made at the biopsy site using a sterile scalpel (Aspen Surgical, Caledonia, MI). Pressure was applied with sterile gauze after the incision was made. A 5 mm biopsy needle was inserted into the incision and into the 'belly' of the vastus lateralis muscle. Once the biopsy needle was pushed through the fascia and settled into the correct location suction was applied using 60 mL syringe, a small muscle sample was collected with the biopsy needle. The biopsy needle was in the muscle for approximately 5 – 20 sec until the procedure was completed.

After the biopsy was obtained, the sample was removed from the needle by forcing air through the syringe connected to the biopsy needle. The muscle was quickly blotted on a sterile cover sponge to remove excess blood and then snap frozen into liquid nitrogen. The sample was then stored at −80 °C for later analysis. Immediately following the biopsy procedure, pressure was applied for at least 10 min to the incision site to halt bleeding. After bleeding had stopped, steristrips (3 M Health Care, St. Paul, MN) were applied to ensure closure of the incision. A tegaderm film (3 M Health Care, St. Paul, MN) was placed over the steristrips, followed by gauze and a self-adherent pressure bandage. Participants were provided with a biopsy care kit including multiple steristrips, tegaderm films, and the contact information of the study coordinator.

Muscle creatine analysis

Muscle samples were analyzed using mass spectrophotometer for muscle creatine (Cr). Samples were analyzed based on methods developed by Harris and colleagues [11, 12, 14]. The previously stored muscle samples were placed in a vacuum centrifuge (Jouan RC1010 SpeedVac Concentrator, Abbott Laboratories, Abbott Park, IL) and centrifuged for approximately 4 h. Following the dehydration process, the samples were powdered using a mortar and pestle and then placed into pre-weight microcentrifuge tubes. Perchloric acid (0.5 M) and a 1 mM ethylenediaminetetraacetic acid (EDTA) solution were used to extract the muscle metabolites. The acid solution was added to microcentrifuge tubes containing the powered muscle. Microcentrifuge tubes were placed on ice for 15 min with periodic vortexing. Samples were centrifuged at 5,000 rpm for 5 min. The supernatant was transferred into a pre-weighed microcentrifuge tube. A 2.1 M $KHCO_3$ solution was used to neutralize the samples. The samples were then centrifuged a second time at 5,000 rpm for 5 min. The supernatant was removed and placed into a label microcentrifuge tube and stored at −80 °C.

The samples were thawed at room temperature with periodic vortexing. Extracts were assayed for Cr in presence of 50 mM imidazole buffer, pH 7.4; 5 mM magnesium chloride; 20 mM potassium chloride; 25 μM phosphoenolpyruvate; 200 μM ATP; 45 μM NADH; 1250 U/mL lactate dehydrogenase; and 2,000 U/mL pyruvate kinase. The reagents were individually added into 1.5 mL cuvettes. The assay was then carried out using 200 μL buffer, 100 μL potassium chloride, 25 μL NADH, 20 μL ATP, 10 μL phosphoenolpyruvate, 2 μL pyruvate kinase, 2 μL lactate dehydrogenase, 150 μL water, and 100 μL of muscle extract. Changes in absorbance were recorded with a Beckman Coulter DU 7400 Diode Array Spectrophotometer (Brea, California, USA) at a wavelength of 339 nm. 20 μL of creatine kinase (25 U/mg) was added after the initial reading. The solution was read every 5 min for 20 min for post-reaction absorbance values. Test-to-test assay variability yielded mean C_V values for muscle creatine (±3.69 %) with a test/retest correlation of $r = 0.946$.

Side effects

The side effects questionnaire was completed after each post-supplementation blood sampling period during Study 1 (acute supplementation). In other words, during Study 1, a side effects questionnaire was completed at 0.5, 1, 2, 3, 4, and 5 h post-supplementation. During Study 2 (chronic supplementation), a side effects questionnaire was completed weekly, at d-7, d-14, d-21, and d-28 of supplementation. The questionnaire was completed to determine how well participants tolerated supplementation; how well participants followed the supplementation protocol; and if participants experienced any adverse symptoms during the supplementation period. Participants were asked to rank the frequency and severity of their symptoms – dizziness, headache, tachycardia, heart skipping or palpitations, shortness of breath, nervousness, blurred vision, and unusual or adverse effects. Participants were requested to rank their symptoms with 0 (none), 1 (minimal: 1-2/wk), 2 (slight: 3-4/wk), 3 (occasional: 5-6/wk), 4 (frequent: 7-8/wk), or 5 (severe: 9 or more/wk).

Strength testing and bench press test

Strength testing was performed on a bench press during the familiarization session when participants completed a 1-repetition maximum (1RM) using standardized isotonic Olympic bench press procedure [21]. Participants warmed-up by performing 10 repetitions at 50 % of their estimated 1RM, 5 repetitions using 70 % of their estimated 1RM, and 1 repetition using 90 % of their estimated 1RM. One RM was determined within 5, one-repetition sets following the warm-up. Our bench press procedures show low day-to-day mean coefficients of variation and high reliability in our lab (1.1 %, intraclass, $r = 0.99$). Bench press testing was performed at baseline and d-28. The bench press test, which only took place at baseline and d-28, consisted of three total sets using a 70 % 1RM load. Two sets of ten repetitions followed by one set of repetitions to failure were performed. Participants had a 2-min rest period between sets. Peak power, average power, and average velocity were measured during each repetition of the three sets with a Tendo Fitrodyne.

Strength training procedures

All participants were required to follow the same resistance training routine. The resistance training routine consisted of exercise 4 d/wk split into two upper and two lower body workouts per week for a total of 6 wk. The 6 wk training protocol was periodized in 3 wk increments consisting of selected exercises for the following muscle groups. Upper body training consisted of two chest exercises, two back exercises, one shoulder exercise, one biceps exercise, one triceps exercise, and one abdominal exercise. Lower body training consisted of two-quadriceps exercises, two hamstring exercises, and one calf exercise. Each exercise consisted of three sets of 10 repetitions (wk 1–3) or 8 repetitions (wk 4–6) performed with as much weight as the participant could perform per set. Individual training logs were maintained throughout the intervention and a training partner or fitness instructor confirmed completion of each training session.

Supplementation protocol

Participants were assigned in a double-blind and counter-balanced manner to ingest [1] PLA (5 g dextrose, 0.5 g flavoring), [2] CrM (3 g CrM, 0.5 g flavoring, 2 g dextrose), [3] CrN-Low (1.5 g CrN, 0.5 g flavoring, 3.5 g dextrose), and [4] CrN-High (3 g CrN, 0.5 g flavoring, 2 g dextrose). Participants were asked to ingest 4 doses per day (at approximately 0800, 1200, 1600, and 2000 h) during the loading phase (d-0 [after baseline testing session] through d-7). During the loading phase participants ingested a total of [1] PLA (26 g dextrose/d), [2] CrM (12 g CrM + 2 g flavoring + 8 g dextrose/d), [3] CrN-Low (6 g CrN + 2 g flavoring + 14 g dextrose/d), and [4] CrN-High (12 g CrN + 2 g flavoring + 8 g dextrose/d). Thereafter, participants ingested supplements one dose daily at 0800 (maintenance phase) for the remainder of the study (d-8 – d-28). During the maintenance phase participants ingested a daily total of [1] PLA (6.5 g dextrose), [2], CrM (3 g CrM + 0.5 g flavoring + 2 g dextrose), [3] CrN-Low (1.5 g CrN + 0.5 g flavoring + 3.5 g dextrose), [4] CrN-High (3 g CrN + 0.5 flavoring + 2 g dextrose). Participants were instructed to take the supplements at the assigned time and to take it as soon as possible if the proper timing was missed. All supplements were provided by Nutrabolt (Bryan, TX).

Total body water

Total body water was determined under standardized conditions using an ImpediMed DF50 bioelectrical impedance analyzer (BIA, ImpediMed, San Diego, CA, USA). Participants were stationed in a supine position with four electrodes placed on the wrists and ankles. Bioelectrical impedance analysis has been shown to be a valid method of determining total body water [29].

Statistical analysis
Data analysis

Prior to initiation of the study, we ran a priori power analysis, which indicated the appropriate sample size estimates for Study 1 and Study 2. All statistical analysis was completed utilizing SPSS 22.0 (IBM Statistics, Chicago, IL). Study data were analyzed using a repeated measured multivariate analysis of variance (MANOVA). Delta and percent change values were calculated and used to determine changes from baseline, which were analyzed by repeated measures analysis of variance (ANOVA). Participant baseline demographic data were analyzed using one-way ANOVA. Overall MANOVA effects were examined as well as MANOVA univariate group effects for certain variables when significant interactions were seen. Greenhouse-Geisser univariate tests of within-subjects time and group x time effects and between-subjects univariate group effects were reported for each variable analyzed within the MANOVA model. Data were considered statistically significant when the probability of type I error was 0.05 or less and statistical trends were considered when the probability of error ranged between $p > 0.05$ to $p < 0.10$. When a significant group, treatment and/or interaction alpha level was observed, Tukey's least significant difference post-hoc analysis was performed to determine where significance was obtained. Lastly, we performed an analysis for relevant clinical chemistries denoting lipids, glucose, muscle and hepatorenal enzyme function changes exceeding normal clinical limits concordant to supplementation for changes from (a) baseline to d-7, (b) baseline to d-28, and (c) d-7 to d-28 using chi-square analyses. Data are presented as mean ± SD, mean change ± 95 % confidence intervals as appropriate and frequency for chi-square analyses.

Results
Study 1: acute supplementation

Twenty-two participants were initially recruited for Study 1, and all completed consent forms, and participated in the required familiarization session. Of the original 22 participants, 13 completed Study 1 (Fig. 1). Seven participants dropped out after the familiarization session due to time constraints and one participant did not pass medical screening due to Crohn's disease. One participant was excluded after being randomized into a treatment group due to missing scheduled testing sessions. None of the participants dropped out of the study due to side effects related to the study protocol or supplementation.

Plasma creatine and nitrate

Figure 2 shows the plasma creatine area under the curve (AUC) after acute supplementation. The plasma creatine AUC for CrM (5,634.4 ± 1,949.8 μmol/L) was significantly greater than PLA (1,012.4 ± 1,882.2 μmol/L, $p = 0.001$), CrN-Low (2,342.0 ± 3,133.3 μmol/L, $p = 0.004$), and CrN-High (1,761.7 ± 3,408.8 μmol/L, $p = 0.007$). There were no significant differences in plasma creatine AUC among PLA, CrN-Low, and CrN-High. Figure 2 also shows the plasma nitrate AUC after acute supplementation. The plasma nitrate AUC for CrN-High (1,988.2 ± 1,618.8 μmol/L) was significantly greater than CrM (48.0 ± 73.1 μmol/L, $p = 0.001$) and PLA (51.4 ± 83.4 μmol/L, $p = 0.001$), but not significantly different than CrN-Low (898.8 ± 1,688.9 μmol/L, $p = 0.10$). Although there was a trend towards a greater AUC with CrN-Low there was no significant difference compared to PLA ($p = 0.099$) or CrM ($p = 0.091$).

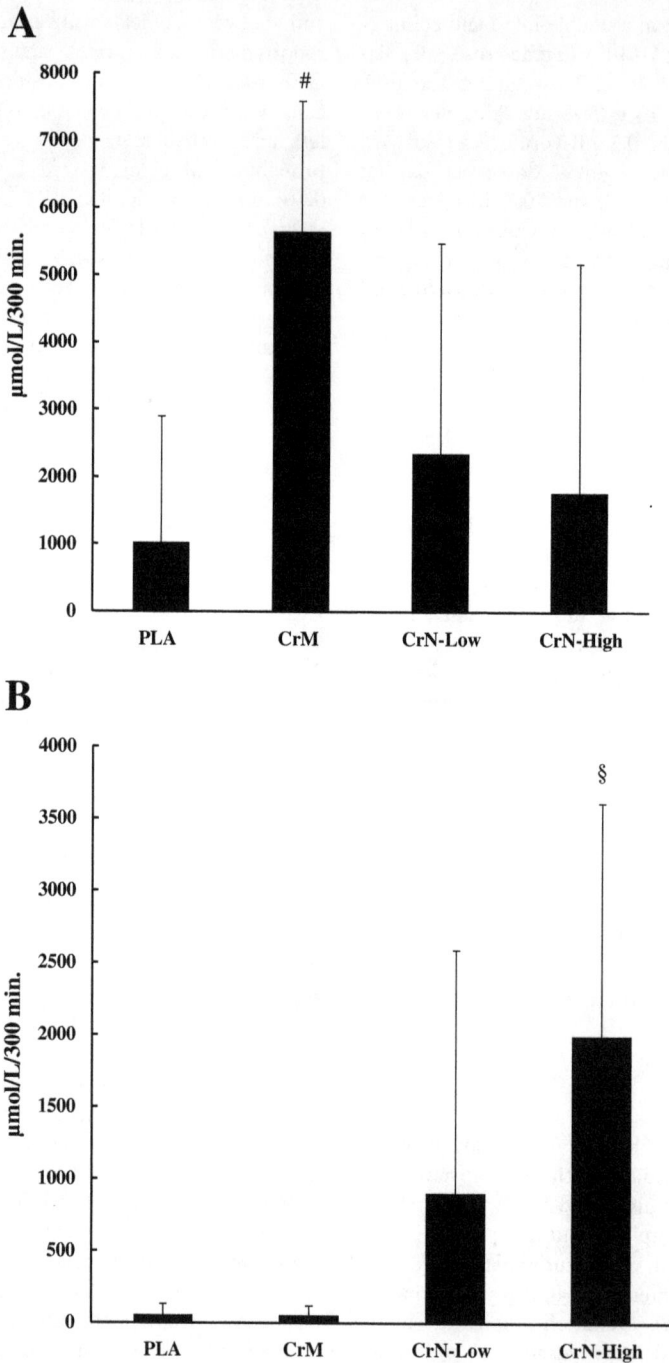

Fig. 2 Data represent mean ± SD plasma creatine (**a**) and plasma nitrate (**b**) area-under-the-curve over 5 h post ingestion. Statistical notations ($p < 0.05$ considered significant): (#) denotes a significant difference from PLA, CrN-Low, and CrN-High. (§) denotes a significant difference from PLA and CrM

Hematologic profile

Findings for participant hepatorenal muscle enzymes, and lipids are presented in Table 1. There were no significant time effects for AST ($p = 0.12$), CK ($p = 0.06$), and LDH ($p = 0.40$). However, there were significant time effects for ALP ($p < 0.001$), ALT ($p = 0.001$), BUN ($p < 0.001$),

Table 1 Hemodynamic and hematological response to supplementation for Study 1

| Group | Time (hours) | | | | | | | Interaction | p-Level |
	0	0.5	1	2	3	4	5		
Hemodynamics									
HR									
(b/min)									
PLA	59.7 ± 8.2	60.1 ± 7.4	58.8 ± 7.7	57.2 ± 5.3	58.0 ± 7.4	54.8 ± 6.4	56.0 ± 7.3	Group	0.23
CrM	63.8 ± 11.8	60.9 ± 5.7	59.9 ± 8.2	58.2 ± 7.0	56.3 ± 6.8	59.6 ± 8.8	58.5 ± 10.0	Time	0.15
CrN-Low	60.0 ± 8.4	57.9 ± 8.3	58.8 ± 9.0	56.3 ± 6.0	56.3 ± 6.0	56.9 ± 5.7	55.1 ± 5.9	Group × Time	0.59
CrN-High	59.1 ± 9.0	56.7 ± 7.4	57.9 ± 5.8	58.6 ± 3.8	58.0 ± 4.1	56.8 ± 4.7	57.5 ± 3.8		
Systolic BP									
(mm Hg)									
PLA	114.8 ± 6.2	113.9 ± 5.6	112.6 ± 4.9	116.5 ± 6.7	116.0 ± 4.8	117.2 ± 8.5	115.5 ± 5.2	Group	0.37
CrM	114.6 ± 5.1	112.6 ± 4.4	112.2 ± 4.2	114.9 ± 5.3	112.9 ± 6.1	113.1 ± 5.8	114.9 ± 3.8	Time	0.02
CrN-Low	115.9 ± 6.1	113.1 ± 4.1	111.9 ± 5.2	113.5 ± 6.9	114.6 ± 6.9	114.62 ± 5.0	112.5 ± 3.5	Group × Time	0.39
CrN-High	115.4 ± 6.7	114.2 ± 5.5	111.4 ± 6.6	112.5 ± 6.0	113.5 ± 6.2	113.7 ± 9.7	114.2 ± 7.0		
Diastolic BP									
(mm Hg)									
PLA	73.1 ± 6.6	71.9 ± 7.5	72.2 ± 6.6	72.3 ± 7.3	73.1 ± 6.6	74.0 ± 5.5	72.3 ± 5.7	Group	0.66
CrM	70.3 ± 6.6	71.5 ± 7.8	72.5 ± 4.1	73.9 ± 5.4	72.8 ± 6.0	73.9 ± 5.0	74.5 ± 4.0	Time	0.29
CrN-Low	72.2 ± 6.5	73.5 ± 5.4	71.9 ± 6.1	75.5 ± 5.4	74.3 ± 6.2	74.5 ± 4.6	73.1 ± 4.1	Group × Time	0.18
CrN-High	73.1 ± 7.9	77.1 ± 4.8	73.9 ± 6.5	74.5 ± 5.2	73.7 ± 6.1	72.2 ± 7.9	72.9 ± 4.8		
Lipids									
Total-C									
(mg/dl)									
PLA	153.8 ± 28.4	156.2 ± 31.1	161.0 ± 31.8	162.5 ± 32.9	164.5 ± 31.2	164.6 ± 36.7	165.0 ± 36.1	Group	0.59
CrM	156.8 ± 29.3	157.2 ± 29.3	160.7 ± 34.3	157.2 ± 31.4	159.3 ± 30.4	160.3 ± 32.8	160.2 ± 28.3	Time	0.06
CrN-Low	154.5 ± 27.6	154.2 ± 28.0	155.7 ± 31.7	156.0 ± 27.8	158.6 ± 28.9	158.5 ± 26.8	159.5 ± 27.9	Group × Time	0.77
CrN-High	158.3 ± 30.0	163.2 ± 27.0	162.3 ± 32.6	159.9 ± 26.9	163.9 ± 32.6	162.9 ± 26.8	163.5 ± 27.9		
HDL-C									
(mg/dl)									
PLA	55.8 ± 15.3	58.2 ± 15.6	58.8 ± 17.4	59.9 ± 16.1	61.0 ± 15.7	61.6 ± 17.0	62.2 ± 17.9	Group	0.29
CrM	53.9 ± 17.1	54.1 ± 16.7	55.6 ± 18.4	55.1 ± 17.2	56.0 ± 17.1	56.9 ± 17.6	56.4 ± 18.8	Time	0.001
CrN-Low	51.0 ± 14.1	50.8 ± 15.6	51.2 ± 15.0	52.1 ± 14.9	53.8 ± 14.5	54.9 ± 15.2	55.3 ± 15.8	Group × Time	0.64
CrN-High	52.9 ± 17.5	54.7 ± 17.0	54.2 ± 16.8	54.2 ± 17.3	55.4 ± 16.9	55.2 ± 16.3	55.4 ± 17.7		
Total-C/HDL-C									
Ratio									
(mg/dl)									
PLA	2.9 ± 0.8	2.8 ± 0.8	2.9 ± 0.8	2.8 ± 0.8	2.8 ± 0.8	2.8 ± 0.8	2.8 ± 0.8	Group	0.40
CrM	3.1 ± 1.0	3.1 ± 0.9	3.1 ± 0.9	3.0 ± 0.8	3.0 ± 0.8	3.0 ± 0.8	3.1 ± 0.9	Time	0.09
CrN-Low	3.3 ± 1.2	3.3 ± 1.1	3.3 ± 1.0	3.2 ± 1.0	3.2 ± 1.0	3.1 ± 1.0	3.1 ± 1.0	Group × Time	0.62
CrN-High	3.3 ± 1.4	3.3 ± 1.4	3.3 ± 1.4	3.3 ± 1.4	3.3 ± 1.4	3.3 ± 1.5	3.3 ± 1.5		
LDL-C									
(mg/dl)									
PLA	94.0 ± 26.3	96.5 ± 27.6	98.1 ± 28.1	100.1 ± 29.1	102.4 ± 32.6	102.5 ± 32.3	102.2 ± 32.0	Group	0.72
CrM	99.1 ± 25.6	99.0 ± 24.1	102.5 ± 27.7	101.1 ± 24.7	102.0 ± 23.7	103.8 ± 26.5	102.5 ± 22.9	Time	0.06
CrN-Low	97.2 ± 23.0	97.1 ± 22.4	98.8 ± 24.0	100.0 ± 22.4	102.4 ± 23.1	102.6 ± 21.6	104.4 ± 22.5	Group × Time	0.67
CrN-High	102.7 ± 27.1	105.3 ± 25.8	105.0 ± 29.8	104.1 ± 26.6	101.5 ± 43.7	106.0 ± 27.0	105.4 ± 25.8		
Triglyceride									
PLA	79.2 ± 26.2	82.1 ± 27.9	78.8 ± 24.8	73.9 ± 23.5	72.6 ± 21.0	71.8 ± 22.1	71.1 ± 22.6	Group	0.60

Table 1 Hemodynamic and hematological response to supplementation for Study 1 (Continued)

	Group								Effect	p
(mg/dl)	CrM	90.7 ± 33.1	88.1 ± 34.1	86.6 ± 30.9	76.2 ± 27.3	72.5 ± 25.9	73.7 ± 27.2	68.9 ± 22.6	Time	0.01
	CrN-Low	88.3 ± 36.9	94.5 ± 37.9	90.6 ± 34.7	79.4 ± 25.3	75.4 ± 20.4	73.2 ± 18.3	72.8 ± 17.9	Group × Time	0.66
	CrN-High	79.4 ± 25.6	86.1 ± 34.1	81.8 ± 29.1	73.0 ± 18.3	70.9 ± 19.5	71.9 ± 19.4	70.2 ± 20.3		
Glucose	PLA	95.8 ± 10.3	103.0 ± 10.4	92.1 ± 8.0	92.2 ± 5.5	91.5 ± 4.0	85.9 ± 26.1	91.9 ± 4.3	Group	0.33
(mg/dl)	CrM	96.3 ± 9.9	85.3 ± 27.0	91.4 ± 6.0	89.8 ± 5.1	91.4 ± 5.4	91.6 ± 5.6	91.2 ± 4.9	Time	0.01
	CrN-Low	96.3 ± 5.5	102.6 ± 8.1	94.1 ± 5.9	91.8 ± 6.5	91.2 ± 6.8	92.9 ± 6.7	92.1 ± 6.2	Group × Time	0.12
	CrN-High	94.7 ± 7.5	96.1 ± 6.4	91.4 ± 6.2	91.1 ± 4.0	90.6 ± 5.4	91.3 ± 4.2	83.8 ± 25.3		
Hepatorenal function										
ALP	PLA	7.9 ± 6.5	11.5 ± 8.0	11.9 ± 8.8	13.3 ± 9.1	13.9 ± 9.9	14.3 ± 9.4	16.9 ± 14.1	Group	0.23
(U/L)	CrM	14.7 ± 9.1	15.9 ± 11.7	15.9 ± 10.4	16.8 ± 12.9	20.5 ± 14.4	25.4 ± 15.3	24.6 ± 14.9	Time	0.001
	CrN-Low	12.3 ± 9.3	16.3 ± 10.3	20.3 ± 10.8	18.7 ± 11.5	21.7 ± 10.9	20.6 ± 10.2	22.8 ± 10.5	Group × Time	0.65
	CrN-High	12.8 ± 8.1	17.5 ± 9.5	16.1 ± 8.2	17.2 ± 11.2	16.2 ± 9.7	17.2 ± 15.6	20.1 ± 18.1		
ALT	PLA	19 ± 8.2	19.5 ± 9.1	20.2 ± 9.6	19.6 ± 8.5	20.2 ± 9.7	20.3 ± 9.3	20.2 ± 9.3	Group	0.70
(U/L)	CrM	20.3 ± 7.3	20.5 ± 7.7	21.4 ± 7.8	21.1 ± 8.4	21.1 ± 8.4	21.0 ± 7.9	21.2 ± 8.7	Time	0.001
	CrN-Low	20.1 ± 7.7	20.63 ± 8.4	20.7 ± 8.5	20.8 ± 8.1	21.3 ± 8.2	21.0 ± 8.3	21.1 ± 8.0	Group × Time	0.66
	CrN-High	21.2 ± 8.5	21.3 ± 8.3	21.5 ± 8.7	21.9 ± 8.6	21.1 ± 8.5	22.6 ± 8.8	22.7 ± 8.8		
AST	PLA	24.7 ± 4.9	23.8 ± 5.3	25.1 ± 4.7	25.4 ± 5.8	25.5 ± 5.8	25.2 ± 6.2	25.5 ± 6.1	Group	0.40
(U/L)	CrM	25.9 ± 7.9	26.5 ± 8.8	27.1 ± 8.9	26.0 ± 9.1	26.3 ± 8.8	26.5 ± 8.6	27.0 ± 9.5	Time	0.12
	CrN-Low	24.1 ± 6.1	24.6 ± 6.3	23.9 ± 5.9	24.7 ± 6.1	24.8 ± 5.3	24.3 ± 5.6	24.6 ± 5.4	Group × Time	0.64
	CrN-High	28.0 ± 15.6	28.8 ± 16.3	28.7 ± 16.4	28.8 ± 14.8	29.6 ± 15.2	28.9 ± 14.8	29.8 ± 16.0		
CK	PLA	260 ± 222	264 ± 231	266 ± 219	262 ± 210	259 ± 211	254 ± 200	247 ± 193	Group	0.40
(U/L)	CrM	160 ± 220	262 ± 222	263 ± 212	240 ± 207	249 ± 195	242 ± 189	237 ± 185	Time	0.06
	CrN-Low	265 ± 275	270 ± 273	272 ± 287	267 ± 271	266 ± 273	256 ± 250	255 ± 252	Group × Time	0.51
	CrN-High	490 ± 931	505 ± 958	497 ± 940	475 ± 864	470 ± 863	453 ± 809	470 ± 894		
LDH	PLA	168 ± 40	158 ± 24	170 ± 27	172 ± 26	169 ± 22	171 ± 30	171 ± 27	Group	0.08
(U/L)	CrM	168 ± 21	164 ± 31	168 ± 31	162 ± 23	164 ± 28	165 ± 31	172 ± 29	Time	0.39
	CrN-Low	146 ± 25	165 ± 31	155 ± 19	161 ± 23	160 ± 18	158 ± 22	159 ± 18	Group × Time	0.40
	CrN-High	169 ± 36	179 ± 42	183 ± 40	167 ± 47	196 ± 74	176 ± 32	180 ± 27		
BUN	PLA	14.4 ± 4.8	14.0 ± 4.2	14.0 ± 4.3	13.4 ± 4.5	13.2 ± 4.2	12.8 ± 4.1	12.3 ± 3.8	Group	0.28
(mg/dl)	CrM	15.2 ± 5.0	14.8 ± 4.6	14.6 ± 4.7	13.7 ± 4.5	13.4 ± 4.3	13.1 ± 4.3	12.6 ± 4.0	Time	0.001
	CrN-Low	13.5 ± 4.8	13.0 ± 4.5	12.8 ± 4.5	12.2 ± 4.1	12.1 ± 4.1	11.6 ± 3.8	11.4 ± 3.8	Group × Time	0.76
	CrN-High	14.6 ± 5.1	14.5 ± 5.22	14.1 ± 4.9	13.7 ± 5.1	13.2 ± 4.6	12.9 ± 4.3	12.7 ± 4.3		

Table 1 Hemodynamic and hematological response to supplementation for Study 1 (*Continued*)

Creatinine									
(mg/dl)	PLA	1.00 ± 0.15	0.99 ± 0.16	0.99 ± 0.15	0.98 ± 0.15	0.98 ± 0.17	0.95 ± 0.14[d]	Group	0.001
	CrM	0.99 ± 0.18	1.04 ± 0.17	1.04 ± 0.19	1.01 ± 0.19	0.99 ± 0.17	1.00 ± 0.17	Time	0.001
	CrN-Low	1.01 ± 0.19	1.08 ± 0.18	1.09 ± 0.17[a,d]	1.05 ± 0.17[a]	1.05 ± 0.17[a]	1.01 ± 1.16	Group × Time	0.001
	CrN-High	1.05 ± 0.14[a]	1.11 ± 0.15[a,b]	1.17 ± 0.14[a,b,c]	1.12 ± 0.16[a,b,c]	1.06 ± 0.16[a]	1.02 ± 0.14		
BUN: Creatinine	PLA	14.4 ± 4.2	14.2 ± 4.1	14.3 ± 4.1	13.7 ± 3.9	13.5 ± 3.6	12.9 ± 3.2	Group	0.11
(mg/dl)	CrM	15.3 ± 4.3	14.5 ± 4.3	14.2 ± 3.9	13.7 ± 4.1	13.6 ± 4.2	12.7 ± 3.5	Time	0.001
	CrN-Low	13.7 ± 5.4	12.2 ± 4.6	11.9 ± 4.6	11.8 ± 4.3	11.8 ± 4.4	11.5 ± 4.0	Group × Time	0.08
	CrN-High	14.0 ± 4.8	13.2 ± 4.6	12.0 ± 3.9	12.3 ± 4.0	12.6 ± 3.9	12.5 ± 3.8		

Data are mean ± SD. To convert respective values to mmol/L multiply total cholesterol, HDL-C and LDL-C to mmol/L multiply by 0.0259; triglycerides by 0.0113, BUN by 0.357 and glucose by 0.0555. To convert ALP, ALT, AST, CK, LDH, to µkat/L multiply by 0.0167. To convert creatinine to µmol/L multiply by 88.54. $p < 0.05$ is considered significant

Statistical notations. [a]denotes a significant difference from PLA. [b]denotes a significant difference from CrM. [c]denotes a significant difference from CrN-Low. [d]denotes a significant difference from CrM, CrN-Low, and CrN-High

Table 2 Anthropometry and blood lipid, glucose, nitrate, and creatine characteristics of Study 2 participants

Variable	Group	Baseline	7	28		p-level
Body Weight	PLA	77.3 ± 11.9	77.6 ± 12.1	77.4 ± 12.7	Group	0.003
(kg)	CrM	81.7 ± 13.2	82.4 ± 13.4	82.6 ± 14.0	Time	0.002
	CrN-Low	72.0 ± 9.7	72.2 ± 9.9	72.7 ± 10.0	Group × Time	0.29
	CrN-High	90.8 ± 13.4	90.8 ± 13.2	92.0 ± 14.3		
Fat Mass	PLA	12.7 ± 6.3	12.6 ± 6.3	12.7 ± 6.3	Group	0.02
(kg)	CrM	12.9 ± 5.3	13.0 ± 5.5	13.2 ± 5.2	Time	0.17
	CrN-Low	8.9 ± 4.7	8.7 ± 4.6	9.1 ± 4.7	Group × Time	0.90
	CrN-High	16.5 ± 6.9	16.2 ± 6.4	16.6 ± 7.4		
Fat-Free Mass	PLA	58.1 ± 8.0	58.5 ± 8.0	58.3 ± 8.3	Group	0.01
(kg)	CrM	62.4 ± 8.7	62.5 ± 8.8	62.9 ± 9.2	Time	0.02
	CrN-Low	56.9 ± 7.4	57.4 ± 7.3	57.3 ± 7.3	Group × Time	0.50
	CrN-High	67.4 ± 8.1	67.7 ± 8.2	68.5 ± 8.2		
Body Fat	PLA	17.8 ± 6.9	17.1 ± 6.7	17.2 ± 6.7	Group	0.07
(%)	CrM	16.7 ± 4.0	16.8 ± 4.3	16.8 ± 3.7	Time	0.24
	CrN-Low	13.1 ± 5.4	12.8 ± 5.2	13.2 ± 5.2	Group × Time	0.78
	CrN-High	19.2 ± 5.9	18.7 ± 5.5	18.8 ± 6.3		
Total Body Water	PLA	51.3 ± 4.5	50.6 ± 5.1	52.5 ± 6.9	Group	0.18
(%)	CrM	51.4 ± 3.3	50.8 ± 3.7	49.4 ± 8.4	Time	0.64
	CrN-Low	52.9 ± 4.6	54.1 ± 5.1	52.7 ± 4.2	Group × Time	0.47
	CrN-High	50.6 ± 6.5	48.8 ± 4.1	49.0 ± 4.7		
Lipids, Glucose, Nitrate, and Creatine						
Total-C	PLA	165.0 ± 33.4	161.5 ± 38.8	164.6 ± 38.8	Group	0.19
(mg/dl)	CrM	174.4 ± 25.5	175.4 ± 27.8	183.4 ± 41.1	Time	0.38
	CrN-Low	151.9 ± 35.8	149.7 ± 29.5	150.0 ± 37.5	Group × Time	0.83
	CrN-High	162.7 ± 25.1	155.9 ± 23.8	160.7 ± 29.1		
HDL-C	PLA	49.2 ± 11.4	50.6 ± 10.2	50.3 ± 12.8	Group	0.62
(mg/dl)	CrM	51.8 ± 15.2	54.7 ± 15.5	55.2 ± 17.4	Time	0.36
	CrN-Low	48.6 ± 15.7	48.3 ± 15.1	47.9 ± 12.8	Group × Time	0.85
	CrN-High	46.7 ± 10.7	47.2 ± 12.3	48.7 ± 10.6		
Total-C/HDL-C	PL	3.45 ± 0.71	3.23 ± 0.64	3.30 ± 0.59	Group	0.82
Ratio	CrM	3.70 ± 1.46	3.50 ± 1.34	3.69 ± 1.58	Time	0.24
(mg/dl)	CrN-Low	3.26 ± 0.81	3.32 ± 1.04	3.29 ± 1.05	Group × Time	0.74
	CrN-High	3.62 ± 0.82	3.47 ± 0.88	3.44 ± 0.94		
LDL-C	PLA	93.4 ± 23.4	91.7 ± 29.6	95.8 ± 34.6	Group	0.34
(mg/dl)	CrM	103.8 ± 33.3	106.6 ± 33.5	112.2 ± 49.0	Time	0.36
	CrN-Low	86.3 ± 22.6	84.8 ± 23.7	87.3 ± 28.7	Group × Time	0.88
	CrN-High	95.2 ± 25.0	93.4 ± 22.9	94.3 ± 28.4		
Triglyceride	PLA	109.1 ± 52.5	98.2 ± 36.9	94.2 ± 19.1	Group	0.63
(mg/dl)	CrM	114.5 ± 60.6	93.1 ± 30.9	112.0 ± 42.6	Time	0.16
	CrN-Low	87.5 ± 43.2	90.7 ± 49.1	85.8 ± 30.7	Group × Time	0.69
	CrN-High	104.8 ± 47.1	85.6 ± 39.2	97.2 ± 49.8		
Glucose	PLA	102.0 ± 18.6	102.1 ± 15.3	94.9 ± 12.6	Group	0.74
(mg/dl)	CrM	97.5 ± 13.9	99.7 ± 15.1	100.4 ± 16.8	Time	0.70

Table 2 Anthropometry and blood lipid, glucose, nitrate, and creatine characteristics of Study 2 participants *(Continued)*

	CrN-Low	96.1 ± 8.5	96.1 ± 7.9	96.4 ± 17.9	Group × Time	0.27
	CrN-High	97.1 ± 9.4	93.2 ± 5.2	96.0 ± 9.4		
Nitrate	PLA	4.5 ± 2.0	5.1 ± 3.3	9.0 ± 15.3	Group	0.001
(µmol/L)	CrM	4.9 ± 3.6	3.8 ± 1.8	4.5 ± 1.8	Time	0.001
	CrN-Low	5.6 ± 3.1	64.8 ± 30.9[a,b]	13.9 ± 13.9	Group × Time	0.001
	CrN-High	4.3 ± 1.6	72.0 ± 47.3[a,b]	21.5 ± 28.9[b]		
Creatine	PLA	131.1 ± 92.2	143.5 ± 131.9	150.6 ± 152.0	Group	0.04
(µmol/L)	CrM	165.2 ± 94.4[c]	504.9 ± 422.8[d]	231.2 ± 126.1	Time	0.001
	CrN-Low	73.0 ± 56.4	170.4 ± 153.7	147.9 ± 95.3	Group × Time	0.01
	CrN-High	120.3 ± 99.8	241.3 ± 131.9	251.9 ± 406.4		

Data are mean ± SD. To convert respective values to mmol/L multiply total cholesterol, HDL-C and LDL-C multiply by 0.0259; triglycerides by 0.0113, BUN by 0.357 and glucose by 0.0555. To convert creatinine to µmol/L multiply by 88.54. $p < 0.05$ considered significant
Statistical notations. [a]denotes a significant difference from PLA. [b]denotes a significant difference from CrM. [c]denotes a significant difference from CrN-Low. [d]denotes a significant difference from PLA, CrN-Low, and CrN-High

BUN: Creatinine ratio ($p < 0.001$), and glucose ($p = 0.009$). No significant group x time interactions were observed for ALP ($p = 0.65$), ALT ($p = 0.66$), AST ($p = 0.64$), CK ($p = 0.51$), LDH ($p = 0.40$), BUN ($p = 0.76$), BUN: Creatinine ratio ($p = 0.08$), and glucose ($p = 0.12$). Significant time ($p = 0.001$) and group × time effects ($p = 0.001$) were only observed for creatinine. Specifically, CrN-High had significantly greater creatinine concentration than PLA at time 0. The PLA group had significantly lower creatinine concentration than CrN-Low and CrN-High at 0.5 h. CrN-High had significantly greater creatinine concentration than CrM at 0.5 h. CrN-Low had significantly greater creatinine concentration than PLA and CrM, but significantly lower concentrations than CrN-High at 1 h. Concentrations of creatinine in CrN-High were significantly greater than PLA, CrM, and CrN-Low at 1 h and at 2 h. CrN-Low had significantly lower creatinine concentration than PLA at 2, 3, 4, and 5 h. Creatinine concentrations in CrN-High were significantly greater than PLA at 4 and 5 h. No significant time effects were observed for TC ($p = 0.06$), or the ratio ($p = 0.09$), and LDL ($p = 0.06$). While we did observe a significant time effect for HDL-C ($p = 0.001$) and TG ($p = 0.007$), no significant group × time interactions were noted for any lipid variable.

Hemodynamic profile
Findings for heart rate (HR), systolic blood pressure (SBP), and diastolic blood pressure (DBP) data are presented in Table 1. Overall, we observed a significant trend for time as systolic blood pressure changed throughout the study so that time 0 was greater than 0.5 h and 1 h post supplementation ($p < 0.05$). Further, the 1 h assessment was significantly lower than SBP at 0, 2, 3, 4, and 5 h post-supplementation (*all*, $p < 0.01$). We

did not observe any significant trends for DBP and no between group effects were noted for SBP or DBP at any time point.

Study 2: chronic supplementation
Seventy-one participants were initially recruited for Study 2 and completed consent forms, and all participated in the required familiarization session. Of the original 71 participants, 48 completed the study. Twenty-three participants dropped out after the familiarization, 22 due to time constraints and one due to apprehension of the muscle biopsy procedure. Fifty-three participants were randomized to the four treatment groups. Twelve participants were initially randomized to the PLA group, but one participant was dropped due to missed scheduled laboratory visits. Fifteen were initially randomized to the CrM group. Four participants dropped out of this group, one due to missed scheduled laboratory visits, one developed abdominal pains after the second day of supplementation, one due to a family emergency, and one withdrew due to time constraints. There were no withdraws from either creatine nitrate (CrN) group.

Compliance, side effects, training, and diet
All participants were 100 % compliant with the ingestion of the supplements and 99.4 % were compliant with the proper timing of the supplements.
Our analysis of side effects examining the frequency and severity of dizziness, headache, tachycardia, heart skipping or palpitations, shortness of breath, nervousness, blurred vision, and any other unusual or adverse effects demonstrated no time ($p = 0.35$) or group × time ($p = 0.34$) effects for any variable. However, some participants reported minimal (no greater than 1 in severity)

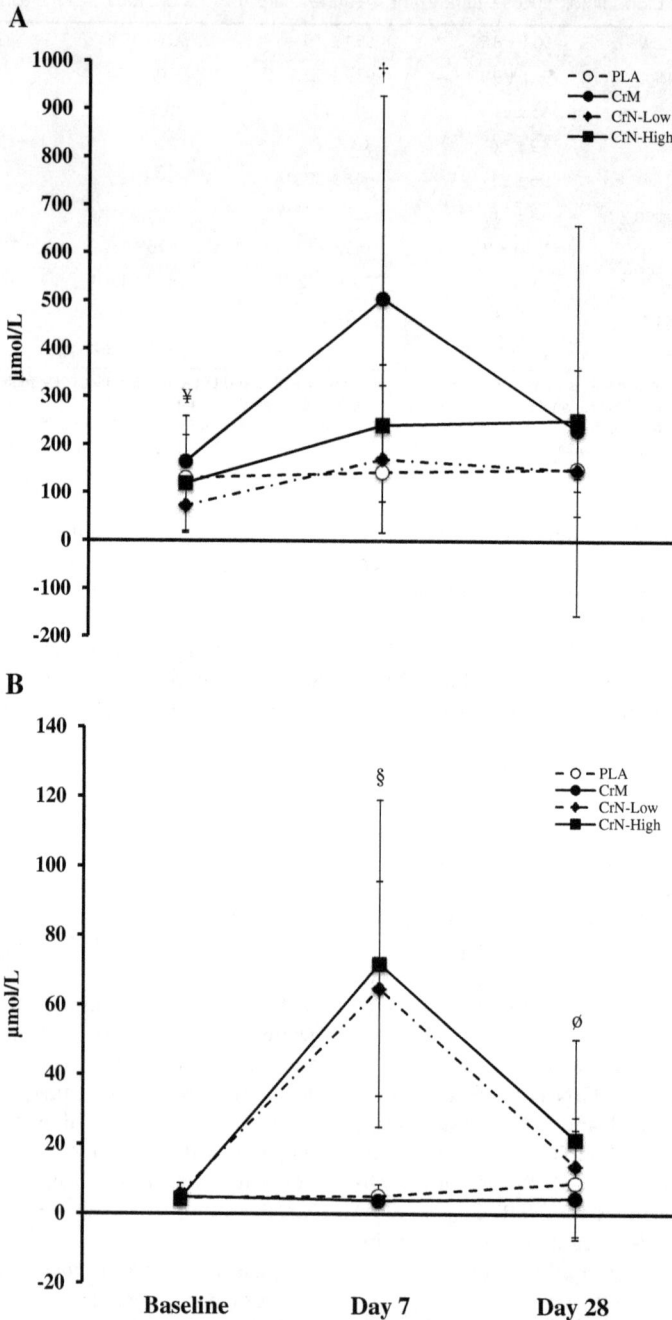

Fig. 3 Data represent mean ± SD plasma creatine (**a**) and plasma nitrate (**b**) concentrations following 7 and 28 days supplementation. Statistical notations ($p < 0.05$ considered significant): (¥) denotes CrM significantly greater than CrN-Low. (†) denotes CrM significantly greater than PLA, CrN-Low, and CrN-High. (§) denotes CrN-Low and CrN-High significantly greater than PLA and CrM. (Ø) denotes CrN-High significantly greater than CrM

side effects such as dizziness, headache, tachycardia, heart skipping or palpitations, shortness of breath, nervousness, and blurred vision; however, these symptoms where similar amongst the treatment groups over the 28-d period (PLA = 11, CrM = 11, CrN-Low = 13, CrN-High = 13).

Table 3 Hepatorenal and blood cell characteristics of Study 2 participants

Marker	Group	Day 0	7	28		p-level
Hepatorenal						
ALPS	PLA	11.2 ± 14.6	10.5 ± 10.7	12.4 ± 10.9	Group	0.44
(U/L)	CrM	11.4 ± 9.5	12.0 ± 10.4	11.0 ± 7.8	Time	0.36
	CrN-Low	15.5 ± 11.4	16.2 ± 11.9	19.5 ± 15.9	Group × Time	0.85
	CrN-High	12.0 ± 7.1	13.6 ± 6.1	14.3 ± 11.7		
ALT	PLA	27.2 ± 8.6	30.2 ± 13.8	32.1 ± 30.6	Group	0.24
(U/L)	CrM	28.9 ± 16.6	25.1 ± 10.0	32.7 ± 22.9	Time	0.06
	CrN-Low	21.3 ± 6.7	19.9 ± 4.4	22.4 ± 6.7	Group × Time	0.70
	CrN-High	28.7 ± 13.2	30.0 ± 15.7	36.8 ± 23.2		
AST	PLA	31.2 ± 13.3	30.1 ± 11.6	29.5 ± 13.4	Group	0.90
(U/L)	CrM	28.3 ± 10.2	26.4 ± 7.7	32.5 ± 12.3	Time	0.56
	CrN-Low	26.0 ± 7.0	30.6 ± 25.3	26.0 ± 6.0	Group × Time	0.47
	CrN-High	26.4 ± 5.9	28.7 ± 7.0	32.0 ± 7.6		
CK	PLA	252 ± 128	294 ± 399	206 ± 161	Group	0.79
(U/L)	CrM	285 ± 169	345 ± 319	409 ± 373	Time	0.35
	CrN-Low	283 ± 169	480 ± 987	243 ± 136	Group × Time	0.56
	CrN-High	284 ± 171	349 ± 203	424 ± 287		
LDH	PLA	226 ± 180	167 ± 29	158 ± 34	Group	0.93
(U/L)	CrM	185 ± 62	172 ± 39	184 ± 48	Time	0.20
	CrN-Low	175 ± 50	173 ± 41	166 ± 29	Group × Time	0.23
	CrN-High	173 ± 29	176 ± 30	182 ± 39		
BUN	PLA	16.3 ± 3.6	15.6 ± 5.2	15.7 ± 4.9	Group	0.64
(mg/dl)	CrM	15.3 ± 5.5	15.2 ± 4.9	16.3 ± 6.1	Time	0.48
	CrN-Low	14.9 ± 3.8	13.3 ± 3.9	13.5 ± 4.6	Group × Time	0.64
	CrN-High	14.6 ± 3.2	14.8 ± 2.7	15.7 ± 5.8		
Creatinine	PLA	1.18 ± 0.26	1.19 ± 0.33	1.15 ± 0.27	Group	0.97
(mg/dl)	CrM	1.15 ± 0.46	1.26 ± 0.36	1.23 ± 0.39	Time	0.001
	CrN-Low	1.09 ± 0.25	1.21 ± 0.31	1.23 ± 0.31	Group × Time	0.12
	CrN-High	1.12 ± 0.18	1.15 ± 0.23	1.20 ± 0.23		
BUN: Creatinine	PLA	14.2 ± 3.7	13.9 ± 6.8	13.6 ± 3.1	Group	0.78
(mg/dl)	CrM	13.7 ± 3.6	12.8 ± 5.3	14.0 ± 6.1	Time	0.07
	CrN-Low	14.1 ± 4.2	11.4 ± 3.8	11.3 ± 3.4	Group × Time	0.13
	CrN-High	13.3 ± 3.8	13.3 ± 3.3	13.4 ± 4.8		
Blood cell characteristics						
MCV	PLA	92.2 ± 3.1	91.7 ± 3.7	91.6 ± 3.8	Group	0.79
(fL)	CrM	93.0 ± 3.9	93.7 ± 3.9	93.6 ± 4.7	Time	0.47
	CrN-Low	91.7 ± 3.8	91.8 ± 4.0	92.3 ± 4.2	Group × Time	0.49
	CrN-High	93.3 ± 3.0	93.4 ± 3.1	88.7 ± 17.7		
MCH	PLA	30.4 ± 1.7	30.5 ± 1.3	31.0 ± 2.3	Group	0.45
(pg/cell)	CrM	30.6 ± 1.4	31.2 ± 1.5	31.0 ± 2.6	Time	0.23
	CrN-Low	30.6 ± 1.7	31.6 ± 2.1	31.3 ± 2.2	Group × Time	0.92
	CrN-High	31.2 ± 0.9	31.3 ± 1.4	31.5 ± 1.2		

Table 3 Hepatorenal and blood cell characteristics of Study 2 participants *(Continued)*

MCHC	PLA	32.9 ± 1.2	33.3 ± 1.7	33.8 ± 1.8	Group	0.40
(g/dl)	CrM	32.9 ± 0.7	33.3 ± 1.5	33.1 ± 1.9	Time	0.53
	CrN-Low	33.3 ± 0.8	34.5 ± 3.4	33.9 ± 1.7	Group × Time	0.66
	CrN-High	33.5 ± 0.7	33.5 ± 1.6	32.2 ± 6.0		
RBCDW	PLA	13.2 ± 0.5	13.1 ± 0.9	13.1 ± 0.3	Group	0.02
(%)	CrM	13.5 ± 0.9	13.7 ± 0.9	13.9 ± 0.8	Time	0.11
	CrN-Low	13.6 ± 0.6	13.4 ± 0.6	13.5 ± 0.7	Group × Time	0.66
	CrN-High	12.8 ± 0.6	13.2 ± 0.6	13.1 ± 0.4		
Platelet Count	PLA	206 ± 36	188 ± 32	208 ± 70	Group	0.35
($\times 10^3/\mu L$)	CrM	234 ± 57	226 ± 91	255 ± 51	Time	0.56
	CrN-Low	218 ± 69	183 ± 50	194 ± 68	Group × Time	0.39
	CrN-High	220 ± 61	412 ± 713	224 ± 59		
WBC	PLA	6.2 ± 1.7	5.3 ± 1.5	6.2 ± 1.1	Group	0.72
($\times 10^3/\mu L$)	CrM	6.0 ± 1.7	6.6 ± 1.3	6.4 ± 1.3	Time	0.58
	CrN-Low	6.2 ± 1.6	5.9 ± 1.8	5.4 ± 1.3	Group × Time	0.18
	CrN-High	5.9 ± 1.4	5.5 ± 1.6	6.1 ± 1.6		
RBC	PLA	5.2 ± 0.8	5.01 ± 0.83	4.8 ± 0.6	Group	0.25
($\times 10^6/\mu L$)	CrM	5.3 ± 0.6	5.60 ± 0.97	5.1 ± 0.8	Time	0.09
	CrN-Low	5.0 ± 0.5	5.11 ± 0.95	4.9 ± 0.7	Group × Time	0.65
	CrN-High	5.5 ± 0.8	5.08 ± 0.51	5.1 ± 0.5		
Hematocrit	PLA	47.7 ± 7.1	46.0 ± 8.2	44.0 ± 4.5	Group	0.16
(%)	CrM	49.5 ± 6.7	52.5 ± 9.7	47.6 ± 8.4	Time	0.51
	CrN-Low	46.2 ± 5.5	47.1 ± 10.3	44.8 ± 7.1	Group × Time	0.44
	CrN-High	51.2 ± 7.8	47.5 ± 5.2	51.7 ± 15.4		
Hemoglobin	PLA	15.7 ± 2.5	15.3 ± 2.7	14.8 ± 1.2	Group	0.17
(g/dl)	CrM	16.3 ± 2.1	20.1 ± 10.2	15.7 ± 2.8	Time	0.63
	CrN-Low	15.4 ± 2.1	16.1 ± 3.1	15.2 ± 2.3	Group × Time	0.19
	CrN-High	17.2 ± 2.7	15.9 ± 1.4	18.7 ± 9.5		

Data are mean ± SD

Dietary characteristics

We observed no significant time effects for daily caloric (absolute: $p = 0.38$; relative: $p = 0.37$), protein (absolute: $p = 0.74$; relative: $p = 0.77$), carbohydrate (absolute: $p = 0.23$; relative: $p = 0.15$), and fat (absolute: $p = 0.41$; relative: $p = 0.57$) intake. There were also no significant group × time effects for daily caloric (absolute: $p = 0.89$; relative: $p = 0.94$), protein (absolute: $p = 0.40$; relative: $p = 0.39$), carbohydrate (absolute: $p = 0.31$; relative: $p = 0.33$), and fat (absolute: $p = 0.64$; relative: $p = 0.54$) intake.

Clinical chemistry panels, plasma creatine plasma nitrates, muscle creatine

Results for the plasma lipid, glucose, nitrate and creatine are presented in Table 2 and Fig. 3 while corresponding hepatorenal and blood cell characteristics are presented in Table 3. As a whole, there were no significant time or group × time effects for any blood safety marker. There were significant group, time, and group x time interactions for plasma nitrate and plasma and intramuscular creatine concentrations (*all*, $P < 0.04$). After 7-d of supplementation, there was a significant increase in plasma nitrates in CrN-Low (59.5 µmol/L, 95 % CI 42.6, 76.4) and CrN-High (76.5 µmol/L, 95 % CI 50.7, 84.3) groups, with no concomitant increase observed for the PLA (0.49 µmol/L, 95 % CI –17.7, 18.6) and CrM groups (–1.1 µmol/L, 95 % CI –19.2, 17.1, $p < 0.001$). By d-28, nitrate levels had dropped for the CrN-Low group to a non-significant level relative to baseline (8.52 µmol/L, 95 % CI, –1.9, 18.9), while the CrN-High group remained elevated relative to baseline, but at a concentration ~25 % of the d-7 value (17.09 µmol/L, 95 % CI, 6.7, 27.4). Between group analysis further demonstrated that while the CrN-High condition remained significant relative to the CrM treatment (*P* <

Table 4 Assessment of blood chemistry changes denoting lipids, glucose, muscle and hepatorenal function concordant to supplementation

			Treatment				
			PLA	CrM	CrN-Low	CrN-High	Chi-Square
Lipids & glucose	Cholesterol	No Change	0	0	0	0	0.33
		Normal Base; Exceed Day 7	10	8	12	13	
		Normal Base; Exceed Day 28	1	1	0	0	
		Normal Day7; Exceed Day 28	0	2	1	0	
	HDL-C	No Change	6	9	10	10	0.72
		Normal Base; Exceed Day 7	2	1	0	0	
		Normal Base; Exceed Day 28	1	0	1	1	
		Normal Day7; Exceed Day 28	2	1	2	2	
	LDL-C	No Change	9	10	13	12	0.30
		Normal Base; Exceed Day 7	0	0	0	0	
		Normal Base; Exceed Day 28	2	1	0	0	
		Normal Day7; Exceed Day 28	0	0	0	1	
	Triglycerides	No Change	11	11	13	13	0.31
		Normal Base; Exceed Day7	0	0	0	0	
		Normal Base; Exceed Day28	0	0	0	0	
		Normal Day7; Exceed Day28	0	0	0	0	
	Glucose	No Change	10	9	11	11	0.56
		Normal Base; Exceed Day 7	1	1	1	0	
		Normal Base; Exceed Day 28	0	1	0	0	
		Normal Day7; Exceed Day 28	0	0	1	2	
Muscle	LDH	No Change	9	9	12	11	0.26
		Normal Base; Exceed Day 7	1	0	0	0	
		Normal Base; Exceed Day 28	0	0	0	2	
		Normal Day7; Exceed Day 28	1	2	1	0	
	Creatine Kinase	No Change	7	7	10	11	0.75
		Normal Base; Exceed Day 7	2	1	1	0	
		Normal Base; Exceed Day 28	0	0	0	0	
		Normal Day7, Exceed Day 28	2	3	2	2	
	Creatinine	No Change	11	9	11	11	0.32
		Normal Base; Exceed Day 7	0	0	0	0	
		Normal Base; Exceed Day 28	0	1	0	2	
		Normal Day7; Exceed Day 28	0	1	2	0	
Kidney	BUN	No Change	10	8	11	12	0.37
		Normal Base; Exceed Day 7	0	0	1	0	
		Normal Base; Exceed Day 28	0	2	0	0	
		Normal Day7; Exceed Day 28	1	1	1	1	
	ALP	No Change	11	11	13	13	0.32
		Normal Base; Exceed Day 7	0	0	0	0	
		Normal Base; Exceed Day 28	0	0	0	0	
		Normal Day7; Exceed Day 28	0	0	0	0	

Table 4 Assessment of blood chemistry changes denoting lipids, glucose, muscle and hepatorenal function concordant to supplementation *(Continued)*

Liver	ALT	No Change	11	9	12	11	0.49
		Normal Base; Exceed Day 7	0	0	0	0	
		Normal Base; Exceed Day 28	0	2	1	2	
		Normal Day7; Exceed Day 28	0	0	0	0	
	AST	No Change	8	8	12	8	0.54
		Normal Base; Exceed Day 7	1	0	1	0	
		Normal Base; Exceed Day 28	1	1	0	2	
		Normal Day7; Exceed Day 28	1	2	0	3	

Data are presented as frequency. Statistical significance is detailed from chi-square analyses

0.03), it no longer remained significant relative to the PLA treatment (Table 2). Table 4 presents the assessment of the blood chemistry changes in serum lipids, glucose, muscle and hepatorenal function associated with supplementation. No significant differences were noted between groups for any analyte.

There was a significant increase in plasma creatine for the CrM (312.0 µmol/L, 95 % CI 192.1, 432.0), CrN-Low (126.5 µmol/L, 95 % CI, 15.1, 238.0), and CrN-High groups at d-7 (120.9 µmol/L, 95 % CI 14.1, 227.8), all three of which were significant relative to the PLA group (7.7 µmol/L, 95 % CI, −110.0, 131.7, $p < 0.03$). By d-28, only the CrN-High plasma creatine remained significantly elevated relative to baseline (131.5 µmol/L, 95 % CI, 22.5, 240.5) while the CrM (39.0 µmol/L, 95 % CI, −83.4, 161.0) and CrN-Low (103.2 µmol/L, 95 % CI −10.5, 216.9) groups no longer demonstrated a significant elevation. No between group differences at d-28 were otherwise noted.

Intramuscular creatine was significantly increased in the CrM (7.1 mmol/kg DW, 95 % CI, 3.1, 11.0) and CrN-High (4.6 mmol/kg DW, 95 % CI, 0.8, 8.4) groups and significantly decreased in the CrN-Low group (−4.0 mmol/kg DW, 95 % CI −7.7, −0.3) while no significant change was noted for the PLA group (−2.5 mmol/kg DW, 95 % CI, −6.7, 1.7). Between group post-hoc comparisons showed that the CrM and CrN-High groups had significantly greater concentrations relative to the PLA ($p = 0.002$) and CrN-Low groups ($p = 0.001$). On d 28, the CrM group remained the only group to have significantly elevated muscle creatine (8.8 mmol/kg DW, 95 % CI, 5.5, 12.2), while the CrN-High group initial 7-d concentrations abated to a lower concentration (1.4, 95 % CI, −1.8, 4.7 mmol/kg DW). Both the CrN-Low and PLA groups remained relatively unchanged.

Anthropometry
While body mass increased over time in all groups by d-28, only the CrM and CrN-High groups had a significant increase in FFM and lean mass, with the CrN-High group significantly greater than the CrN-Low group for both variables (Fig. 5).

Bench press performance, anaerobic sprint and Wingate test
Results for all exercise performance variables are presented in Table 5. Overall, we observed significant time effects and group × time effects for several strength testing variables. Specifically, we observed significant increases in bench press lifting volume (kg) to fatigue for all groups over the 28-d testing period. Only the CrN-High group demonstrated significance differences relative to the PLA group (Fig. 4). Similar findings were noted for peak and average bench press power output as determined by the Tendo™ assessment. Interestingly, post-hoc analyses demonstrated that the CrN-High changes were significantly greater than PLA and CrN-Low (Fig. 4). No significant treatment effects were observed for the Wingate or anaerobic sprint tests.

Discussion and conclusions
The primary aim of our studies was to examine the dose-dependent effects of CrN on acute and chronic indices of safety and exercise performance. Accordingly, we performed an acute safety study to assess basic hematologic variables attesting to hepatorenal and muscle enzyme function, blood glucose, lipids, and hemodynamic variables, followed by 28-d of chronic supplementation to examine safety and exercise performance. In Study 1, there were no significant changes in any blood marker or hemodynamic function for any treatment group throughout 5 h of post-ingestion follow-up (Table 1). Study 2 also included a 7-d loading schema. Similar safety findings were observed in Study 2, with two exceptions: ALP and creatine kinase (*see below*). While some side effects were reported, they were distributed amongst all groups, including the PLA group, and were reported to be minimal in regard to severity. There also was a significant increase in several

Table 5 Bench press and anaerobic sprint performance characteristics of Study 2 participants

	Group	Day 0	Day 28	Interactions	p-level
Bench press performance					
Max reps	PLA	10.8 ± 2.9	13.0 ± 4.8	Group	0.83
(@70 % 1RM)	CrM	12.0 ± 5.5	15.0 ± 7.1	Time	0.001
	CrN-Low	11.9 ± 2.7	14.0 ± 3.7	Group × Time	0.55
	CrN-High	11.5 ± 3.6	14.8 ± 3.7		
Workload [kg]	PLA	1474.1 ± 373.6	1753.2 ± 548.5	Group	0.17
(wt x reps)	CrM	1827.0 ± 926.3	2255.0 ± 1121.5	Time	0.001
	CrN-Low	1616.5 ± 491.3	1877.3 ± 535.4	Group × Time	0.10
	CrN-High	1927.3 ± 830.2	2516.5 ± 867.2		
Peak power	PLA	425.5 ± 101.1	443.3 ± 107.1	Group	0.10
(W)	CrM	452.9 ± 113.7	521.5 ± 119.9	Time	0.001
	CrN-Low	440.2 ± 76.0	481.1 ± 88.4	Group × Time	0.57
	CrN-High	492.4 ± 95.0	553.3 ± 98.4		
Average power	PLA	357.7 ± 88.4	382.4 ± 93.2	Group	0.03
(W)	CrM	423.8 ± 120.5	456.4 ± 105.0	Time	0.001
	CrN-Low	371.6 ± 70.4	396.4 ± 73.4	Group × Time	0.82
	CrN-High	451.2 ± 91.8	489.4 ± 89.7		
Average velocity	PLA	0.50 ± 0.09	0.53 ± 0.11	Group	0.10
(m/s)	CrM	0.55 ± 0.09	0.62 ± 0.11	Time	0.001
	CrN-Low	0.61 ± 0.83	0.65 ± 0.12	Group × Time	0.74
	CrN-High	0.54 ± 0.11	0.61 ± 0.15		
Anaerobic sprint performance					
Mean power	PLA	668.1 ± 172.0	682.7 ± 142.3	Group	0.03
(W)	CrM	684.2 ± 129.2	720.5 ± 141.5	Time	0.12
	CrN-Low	670.8 ± 124.8	708.9 ± 106.9	Group × Time	0.46
	CrN-High	807.9 ± 91.0	797.7 ± 61.4		
Peak power	PLA	1,464.4 ± 379.7	1,486.8 ± 322.5	Group	0.13
(W)	CrM	1,548.4 ± 351.6	1,611.4 ± 440.5	Time	0.11
	CrN-Low	1,497.4 ± 270.1	1,565.0 ± 278.1	Group × Time	0.95
	CrN-High	1,739.0 ± 275.5	1,783.7 ± 306.8		
Total work	PLA	6,119.6 ± 991.9	6,423.7 ± 896.4	Group	0.55
(J)	CrM	7,188.1 ± 2195.3	6,886.7 ± 744.7	Time	0.76
	CrN-Low	6,760.7 ± 1618.4	6,817.5 ± 1290.8	Group × Time	0.71
	CrN-High	6,716.3 ± 1532.6	6,884.4 ± 1495.3		

Data are mean ± SD

strength parameters for the CrM and CrN-High groups in Study 2. Though the changes associated with CrM and CrN-High were similar, the CrN-High group reached significance when compared to the PLA group for total lifting volume and Tendo™ average power output (Fig. 4). A similar pattern for improvement was also observed for FFM and lean mass (Fig. 5). The differences observed, however, could not be attributed to greater muscle creatine content in the CrN groups compared to CrM. Based on these findings we accept both our

hypotheses that CrN is safe when provided up to 3 g/d and is efficacious with regard to changes in strength and body composition.

Several investigations have reported the effects of nitrate supplementation on blood pressure and heart rate [23, 25, 31]. Though we observed a slight trend for a decrease in systolic blood pressure (SBP) (~3 mmHg) in all treatment groups with no significant difference observed among groups. No similar trend was noted for diastolic blood pressure (DBP) or heart rate (HR), nor did we

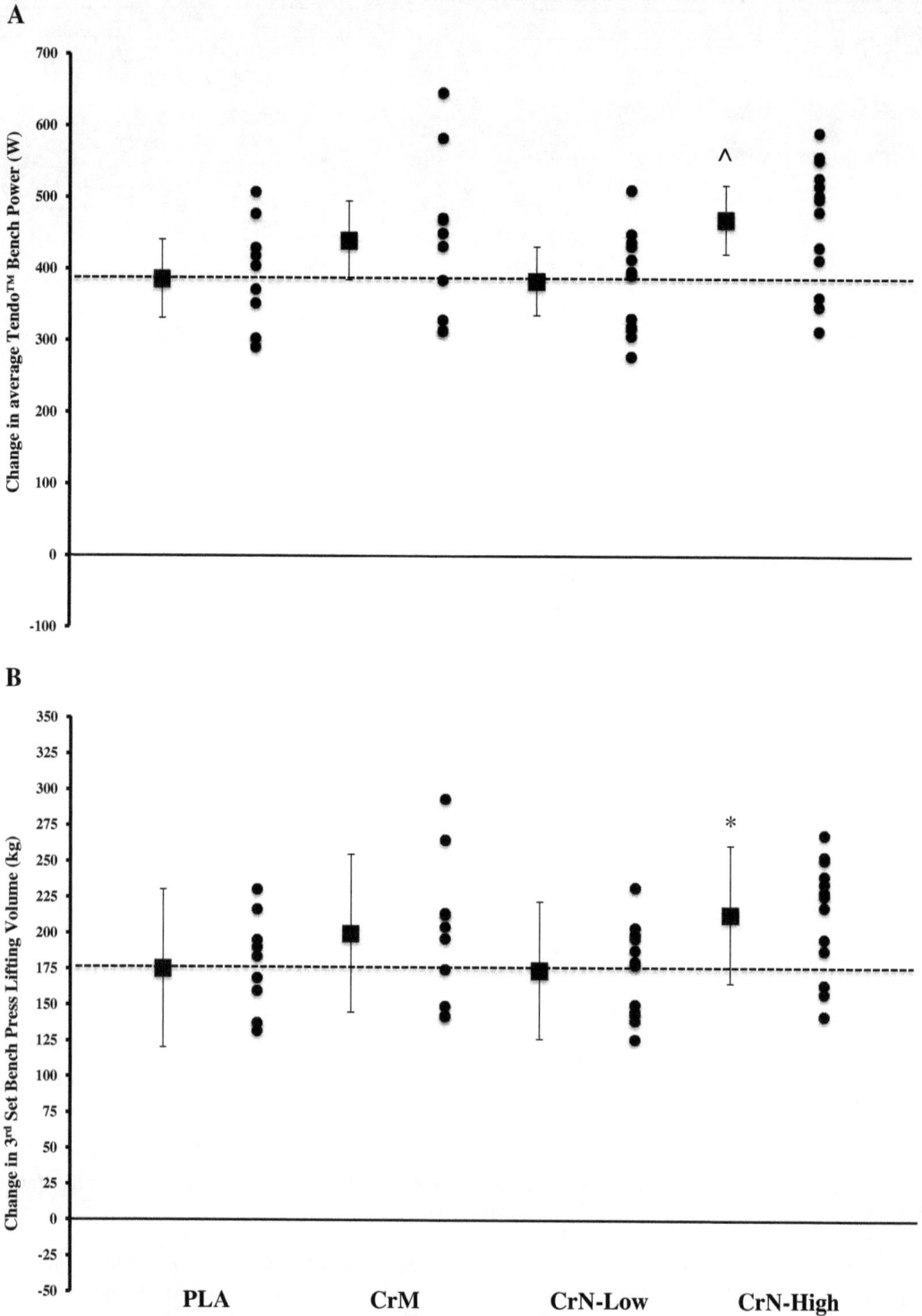

Fig. 4 Data represent mean ± 95 % CI change in average Tendo™ bench press power (**a**) and lifting volume based on reps to fatigue during set 3 at 70 % of 1RM bench press (**b**) following 28 days of supplementation. Statistical notations ($p < 0.05$ considered significant): (^) denotes significantly greater than PLA and CrN-Low. (*) denotes significantly greater than PLA

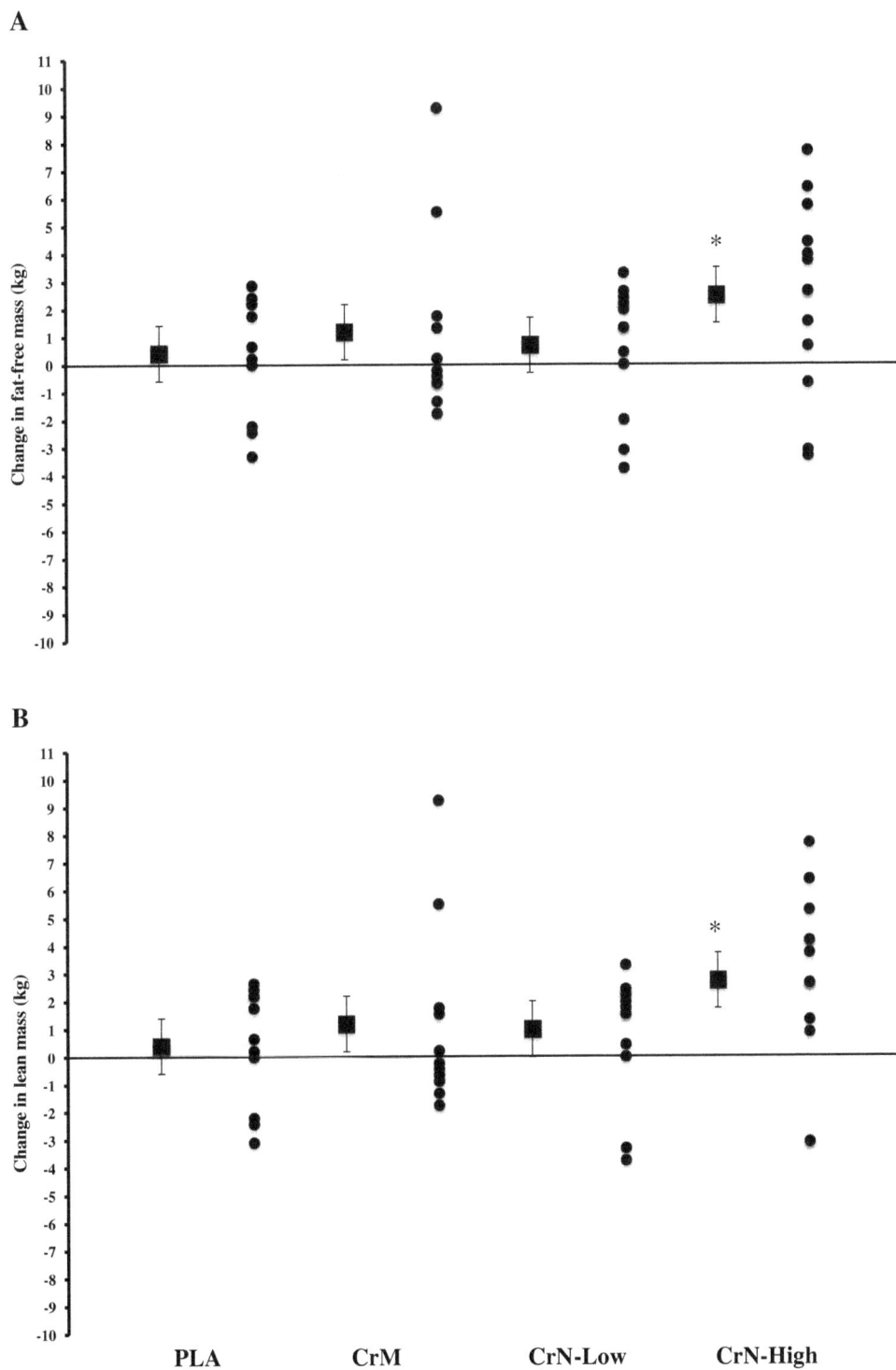

Fig. 5 Data represent mean ± 95 % CI change in fat free mass (**a**) and lean body mass (**b**) following 28 days of supplementation. Statistical notations ($p < 0.05$ considered significant): (*) denotes significantly greater than PLA

observe any between group differences for the same parameters. Others using beetroot juice as a vehicle for nitrate delivery have reported similar findings. For
example, Larsen et al., reported no change in blood pressure following 3-d of ~430 mg nitrate/d [23]. Murphy
and colleagues reported similar findings [25]. To the
contrary, Webb et al., observed a ~10 mmHg decrease
in SBP 2.5 h after ~1,400 mg of nitrate ingestion [31]. In
Study 1 we provided 0.5 g nitrate (CrN-Low) and 1 g
(CrN-High) and found no evidence that CrN reduced
blood pressure or affected HR in comparison to PLA or
CrM. Additionally, no participant had a hypotensive response (SBP < 90 mmHg, DBP < 60 mmHg) to either
dose of CrN studied. It is therefore conceivable that a
dose threshold exists for a single dose of nitrate ingestion as it pertains to hemodynamic alterations. Based on
our findings, CrN appears to be well tolerated up to 3 g
per serving, yielding 1 g of nitrate, whether ingested
acutely or chronically. Adding to these finding is our observation of minimal self-reported side effects associated
with acute and chronic CrN ingestion.

During each study we observed a small number of
side effects that were rated as minimal in frequency
and severity. Collectively, the total number of reported side effects was distributed evenly amongst all
treatment groups whereby each treatment group was
no different than the PLA group. These findings are
similar to previous creatine research investigations.
Moreover, creatine supplementation and a diet rich in
nitrates have been shown to have a beneficial influence on health [4, 34], either of which may explain
the minor, yet positive perturbations of blood lipids
observed in Study 1. It should also be noted that
changes in lipid fractions have been observed previously accompanying creatine ingestion [9, 26]. There
were no consistent, significant effects on any blood
variable related hepatorenal or muscle enzyme function. While there were some between group differences, the pattern for these changes was stochastic
and inconsistent for any treatment group. For example, there were significant changes across time for
high-density lipoprotein (HDL), triglyceride (TG), alkaline phosphatase (ALP), alanine transaminase (ALT),
blood urea nitrogen (BUN), BUN-to-creatinine ratio,
and glucose. Also, CK values for CrN-High (453 – 505
U/L) were elevated above expected normal ranges
(50 – 398 U/L) at baseline and after ingested acutely
[28]. However, similar elevations were not observed
in CK after 28-d of supplements.

The results of the chronic supplementation trial are
intriguing owing to a dichotomy of results suggesting an
improvement in exercise performance unmatched by a
distinct mechanism of action. While we did observed a
significant increase in performance and body composition

characteristics generally favoring the CrM and CrN-High
groups, these results were not associated with a significant
increase in muscle creatine concentrations. In both cases,
CrN-High was significantly greater than the PLA group
and in the latter example, also greater than the CrN-Low.
Despite these differences, only the CrM caused a significant increase in muscle creatine at follow-up.

There was no improvement in cycling anaerobic power
output for our assessments despite the CrM group having significantly greater creatine stores than CrN-Low,
CrN-High, and PLA groups. It is possible that the dose
of CrM used in Study 2 was too low as compared to
more typical doses of 5 g. This higher dosing pattern
generally yields more consistent results versus studies
using 3 g of CrM [5, 14, 27, 32, 33]. These findings contrast claims that there is no need to load when taking
CrN due to greater solubility and retention. The effects
of nitrate as a precursor to nitric oxide may have also
played a role in the development of muscle whereby the
acute effects of nitrates increase exercise performance
directly, while the chronic effects associated with nitrate
supplementation may result from an increase in muscle
protein synthesis [6, 13, 30, 35]. While the former point
has been demonstrated with endurance exercise, the latter point has recently been hypothesized relative to nitric
oxide's potential role in protein synthesis and is currently under investigation by others [6, 30, 35]. Therefore, it is possible that creatine and nitrate work
synergistically, rather than independently, though the
mechanism of action is currently unknown.

A strength of this research is that we examined CrN at
a supplementation dose that is currently recommended,
as well as at a dose twice that, by first performing a general safety assessment, followed by a longer study to
monitor chronic safety parameters and exercise performance. A limitation this research is that we did not examine a more typical CrM loading schema using 5 g per
serving. We did, however, give this a great deal of consideration and ultimately decided to examine a dose
equivalent to those used in the highest CrN group. The
decision to use a lower dose partially was based on certain ingredient manufactures assertions that the increased solubility of CrN would increase intramuscular
creatine concentrations at a lower dose. This apparently
was not the case. However, strength and body composition changes were similar between the CrN-High and
CrM groups. It is important to understand that study 2
was not a CrM efficacy study, but rather an assessment
of CrN. Future research should examine typically used
creatine dosing and/or CrN-High for longer periods of
time to better understand the mechanisms of action associated with CrN ingestion. To our knowledge, this is
the first study examining the efficacy of CrN in strength
training individuals. Although Joy et al. [20] have examined

the safety of CrN up to 2 g, we have extended the current body of knowledge to 3 g/d, inclusive of a 7-d loading sequence at four times per day. Creatine nitrate delivered at 3 g was well-tolerated, demonstrated similar performance benefits to 3 g CrM, in addition, within the confines of this study, there were no safety concerns. However, there was no evidence that CrN at recommended or twice recommended doses is more efficacious than CrM at the doses studied.

Competing interests

This study was supported by Nutrabolt (Bryan, TX) through an unrestricted research grant provided to Texas A&M University. CP Earnest serves as a Director of Clinical Sciences for Nutrabolt and is a Research Associate in the ESNL. RB Kreider serves as a university approved scientific advisor for Nutrabolt International. PS Murano served as quality assurance supervisor. Remaining investigators have no competing interest to declare. The results from this study do no constitute endorsement by the authors/and or institution concerning the nutrients investigated.

Authors' contributions

EG served as study coordinator and assisted with data collection, data analysis, and manuscript preparation. DKW, SYS, RD, KL, NDB, AO, and CG, assisted in data collection and sample analysis. CR is the director of the Exercise and Sport Nutrition Laboratory. SBS, SER, JDF, PSM, MG, and CPE assisted in research design and consultation. RBK (corresponding author) assisted in the design of the study, data analysis, manuscript preparation, obtained the grant, and served as the study PI. All authors read and approved the final manuscript.

Acknowledgements

We would like to thank the subjects that participated in this study as well as all the students and laboratory assistants in the Exercise & Sport Nutrition Laboratory at Texas A&M University who assisted with data collected. We would also like to thank Dr. Jonathan Oliver and Katherine Kelly for their valuable assistance in sample analysis.

Author details

[1]Department of Health and Kinesiology, Exercise and Sport Nutrition Laboratory, Texas A&M University, College Station, TX 77843-4243, USA. [2]Department of Health and Kinesiology, Center for Translational Research in Aging and Longevity, Texas A&M University, College Station, TX 77843-4243, USA. [3]United States Military-Baylor University Graduate Program in Nutrition, Joint Base, San Antonio, TX 78234, USA. [4]Department of Animal Science, Texas A&M University, College Station, TX 77843-4243, USA. [5]Department of Health and Kinesiology, Human Countermeasures Laboratory, Texas A&M University, College Station, TX 77843-4243, USA. [6]Department of Health and Kinesiology, Muscle Biology Laboratory, Texas A&M University, College Station, TX 77843-4243, USA. [7]Department of Nutrition and Food Science, Texas A&M University, College Station, TX 77843-4243, USA. [8]Nutrabolt, Bryan, TX 77807, USA.

References

1.   Almada A, Kreider R, Ransom J, Rasmussen C. Comparison of the reliability of repeated whole body DEXA scans to repeated spine and hip scans. J Bone Miner Res. 1999;14:S369.
2.   Bailey SJ, Winyard P, Vanhatalo A, Blackwell JR, DiMenna FJ, Wilkerson DP, Tarr J, Benjamin N, Jones AM. Dietary nitrate supplementation reduces the O2 cost of low-intensity exercise and enhances tolerance to high-intensity exercise in humans. J Appl Physiol. 2009;107:1144–55.
3.   Bescós R, Rodríguez FA, Iglesias X, Ferrer MD, Iborra E, Pons A. Acute administration of inorganic nitrate reduces VO2peak in endurance athletes. Med Sci Sports Exerc. 2011;43:1979–86.
4.   Blumenthal JA, Babyak MA, Hinderliter A, Watkins LL, Craighead L, Lin P-H, Caccia C, Johnson J, Waugh R, Sherwood A. Effects of the DASH diet alone and in combination with exercise and weight loss on blood pressure and

5.   cardiovascular biomarkers in men and women with high blood pressure: the ENCORE study. Arch Intern Med. 2010;170:126–35.
5.   Buford TW, Kreider RB, Stout JR, Greenwood M, Campbell B, Spano M, Ziegenfuss T, Lopez H, Landis J, Antonio J. International Society of Sports Nutrition position stand: creatine supplementation and exercise. J Int Soc Sports Nutr. 2007;4:6.
6.   Campbell B, Roberts M, Kerksick C, Wilborn C, Marcello B, Taylor L, Nassar E, Leutholtz B, Bowden R, Rasmussen C. Pharmacokinetics, safety, and effects on exercise performance of L-arginine α-ketoglutarate in trained adult men. Nutrition. 2006;22:872–81.
7.   Cooper R, Naclerio F, Allgrove J, Jimenez A. Creatine supplementation with specific view to exercise/sports performance: an update. Sports Nutr Rev J. 2012;9:33.
8.   Dalbo VJ, Roberts MD, Stout JR, Kerksick CM. Putting to rest the myth of creatine supplementation leading to muscle cramps and dehydration. Br J Sports Med. 2008;42:567–73.
9.   Earnest CP, Almada AL, Mitchell TL. High-performance capillary electrophoresis-pure creatine monohydrate reduces blood lipids in men and women. Clin Sci (Lond). 1996;91:113–8.
10. Evans W, Phinney S, Young V. Suction applied to a muscle biopsy maximizes sample size. Med Sci Sports Exerc. 1981;14:101–2.
11. Harris R, Hultman E, Nordesjö L-O. Glycogen, glycolytic intermediates and high-energy phosphates determined in biopsy samples of musculus quadriceps femoris of man at rest. Methods and variance of values. Scand J Clin Lab Invest. 1974;33:109–20.
12. Harris RC, Soderlund K, Hultman E. Elevation of creatine in resting and exercised muscle of normal subjects by creatine supplementation. Clin Sci. 1992;83:367–74.
13. Hord NG, Tang Y, Bryan NS. Food sources of nitrates and nitrites: the physiologic context for potential health benefits. Am J Clin nutr. 2009;90:1–10.
14. Hultman E, Soderlund K, Timmons J, Cederblad G, Greenhaff P. Muscle creatine loading in men. J Appl Physiol. 1996;81:232–7.
15. Bowling JL, Katayev A. An evaluation of the Roche Cobas c 111. Lab Medicine. 2010;41:398–402.
16. Jones AM. Dietary nitrate supplementation and exercise performance. Sports Med. 2014;44(Suppl 1): S35-45.
17. Jones AM. Influence of dietary nitrate on the physiological determinants of exercise performance: a critical review. Appl Physiol Nutr Metab. 2014;39:1019–28.
18. Jones AM, Grassi B, Christensen PM, Krustrup P, Bangsbo J, Poole DC. Slow component of VO2 kinetics: mechanistic bases and practical applications. Med Sci Sports Exerc. 2011;43:2046–62.
19. Jones AM, Vanhatalo A, Bailey SJ. Influence of dietary nitrate supplementation on exercise tolerance and performance. Nestle Nutr Inst Workshop Ser. 2013;75:27–40.
20. Joy JM, Lowery RP, Falcone PH, Mosman M, Vogel RM, Carson LR, Tai C-Y, Choate D, Kimber D, Ormes JA, Wilson JM, and Moon JR. 28 days of creatine nitrate supplementation is apparently safe in healthy individuals. J Int Soc Sports Nutr. 2014;11:60.
21. Kerksick CM, Wilborn CD, Campbell BI, Roberts MD, Rasmussen CJ, Greenwood M, Kreider RB. Early-phase adaptations to a split-body, linear periodization resistance training program in college-aged and middle-aged men. J Strength Condit Res. 2009;23:962–71.
22. Larsen F, Weitzberg E, Lundberg J, Ekblom B. Effects of dietary nitrate on oxygen cost during exercise. Acta physiologica. 2007;191:59–66.
23. Larsen FJ, Ekblom B, Sahlin K, Lundberg JO, Weitzberg E. Effects of dietary nitrate on blood pressure in healthy volunteers. N Engl J Med. 2006;355:2792–3.
24. Larsen FJ, Weitzberg E, Lundberg JO, Ekblom B. Dietary nitrate reduces maximal oxygen consumption while maintaining work performance in maximal exercise. Free Radic Biol Med. 2010;48:342–7.
25. Murphy M, Eliot K, Heuertz RM, Weiss E. Whole beetroot consumption acutely improves running performance. J Acad Nutr Diet. 2012;112:548–52.
26. Polyviou TP, Pitsiladis YP, Celis-Morales C, Brown B, Speakman JR, Malkova D. The effects of hyperhydrating supplements containing creatine and glucose on plasma lipids and insulin sensitivity in endurance-trained athletes. J Amino Acids. 2015;2015:352458.
27. Rawson ES, Stec MJ, Frederickson SJ, Miles MP. Low-dose creatine supplementation enhances fatigue resistance in the absence of weight gain. Nutrition. 2011;27:451–5.

28. Stomme J, Rustad P, Steensland H, Theodorsen L, Urdal P. Reference
intervals for eight enzymes in blood of adult females and males measured
in accordance with the international Federation of Clinical Chemistry
reference system at 378C: part of the Nordic Reference Interval Project.
Scand J Clin Lab Invest. 2004;64:371–84.
29. Van Loan MD. Bioelectrical impedance analysis to determine fat-free mass,
total body water and body fat. Sports Medicine (Auckland). 1990;10:205–17.
30. van Loon L. Impact of Nitrate Ingestion on Protein Synthesis (PRO-Nitrate).
In: ClinicalTrialsgovU.S. National Institutes of Health, 2012.
31. Webb AJ, Patel N, Loukogeorgakis S, Okorie M, Aboud Z, Misra S, Rashid R,
Miall P, Deanfield J, Benjamin N. Acute blood pressure lowering,
vasoprotective, and antiplatelet properties of dietary nitrate via
bioconversion to nitrite. Hypertension. 2008;51:784–90.
32. Wilder N, Deivert RG, Hagerman F, Gilders R. The effects of low-dose
creatine supplementation versus creatine loading in collegiate football
players. Journal of athletic training. 2001;36:124.
33. Wilder N, Gilders R, Hagerman F, Deivert RG. The effects of a 10-week,
periodized, off-season resistance-training program and creatine
supplementation among collegiate football players. J Strength Cond Res.
2002;16:343–52.
34. Wyss M, Kaddurah-Daouk R. Creatine and creatinine metabolism. Physiol
Rev. 2000;80:1107–213.
35. Zhang XJ, Chinkes DL, Wolfe RR. The anabolic effect of arginine on proteins
in skin wound and muscle is independent of nitric oxide production. Clin
Nutr. 2008;27:649–56.

## 12

Evaluation of congruence among dietary supplement use and motivation for supplementation in young, Canadian athletes

Jill A. Parnell[1][*], Kristin Wiens[2] and Kelly Anne Erdman[3]

Abstract

Background: Dietary supplement use is endemic in young athletes; however, it is unclear if their choices are congruent with their motivation for supplementation and the established benefits of the dietary supplements. The aim of this study was to evaluate the relationships between dietary supplement use and self-reported rationale in young athletes.

Methods: Canadian athletes ($n = 567$; 11–25 years; 76 % club or provincial level, 24 % national or higher) completed a questionnaire designed to assess supplementation patterns and motivation for supplementation. Chi square tests examined associations between dietary supplements and self-reported rationale for use.

Results: Vitamin and mineral supplements, including vitamin-enriched water, were associated with several health- and performance- related reasons ($p < 0.001$). Branched chain amino acids (BCAA) and glutamine were linked to improving diet and immune function ($p < 0.01$), but were more strongly associated with performance reasons, as were performance foods (protein powder, sport bars, sport gels, etc.). Plant extracts and fatty acids were primarily associated with health reasons, particularly immune support ($p < 0.001$).

Conclusions: Congruencies exist between performance rationales and supplementation for common ergogenic aids, however, less so for vitamin and mineral supplements, vitamin-enriched water, and plant extracts. Incongruences were found between fatty acids, protein supplements, vitamin and mineral supplements, vitamin-enriched water, and plant extracts and health motivators for supplementation. Educational interventions are essential to ensure young athletes are using dietary supplements safely and effectively.

Keywords: Sport supplements, Dietary ergogenic aids, Supplementation rationale, Dietary supplements

Background

Athletes experience significant internal and external pressures inspiring them to set high performance goals. Young athletes have the added requirement of supporting growth and promoting healthy maturation, which can be especially difficult in sports encouraging low body weight or body fat. Further, challenges identified as unique to young athletes include: decreased metabolic efficiency (increased energy requirements per kilogram of body weight as compared to adults performing the same type of exercise), preferential fat oxidation, and reduced ability to thermo-regulate while exercising [1].

In order to maximize performance, athletes often turn to supplements in the belief they will help them stay competitive and healthy. Petroczi et al. [2] report 78 % of young athletes thought nutritional supplementation was not essential for athlete success; however, note the contradiction in actual habits, where 48 % of these same athletes were using nutritional supplements. In this case, the most common reasons for supplement use included "maintaining strength", "avoiding sickness" and "endurance enhancement". Recent work in young, Canadian athletes found the

* Correspondence: jparnell@mtroyal.ca
[1]Department of Physical Education and Recreation Studies, Mount Royal University, 4825 Mount Royal Gate SW, Calgary, Alberta T3E 6K6, Canada
Full list of author information is available at the end of the article

top five reasons for supplement use were "stay healthy", "increase energy", "immune system", "recovery" and "overall athletic performance" [3].

Supplementation is common in young athletes with prevalence estimates varying depending on the specific population and dietary supplements included in the assessment. We report one of the highest rates of supplement use at 98 % in young, Canadian athletes [3]. The reason for higher rates in young, Canadian athletes is unclear; however, is likely due to the broad definition of dietary supplements based on the Dietary Supplement Health and Education Act in the United States [4] and the Canadian Natural Health Products Regulations [5]. Popular supplements consumed by young athletes include, but are not restricted to: sport drinks (i.e., carbohydrate electrolyte solutions), energy drinks (i.e., caffeinated beverages), vitamin-enriched water, vitamin or minerals either individually or in combination, sport bars, protein powders, creatine, fatty acid preparations (i.e. omega-3 supplements, fish oil, flax seed oil, cod liver oil), and plant extracts [2, 3, 6].

Dietary supplement patterns and motivations for supplement use in young athletes have been established. What remains to be determined is if there is a link between the purported functions of the dietary supplements athletes are consuming and their self-reported rationale(s) for supplement use. One study, among youth, reports perceived associations between energy drinks and enhanced endurance, as well as maintaining strength and creatine and whey protein [2]. Conversely, overall there was significant incongruence between rationale for supplement use and actual practice in these athletes [2]. The same group reported a high degree of incongruence between supplementation and performance-related rationales in athletes who were primarily between 19 and 29 years of age [7]. Notable exceptions include the associations between creatine, whey protein and strength maintenance, as well as creatine and the ability to train longer. Conversely, the authors single out iron, vitamin C and ginseng as particularly problematic when it comes to the athletes' perception of the potential performance benefits of these supplements as compared to their actual benefits [7].

The aim of the present study was to assess the relationship between supplementation and self-reported rationale for supplement use with the goal of developing a better understanding of the knowledge and practices of young athletes. There is currently very little information available in this area, and even less so in developing, Canadian athletes competing primarily at lower performance levels. The focus on club and provincial level athletes is crucial, as this is the extent at which most youth compete. This research will contribute to the field, as it will identify knowledge gaps that can be addressed by athlete support personnel.

Methods
Participants
Athletes were recruited from the province of Alberta representing a variety of sporting organizations. All athletes were between the ages of 11 and 25 years and participated in structured training for a minimum of five hours per week. Athletes from all levels of competition were included, however, 76 % competed at the provincial level or lower and 24 % competed nationally or internationally. Power calculations using a prior study in high-performance, Canadian athletes and a margin of error (4 % with 95 % confidence and a power of 80 %) established that 567 participants were required [6]. All athletes provided written consent or written assent with written consent from a parent or guardian if they were under the age of 18 years. The study was approved by the Mount Royal University Human Research Ethics Board.

Study design
The athletes completed a paper version of a content validated and reliability tested questionnaire. Detailed information on the questionnaire development and administration has been published previously [3]. Briefly, a panel of experts reviewed all questions for content and clarity and their suggestions were incorporated into a revised version. A second panel of experts reviewed the revised version and all questions were rated using a Likert scale. Test re-test data was collected from 31 participants and analyzed by weighted kappa coefficients to assess reliability. The questionnaire was administered in person by the study investigators. The participants were free to ask the researchers for additional information or to clarify the questions; however, subjects completed the questionnaire without assistance from parents, guardians, coaches, trainers, etc. Further details regarding the administration of the questionnaire are available [3]. The questionnaire asked for information regarding their use of dietary supplements, reason(s) for taking supplements, and sources of information. The questions analyzed here include: 1) "Do you know the kinds of supplements you take? (Do you know what the supplements you take are called or does someone else give you your supplements?)" with "I'm not sure which supplements I take", "I know some of the supplements I take", "I know many of the supplements I take", and "I know all of the supplements I take" as response options. 2) "Do you know why you take each supplement? (Do you know what each supplement is for or do you take the supplement and not question it?)" with "I'm not sure why I take each supplement", "I know why I take some of my supplements", "I know why I take many of my supplements", and "I know why I take all of my supplements" as response options. 3) "How often have you

taken the following dietary supplements in the last 3 months? Please circle Daily, Weekly, Monthly, If I'm Sick or Never in the "How Often" column. If you do take a supplement, please write the exact one in the "Supplement Name" column if you know it". Options for supplements grouped by category can be found in Table 1. 4) "What are your reason(s) for taking dietary supplements? Please check all that apply". Options for reasons for supplement use grouped by category can be found in Table 2. Athletes were not specifically asked to provide a rationale for each supplement they consumed. Relevant information including age, gender, sport type, level of competition, and average number of training hours per week was also collected.

Criteria for evaluating outcome measures

Athletes were categorized by gender, age group (11–13 years, 14–16 years, 17–18 years, and 19–25 years), sport classification (power and strength, endurance, intermittent, and aesthetic), and level of competition (club, provincial, national or higher), as previously described [3]. Rationales for supplementation were grouped into health-related reasons, performance-related reasons, or influence-of-others.

Statistical analyses

Intake for each supplement was categorized into 'Yes or No' based on any reported use. Chi squared tests were used to determine congruency between individual supplements and self-reported rationale for supplement use overall and between gender, age, sport type, and competition level groups. Cramer's V was calculated to describe the magnitude of association between variables and 0.10 was considered a small effect size, 0.30 a medium effect size and 0.50 a large effect size [8]. All analyses were conducted in SPSS Version 22.0 (Armonk, NY: IBM Corp).

Results

Three hundred and thirty five female athletes and 232 male athletes completed the questionnaire. One questionnaire was omitted from the analysis as the respondent reported consuming all supplements on a daily basis. Detailed information regarding the athletes' ages, gender,

sport types, and competition levels have been published previously [3].

Self-evaluation of knowledge for reasons for supplementation

When athletes were asked to evaluate their knowledge of the reasons for taking dietary supplements six percent were "not sure", 22 % said they knew the reasons for "some" of the supplements, 30 % said they knew the purpose of "many" of the supplements they took, and 42 % reported they knew the reasons for taking "all" of their supplements. There were significant differences within age groups ($p = 0.01$; V = 115) with 43 % of those between the ages of 11 and 13 years claiming they knew the purpose of all of their supplements as compared to 60 % of those in the 19–25 age group. No differences were noted in self-evaluated knowledge of the reasons for taking supplements within the gender, sport type, or level of competition groupings.

Supplement choice and health related reasons

Eighty-eight percent of athletes reported at least one health-related reason for supplementation. Vitamin and mineral supplements, either individual or in combinations, were closely associated with all health-related reasons (Table 3). Conversely, vitamin-enriched water was associated with "improve diet" and "stay healthy" but the associations were not as strong as with traditional forms of vitamin and mineral supplements.

Athletes who consumed recovery drinks, sport/protein bars, protein powders, glutamine, and branched chain amino acids (BCAA) were also interested in improving their diet and supporting their immune system. Fatty acid supplementation was linked to all health-related reasons (Table 3).

Creatine, sport drinks, energy drinks, and sport gels and gummies were rarely associated with health-related reasons. Conversely, plant extracts were related to all health reasons for supplementation (Table 3). Plant extracts athletes consumed included: oil of oregano, ginseng, green tea pills, garlic, herbs, St John's Wart, echinacea, and Cold FX (™).

Table 1 Supplements listed on the questionnaire

Supplement Category	Individual Supplements Listed
Dietary/Medical	Multi-vitamin/Multi-mineralVitamin CB-VitaminsVitamin DVitamin EVitamin-enriched waterCalciumIronMagnesium
Other Supplements	Fatty acid preparationsPlant/herbal extracts
Ergogenic Aids (Muscle Building/Increased Energy)	Branched chain amino acidsBeta-alanineGlutamineCreatineEnergy drinks
Performance Foods	Protein powderSport/electrolyte drinksRecovery drinksProtein/sport barSport gelsGummy/bean

Table 2 Reasons for supplementation listed on the questionnaire

Reason Category	Individual Reasons Listed
Health-Related	Medical (your doctor told you to)To improve your diet (food you eat everyday)Stay healthyEnhance immune system (so you don't get sick)
Performance-Related	Increase or maintain muscle mass, strength, and/or powerIncrease endurance (how long you can exercise)Increase energy (so you don't feel tired)Enhance overall athletic performanceImprove exercise recovery (after exercise)
Influence of Others	Because others (friends, family, teammates) doSomeone told you to (coach, parent, friend etc.)

Table 3 Associations between supplement use and health-related reasons for supplementation

Supplement	Medical (19 %)	Improve Diet (43 %)	Stay Healthy (81 %)	Support Immune System (52 %)
Multi-vitamin/Multi-mineral (67 %)	$\chi^2 = 12.576$ $p < 0.001$ $V = 0.150$	$\chi^2 = 7.057$ $p = 0.008$ $V = 0.112$	$\chi^2 = 32.679$ $p < 0.001$ $V = 0.241$	$\chi^2 = 41.807$ $p < 0.001$ $V = 0.273$
Vitamin C (66 %)	$\chi^2 = 5.825$ $p = 0.016$ $V = 0.102$	$\chi^2 = 15.603$ $p < 0.001$ $V = 0.166$	$\chi^2 = 35.707$ $p < 0.001$ $V = 0.252$	$\chi^2 = 32.878$ $p < 0.001$ $V = 0.241$
B Vitamins (32 %)	$\chi^2 = 3.623$ $p = 0.057$ $V = 0.080$	$\chi^2 = 12.740$ $p < 0.001$ $V = 0.150$	$\chi^2 = 14.195$ $p < 0.001$ $V = 0.159$	$\chi^2 = 17.709$ $p < 0.001$ $V = 0.177$
Vitamin E (26 %)	$\chi^2 = 2.136$ $p = 0.144$ $V = 0.062$	$\chi^2 = 8.109$ $p = 0.004$ $V = 0.120$	$\chi^2 = 8.428$ $p = 0.004$ $V = 0.122$	$\chi^2 = 10.368$ $p = 0.001$ $V = 0.136$
Vitamin D (48 %)	$\chi^2 = 15.691$ $p < 0.001$ $V = 0.167$	$\chi^2 = 12.615$ $p < 0.001$ $V = 0.150$	$\chi^2 = 32.496$ $p < 0.001$ $V = 0.240$	$\chi^2 = 22.208$ $p < 0.001$ $V = 0.199$
Vitamin-enriched Water (65 %)	$\chi^2 = 3.386$ $p = 0.066$ $V = 0.077$	$\chi^2 = 4.664$ $p = 0.031$ $V = 0.091$	$\chi^2 = 5.183$ $p = 0.023$ $V = 0.096$	$\chi^2 = 2.510$ $p = 0.113$ $V = 0.067$
Iron (27 %)	$\chi^2 = 17.142$ $p < 0.001$ $V = 0.174$	$\chi^2 = 20.320$ $p < 0.001$ $V = 0.190$	$\chi^2 = 13.759$ $p < 0.001$ $V = 0.156$	$\chi^2 = 16.803$ $p < 0.001$ $V = 0.172$
Calcium (43 %)	$\chi^2 = 22.947$ $p < 0.001$ $V = 0.202$	$\chi^2 = 30.458$ $p < 0.001$ $V = 0.232$	$\chi^2 = 31.370$ $p < 0.001$ $V = 0.236$	$\chi^2 = 26.782$ $p < 0.001$ $V = 0.218$
Magnesium (17 %)	$\chi^2 = 1.001$ $p = 0.317$ $V = 0.042$	$\chi^2 = 9.440$ $p = 0.002$ $V = 0.129$	$\chi^2 = 8.538$ $p = 0.003$ $V = 0.123$	$\chi^2 = 12.815$ $p < 0.001$ $V = 0.151$
Protein Powder (51 %)	$\chi^2 = 1.692$ $p = 0.193$ $V = 0.055$	$\chi^2 = 14.825$ $p < 0.001$ $V = 0.162$	$\chi^2 = 5.085$ $p = 0.024$ $V = 0.095$	$\chi^2 = 16.882$ $p < 0.001$ $V = 0.173$
BCAA (8 %)	$\chi^2 = 0.233$ $p = 0.629$ $V = 0.020$	$\chi^2 = 9.765$ $p = 0.002$ $V = 0.132$	$\chi^2 = 2.415$ $p = 0.120$ $V = 0.065$	$\chi^2 = 7.317$ $p = 0.007$ $V = 0.114$
Beta-alanine (4 %)	$\chi^2 = 5.191$ $p = 0.023$ $V = 0.096$	$\chi^2 = 3.369$ $p = 0.066$ $V = 0.077$	$\chi^2 = 0.871$ $p = 0.351$ $V = 0.039$	$\chi^2 = 0.228$ $p = 0.633$ $V = 0.020$
Glutamine (8 %)	$\chi^2 = 0.260$ $p = 0.610$ $V = 0.021$	$\chi^2 = 13.015$ $p < 0.001$ $V = 0.152$	$\chi^2 = 4.687$ $p = 0.030$ $V = 0.091$	$\chi^2 = 6.923$ $p = 0.009$ $V = 0.111$
Fatty Acids (40 %)	$\chi^2 = 13.960$ $p < 0.001$ $V = 0.157$	$\chi^2 = 9.602$ $p = 0.002$ $V = 0.130$	$\chi^2 = 21.589$ $p < 0.001$ $V = 0.196$	$\chi^2 = 34.971$ $p < 0.001$ $V = 0.249$
Energy Drinks (27 %)	$\chi^2 = 4.642$ $p = 0.031$ $V = 0.091$	$\chi^2 = 8.362$ $p = 0.004$ $V = 0.122$	$\chi^2 = 0.757$ $p = 0.384$ $V = 0.037$	$\chi^2 = 0.285$ $p = 0.593$ $V = 0.022$

Table 3 Associations between supplement use and health-related reasons for supplementation *(Continued)*

Sport/Electrolyte Drinks (90 %)	$x^2 = 0.817$	$x^2 = 1.164$	$x^2 = 5.081$	$x^2 = 1.172$
	$p = 0.366$	$p = 0.281$	$p = 0.024$	$p = 0.279$
	$V = 0.038$	$V = 0.045$	$V = 0.095$	$V = 0.046$
Sport Gels/Gummies (26 %)	$x^2 = 1.315$	$x^2 = 0.555$	$x^2 = 5.810$	$x^2 = 3.462$
	$p = 0.251$	$p = 0.456$	$p = 0.016$	$p = 0.063$
	$V = 0.048$	$V = 0.031$	$V = 0.101$	$V = 0.078$
Sport/Protein Bar (71 %)	$x^2 = 0.961$	$\mathbf{x^2 = 10.708}$	$\mathbf{x^2 = 11.233}$	$\mathbf{x^2 = 10.456}$
	$p = 0.327$	$\mathbf{p = 0.001}$	$\mathbf{p = 0.001}$	$\mathbf{p = 0.001}$
	$V = 0.041$	$\mathbf{V = 0.138}$	$\mathbf{V = 0.141}$	$\mathbf{V = 0.136}$
Recovery Drinks (31 %)	$x^2 = 0.166$	$\mathbf{x^2 = 10.532}$	$x^2 = 6.735$	$x^2 = 9.528$
	$p = 0.684$	$\mathbf{p = 0.001}$	$p = 0.009$	$p = 0.002$
	$V = 0.017$	$\mathbf{V = 0.137}$	$V = 0.109$	$V = 0.130$
Creatine (7 %)	$x^2 = 0.015$	$x^2 = 1.416$	$x^2 = 0.123$	$x^2 = 1.617$
	$p = 0.903$	$p = 0.234$	$p = 0.726$	$p = 0.204$
	$V = 0.005$	$V = 0.050$	$V = 0.015$	$V = 0.054$
Plant Extracts (47 %)	$x^2 = 9.536$	$x^2 = 7.859$	$x^2 = 9.864$	$\mathbf{x^2 = 49.130}$
	$p = 0.002$	$p = 0.005$	$p = 0.002$	$\mathbf{p < 0.001}$
	$V = 0.130$	$V = 0.118$	$V = 0.132$	$\mathbf{V = 0.295}$

Statistically significant associations at $p \leq 0.001$ are in bold. Percentages after the supplement type represent the percent of total athletes consuming the supplements listed. Percentages after the health-related reasons represent the percent of total athletes supplementing for the reasons listed

Age did not have an effect on health-related reasons for choosing supplementation as the percentage of athletes choosing supplements for health-related reasons ranged from 87 to 89 % in the various age groups ($p = 0.94$; V = 0.026). Gender, level of competition or sport type did not impact health reasons for supplement choice.

Supplement choice and performance related reasons

In total, 81 % of athletes reported performance reasons as a rationale for supplementation. Generally, vitamin supplements were associated with all performance reasons with the exception of recovery. There were variations depending on the specific vitamin; however, the strongest associations were found with the B vitamins and vitamin E. Vitamin-enriched water was associated with all performance-related reasons for choosing supplements (Table 4). Minerals followed a similar trend with associations between iron, calcium, and magnesium and all performance-related reasons with the exception of recovery, for which only magnesium showed an association (Table 4).

Protein powders, BCAA, and glutamine were strongly linked to performance reasons for supplementation; however, beta-alanine was not. Energy drinks were associated with muscle mass/strength, endurance, increase energy, and recovery but not overall athletic performance. Sport/electrolyte drinks, sport gels and gummies, sport/protein bars, and recovery drinks were associated with all performance reasons as was creatine, with the exception of increase energy (Table 4). Plant extracts were associated with muscle mass/strength, increase energy, overall athletic performance, however, the association was not as strong as with many other supplements (Table 4).

There were noticeable differences within the age groups in performance reasons for supplementation.

The 11–13 year olds were the least likely to choose supplementation for performance reasons at 73 % and the 19–25 year olds the most likely at 94 % ($p < 0.01$; V = 0.144). Males had a higher use of supplements for performance reasons at 87 % as compared to females at 76 % ($p < 0.01$; V = 0.144). Level of competition did not influence supplement usage for performance-related reasons with all groups at approximately 80 %; however, aesthetic athletes were the least likely to use supplements for performance reasons at 64 % as compared to 77 % for intermittent athletes, 82 % for endurance athletes and 90 % for strength athletes ($p < 0.01$; V = 0.174).

Supplement choice and influence of others

Reasons for supplementation under the purview of others included "because others (family/friends/teammates) do" and "someone told you to". Although 44 % of athletes report others influenced their decision to use supplements, this category was the lowest ranking. Calcium and performance foods were associated with family/friends/teammates. Those athletes who reported taking supplements because "someone told them to" were also more likely to use multi-vitamin/multi-minerals, vitamin D, iron, calcium, fatty acids, and energy drinks (Table 5). Notably, supplement usage for reasons classified as due to the influence of others was 46 % in the 11–13 year olds and 50 % in the 14–16 year olds, whereas, it dropped to 35 % in 17–18 year olds and 30 % in 19–25 year olds ($p < 0.01$; V = 0.144). Gender, level of competition or sport type did not impact supplementation due to the influence of others.

Discussion

The current study highlights the links between dietary supplement consumption and motivation for supplement

Table 4 Associations between supplement use and performance-related reasons for supplementation

Supplement	Muscle Mass/Strength (38 %)	Endurance (31 %)	Increase Energy (55 %)	Overall Athletic Performance (49 %)	Recovery (49 %)
Multi-vitamin/Multi-mineral (67 %)	$\chi^2 = 11.965$ $p = 0.001$ $V = 0.146$	$\chi^2 = 8.469$ $p = 0.004$ $V = 0.123$	$\chi^2 = 0.203$ $p = 0.652$ $V = 0.019$	$\chi^2 = 6.370$ $p = 0.012$ $V = 0.106$	$\chi^2 = 5.773$ $p = 0.016$ $V = 0.101$
Vitamin C (66 %)	$\chi^2 = 7.688$ $p = 0.006$ $V = 0.117$	$\chi^2 = 5.278$ $p = 0.022$ $V = 0.097$	$\chi^2 = 2.580$ $p = 0.108$ $V = 0.068$	$\chi^2 = 4.662$ $p = 0.031$ $V = 0.091$	$\chi^2 = 3.046$ p = 0.081 $V = 0.073$
B Vitamins (32 %)	$\chi^2 = 11.002$ $p = 0.001$ $V = 0.140$	$\chi^2 = 20.610$ $p < 0.001$ $V = 0.191$	$\chi^2 = 6.675$ $p = 0.010$ $V = 0.109$	$\chi^2 = 11.867$ $p = 0.001$ $V = 0.145$	$\chi^2 = 1.487$ $p = 0.223$ $V = 0.051$
Vitamin E (26 %)	$\chi^2 = 25.084$ $p < 0.001$ $V = 0.211$	$\chi^2 = 27.410$ $p < 0.001$ $V = 0.221$	$\chi^2 = 10.883$ $p < 0.001$ $V = 0.139$	$\chi^2 = 18.510$ $p < 0.001$ $V = 0.181$	$\chi^2 = 2.257$ $p = 0.133$ $V = 0.063$
Vitamin D (48 %)	$\chi^2 = 9.013$ $p = 0.003$ $V = 0.127$	$\chi^2 = 12.488$ $p < 0.001$ $V = 0.149$	$\chi^2 = 0.619$ $p = 0.431$ $V = 0.033$	$\chi^2 = 2.629$ $p = 0.105$ $V = 0.068$	$\chi^2 = 0.616$ $p = 0.433$ $V = 0.033$
Vitamin- enriched Water (65 %)	$\chi^2 = 5.594$ $p = 0.018$ $V = 0.100$	$\chi^2 = 10.919$ $p = 0.001$ $V = 0.139$	$\chi^2 = 13.372$ $p < 0.001$ $V = 0.154$	$\chi^2 = 17.511$ $p < 0.001$ $V = 0.176$	$\chi^2 = 4.535$ $p = 0.033$ $V = 0.090$
Iron (27 %)	$\chi^2 = 6.234$ $p = 0.013$ $V = 0.105$	$\chi^2 = 7.387$ $p = 0.007$ $V = 0.114$	$\chi^2 = 6.574$ $p = 0.010$ $V = 0.108$	$\chi^2 = 7.795$ $p = 0.005$ $V = 0.117$	$\chi^2 = 0.223$ $p = 0.637$ $V = 0.020$
Calcium (43 %)	$\chi^2 = 25.438$ $p < 0.001$ $V = 0.212$	$\chi^2 = 10.571$ $p = 0.001$ $V = 0.137$	$\chi^2 = 9.816$ $p = 0.002$ $V = 0.132$	$\chi^2 = 10.204$ $p = 0.001$ $V = 0.134$	$\chi^2 = 3.097$ $p = 0.078$ $V = 0.074$
Magnesium (17 %)	$\chi^2 = 11.060$ $p = 0.001$ $V = 0.140$	$\chi^2 = 16.037$ $p < 0.001$ $V = 0.169$	$\chi^2 = 7.193$ $p = 0.007$ $V = 0.113$	$\chi^2 = 7.827$ $p = 0.005$ $V = 0.118$	$\chi^2 = 5.510$ $p = 0.019$ $V = 0.099$
Protein Powder (51 %)	$\chi^2 = 120.609$ $p < 0.001$ $V = 0.462$	$\chi^2 = 27.927$ $p < 0.001$ $V = 0.223$	$\chi^2 = 12.172$ $p < 0.001$ $V = 0.147$	$\chi^2 = 47.946$ $p < 0.001$ $V = 0.292$	$\chi^2 = 51.470$ $p < 0.001$ $V = 0.302$
BCAA (8 %)	$\chi^2 = 21.995$ $p < 0.001$ $V = 0.198$	$\chi^2 = 14.313$ $p < 0.001$ $V = 0.159$	$\chi^2 = 7.943$ $p = 0.005$ $V = 0.119$	$\chi^2 = 16.010$ $p < 0.001$ $V = 0.169$	$\chi^2 = 3.392$ $p = 0.065$ $V = 0.078$
Beta-alanine (4 %)	$\chi^2 = 3.440$ $p = 0.064$ $V = 0.078$	$\chi^2 = 5.451$ $p = 0.020$ $V = 0.098$	$\chi^2 = 3.095$ $p = 0.079$ $V = 0.074$	$\chi^2 = 2.462$ $p = 0.117$ $V = 0.066$	$\chi^2 = 0.536$ $p = 0.464$ $V = 0.031$
Glutamine (8 %)	$\chi^2 = 26.895$ $p < 0.001$ $V = 0.218$	$\chi^2 = 27.131$ $p < 0.001$ $V = 0.219$	$\chi^2 = 9.594$ $p = 0.002$ $V = 0.130$	$\chi^2 = 15.530$ $p < 0.001$ $V = 0.166$	$\chi^2 = 15.335$ $p < 0.001$ $V = 0.165$
Fatty Acids (40 %)	$\chi^2 = 12.534$ $p < 0.001$ $V = 0.149$	$\chi^2 = 4.866$ $p = 0.027$ $V = 0.093$	$\chi^2 = 0.302$ $p = 0.583$ $V = 0.023$	$\chi^2 = 2.087$ $p = 0.149$ $V = 0.061$	$\chi^2 = 0.267$ $p = 0.606$ $V = 0.022$
Energy Drinks (27 %)	$\chi^2 = 14.246$ $p < 0.001$ $V = 0.159$	$\chi^2 = 5.024$ $p = 0.025$ $V = 0.094$	$\chi^2 = 22.360$ $p < 0.001$ $V = 0.199$	$\chi^2 = 0.653$ $p = 0.419$ $V = 0.034$	$\chi^2 = 4.312$ $p = 0.038$ $V = 0.087$
Sport/Electrolyte Drinks (90 %)	$\chi^2 = 17.637$ $p < 0.001$ $V = 0.177$	$\chi^2 = 9.922$ $p = 0.002$ $V = 0.133$	$\chi^2 = 19.795$ $p < 0.001$ $V = 0.187$	$\chi^2 = 16.349$ $p < 0.001$ $V = 0.170$	$\chi^2 = 18.945$ $p < 0.001$ $V = 0.183$
Sport Gels/Gummies (26 %)	$\chi^2 = 14.132$ $p < 0.001$ $V = 0.158$	$\chi^2 = 8.300$ $p = 0.004$ $V = 0.121$	$\chi^2 = 12.120$ $p < 0.001$ $V = 0.146$	$\chi^2 = 8.098$ $p = 0.004$ $V = 0.120$	$\chi^2 = 18.349$ $p < 0.001$ $V = 0.180$
Sport/Protein Bar (71 %)	$\chi^2 = 27.780$ $p < 0.001$ $V = 0.222$	$\chi^2 = 29.989$ $p < 0.001$ $V = 0.230$	$\chi^2 = 16.794$ $p < 0.001$ $V = 0.172$	$\chi^2 = 28.890$ $p < 0.001$ $V = 0.226$	$\chi^2 = 38.043$ $p < 0.001$ $V = 0.259$
Recovery Drinks (31 %)	$\chi^2 = 57.268$ $p < 0.001$ $V = 0.319$	$\chi^2 = 41.358$ $p < 0.001$ $V = 0.271$	$\chi^2 = 16.384$ $p < 0.001$ $V = 0.171$	$\chi^2 = 41.349$ $p < 0.001$ $V = 0.271$	$\chi^2 = 61.395$ $p < 0.001$ $V = 0.330$

Table 4 Associations between supplement use and performance-related reasons for supplementation *(Continued)*

Creatine (7 %)	$x^2 = 19.434$ $p < 0.001$ $V = 0.186$	$x^2 = 15.634$ $p < 0.001$ $V = 0.166$	$x^2 = 3.173$ $p = 0.075$ $V = 0.075$	$x^2 = 10.546$ $p < 0.001$ $V = 0.137$	$x^2 = 6.629$ $p = 0.010$ $V = 0.108$
Plant Extracts (47 %)	$x^2 = 8.426$ $p = 0.004$ $V = 0.122$	$x^2 = 2.079$ $p = 0.149$ $V = 0.061$	$x^2 = 7.471$ $p = 0.006$ $V = 0.115$	$x^2 = 5.633$ $p = 0.018$ $V = 0.100$	$x^2 = 3.194$ $p = 0.074$ $V = 0.075$

Statistically significant associations at $p \le 0.001$ are in bold. Percentages after the supplement type represent the percent of total athletes consuming the supplements listed. Percentages after the performance-related reasons represent the percent of total athletes supplementing for the reasons listed

use among young, Canadian athletes. These results are significant as they provide an, albeit indirect, assessment of the athletes' knowledge of the benefits – real or purported – of dietary supplements as they relate to health and performance. Research in this demographic is particularly important, as the group consisted mostly of young, club level athletes who were less likely to have access to sport nutrition professional advisors, yet represent the majority of young athletes. Indeed, fewer than half had ever met with a dietitian and 38 % had previously attended a session on dietary or sport supplements [3]. Furthermore, the high prevalence of dietary supplement use suggests that research in this area is essential to ensure safe and effective supplementation practices.

Athlete self-evaluated perceived knowledge of the reasons for supplement use is generally low, although it does increase with age, whereby 60 % of athletes claim to know the reasons for all of the supplements they are consuming by ages 19–25. Indeed this purported level of knowledge is improved as compared to a 2003 study that found 10 % of Singaporean athletes, 85 % of which were 25 years or younger, self-rated their level of perceived knowledge regarding dietary supplements as good or excellent [9].

Vitamin and mineral supplements were associated with health-related reasons; however, evidence indicates these supplements are only effective in the case of a deficiency [10] suggesting a lack of congruency; with possible exceptions being vitamin D and calcium (females), which are reportedly low in athletes [11, 12]. In the case of micronutrient deficiencies, dietary changes rather than supplementation should be the primary target to bring intakes into the healthy range. The consumption

Table 5 Associations between supplement use and influence-of-others reasons

Supplement	Family/Friends/Teammates (21 %)	Someone Told You To (35 %)
Multi-vitamin/Multi-mineral (67 %)	$x^2 = 1.074 p = 0.300 V = 0.044$	$x^2 = 15.358 p < 0.001 V = 0.165$
Vitamin C (66 %)	$x^2 = 0.522 p = 0.470 V = 0.030$	$x^2 = 1.273 p = 0.259 V = 0.048$
B Vitamins (32 %)	$x^2 = 2.480 p = 0.115 V = 0.066$	$x^2 = 1.255 p = 0.263 V = 0.047$
Vitamin E (26 %)	$x^2 = 1.070 p = 0.301 V = 0.044$	$x^2 = 2.727 p = 0.099 V = 0.070$
Vitamin D (48 %)	$x^2 = 0.014 p = 0.904 V = 0.005$	$x^2 = 9.449 p = 0.002 V = 0.130$
Vitamin-enriched Water (65 %)	$x^2 = 2.108 p = 0.147 V = 0.061$	$x^2 = 0.195 p = 0.659 V = 0.019$
Iron (27 %)	$x^2 = 2.982 p = 0.084 V = 0.073$	$x^2 = 4.773 p = 0.029 V = 0.092$
Calcium (43 %)	$x^2 = 6.104 p = 0.013 V = 0.104$	$x^2 = 7.059 p = 0.008 V = 0.112$
Magnesium (17 %)	$x^2 = 3.587 p = 0.058 V = 0.080$	$x^2 = 1.846 p = 0.174 V = 0.057$
Protein Powder (51 %)	$x^2 = 0.005 p = 0.941 V = 0.003$	$x^2 = 0.003 p = 0.959 V = 0.002$
BCAA (8 %)	$x^2 = 0.051 p = 0.821 V = 0.010$	$x^2 = 0.031 p = 0.859 V = 0.007$
Beta-alanine (4 %)	$x^2 = 0.003 p = 0.957 V = 0.002$	$x^2 = 0.012 p = 0.914 V = 0.005$
Glutamine (8 %)	$x^2 = 1.393 p = 0.238 V = 0.050$	$x^2 = 0.289 p = 0.591 V = 0.023$
Fatty Acids (40 %)	$x^2 = 2.852 p = 0.091 V = 0.071$	$x^2 = 7.947 p = 0.005 V = 0.119$
Energy Drinks (27 %)	$x^2 = 3.643 p = 0.056 V = 0.080$	$x^2 = 5.330 P = 0.021 V = 0.097$
Sport/Electrolyte Drinks (90 %)	$x^2 = 5.129 p = 0.024 V = 0.095$	$x^2 = 0.165 p = 0.685 V = 0.017$
Sport Gels/Gummies (26 %)	$x^2 = 6.952 p = 0.008 V = 0.111$	$x^2 = 0.882 p = 0.348 V = 0.039$
Sport/Protein Bar (71 %)	$x^2 = 6.420 p = 0.011 V = 0.107$	$x^2 = 3.154 p = 0.076 V = 0.075$
Recovery Drinks (31 %)	$x^2 = 0.049 p = 0.826 V = 0.009$	$x^2 = 0.365 p = 0.546 V = 0.025$
Creatine (7 %)	$x^2 = 3.489 p = 0.062 V = 0.079$	$x^2 = 0.012 p = 0.913 V = 0.005$
Plant Extracts (47 %)	$x^2 = 0.376 p = 0.540 V = 0.026$	$x^2 = 0.412 p = 0.521 V = 0.027$

Statistically significant associations at $p \le 0.001$ are in bold. Percentages after the supplement type represent the percent of total athletes consuming the supplements listed. Percentages after the influence-of-others reasons represent the percent of total athletes supplementing for the reasons listed

of sport bars, protein powders, and amino acid supplements was linked to reasons for choosing supplements associated with improved health, particularly immune system enhancement and to improve diet quality. In cases of inadequate dietary intake of protein, performance foods high in protein (protein bars, recovery drinks, protein powders, etc.) would be beneficial, suggesting congruence between the actions and motivation; however, when dietitians observed nutritional habits in young athletes, they found protein intakes to be more than sufficient. Average protein intake in male athletes was 2.3 g/kg body weight, which is significantly higher than the recommended upper intake for athletes of 1.7 g/kg body weight, and 86 % of females met the recommended intake with an average intake of 1.4 g/kg body weight [13]. Furthermore, in Canadian, high-performance athletes, protein intakes were 1.7 g/kg body weight from food alone and 1.8 g/kg body weight from food and supplements in females and 1.9 g/kg body weight from food alone and 2.1 g/kg body weight from food and supplements for males [14], clearly indicating protein is not a nutrient of concern for most athletes.

Evidence of congruence between health-related reasons for supplementation and actual practice also exists in that creatine, energy drinks, sport gels and gummies, and sport drinks were rarely associated with health reasons; indicating athletes are potentially able to distinguish between supplementation for health and performance in these cases. Conversely, it has been suggested that consuming a 6 % or greater carbohydrate beverage, such as a commercial sport drink, during prolonged exercise can reduce the risk of upper respiratory tract infections, potentially creating the case for sport drinks and improved immune function [15]. Fatty acid consumption was associated with health-related reasons and although omega-3 fatty acids are believed to have anti-inflammatory properties, there is currently insufficient evidence to determine if they are capable of altering immune function in athletes [15]. Plant extracts encompass a large group of dietary supplements, however, echinacea and ginseng are consistently popular [16] and these examples were provided in our questionnaire. With respect to motivation for supplementation with plant extracts, health-related reasons such as "prevent or heal illnesses or injuries", "support immune system" and "strengthen overall health" [16] have been reported, which is in agreement with our participants. Unfortunately, there is a paucity of high-quality, human studies to evaluate the effects of herbal supplements on health-related reasons for supplementation in athletes and as such, the potential benefits cannot be confirmed [16]. While the effectiveness of most plant-based natural health products remains to be determined, one should acknowledge these products are generally marketed for health reasons.

The use of dietary supplements to enhance performance in young athletes is controversial. Some experts recommend that athletes under the age of 18 years avoid using dietary supplements unless required for a medical reason and only in cases where they are supervised by a professional [17]. Although this advice is sound in that it errs on the side of safety, it is perhaps not realistic and certainly the high rates of dietary supplement use suggest athletes are not heeding this conservative message. Regardless, if an athlete opts to take supplements, the chosen dietary supplements should be found to be effective in relation to their performance goals.

A large percentage of athletes consumed vitamin or mineral supplements and there was an association with motivation for enhanced performance; however, as with health-related reasons, the conventional thinking is that vitamin and mineral supplements will not improve performance, except in the case of a deficiency, illness or restricted food intake [10]. Vitamin-enriched waters were also associated with performance reasons, however, are unlikely to benefit athletes if dietary intakes are adequate and concerns have been raised regarding the added sugars in some vitamin-enriched water options. Protein powders and various amino acid products were commonly reported in athletes looking to improve performance, a finding supported by others [7, 18]. These products are frequently advertised to increase muscle mass and performance [19], indicating some level of congruence between the performance goals and supplement choice. Protein supplementation has been found to improve muscle hypertrophy and strength, as well as aerobic and anaerobic power, when combined with appropriate training [20], conversely, less support exists for potential benefits with recovery of muscle function, muscle soreness, and muscle damage [19].

Energy drink consumption was also positively associated with performance reasons, notably "increase energy" and "muscle mass/strength" in these athletes. Energy drinks may improve neuromuscular performance, delay central nervous system fatigue, and increase endurance performance [21, 22], however, the optimal dose and their potential superiority to a sport drink is unclear. Furthermore, there are concerns with energy drinks as a hydration choice, in those who are not habituated, as they may increase water and sodium losses and have a mild thermogenic effect [21]. Other potential side effects include: increased sugar intakes, gastrointestinal problems, tachycardia, anxiety, headaches and insomnia [21, 22]. In general, energy drinks are contraindicated for those under the age of 18 years and their consumption should be discouraged except in very specific circumstances and under parental guidance [22–24]. Creatine supplementation was associated with "muscle mass/strength", "endurance", and "overall athletic performance"; indeed there is evidence to suggest creatine may be efficacious in enhancing muscle hypertrophy and performance in short, high-intensity activities, however, the majority of the research has been conducted in adult males [25]. Younger athletes could benefit from creatine supplementation, as their ability to regenerate high energy phosphates is reduced; nonetheless, the International Society of Sports Nutrition only deems creatine supplementation acceptable if the athlete is past puberty, competing at a high level, has parental approval, is supervised by a qualified professional, and uses an appropriate dose [25, 26].

Consuming carbohydrates or carbohydrate-electrolyte combinations during exercise can delay fatigue, thereby improving performance in intermittent and prolonged endurance exercise [27, 28]. Arguably, congruence exists between the use of sport/electrolyte drinks and sport gummies/gels and performance-based motivations for supplement use. Carbohydrate intake during exercise has been identified as an area where young athletes do not meet the recommendation of 30–60 g/h, in at least one study [13], suggesting that this link could be highlighted in sport nutrition education. The use of these products should be carefully considered in the context of the duration and intensity of the exercise, however, as there is a concern with the use of sport drinks and excess calories in the form of added sugars [24]. Plant extracts were also associated with performance reasons, yet controversy exists regarding the potential benefits of common plant extracts such as echinacea [16, 29, 30] and ginseng [31] on athletic performance.

Vitamin and mineral supplements, fatty acids, energy drinks, sport/protein bars, and gels and gummies were associated with "because someone told you to" or "because family/friends/teammates do". These results are in-line with a study in young, elite German athletes that found coaches (37 %), family (30 %), physicians (29 %), and nutritionists (14 %) provided information on dietary supplements. Furthermore, 16 % of athletes learned about dietary supplements from the media and 27 % reported that they did not receive any information about dietary supplements from anyone [32]. As may be expected, the younger the athlete, the more likely they are to consume supplements because others have told them to. Certainly, encouraging young athletes to heed the advice of others, particularly their parents or guardians, is advisable; however, the sport nutrition knowledge of these individuals is uncertain. Influence of others on dietary supplement use, particularly those who may not possess the appropriate knowledge, is a common cause for concern in athlete populations [33, 34]. Clearly education is required not only for the athletes but also their support network, as there is obviously a willingness to try supplements based on the recommendations of others rather than personal knowledge.

Our study is limited in that young participants completed the questionnaire using personal recall and there may be errors due to a lack of understanding. Delivering the questionnaire in a "face-to-face" mode, where they could ask questions and receive explanations minimized this limitation. Additionally, the athletes were not specifically asked the reason for consuming each supplement; rather, the analysis looks at associations within the data, therefore, the magnitude of the association was reported and should be considered in the interpretation of the results. Future research that directly measures athlete knowledge regarding dietary supplements and relates this knowledge to their motivation for supplementation and actual intakes would be valuable to gain a more in-depth understanding.

Conclusions

Young athletes are consuming dietary supplements for reasons related to health, performance, and under the recommendation of others. Although in some cases supplement choices are congruent with the established benefits of the supplement, there are many instances where there is a lack of evidence to support supplementation practices as they relate to their self-reported motivations for supplement use. Additional research into the safety and effectiveness of dietary supplements in this demographic is required. Furthermore, evidence-informed educational programs are required for the athletes and their support personnel to ensure supplements are being used efficaciously to promote health and performance. Current sources of reliable information include on-line resources developed and monitored by sporting organizations or nutrition associations (i.e Coaching Association of Canada coach.ca) and Registered Dietitians who provide training in nutrition and supplement use. A second recommendation would be for sporting organizations to facilitate nutrition sessions for their athlete support personnel, who could then inform the parents and athletes. Future, studies should assess the effectiveness of a variety of educational interventions and their impact on nutrition knowledge and dietary habits and supplement use.

Competing interests
The authors have no financial interests or benefits to declare.

Authors' contributions
JAP oversaw the research study and drafted the manuscript, KW contributed to the study design and data analysis and revised the manuscript, KE contributed to the study design and data collection and revised the manuscript. All authors read and approved the final manuscript.

Acknowledgements
The authors would like to thank Jodi Siever for her assistance with the statistical analyses and Megan Stadnyk for her assistance with data collection.

Funding
This work was supported by the Canadian Foundation for Dietetic Research

Author details
[1]Department of Physical Education and Recreation Studies, Mount Royal University, 4825 Mount Royal Gate SW, Calgary, Alberta T3E 6K6, Canada. [2]Department of Behavioral Health and Nutrition, University of Delaware, 026 North College Avenue, Newark Delaware 19716, USA . [3]Sport Medicine Centre, University of Calgary, 2500 University Drive NW, Calgary, Alberta T2N 1N4, Canada.

References
1. Meyer F, O'Connor H, Shirreffs SM. International Association of Athletics Federations. Nutrition for the young athlete. J Sports Sci. 2007;25 Suppl 1:S73–82.
2. Petroczi A, Naughton DP, Pearce G, Bailey R, Bloodworth A, McNamee M. Nutritional supplement use by elite young UK athletes: fallacies of advice regarding efficacy. J Int Soc Sports Nutr. 2008; doi:10.1186/1550-2783-5-22.
3. Wiens K, Erdman KA, Stadnyk M, Parnell JA. Dietary supplement usage, motivation, and education in young, Canadian athletes. Int J Sport Nutr Exerc Metab. 2014;24:613–22.
4. U. S. Food and Drug Administration. Dietary supplement and Health Education Act of 1994. http://www.fda.gov/regulatoryinformation/legislation/significantamendmentstothefdcact/ucm148003.htm (2009). Accessed 29 May 2015.
5. Government of Canada. Natural Health Products Regulations. http://laws-lois.justice.gc.ca/eng/regulations/SOR-2003-196/page-1.html (2015). Accessed 29 May 2015.
6. Erdman KA, Fung TS, Doyle-Baker PK, Verhoef MJ, Reimer RA. Dietary supplementation of high-performance Canadian athletes by age and gender. Clin J Sport Med. 2007;6:458–64.
7. Petroczi A, Naughton DP, Mazanov J, Holloway A, Bingham J. Performance enhancement with supplements: incongruence between rationale and practice. J Int Soc Sports Nutr. 2007; doi:10.1186/1550-2783-4-19.
8. Kotrlik JW, Williams HA, Jabor MK. Reporting and interpreting effect size in quantitative agricultural education research. J Agric Educ. 2011;52:132–42.
9. Slater G, Tan B, Teh KC. Dietary supplementation practices of Singaporean athletes. Int J Sport Nutr Exerc Metab. 2003;13:320–32.
10. Rodriguez NR, DiMarco NM, Langley S, American Dietetic Association, Dietitians of Canada, American College of Sports Medicine. Position of the American Dietetic Association, Dietitians of Canada, and the American College of Sports Medicine: nutrition and athletic performance. J Am Diet Assoc. 2009;109:509–27.
11. Gibson JC, Stuart-Hill L, Martin S, Gaul C. Nutrition status of junior elite Canadian female soccer athletes. Int J Sport Nutr Exerc Metab. 2011;21:507–14.
12. Farrokhyar F, Tabasinejad R, Dao D, Peterson D, Ayeni OR, Hadioonzadeh R, et al. Prevalence of vitamin D inadequacy in athletes: a systematic-review and meta-analysis. Sports Med. 2015;45:365–78.
13. Baker LB, Heaton LE, Nuccio RP, Stein KW. Dietitian-observed macronutrient intakes of young skill and team-sport athletes: adequacy of pre, during, and postexercise nutrition. Int J Sport Nutr Exerc Metab. 2014;24:166–76.
14. Lun V, Erdman KA, Reimer RA. Evaluation of nutritional intake in Canadian high-performance athletes. Clin J Sport Med. 2009;19:405–11.
15. Gunzer W, Konrad M, Pail E. Exercise-induced immunodepression in endurance athletes and nutritional intervention with carbohydrate, protein and fat-what is possible, what is possible. Nutrients. 2012;4:1187–212.
16. Senchina DS, Shah NB, Doty DM, Sanderson CR, Hallam JE. Herbal supplements and athlete immune function–what's proven, disproven, and unproven? Exerc Immunol Rev. 2009;15:66–106.
17. Maughan RJ, Depiesse F, Geyer H. International Association of Athletics Federations. The use of dietary supplements by athletes. J Sports Sci. 2007;25 Suppl 1:S103–113.
18. Lieberman HR, Stavinoha TB, McGraw SM, White A, Hadden LS, Marriott BP. Use of dietary supplements among active-duty US Army soldiers. Am J Clin Nutr. 2010;92:985–95.
19. Pasiakos SM, Lieberman HR, McLellan TM. Effects of protein supplements on muscle damage, soreness and recovery of muscle function and physical performance: a systematic review. Sports Med. 2014;44:655–70.
20. Pasiakos SM, McLellan TM, Lieberman HR. The effects of protein supplements on muscle mass, strength, and aerobic and anaerobic power in healthy adults: a systematic review. Sports Med. 2015;45:111–31.
21. Mora-Rodriguez R, Pallares JG. Performance outcomes and unwanted side effects associated with energy drinks. Nutr Rev. 2014;72 Suppl 1:108–20.
22. Campbell B, Wilborn C, La Bounty P, Taylor L, Nelson MT, Greenwood M, et al. International Society of Sports Nutrition position stand: energy drinks. J Int Soc Sports Nutr. 2013. doi:10.1186/1550-2783-10-1.
23. Seifert SM, Schaechter JL, Hershorin ER, Lipshultz SE. Health effects of energy drinks on children, adolescents, and young adults. Pediatrics. 2011;127:511–28.
24. Galemore CA. Sports drinks and energy drinks for children and adolescents-are they appropriate? A summary of the clinical report. NASN Sch Nurse. 2011;26:320–1.
25. Cooper R, Naclerio F, Allgrove J, Jimenez A. Creatine supplementation with specific view to exercise/sports performance: an update. J Int Soc Sports Nutr. 2012; doi:10.1186/1550-2783-9-33.
26. Buford TW, Kreider RB, Stout JR, Greenwood M, Campbell B, Spano M, et al. International Society of Sports Nutrition position stand: creatine supplementation and exercise. J Int Soc Sports Nutr. 2007. doi:10.1186/1550-2783-4-6.
27. Phillips SM, Turner AP, Gray S, Sanderson MF, Sproule J. Ingesting a 6% carbohydrate-electrolyte solution improves endurance capacity, but not sprint performance, during intermittent, high-intensity shuttle running in adolescent team games players aged 12-14 years. Eur J Appl Physiol. 2010; 109:811–21.
28. Burke LM, Hawley JA, Wong SH, Jeukendrup AE. Carbohydrates for training and competition. J Sports Sci. 2011;29 Suppl 1:S17–27.
29. Baumann CW, Bond KL, Rupp JC, Ingalls CP, Doyle JA. Echinacea purpurea supplementation does not enhance VO2max in distance runners. J Strength Cond Res. 2014;28:1367–72.
30. Whitehead MT, Martin TD, Scheett TP, Webster MJ. Running economy and maximal oxygen consumption after 4 weeks of oral Echinacea supplementation. J Strength Cond Res. 2012;26:1928–33.
31. Chen CK, Muhamad AS, Ooi FK. Herbs in exercise and sports. J Physiol Anthropol. 2012. doi:10.1186/1880-6805-31-4.
32. Diehl K, Thiel A, Zipfel S, Mayer J, Schnell A, Schneider S. Elite adolescent athletes' use of dietary supplements: characteristics, opinions, and sources of supply and information. Int J Sport Nutr Exerc Metab. 2012;22:165–74.
33. Froiland K, Koszewski W, Hingst J, Kopecky L. Nutritional supplement use among college athletes and their sources of information. Int J Sport Nutr Exerc Metab. 2004;14:104–20.
34. Torres-McGehee TM, Pritchett KL, Zippel D, Minton DM, Cellamare A, Sibilia M. Sports nutrition knowledge among collegiate athletes, coaches, athletic trainers, and strength and conditioning specialists. J Athl Train. 2012;47:205–11.

## 13

The effects PCSO-524®, a patented marine oil lipid and omega-3 PUFA blend derived from the New Zealand green lipped mussel (*Perna canaliculus*), on indirect markers of muscle damage and inflammation after muscle damaging exercise in untrained men: a randomized, placebo controlled trial

Timothy D Mickleborough[*], Jacob A Sinex, David Platt, Robert F Chapman and Molly Hirt

Abstract

Background: The purpose of the present study was to evaluate the effects of PCSO-524®, a marine oil lipid and *n*-3 LC PUFA blend, derived from New Zealand green- lipped mussel (*Perna canaliculus*), on markers of muscle damage and inflammation following muscle damaging exercise in untrained men.

Methods: Thirty two untrained male subjects were randomly assigned to consume 1200 mg/d of PCSO- 524® (a green-lipped mussel oil blend) or placebo for 26 d prior to muscle damaging exercise (downhill running), and continued for 96 h following the muscle damaging exercise bout. Blood markers of muscle damage (skeletal muscle slow troponin I, sTnI; myoglobin, Mb; creatine kinase, CK), and inflammation (tumor necrosis factor, TNF-α), and functional measures of muscle damage (delayed onset muscle soreness, DOMS; pressure pain threshold, PPT; knee extensor joint range of motion, ROM; isometric torque, MVC) were assessed pre- supplementation (baseline), and multiple time points post-supplementation (before and after muscle damaging exercise). At baseline and 24 h following muscle damaging exercise peripheral fatigue was assessed via changes in potentiated quadriceps twitch force ($\Delta Q_{tw,pot}$) from pre- to post-exhaustive cycling ergometer test in response to supra-maximal femoral nerve stimulation.

Results: Compared to placebo, supplementation with the green-lipped mussel oil blend significantly attenuated ($p < 0.05$) sTnI and TNF-α at 2, 24, 48, 72 and 96 h., Mb at 24, 48, 72, 96 h., and CK-MM at all-time points following muscle damaging exercise, significantly reduced ($p < 0.05$) DOMS at 72 and 96 h post-muscle damaging exercise, and resulted in significantly less strength loss (MVC) and provided a protective effect against joint ROM loss at 96 h post- muscle damaging exercise. At 24 h after muscle damaging exercise perceived pain was significantly greater ($p < 0.05$) compared to baseline in the placebo group only. Following muscle damaging exercise $\Delta Q_{tw,pot}$ was significantly less ($p < 0.05$) on the green-lipped mussel oil blend compared to placebo.

(Continued on next page)

* Correspondence: tmickleb@indiana.edu
Department of Kinesiology, Human Performance and Exercise Biochemistry Laboratory, School of Public Health-Bloomington, 1025 E. 7th St. SPH 112, Bloomington, Indiana 47401, USA

(Continued from previous page)

Conclusion: Supplementation with a marine oil lipid and *n*-3 LC PUFA blend (PCSO-524®), derived from the New Zealand green lipped mussel, may represent a useful therapeutic agent for attenuating muscle damage and inflammation following muscle damaging exercise.

Keywords: Omega-3 fatty acids, Green-lipped mussel oil blend, Muscle damage, DOMS, Eccentric

Introduction

Exercise-induced muscle damage (EIMD) can be caused by eccentric type or unaccustomed (novel) exercise, and results in decrements in muscle force production, development of delayed-onset muscle soreness (DOMS) and swelling, rise in passive tension, and an increase in blood intramuscular proteins [1]. Delayed-onset muscle soreness is generally considered a hallmark sign of EIMD [2], and it is thought that DOMS is partially related to direct muscle fiber damage, and its magnitude appears to vary with the type, duration and intensity of exercise [3]. The inflammatory response to EIMD results in the release into blood of reactive species from both neutrophils and macrophages, and an array of cytokines from the injured muscle including tumor necrosis factor (TNF)-α, interleukin (IL)-1β and IL-6, which contribute to a low-grade systemic inflammation and oxidative stress [4]. The pro- inflammatory and pro-oxidant response can provoke secondary tissue damage [5], thus prolonging the regenerative process, which is generally characterized by a restoration of muscle strength and resolution of inflammation [5].

Exercise-induced muscle damage and DOMS can potentially hinder performance in activities ranging from basic physical activity to athletic training and competition. There are a number of strategies that have been used to attenuate EIMD and DOMS such as anti-inflammatory medication, cryotherapy, massage, stretching, hyperbaric oxygen, homeopathy, ultrasound, rest, light exercise and electrotherapeutic modalities [3]. The use of non-steroidal anti- inflammatory drugs (NSAIDs) and continued exercise appear to be the most commonly used methods to treat DOMS [1]. However, while the use of NSAIDs has been shown to decrease perceived muscle soreness and pain associated with DOMS, they fail to impact the length or degree of muscle weakness [6], may be detrimental to muscle cell repair and adaptation by decreasing satellite cell activity [7], and have been shown to suppress the protein synthesis response in skeletal muscle after eccentric resistance exercise [8]. Due to the fact that there appears to be no completely effective treatment for preventing/reducing EIMD and treating DOMS [1,6], the use of complimentary therapy, in particular nutraceuticals (e.g. tart cherry juice [9], curcumin [10], and quercetin [11]) that possess anti-inflammatory properties and have the potential to attenuate EIMD-induced oxidative stress, have become of interest [1].

One class of nutrients that appears to possess both anti-inflammatory and anti-oxidant properties are the long-chain omega (*n*)-3 long chain polyunsaturated fatty acids (LC-PUFA), such as eicosapentaeoic acid (EPA; 20:5 n-3)) and docosahexaenoic acid (DHA; 22:5 n-3), found in fish oil. Numerous studies have shown that *n*-3 LC-PUFA administered at doses greater than one gram per day have beneficial actions in many inflammatory diseases, cancer, and human health in general [12], and that *n*-3 LC-PUFA may act as important energetic molecules that can modulate immune, inflammatory, and oxidative stress responses to exercise [13]. A small number of studies have sought to evaluate whether fish oil supplementation can reduce the degree of skeletal muscle injury, inflammation and oxidative stress following eccentric exercise [13]. Although more studies have demonstrated a positive effect of *n*-3 LC-PUFA in relation to ameliorating muscle damage, DOMS, inflammation, and oxidative stress following eccentric exercise [14-20], some investigations have shown no effect [14,21]. It is likely that the diversity in testing protocols, supplementation dosage and duration, subject population, timing of measurements and selection of biomarkers contribute to the discrepancies in the findings between studies. However, it is possible that different forms of marine oils may have varying effects on these responses, since these oils contain a variety of lipid mediators as well as a different amount of *n*-3 LC-PUFA.

PCSO-524® (Lyprinol®/Omega XL®) is a nutritional supplement comprising of a patented extract of a very condensed form of stabilized marine lipids from the New Zealand green lipped mussel, *Perna canaliculus*, combined with olive oil and vitamin E [22,23]. This marine oil lipid and *n*-3 PUFA blend is a multifarious mixture of sterol esters, sterols, polar lipids, triglycerides, EPA and DHA (split between the triacylglycerol and polar lipid classes), and free fatty acids [24], and has been shown to exert its anti-inflammatory effects via furan fatty acids [25], and inhibition of cyclooxygenase (COX)-2 and 5-lipoxyeganse (LOX) pathways for the metabolism of arachidonic acid, thereby leading to a subsequent reduction in pro-inflammatory leukotriene, prostaglandin, and cytokine production from inflammatory cells [22,26]. A number of human and animal studies have shown that the green-lipped mussel oil blend may have beneficial effects in treating inflammatory diseases such as osteoarthritis, rheumatoid arthritis, inflammatory bowel disease, asthma [22], and exercise- induced bronchoconstriction [27]. These preliminary findings support the potential for supplementation with the green-lipped mussel oil blend in order to attenuate muscle damage and inflammation that can occur following muscle damaging exercise.

Therefore, the primary aim of the present study was to evaluate the effects of supplementation with a green-lipped mussel oil blend on indirect markers of muscle damage, inflammation, and quadriceps fatigue following muscle damaging exercise in untrained men. We hypothesized that supplementation with a green-lipped mussel oil blend, compared to placebo, would significantly reduce blood markers of muscle damage and inflammation, and modulate quadriceps fatigue and functional measures of muscle damage following downhill running designed to induce muscle damage in untrained men.

Methods

Subjects

Forty untrained males volunteered to participate in the study, and of these thirty-two subjects (aged 22.0 ± 2 y, height 176.3 ± 7.0 cm, body mass 70.8 ± 9.8 kg, maximal oxygen consumption (VO_{2peak}) 46.0 ± 6.1 mL·kg^{-1}·min^{-1}) completed the study. Reasons for the non- inclusion of eight subject data sets in the final statistical analysis were (1) subjects failing to show up at testing sessions (incomplete data; n = 3), (2) inability of the investigators to obtain a blood sample (incomplete data; n = 3), and (3) identification of erroneous recordings of data (n = 2). Subjects were classified as 'untrained' if they exercised less than three times per wk for less than 30 min during each session. Subjects were excluded if they had a history of significant pain in hips or knees, had participated in a strength training program within 60 d prior to study participation, or regularly used nutritional supplements and over-the-counter and prescription anti-inflammatory medication. All subjects were screened for coronary artery disease risks factors as per the American College of Sports Medicine guidelines [28]. Subjects were instructed to refrain from downhill running, stair running, resistance training, plyometric or other mode of exercise that could potentially cause muscle damage, and to refrain from modifying their exercise habits during the course of the study. Adherence to these instructions was confirmed at each visit to the laboratory. The study was approved by the Indiana University Institutional Review Board for Human Subjects, and written informed consent for all subjects was obtained prior to participation in the study.

Study design

The study was conducted as a randomized, double-blind, placebo-controlled parallel group trial over 30 days. This design was chosen over a crossover design in order to avoid the repeated-bout effect acting as a confounding variable [1]. Subjects were randomly assigned to either a green-lipped mussel oil blend (PCSO-524®) supplementation group (n = 16) or a placebo group (n = 16). Supplementation with the green-lipped mussel oil blend and placebo began 26 days before an eccentric exercise bout (downhill running, designed to induce muscle damage) and continued for 4 days following the muscle damaging exercise bout. An activity diary and food frequency questionnaire was completed by each subject during the course of the study.

Pre-supplementation measures

After subjects provided written informed consent for participation and the investigators explained the study protocol, all subjects underwent an exhaustive 20-min cycle ergometer familiarization test (T1 day −21), followed one week later (T2 day −14) by an incremental treadmill load test of their maximal oxygen uptake (VO_{2max}), in order to determine the intensity (70% VO_{2peak}) the subjects will exercise at for the eccentric exercise test. One week (T3 day −7) following the VO_{2peak} test an initial (baseline) blood draw was taken in order to measure baseline blood markers of muscle damage, inflammation and DNA oxidative stress, along with baseline functional measures of muscle damage [i.e. isometric torque (MVC), knee flexion (joint range of motion), limb girth (swelling), muscle soreness, and muscle pain], which were followed one week later (T4 day 0) by measures of quadriceps muscle fatigue (quadriceps twitch force measured via femoral magnetic nerve stimulation before and after a 20-min exhaustive cycle ergometer test).

Post-supplementation measures

Following the 26 days of supplementation a venous blood draw was taken and functional measures of muscle damage conducted (T5 day 26), which was directly followed by the downhill running protocol specifically designed to induce muscle damage [29,30] (T6 day 26). Immediately (T7 day 26) and 2 h following the muscle damaging exercise a venous blood draw was taken (T8 day 26), followed by additional blood draws and functional measures of muscle damage at 24 h (T9 day 27), 48 h (T10 day 28), 72 h (T11 day 29) and 96 h (T12 day 30) post-muscle damaging exercise. Quadriceps muscle fatigue was measured 24 h following the muscle damaging exercise bout (T8 day 27). The timing of this measurement was chosen in order to correspond with expected decrements in muscle strength, range of motion and significant increases in swelling, tenderness and soreness. On testing days T3 day −7, T5 day 26, T9 day 27, T10 day 28, T11 day 29 and T12 day

30 the sequence of procedures comprised the following order: blood draws, DOMS, range of motion, pressure pain threshold, thigh girth (swelling) and isometric torque (MVC). On testing T9 day 27 only, subjects underwent the protocol for the measurement of quadriceps muscle fatigue before and after the 20-min exhaustive cycle ergometer trial.

Supplementation

Subjects ingested either 8 capsules per d of PCSO-524® (Lyprinol®/Omega XL®; Pharmalink International Ltd, Hong Kong) (n = 16), which equaled 800 mg olive oil, 400 mg lipid extract (~58 mg EPA and 44 mg DHA) and 1.8 mg vitamin E (d-alpha-tocopherol) or 8 placebo capsules containing olive oil (1200 mg olive oil) (n = 16) for 30 d. Each PCSO-524® capsule contains 50 mg lipid extract (fatty acids), 7.3 mg (14%) EPA, 5.5 mg (11%) DHA, 100 mg olive oil and 0.225 mg vitamin E, and 1 placebo capsule contains 150 mg olive oil. The active PCSO-524® capsules containing the green-lipped mussel oil blend were identical in size, color, texture and taste to their respective placebo counterpart. Product specification was provided to the investigators by the trial sponsor (Pharmalink). Cawthron Laboratories (Nelson, NZ), an independent laboratory, completed the fatty acid analysis of the raw material, and Chemisches Labor (Hannover, Germany) conducted the final fatty acid testing of the finished PCSO-524 ® capsuled product. Alpha laboratories (Auckland, NZ) conduced the fatty acid analysis on the placebo (olive oil) capsules. While Table 1 presents the fatty acid analysis conducted on the PCSO-524® (Batch No. A6530-01) and placebo (Batch No. 7820) capsules used in the present study, a detailed fatty acid analysis of the PCSO-524® and placebo capsules has been published elsewhere [31,32]. Wolyniak et al. [23] have shown that the 'lipid extract' portion of the green-lipped mussel oil blend contains up to 91 fatty acids (including EPA and DHA). Of the 91 fatty acids reported [23], 16 represented more than 1% of the total FA. In decreasing order of abundance, these were EPA, C16:0 (Palmitic acid), DHA, C14:0 (Myristic acid), C16:1n-7 (Palmitoleic acid), C18:0 (Steroic acid), C18:1n-5, C18:4n-3 (Stearidonic acid), C18:2n-6 (Linoleic acid), C20:4n-6 (Arachidonic acid), C18:3n- 3 (Alpha-linoleic acid), C16:1n-5, C20:1n-9 (Eicosenoic acid), C18:1n-9 (Oleic acid), C15:0 (Pentadecanoic acid), and C16:1n-9 (7-(hexadecenoic acid). PCSO-524® is a natural product subject to variations in the New Zealand Marlborough Sounds ecosystems. Values in the specification of this organic compound can vary according to season and climate temperatures, and therefore, during the manufacturing process a variance of +/– 10% in the saturated, monounsaturated and PUFA composition of PCSO-524® is deemed acceptable.

Table 1 Fatty acid composition (%) of PCSO-524®, a marine oil extract of the New Zealand green-lipped mussel (*Perna canaliculus*) * and placebo (olive oil) ** capsules

FA nomenclature	Fatty acid name	PCSO-524® capsules (Weight, %)	Placebo (Olive oil) capsules (Weight, %)
14:0	Myristic acid	1.7	
16:0	Palmitic acid	13.4	9.2
16:1	Palmitoleic acid	3.6	3.0
18:0	Stearic acid	3.6	3.5
18:1	Oleic acid	58.2	81.0
18:2n-6	Linoleic acid	5.7	2.6
18:3n-3	Alpha-linolenic acid	0.9	0.4
18:4n-3	Octadecatetraenoic acid	1.0	
20:0	Arachidic acid	0.4	0.3
20:1	Eicosamonoenoic acid	0.7	
20:4n-6	Arachidonic acid	0.1	
20:4n-3	Eicosatetraenoic acid	0.3	
20:5n-3	Eicosapentaenoic acid	5.8	
22:5n-3	Docosapentaenoic acid	0.3	
22:6n-3	Docosahexaenoic acid	3.0	
Others		1.3	

*Batch number: A6530-01. **Batch number: 7820. FA nomenclature: number of carbon atoms (chain length), number of double bonds, and position of the last double bond from the methyl (omega) end.

Experimental measures

Peak aerobic exercise capacity (VO$_{2peak}$)

Subjects performed a peak aerobic exercise capacity test, adapted from a previously published protocol from our laboratory [33], on a motor driven treadmill (Model 18–60, Quinton, Seattle, WA), while fitted with a heart rate monitor (Polar Electro Inc., Lake Success, NY) and breathing mask (7450 Series V2, Hans Rudolph, Shawnee, KS USA). The protocol started with a warm-up period of 5 min, in which subjects chose a comfortable running speed that they would be expected to be able to continue on a level treadmill for 15 min; selected speeds ranged from 7.2 – 13.8 km/h. After 5 min of seated rest, the exercise portion of the test began with each subject running at 0% grade at a speed of 1.6 k/h less than the selected (warm-up) speed for 2 min. Following the initial stage, the speed was increased to the predetermined speed. After 3 min, the slope of the treadmill was increased to 4% for 3 min, and then increased an additional 2% every 3 min until volitional exhaustion or valid test criteria were met. Ventilatory and metabolic data were collected using open-circuit, indirect calorimetry. Dried expired gases were sampled at a rate of 300 mL·min^{-1} for fractional concentrations of O_2 and CO_2 using an Applied Electrochemistry S-3A oxygen analyzer and a CD-3A carbon dioxide analyzer (Ametek, Thermox Instruments, Pittsburgh, PA). Inspired ventilation was measured with a pneumotachometer (Hans Rudolph 3813).

Eccentric muscle damaging exercise

All subjects performed a 20-min downhill running bout on a motorized treadmill (A.R. Young Company, Indianapolis) modified to run in reverse at a −16% grade, which is a protocol that has previously been shown to elicit a significant degree of muscle damage following downhill running [29,30]. Once the test commenced subjects were not allowed to stop, and treadmill speed was adjusted so that the subjects maintained a heart rate that corresponded to 70% VO_{2max}. It has been shown that downhill running is effective in causing skeletal muscle damage, symptoms of DOMS, and loss of muscle force [34].

Delayed onset muscle soreness and pain threshold

Lower limb soreness was assessed using a visual analog (numeric) rating pain scale with "no soreness" indicated at one end (score 0) and "unbearably painful" at the other (score 10) Subjects stood with hands on hips and feet approximately shoulder width apart. The subject was asked to squat down to 90° (internal angle), rise to the start position and then indicate on the numeric scale the soreness felt in the lower limbs.

The pressure pain threshold was measured at five specific sites on the quadriceps with a digital algometer (Force One, Wagner Instruments, Greenwich, CT.) to quantify muscle tenderness. The same investigator performed all measurements throughout the study. Specific sites for assessment were determined using established literature and landmarks [32], involving two anatomical points (anterior superior iliac spine (ASIS) and superior pole of the patella (SPP)). All measurements were taken on the right side with the subject in the supine position. A longitudinal axis was created between the ASIS and the SPP from which the sites were marked with a permanent marker to ensure accuracy at each time point. The measured sites were: 15 cm distal to the ASIS, 4 cm proximal to the SPP, midpoint of the ASIS and SPP along the axis, then 2 cm lateral and 2 cm medial of this midpoint. Subjects were instructed to let the investigator know when the pressure transformed into pain at which point the amount of force was recorded in newtons (N).

Range of motion (knee flexion), swelling (thigh girth) and isometric strength (torque)

Range of motion has been shown to be an accurate method of determining the extent of muscle damage [35]. Subjects were instructed to lay prone on a massage table with both knees fully extended. Subjects flexed their left knee with no assistance from the investigator, and the angle measured with a goniometer (Prestige Medical, Northridge, CA) using universal landmarks (lateral epicondyle of the femur, lateral malleolus and greater trochanter) that were marked with a permanent marker to ensure consistency on subsequent measures. Three measurements were averaged and reported in degrees. This method for a assessing ROM has been validated previously [36].

In order to determine the presence of swelling/edema within a muscle thigh circumference was assessed at the midpoint of the ASIS and SPP of the right leg with an anthropometric tape (Idass, Glastonbury, UK). Subjects were standing fully relaxed in the anatomical position. Subjects were instructed to put all their weight on the opposite leg and 3 measurements were taken. Measurement sites were marked to ensure consistent measurements and the average was reported.

Isometric torque was assessed at a knee angle of 80° using previously described protocol [37]. Subjects were seated in a chair, secured with a belt across the legs and chest, and their left leg secured to a force transducer (Model Z Tension Load Cell, Dillon, Fairmont, MN) with a non-compliant strap. Subjects were familiarized with the equipment by performing three warm-up contractions (two submaximal, 1 maximal) separated by 10 seconds of rest, followed by a 5 min recovery. After the recovery period, subjects performed 3 maximum voluntary contractions (MVCs) of the quadriceps, interspersed with a 10 s recovery interval between contractions. The highest peak torque from the 3 contractions was recorded. Subjects were verbally encouraged during the contractions to produce a maximum effort.

Quadriceps muscle fatigue

Potentiated quadriceps twitch force was measured in the subject's left leg to quantify an index of muscle fatigue following a 20 min exhaustive cycle ergometer test. Subjects lay semirecumbent on a table with a left knee joint angle of 90 degrees. The subject's ankle was wrapped in a non-compliant strap, placed just superior to the ankle malleoli. The strap was attached to a calibrated load cell (Model Z Tension Load Cell, Dillon, Fairmont, MN) for the measurement of force connected to a custom amplifier (Hector Engineering Co. Inc., Ellettsville, IN). A magnetic stimulator (Magstim 200, Magstim, Whitland, UK) connected to a double 70 mm coil was used to stimulate the femoral nerve, causing an involuntary contraction of the quadriceps muscle. Nerve stimulation followed two protocols, which have been described previously [38].

Assessment of maximal nerve stimulation

Prior to the exhaustive 20 min cycle ergometer test, a series of single twitches were obtained at varying levels of stimulator intensity (80%, 85%, 90%, 95%, and 100% of maximal stimulator power output) to determine when supramaximal stimulation had been reached. The position of the stimulator coil was placed over the femoral triangle and adjusted to determine an acceptable location for each subject. Stimulator placement was determined to be acceptable when repeatable and measurable quadriceps contractions were obtained. Stimulator placement was marked on the subject's skin with an indelible marker to insure repeatability of the location and measurement. Typical stimulator output required to achieve supramaximal stimulation has been found to be a mean of approximately 83% of stimulator output [39].

Exhaustive 20 min cycle ergometer test

Following a 5 min warm up at a self-selected intensity, subjects completed a 20 min exercise task on a cycle ergometer (Velotron, RacerMate Inc., Seattle, Washington, USA). Subjects were allowed to change resistance freely and were asked to complete the furthest possible distance, and to achieve the highest possible power output, during the 20 min ergometer test.

Assessment of fatigue

Prior to and immediately following the exhaustive cycle ergometer test, an assessment of quadriceps twitch force ($Q_{tw,pot}$) was performed. Twitch force prior to the 20 min cycle ergometer test was used as a baseline for twitch force obtained after the time trial. The assessment of fatigue protocol consisted of six repetitions of potentiation and magnetic stimulation with 30 s of rest between repetitions. For each repetition, subjects performed a maximal voluntary isometric contraction (MVC) of the quadriceps muscle for 5 s. At the end of the 5 s MVC, the subject received a supra-maximal magnetic stimulation of the femoral nerve, and a second stimulation after 5 seconds of rest [40]. The force produced during the second twitch of each repetition was recorded as $Q_{tw,pot}$. Force values from the first two repetitions were discarded based on previous findings that the degree of potentiation is smaller after the first two measurements [38]. Force values from the final four repetitions were averaged to produce a $Q_{tw,pot}$ force value for each trial.

Blood sampling and analysis

All blood draws were taken from the antecubital vein and collected into 10 ml plain Vacutainer® clot tubes

(PulmoLab, Porter Ranch, CA). The tubes were gently inverted five times after collection to mix the clot activator with blood, and then placed on ice for at least 30 minutes before centrifugation (Allegra ™ X-22R Centrifuge, Beckman Coulter, Inc., Brea, CA) at 20°C at 3000 RPM for 15 min. Serum was removed after spinning and allocated to storage tubes and stored immediately at –80°C until later analysis of muscle damage, inflammation and oxidative stress markers using enzyme immunoassay techniques [Powerwave XS™ Spectrophotometer (Bio-Tek Instruments, Winooski, VT)] according to manufacturer's instructions.

Skeletal and cardiac muscle damage

Creatine kinase, muscle (CK-MM) was assessed using a sandwich enzyme linked immunoassay test (sensitivity: 12.8 U/L; Detection range: 31.2 – 2,000 U/L. Intra-assay precision: $CV < 10\%$; Inter-assay precision: $CV < 12\%$ as per the manufacturer's (Caltag Medsystems Ltd, Milton Keynes, UK) protocol. Skeletal muscle slow troponin I (sTnI) was assessed using a sandwich enzyme linked immunoassay test (Minimum detectable concentration typically 5.4 pg/ml; Detection range: 15.6-1,000 pg/ml; Intra-assay precision: $CV < 10\%$; Inter-assay precision: $CV < 12\%$ as per the manufacturer's (USCN Life Science Inc., Hubei, Peoples Republic of China) protocol. Myoglobin (Mb) was assessed using an enzyme-linked immunoassay test (minimum detectable concentration: 5.0 ng/ml; sensitivity: 25 ng/ml; Detection range: 25.0-1,000 ng/ml) following the manufacturer's recommendations (Calbiotech, Spring Valley, CA, USA). Cardiac troponin I (CTnI) was analyzed a using sandwich enzyme-linked immunoassay test (minimum detectable concentration: 0.45 ng/ml; Detection range: 0.48-5.0 ng/ml; inter-assay precision: $<10\%$) as per the manufacturer's (Abnova, Taipei, Taiwan) recommendations. Human heart fatty acid binding protein (hFABP) was assessed using a sandwich enzyme linked immunoassay test (minimum detectable concentration: 156 pg/ml; Detection range: 312 – 20,000 pg/ml. Intra-assay precision: $CV < 4\text{-}6\%$; Inter-assay precision: $CV < 8\text{-}10\%$) following the manufacturer's (Innovative Research, Novi, MI, USA) recommendations.

Inflammatory and DNA oxidative stress markers

Tumor necrosis factor (TNF)-α was assessed using a sandwich enzyme linked immunoassay test (sensitivity: 1.7 pg/ml; Detection range: 15.6 – 1,000 pg/ml. Intra-assay precision: $CV < 4.4\%$; Inter-assay precision: $CV < 7.5\%$ as per the manufacturer's (Invitrogen Corp., Camarillo, CA, USA) protocol. 8-Oxo-2'-deoxyguanosine (8-OhdG) was analyzed using a competitive enzyme linked immunoassay test (Detection range: 100 pg/ml – 20 ng/ml) as per the manufacturer's (Cell Biolabs Inc., San Diego, CA, USA) recommendations.

Nutrient intake and compliance

All subjects were given an activity diary to record frequency, mode and duration of exercise. Nutrient intake was monitored to ensure that dietary factors would do not change through the course of the study, and potentially affect the dependent measures. Nutrient data was collected using the GSEL food frequency questionnaire (FFQ) developed by the Nutrition Assessment Shared Resource (NASR) of Fred Hutchinson Cancer Research Center. Subjects completed the GSEL version of the questionnaire before supplementation and at the end of the 30 day supplementation period. Analysis of GSEL for nutrient intake was conducted at the Fred Hutchinson Cancer Research Center. Nutrients of interest obtained from the GSEL analysis included macronutrient composition, antioxidants (α-tocopherol, β-carotene, lycopene, Vitamin C), certain minerals (magnesium, sodium, zinc), and types of dietary fatty acids (omega-3, total polyunsaturated fatty acids, saturated fatty acids). While the FFQ has been shown to be valid and reliable in the collection of dietary data [41], we acknowledge that diet may act as confounding factor, since it was not directly controlled for in our study. Adherence to the treatment regimen was monitored by asking the subjects to document the dose of capsules consumed daily and to return any unused capsules. For the purpose of the present study a compliance of ≥90% was considered acceptable.

Data analysis

The data were analyzed using a two-way (group, 2; time, 6–8) split-plot repeated measures ANOVA using SPSS version 20.0 (IBM Corporation, Chicago, IL, USA) statistical software. The data was assessed for normality using the Kolmogorov–Smirnov test, and Levene's test was used to test for homogeneity of variance between groups. Mauchly's test was be conducted to determine whether sphericity is violated. If sphericity is violated, the repeated-measures ANOVA was corrected using the Greenhouse–Geiser correction factor. A fisher's protected least-square difference post-hoc test was used *a priori* to determine differences in dependent measures within and between groups. Statistical significance was set at $p \leq 0.05$. Data are expressed as mean ± SD.

To determine an appropriate sample size for present study, a post-hoc power analysis of existing literature was conducted using G*Power version 3.0.5 (Universität Kiel, Germany). Based on two studies [19,20] investigating the efficacy of *n*-3 LC-PUFA on DOMS, and blood markers of muscle damage and inflammation following eccentric exercise, achieving an experiment-wise error rate of 0.05 required 15 subjects within each treatment group. In these studies, Tartibian et al. [19,20] has shown that ingestion of *n*-3 LC-PUFA (n = 9–15) for 30 days compared to placebo/control (n = 9–15) significantly

reduced inflammatory markers, and perceived pain and symptoms, following eccentric exercise, with effect sizes ranging from 0.64-0.75 for a study power of 0.82 and 0.84 respectively.

Results

Subject characteristics

There were no significant differences ($p > 0.05$) for age, height, BMI, VO_{2max} (L) and VO_{2peak} (mL/kg/min) between the green-lipped mussel oil blend (PCSO-524™) and placebo group (Table 2). However, body mass (kg) was significantly different ($p < 0.05$) between groups.

Delayed onset muscle soreness and pain threshold

Muscle soreness significantly increased ($p < 0.05$) in both groups after the muscle damaging exercise protocol, peaking between 24 and 48 h and declining toward baseline at 72 and 96 h (Table 3). Significant effects for time were found in the green-lipped mussel oil blend group ($p < 0.001$) and placebo group ($p < 0.001$). Post-hoc pairwise comparisons between groups at each time point revealed significantly lower DOMS in the treatment group, compared to placebo, at 72 h [$p = 0.027$; mean difference (Δ), 1.25 ± 2.41; 95% CI (difference of means), 0.08 to 2.52] and 96 h ($p = 0.037$; Δ, 1.25 ± 1.95; 95% CI, 0.13 to 2.63) following muscle damaging exercise. However, there were no significant differences ($p > 0.05$) between groups prior to supplementation (baseline) and following supplementation (before, and at 24 and 48 h following muscle damaging exercise).

The test of within-subject effects indicated that there was no significant effect ($p > 0.05$) of time on percent change from baseline in all post-supplementation time points for pressure pain threshold (PPT) values within the green-lipped mussel oil blend group. Post-hoc pairwise comparisons within the placebo group revealed a significant increase ($p = 0.034$; Δ, 0.12 ± 0.25%; 95% CI, 0.01 to 0.26%) in muscle tenderness at 24 h post-muscle damaging exercise only compared to before muscle damaging exercise in the placebo group (Table 3).

Table 2 Subjects' baseline characteristics

	Green-lipped mussel oil blend (n = 16)	Placebo (n = 16)	p-value
Age (years)	21.7 + 1.7	21.5 + 2.4	0.803
Height (cm)	178.1 + 5.8	174.2 + 6.7	0.091
Body mass (kg)	74.8 + 8.8	66.6 + 9.7	0.018*
BMI (kg/m^2)	23.6 + 2.9	21.9 + 2.8	0.102
VO_{2peak} (L)	3.4 + 0.5	3.0 + 0.6	0.073
VO_{2peak} (ml/kg/min)	46.4 + 6.2	45.6 + 6.1	0.732

*Significantly different ($p < 0.05$) between groups. BMI, body mass index. VO2peak, peak oxygen consumption. Values are expressed as mean ± SD.

Table 3 Effect of supplementation on functional measures of muscle damage and fatigue following eccentric exercise

Variables/ Groups	Pre-supplementation (Baseline)	Post-supplementation Before muscle damaging exercise	24 h after muscle damaging exercise	48 h after muscle damaging exercise	72 h after muscle damaging exercise	96 h after muscle damaging exercise
DOMS (arbitrary units)						
Green-lipped mussel oil blend	2.3 ± 1.7	2.0 ± 2.0	4.9 ± 2.7[¥,#]	4.6 ± 2.2[¥]	2.7 ± 1.7[#]	1.8 ± 1.6[#]
Placebo	1.9 ± 1.6	1.4 ± 1.5	4.4 ± 2.1[¥, #]	4.8 ± 1.8[¥]	3.9 ± 1.8[¥,#]	3.0 ± 2.2[¥,#]
p-value*	0.700	0.563	0.847	0.441	0.029*	0.037*
Pressure Pain Threshold (% Δ from baseline)						
Green-lipped mussel oil blend	-	−0.08 ± 0.32%	−0.13 ± 0.26%	−0.12 ± 0.28%	−0.07 ± 0.34%	−0.01 ± 0.34%
Placebo	-	−0.03 ± 0.35%	−0.15 ± 0.27%[#]	−0.10 ± 0.39%	−0.07 ± 0.41%	0.01 ± 0.50%
p-value*	-	0.643	0.844	0.824	0.978	0.896
Knee Flexion Range of Motion (degrees)						
Green-lipped mussel oil blend	47.5 ± 6.1	46.7 ± 5.0	47.4 ± 5.2	44.6 ± 5.9[#]	45.7 ± 5.4	46.7 ± 4.4
Placebo	45.8 ± 8.4	46.9 ± 9.8	47.3 ± 9.0	43.4 ± 7.1[#]	44.9 ± 8.5	41.8 ± 5.3[¥]
p-value*	0.476	0.939	0.980	0.628	0.760	0.007*
Thigh Girth (swelling) (% Δ from baseline)						
Green-lipped mussel oil blend	-	0.01 ± 0.02%	0.02 ± 0.02%	0.01 ± 0.02%	0.01 ± 0.02%	0.02 ± 0.04%
Placebo	-	0.00 ± 0.02%	0.02 ± 0.02%	0.01 ± 0.02%	0.02 ± 0.02%	0.02 ± 0.06%
p-value*	-	0.631	0.970	0.953	0.582	0.971
Maximum Voluntary Isometric torque (Strength) (Nm)						
Green-lipped mussel oil blend	72.8 ± 22.2	82.1 ± 19.7[#]	76.2 ± 19.8[#]	78.7 ± 21.5	79.9 ± 20.2	84.6 ± 22.4[¥,#]
Placebo	75.4 ± 19.3	82.1 ± 22.4[#]	74.9 ± 19.4[#]	74.6 ± 22.5	76.2 ± 20.8	83.9 ± 14.4
p-value*	0.721	0.843	0.987	0.569	0.608	0.872
%ΔQ$_{tw,pot}$						
Green-lipped mussel oil blend	−27.8 ± 26.2	-	−30.4 ± 14.3	-	-	-
Placebo	−23.9 ± 24.0	-	−39.5 ± 24.3[¥]	-	-	-
p-value*	0.669	-	0.039	-	-	-

*, p-value between groups at distinct time points (p < 0.05 denotes statistical significance between groups; p > 0.05 denotes no statistical significance between groups); ¥, significantly different (p < 0.05) to pre- supplementation (baseline) within group; #, significantly different (p < 0.05) from previous time point within group. Pressure pain threshold and thigh girth (swelling) are expressed as % change (Δ) from the pre- supplementation (baseline) value within group, since baseline values were significantly different (p < 0.05) between groups. DOMS, delayed onset muscle soreness; % ΔQ$_{tw,pot}$, % change in potentiated quadriceps twitch force from pre- to post-exercise (cycling time trial). Values expressed as mean ± SD.

Range of motion (knee flexion), swelling (thigh Girth) and isometric strength (torque)

The test of within-subject effects indicated that there was a significant effect (p < 0.01) of time on ROM within each group. Range of motion was significantly reduced (p < 0.05) at 48 h compared to 24 h post-muscle damaging exercise within the green-lipped mussel oil blend and placebo group. However, while no significant difference (p > 0.05) was found between groups for ROM values at baseline and post-supplementation (prior to, and at 24, 48 and 72 h post-muscle damaging exercise) a

significant reduction (p < 0.05) in ROM occurred in the placebo group compared to the green-lipped mussel oil blend group at 96 h post-muscle damaging exercise (p = 0.007; Δ, −4.94 ± 8.10 degrees; 95% CI, −1.42 to −8.45 degrees) (Table 2). No significant difference (p > 0.05) was observed for the percent change from baseline in thigh girth (swelling) within or between groups at all-time points (Table 3).

The test of within-subject effects revealed that there was a significant effect (p < 0.01) of time on MVC (torque) within the both groups (Table 3). For both groups post- supplementation MVC significantly increased immediately prior to muscle damaging exercise compared to the baseline value (Placebo: p = 0.009; Δ, 6.68 ± 10.1 Nm; 95% CI, 1.30 to 12.10 Nm. Green-lipped mussel oil blend: p = 0.014; Δ, 9.41 ± 15.48 Nm; 95% CI, 1.16 to 17.66 Nm), and was significantly reduced at 24 h post-muscle damaging exercise compared to the MVC value obtained immediately prior to muscle damaging exercise (Placebo: p = 0.002; Δ, 7.13 ± 8.4 Nm; 95% CI, −2.65 to −11.61 Nm. Green-lipped mussel oil blend: p = 0.022, Δ, 6.02 + 11.00 Nm; 95% CI, −0.16 to −11.89 Nm). In addition, within the green-lipped mussel oil blend group only, MVC increased significantly at 96 h compared to 72 h post-muscle damaging exercise (p = 0.014; Δ, 4.67 ± 7.69 Nm; 95% CI, 0.57 to 8.77 Nm) and baseline (p = 0.003; Δ, 11.83 ± 15.24 Nm; 95% CI, 3.71 to 19.95 Nm). No significant difference (p > 0.05) in MVC was observed at any time point between groups.

Quadriceps muscle fatigue

There was no significant difference (p > 0.05) in the percent change (%Δ) in $Q_{tw, pot}$ between groups at baseline, or within the green-lipped mussel oil blend group when comparing the %$\Delta Q_{tw,pot}$ at baseline with 24 h following muscle damaging exercise. However, %$\Delta Q_{tw,pot}$ was significantly greater at 24 h following muscle damaging exercise compared to baseline within the placebo group (p = 0.018 Δ, −11.4 ± 23.3%, 95% CI, −2.7 to −25.4%), and %$\Delta Q_{tw,pot}$ was significantly greater for the placebo group compared with the green-lipped mussel oil blend group at 24 h following muscle damaging exercise (p = 0.039; Δ, −10.1 ± 24.7%; 95% CI, −4.3 to −29.1%) (Table 3), indicating greater muscle quadriceps fatigue in the placebo group.

Skeletal and cardiac muscle damage blood markers

Serum sTnI levels were not significantly different (p > 0.05) for baseline (pre- supplementation), immediately prior to, and immediately following (0 h) muscle damaging exercise (post-supplementation) either within or between groups (Figure 1). However, a significant increase (p < 0.05) in serum sTnI concentration, compared to baseline, was observed at 2, 24, 48, 72, and 96 h post- muscle damaging exercise within each group. Serum sTnI concentration peaked at 24 h following muscle damaging exercise, and compared to baseline increased by 260.2 ± 170.6% in the placebo group and by 165.1 ± 139.1% in the green-lipped mussel oil blend group. There was a significant reduction in the green-lipped mussel oil blend mean serum sTnI concentration compared to the placebo group at 2 h (p = 0.007; Δ, −4.5 ± 5.8 ng/ml; 95% CI, −0.9 to −8.0 ng/ml), 24 h (p < 0.001; Δ, −9.9 ± 10.1 ng/ml; 95% CI, −4.4 to −15.4 ng/ml), 48 hr. (p < 0.001, Δ, −9.4 ± 10.0 ng/ml; 95% CI, −4.7 to −14.0 ng/ml), 72 h (p = 0.003; Δ, −6.8 ± 9.1 ng/ml; 95% CI, −2.5 to −11.1 ng/ml), and 96 h (p = 0.02, Δ, −5.4 ± 10.5 ng/ml; 95% CI, −0.3 to −10.4 ng/ml) (Figure 1) following muscle damaging exercise.

Serum CK-MM levels were not significantly different (p > 0.05) for baseline, and immediately prior to muscle damaging exercise either within or between groups (Figure 2). However, a significant increase (p < 0.05) in serum CK-MM concentration, compared to baseline, was observed at 0, 2, 24, 48, 72, and 96 h post-muscle damaging exercise within each group. Serum CK-MM

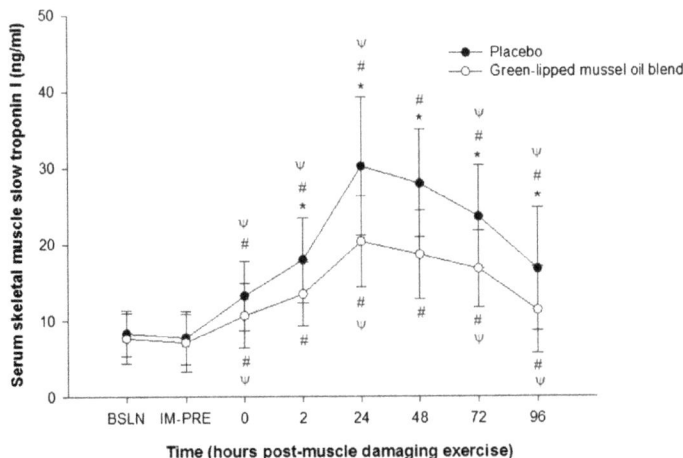

Figure 1 Effect of supplementation on mean serum skeletal muscle slow troponin I concentration (ng/ml) pre- and post-eccentric exercise. *, designates a statistical difference (p < 0.05) between groups at distinct time points. #, designates a significant difference (p < 0.05) compared to baseline (BSLN; pre-supplementation before eccentric exercise).ψ, designates a significant difference (p < 0.05) from previous time point within group. IM-PRE, immediately prior to eccentric exercise (post-supplementation). Data are expressed as mean ± SD.

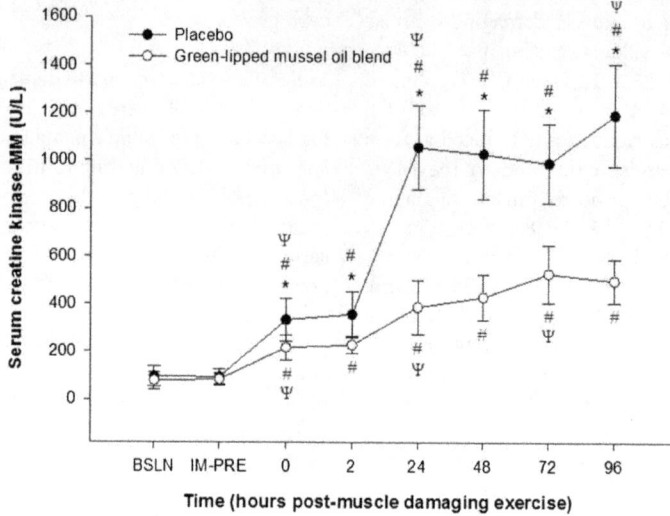

Figure 2 Effect of supplementation on mean serum creatine kinase-MM concentration (ng/ml) pre- and post-eccentric exercise. *, designates a statistical difference ($p < 0.05$) between groups at distinct time points. #, designates a significant difference ($p < 0.05$) compared to baseline (BSLN; pre-supplementation before eccentric exercise).ψ, designates a significant difference ($p < 0.05$) from previous time point within group. IM-PRE, immediately prior to eccentric exercise (post-supplementation). Data are expressed as mean ± SD.

concentration peaked at 24 h following muscle damaging exercise for the placebo group and 72 h for the green-lipped mussel oil blend group, and compared to baseline increased by 1006.5 ± 631.2% in the placebo group and by 579.8 ± 287.4% in the green-lipped mussel oil blend group. A significant attenuation in the green- lipped mussel oil blend mean serum CK-MM concentration, compared to the placebo group, was detected at 0 h ($p < 0.001$; Δ, −116.1 ± 112.0 ng/ml; 95% CI, − 63.0 to −169.2 ng/ml), 2 h ($p < 0.001$; Δ, −127.3 + 101.7 ng/ml; 95% CI, −76.0 to −178.6 ng/ml), 24 hr. ($p < 0.001$; Δ, −386.1 ± 201.0 ng/ml; 95% CI, −562.6 to −775.6 ng.ml), 48 h ($p < 0.001$; Δ, −600.0 ± 208.5 ng/ml; 95% CI, −493.2 to −706.7 ng/ml), 72 h ($p < 0.001$; Δ, −463.7 ± 221.8 ng/ml; 95% CI, −360.0 to −568.0 ng/ml) and 96 h ($p < 0.001$; Δ, −693.0 ± 243.0 ng/ml; 95% CI, − 564.0 to −822.4 ng/ml) following muscle damaging exercise (Figure 2).

Serum Mb levels were not significantly different ($p > 0.05$) when comparing baseline, and immediately prior to and at 0 h and 2 h muscle damaging eccentric exercise either within or between groups. However, a significant increase ($p < 0.05$) in serum Mb concentration, compared to baseline, was observed at 24, 48, 72, and 96 h post-muscle damaging exercise within each group. Serum Mb concentration peaked at 72 h following muscle damaging exercise (post-supplementation) for both groups, and compared to baseline increased by 1917.6 ± 876.3% in the placebo group and by 1109.5 ± 496.2% in the green-lipped mussel oil blend group. A significant attenuation in the green-lipped mussel oil blend mean serum Mb concentration

compared to the placebo group was observed at 24 h ($p < 0.001$; Δ, −43.3 ± 37.1 ng/ml; 95% CI, −22.9 to −63.7 ng. ml), 48 hr. ($p < 0.001$; Δ, −99.4 ± 58.7 ng/ml; 95% CI, −67.7 to −131.2 ng/ml), 72 h ($p < 0.001$; Δ, −192.6 ± 159.8 ng/ml; 95% CI, −119.0 to −226.3 ng/ml) and 96 h ($p = 0.001$; Δ, −130.7 ± 161 ng/ml; 95% CI, − 49.1 to −212.2 ng/ml) following muscle damaging exercise (post-supplementation) (Figure 3). For serum cTnI and h-FABP concentration no significant differences ($p > 0.05$) were observed for all time points either within or between groups.

Inflammatory and DNA oxidative stress markers

Mean serum TNF-α concentration did not significantly differ ($p > 0.05$) for baseline, immediately prior to, and at 0 h following muscle damaging exercise either within or between groups. However, a significant increase ($p < 0.05$) in serum TNF-α concentration, compared to baseline, was observed at 2, 24, 48, 72, and 96 h post-muscle damaging exercise within each group. Serum TNF-α levels peaked at 24 h following muscle damaging exercise, and compared to baseline increased by 156.2 ± 65.7% in the placebo group and by 93.3 ± 49.4% in the green-lipped mussel oil blend group. There was a significant reduction in mean serum TNF-α concentration for the green-lipped mussel oil blend group compared to the placebo group at 2 h ($p = 0.042$; Δ, −4.9 ± 8.1 pg/ml; 95% CI, −0.4 to −10.6 pg/ml), 24 h ($p < 0.001$; Δ, −19.8 ± 13.4 ng/ml; 95% CI, −11.1 to −28.5 pg/ml), 48 hr. ($p < 0.001$, Δ, −18.1 ± 12.7 pg/ml; 95% CI, −10.7 to −25.7 pg/ml), 72 h ($p = 0.003$; Δ, −19.9 ± 13.0 pg/ml; 95% CI, −11.3 to −28.5 pg/ml), and 96 h

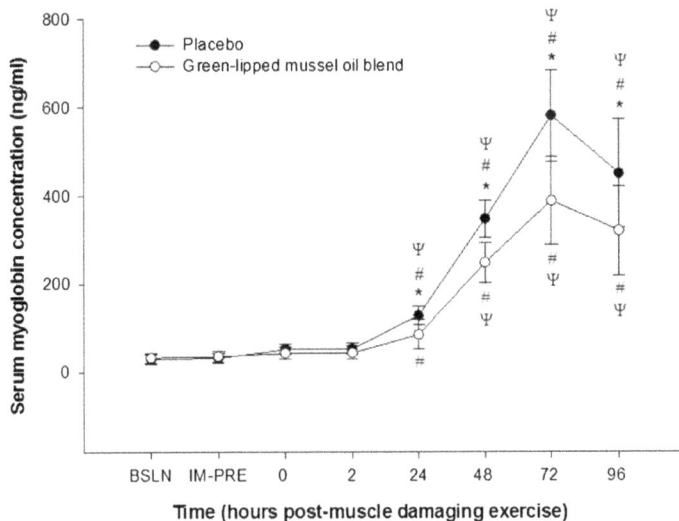

Figure 3 Effect of supplementation on mean serum myoglobin concentration (ng/ml) pre- and post-eccentric exercise. *, designates a statistical difference (p < 0.05) between groups at distinct time points. #, designates a significant difference (p < 0.05) compared to baseline (BSLN; pre-supplementation before eccentric exercise).ψ, designates a significant difference (p < 0.05) from previous time point within group. IM-PRE, immediately prior to eccentric exercise (post-supplementation). Data are expressed as mean ± SD.

(p < 0.001, Δ, −24.8 ± 15.1 pg/ml; 95% CI, −16.8 to −32.8 pg/ml) following muscle damaging exercise (Figure 4).

Mean serum 8-OHdG concentration was not significantly changed (p > 0.05) either within or between groups for all time points.

Nutrient intake and compliance

Mean daily nutrient intake, such as, for example, α-tocopherol, β-carotene, lycopene, vitamin C, magnesium, sodium, zinc, omega-3, total polyunsaturated fatty acids and saturated fatty acids did not differ

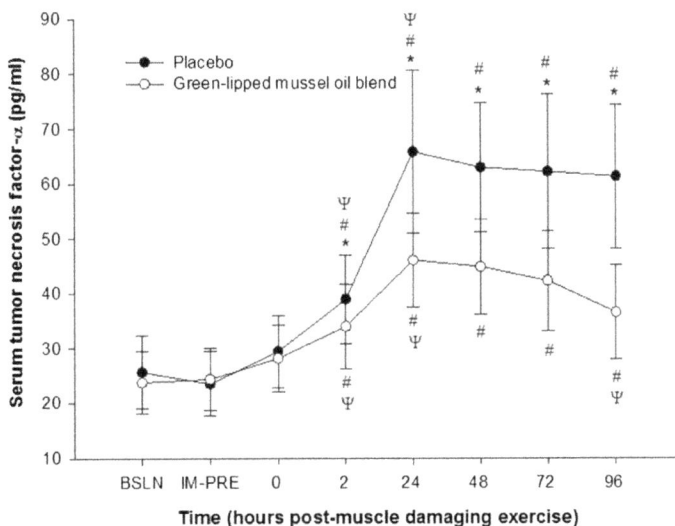

Figure 4 Effect of supplementation on mean serum tumor-necrosis factor-α concentration (pg/ml) pre- and post-eccentric exercise. *, designates a statistical difference (p < 0.05) between groups at distinct time points. #, designates a significant difference (p < 0.05) compared to baseline (BSLN; pre-supplementation before eccentric exercise).ψ, designates a significant difference (p < 0.05) from previous time point within group. IM-PRE, immediately prior to eccentric exercise (post-supplementation). Data are expressed as mean ± SD.

significantly (p > 0.05) between groups during the course of the study. Compliance as estimated from return-capsule count was high (median, 99%).

Discussion

The present study has shown that supplementing the diet of untrained men for 4 wk with a marine oil lipid and n-3 LC PUFA blend (PCSO-524®), derived from the New Zealand green lipped mussel (*P. canaliculus*), significantly reduced lower limb DOMS, quadriceps pain (tenderness), and peripheral muscle fatigue, and provided a protective effect against ROM (knee flexion) and isometric strength (torque) loss that can occur following downhill running designed to induce muscle damage. In addition, although blood markers of muscle damage and inflammation, sTnI, CK-MM, MB, and TNF-α, significantly increased following eccentric exercise in both groups, the rise in these blood markers were significantly suppressed on the green-lipped mussel oil blend supplemented diet compared to the placebo diet at most time points following muscle damaging exercise. No significant changes occurred between the green-lipped mussel oil blend and placebo group following eccentric exercise for swelling (thigh girth), and serum h-FABP, cTnI and 8-OHdG concentrations. Our findings may have implications for those who train regularly, especially since it has recently been shown that EPA and DHA levels (Omega-3 Index: percentage of EPA and DHA in total erythrocyte fatty acids) were low in a cohort of German elite winter endurance athletes [42], and importantly that n-3 LC-PUFA supplementation leads to a higher Omega-3 index level and decreased incidence of DOMS in healthy college aged individuals [43].

To date only two studies have been conducted in order to determine the efficacy of supplementation with this specific green-lipped mussel oil blend (PCSO-524®) on markers of EIMD and DOMS following muscle damaging [32] and exhaustive exercise [31]. While Baum et al. [31] found that 11 wk. of the green-lipped mussel oil blend supplemented diet reduced DOMS following an exhaustive 30 km run in male and female trained distance runners, Pumpa et al. [32] found no effect of 8 wk of supplementation with this specific green-lipped mussel oil blend on DOMS and functional and blood markers of EIMD following downhill running in trained men from a variety of sports. The divergent findings between the present study and the Pumpa et al. study [32] are difficult to reconcile, but is likely related to Pumpa and colleagues [32] using a lower dose (600 mg/day) of green-lipped mussel oil blend supplementation compared to the present study (1200 mg/day), and using a downhill running protocol of insufficient intensity to promote muscle damage and a robust inflammatory response in trained individuals.

Effect of green-lipped mussel oil blend supplementation on delayed onset muscle soreness and pain threshold

We observed a significant decrease in DOMS at 96 h following muscle damaging exercise on the green-lipped mussel oil blend supplemented diet compared to the placebo diet, which is in agreement with some studies [15,17,19], but not all [14,21,32], that have shown that supplementing the diet with n-3 LC-PUFA prior to muscle damage attenuates DOMS following eccentric exercise and a 30 km run [31]. Delayed-onset muscle soreness appears many hours after muscle damaging exercise and peaks 24–72 h post-eccentric exercise [5], as was observed in both groups in the present study. What is clear is that while DOMS is not considered a disease or a disorder, it can limit further exercise in the days following an initial training bout [3].

In the present study the quadriceps pressure pain threshold (PPT) was used as an additional measure of muscle soreness in an attempt to ameliorate the subjective nature of the visual analog scale measure of soreness. We observed no change in the PPT for all time points within the green-lipped mussel oil blend group or between groups. However, in the placebo group perceived pain increased significantly 24 h following muscle damaging exercise compared to before muscle damaging exercise. These data seem to suggest that the green-lipped mussel oil blend supplemented diet may have afforded a protective effect against perceived pain developing in the quadriceps, and may be partially explained by the attenuation in muscle damage and the inflammatory response that occurred in this group [5]. While Tartibian et al. [19] have demonstrated that n-3 LC-PUFA supplementation for 30 days reduced perceived pain 48 hr. following eccentric exercise compared to placebo, other studies [16,21,32] have found no change in perceived pain following eccentric exercise when pre- treated with n-3 LC-PUFA.

Effect of green-lipped mussel oil blend supplementation on range of motion (knee flexion), swelling (thigh Girth) and isometric strength (torque)

Among the numerous indirect markers of EIMD, muscle function measures such as muscle strength (MVC torque) and ROM are considered the best tools for quantifying muscle damage [2]. Eccentric-biased downhill running protocols typically generate 10-30% force loss after exercise, and that the reduction in MVC torque resulting from injury persists until the muscle function returns to its pre-injury condition (~24 h) [2]. Strength losses following eccentric exercise are likely due to the effects of muscle damage, and evidence suggests that excitation-contraction coupling failure plays a role [44]. In the present study there were no significant change observed for MVC torque at all-time points between groups or within the placebo group. However,

MVC torque significantly increased compared to baseline (pre- supplementation) at 96 h following muscle damaging exercise on the green-lipped mussel oil blend supplemented diet. In support of this finding of an increase in muscle strength, Rajabi et al. [17] observed a significant increase in isotonic voluntary contractile strength of the quadriceps 24, 48 and 72 h following leg press eccentric exercise on a 30 day n-3 LC-PUFA supplemented diet compared to a placebo diet. Conversely, Gray et al. [14] observed no changes in MVC torque following 200 eccentric knee contractions, while Pumpa et al. [32] and Lenn et al. [21] observed no difference in muscle strength of the right and left quadriceps and non-dominant arm respectively between a placebo and n-3 LC-PUFA supplemented diet.

Many studies have documented decreases in the voluntary ROM (~20-45 degrees) following eccentric exercise, with full recovery not achieved until 10 days after exercise [44]. The mechanism to explain this decrease has been attributed to an increase in resting cytosol calcium levels, ultrastructure damage and/or an increase in fluid accumulation (swelling), and the measurement of joint ROM in muscle damage studies has been used as an indicator of passive muscle stiffness and soreness [45]. Our data indicate that muscle damaging exercise induced no loss of ROM in the green-lipped mussel oil blend group. However, within the placebo group ROM was significantly reduced (~4 deg) at 96 h post-muscle damaging exercise compared to baseline, and was significantly less (~4.9 deg) at 96 h following muscle damaging exercise on the placebo diet compared to the green-lipped mussel oil blend supplemented diet*. The protective effect provided by the n-3 LC-PUFA rich diet against ROM loss in the present study is similar to Tartibian et al. [19] and Rajabi et al. [17] who observed that on a n-3 LC-PUFA supplemented diet, compared to a placebo diet, the loss of knee ROM was significantly less post-eccentric bench stepping exercise and leg press eccentric exercise respectively, but are in contrast to the findings of Lenn et al. [21] and Phillips et al. [21] who observed no change in joint ROM following eccentric elbow flexion exercise.

Although swelling has been shown to occur following eccentric exercise and to be associated with the mechanisms of DOMS induced by eccentric exercise [46], there are studies that have shown a dissociation between when swelling and DOMS occur following eccentric exercise. Rodenburg et al. [47] have shown that MRI changes indicating the presence of edema do not to coincide with soreness following eccentric exercise (left forearm flexors) [47], while Clarkson et al. [35] noted that peak soreness occurred 2–3 d post-eccentric exercise (forearm flexor muscles) while peak swelling occurred 5 d following maximal effort eccentric actions of the forearm flexor muscles, while Yu et al. [48] has demonstrated that eccentric exercise (downstairs running) does induce muscle fiber swelling (soleus muscle), but it emerges at 7–8 d, and not at 2–3 d post-eccentric exercise when DOMS peaked. Based on the data from these studies [35,47,48] it is possible that we missed a potential effect of treatment on limb girth (swelling) since our final measurement of limb girth was at 96 h post-muscle damaging exercise.

Effect of green-lipped mussel oil blend supplementation on quadriceps muscle fatigue

Potentiated quadriceps twitch force ($Q_{tw,pot}$) assessed via magnetic stimulation before and after a 20-min cycling time trial pre- and post-supplementation (24 h following muscle damaging exercise) was used to quantify the degree of quadriceps muscle fatigue ($\Delta Q_{tw,pot}$). The measurement of quadriceps twitch force produced by supramaximal magnetic stimulation of the femoral nerve has been shown to be a reliable method to detect quadriceps fatigue following loading [38,40,49]. This study has shown for the first time in humans that n-3 LC-PUFA supplementation provided a protective effect against the development of quadriceps muscle fatigue following a 20 min exhaustive cycling ergometer test compared to placebo supplementation. While the $\%\Delta Q_{tw,pot}$ was unaltered between pre- and post- supplementation (24 h following muscle damaging exercise) for the green-lipped mussel oil blend group, there was a significant decline (~65%) in the $\%\Delta Q_{tw,pot}$ post-supplementation compared to pre-supplementation for the placebo group. Our data are in agreement with animal studies [50,51] that have shown that rats fed fish oil, hindlimb skeletal muscle were more resistant to fatigue during continuous muscle twitch contractions, and recovered contractile force better between repeat bouts, compared to an n-6 LC-PUFA or saturated fat enriched diet.

Effect of green-lipped mussel oil blend supplementation on blood markers of muscle damage, inflammation and DNA oxidative stress

Although a few studies have shown that eccentric exercise leads to myofibrillar remodeling specifically through Z-band related proteins, rather than muscle necrosis and inflammation [48,52], we have shown that supplementing the diet with a green-lipped mussel oil blend can mitigate the rise in a number of indirect markers of skeletal muscle damage and inflammation, and this effect persists for up to 96 h following muscle damaging exercise.

Slow skeletal troponin I is considered an early marker of EIMD, since it is particularly susceptible to calpain digestion, which may contribute to the early rise in plasma sTnI levels following eccentric exercise [53]. Our data are in agreement with Sorichter et al. [29] and Willoughby et al. [54] that a significant increase in serum sTnI can be detected within 2 h following muscle damaging exercise, and peaks within 24 h after the muscle injury- inducing sessions. In addition, we have shown for the first time that n-3 LC-PUFA supplementation can mitigate the increase in serum sTnI following muscle damaging exercise.

We observed a significant attenuation in serum Mb concentration in the green-lipped mussel oil blend group, compared to the placebo group, at 24, 48, 72 and 96 h following muscle damaging exercise, which is similar to the findings from a previous study [20] that showed that 30 d of n-3 LC-PUFA supplementation can moderate the rise in serum Mb at 24 and 48 h after eccentric exercise in untrained men. Myoglobin is an oxygen-binding heme protein found in skeletal and cardiac muscle, and thus is not specific for skeletal muscle, and h- FABP, which is involved in the transport and metabolism of fatty acids, is found in higher concentrations in the heart compared to human skeletal muscle [53]. However, both myoglobin and h-FABP have been proposed as useful markers of skeletal muscle injury in the absence of cardiac damage [30]. In the present study we did not observe any significant change in serum cTnI or h-FABP following muscle damaging exercise at any time point within either group, which suggests that the increase in serum myoglobin following muscle damaging exercise was likely the result of skeletal and not cardiac muscle damage.

Myofibrillar CK-MM is a cytosolic enzyme specifically bound to the myofibrillar M-line structure located in the sarcomere, and is also found in the space of the I-band sarcomeres where it provides support for muscle energy requirements. Whist we found that serum CK- MM significantly increased immediately following muscle damaging exercise and remained elevated in both groups for a further 96 h, there was a significant attenuation in serum CK- MM in the green-lipped mussel oil blend group, compared to the placebo group, for all-time points following muscle damaging exercise. A number of studies assessing the efficacy of n-3 LC-PUFA supplementation on EIMD and DOMS have not used serum CK-MM, but rather total serum CK concentration as an indirect marker of muscle damage. Given that total serum CK has not been shown to correlate with histological evidence of skeletal muscle damage [55] it is not surprising that considerable variability is observed in this blood marker among studies assessing the impact of n-3 LC-PUFA supplementation on muscle damage and DOMS following eccentric exercise [14,16,17,20,21,32].

An important aspect associated with the initiation and amplification of acute inflammation is the production of cytokines that are synthesized de nova by lymphocyte's and monocytes at the site of muscle injury, and aid in directing inflammatory-related events [56]. At the onset of inflammation there is an upregulation of the pro-inflammatory cytokines interleukin-1β, and tumor-necrosis factor (TNF)-α. While IL-1β and TNF-α are most likely released by resident macrophages at the site of injury [56], and initiate the inflammatory response, TNF- α, in particular, has been shown to play a significant role in the muscle regeneration phase following muscle injury [57,58]. While we observed a significant increase in TNF-α for both groups following muscle damaging exercise, with serum TNF-α peaking at 24 h post-muscle damaging exercise, and remaining elevated for up to 96 h, the serum concentration of TNF-α was significantly lower in the green-lipped mussel oil blend group compared to the placebo group. At present the data are conflicting as to whether n-3 LC-PUFA can suppress the inflammatory response following eccentric exercise [16,20,21,32].

Oxidative stress-induced muscle damage has been shown to be associated with muscle soreness, and the resultant generation of free radicals causes oxidative damage to cellular DNA [59]. 8-hydroxy-2' –deoxyguanosine (8-OHdG) is a product of oxidative DNA damage induced by the action of hydroxyl radicals on the DNA base deoxyguanosine (dG) and DNA single-strand breakage, and represents the most frequently used marker to assess DNA damage. Serum 8-OHdG has been shown to increase following eccentric isokinetic exercise in humans [59], but not after downhill running in rats [60] or humans [61]. In the present study we observed no significant increase in serum 8-OHdG following muscle damaging exercise in both groups compared to baseline, and no significant difference in serum 8-OHdG between groups at any time point. The lack of change in serum 8-OHdG following muscle damaging exercise does not exclude the possibility that changes in this marker were present in the active skeletal muscle, as the serum concentration 8-OHdG may be diluted in comparison with the actual site of generation (within muscle). In addition, the intensity/duration of the stimulus may not have been sufficient to overwhelm the body's endogenous antioxidant system, and/or an upregulation of protective mechanisms against DNA damage developing [59], may have also played a role. It is surprising that serum 8- OhdG was not increased following muscle damaging exercise, especially given that structural protein within skeletal muscle was damaged (i.e. increase in serum sTnI). Changes in oxidative stress observed following muscle damaging exercise may not be the same when comparing blood and skeletal muscle, and thus we acknowledge that a limitation to our study is that we did not include additional biomarkers of oxidative stress.

While inflammation contributes to fibrosis, and causes pain and may well impair skeletal muscle function it does appear that inflammation represents a critical aspect of skeletal muscle repair and regeneration, and therefore blocking the inflammatory response with either pharmacological drugs or nutraceuticals may well hinder recovery [62]. With this in mind an important question that needs to be resolved is whether the most beneficial course of treatment should be to inhibit the inflammatory response or to let it progress naturally. Therefore, if there is a benefit in blocking inflammation, when is the appropriate time to do so and for how long post-muscle injury? While post-treatment of skeletal muscle injury is likely a more practical tactic, regardless of whether the injury is acute or slower to materialize such as with repetitive use injuries, it is not known at present whether n-3 LC-PUFA supplementation would be as effective in ameliorating EIMD and the inflammatory response if delivered post-injury only. This is an important question to answer since in some cases of skeletal muscle injury pre-treatment with anti-inflammatory agents for long periods of time is not always a realistic option for an individual.

Anti-inflammatory mechanisms of action of PCSO-524®

In the present study the attenuation of a number of indirect markers of EIMD and inflammation cannot be explained entirely by the EPA and DHA content of PCSO-524®, since the total amount of EPA and DHA content consumed daily was 58 mg and 44 mg respectively, which are considerably lower amounts than previous studies [14-20] that have demonstrated a positive effect of n-3 LC-PUFA supplementation (0.3 - 2.0 g EPA/day and 0.2 – 1.0 g DHA/day) on mitigating EIMD, DOMS and inflammation. It has been shown the green-lipped mussel oil blend used in the present study, which contains up to 91 fatty acid components [23], has more potent anti-inflammatory activity than fish oil, which contains abundant EPA, in various animal models of arthritis, and inflammatory bowel disease [22]. Therefore, it is possible that additional constituents of the green-lipped mussel oil blend, which may act synergistically with the n-3 LC-PUFA, may also be partially responsible for its anti-inflammatory effects. The green-lipped mussel oil blend contains polyphenols (oleuropein and hydroxtyrosol) and oleic acid, which are anti-inflammatory, and postulated to reduce risk factors for heart disease, lower cancer mortality, and reduce inflammation [22,63]. It has been shown that furan fatty acids, which are a minor component of the green- lipped mussel oil blend, exhibit more potent anti-inflammatory activity than EPA in a rat model of adjuvant-induced arthritis [25], and which possess potent free-radical scavenging abilities [64], may explain, at least in part, why in the present study the green-lipped mussel oil blend was effective in attenuating EIMD, DOMS and inflammation, given the very low dose of EPA and DHA.

Conclusion

In conclusion, the present study has shown that supplementing the diet of untrained men for 30 days with 1200 mg/d of a marine oil lipid and n-3 LC PUFA blend (PCSO-524®), derived from the New Zealand green lipped mussel, attenuated indirect markers of muscle damage and inflammation following downhill running designed to induce muscle damage, and may represent a useful therapeutic agent for mitigating muscle damage and inflammation following unaccustomed and/or eccentric exercise.

Competing interests

The authors declare that they have no competing interests.

Authors' contributions

JS, DP collected the study data, contributed to data interpretation and assisted in the drafting the manuscript. MH assisted in data collection. TM and RC designed the study and drafted the manuscript. All authors read and approved the final manuscript.

Acknowledgments

This work was supported by a grant from Pharmalink International Ltd, Hong Kong. The funders had no role in study design, data collection and analysis, in writing the manuscript, or decision to publish.

References

1. Howatson G, van Someren KA. The prevention and treatment of exercise-induced muscle damage. Sports Med. 2008;38(6):483–503.
2. Warren GL, Lowe DA, Armstrong RB. Measurement tools used in the study of eccentric contraction-induced injury. Sports Med. 1999;27(1):43–59.
3. Cheung K, Hume P, Maxwell L. Delayed onset muscle soreness: treatment strategies and performance factors. Sports Med. 2003;33(2):145–64.
4. Hirose L, Nosaka K, Newton M, Laveder A, Kano M, Peake JM, et al. Changes in inflammatory mediators following eccentric exercise of the elbow flexors. Exerc Immunol Rev. 2004;10:75–90.
5. Clarkson PM, Hubal MJ. Exercise-induced muscle damage in humans. Am J Phys Med Rehabil. 2002;81(11 Suppl):S52–69.
6. Lewis PB, Ruby D, Bush-Joseph CA. Muscle soreness and delayed-onset muscle soreness. Clin Sports Med. 2012;31(2):255–62.
7. Mikkelsen UR, Langberg H, Helmark IC, Skovgaard D, Andersen LL, Kjaer M, et al. Local NSAID infusion inhibits satellite cell proliferation in human skeletal muscle after eccentric exercise. J Appl Physiol. 2009;107(5):1600–11.
8. Trappe TA, White F, Lambert CP, Cesar D, Hellerstein M, Evans WJ. Effect of ibuprofen and acetaminophen on postexercise muscle protein synthesis. Am J Physiol Endocrinol Metab. 2002;282(3):E551–6.
9. Connolly DA, McHugh MP, Padilla-Zakour OI, Carlson L, Sayers SP. Efficacy of a tart cherry juice blend in preventing the symptoms of muscle damage. Br J Sports Med. 2006;40(8):679–83. discussion 683.
10. Drobnic F, Riera J, Appendino G, Togni S, Franceschi F, Valle X, et al. Reduction of delayed onset muscle soreness by a novel curcumin delivery system (Meriva(R)): a randomised, placebo-controlled trial. J Int Soc Sports Nutr. 2014;11:31.
11. O'Fallon KS, Kaushik D, Michniak-Kohn B, Dunne CP, Zambraski EJ, Clarkson PM. Effects of quercetin supplementation on markers of muscle damage and inflammation after eccentric exercise. Int J Sport Nutr Exerc Metab. 2012;22(6):430–7.
12. Serhan CN, Chiang N, Van Dyke TE. Resolving inflammation: dual anti-inflammatory and pro-resolution lipid mediators. Nat Rev Immunol. 2008;8(5):349–61.

13. Mickleborough TD. Omega-3 polyunsaturated fatty acids in physical performance optimization. Int J Sport Nutr Exerc Metabol. 2012;23(1):83–96.

14. Gray P, Chappell A, Jenkinson AM, Thies F, Gray SR. Fish oil supplementation reduces markers of oxidative stress but not muscle soreness after eccentric exercise. Int J Sport Nutr Exerc Metab. 2014;24(2):206–14.

15. Jouris KB, McDaniel JL, Weiss EP. The effect of omega-3 fatty acid supplemntation on the inflammatory response to eccentric strength exercise. J Sports Sci Med. 2011;10:432–8.

16. Phillips T, Childs AC, Dreon DM, Phinney S, Leeuwenburgh C. A dietary supplement attenuates IL-6 and CRP after eccentric exercise in untrained males. Med Sci Sports Exerc. 2003;35(12):2032–7.

17. Rajabi A, Lotfi N, Abdolmaleki A, Rashid-Amiri S. The effects of omega-3 intake on delayed onset muscle soreness in non-athletic men. Pedagogies, Psychology, Medical- Biological Problems of Physical Training and Sport. 2013;1:91–5.

18. Santos EP, Silva AS, Costa MJC, Moura Junior JS, Quirino ELO, Franca GAM, et al. Omega-3 supplementation attenuates the production of c-reactive protein in military personnel during 5 days of intense phsyical stress and nutritional restriction. Biol Sport. 2012;29:93–9.

19. Tartibian B, Maleki BH, Abbasi A. The effects of ingestion of omega-3 fatty acids on perceived pain and external symptoms of delayed onset muscle soreness in untrained men. Clin J Sport Med. 2009;19(2):115–9.

20. Tartibian B, Maleki BH, Abbasi A. Omega-3 fatty acids supplementation attenuates inflammatory markers after eccentric exercise in untrained men. Clin J Sport Med. 2011;21(2):131–7.

21. Lenn J, Uhl T, Mattacola C, Boissonneault G, Yates J, Ibrahim W, et al. The effects of fish oil and isoflavones on delayed onset muscle soreness. Med Sci Sports Exerc. 2002;34(10):1605–13.

22. Doggrell SA. Lyprinol - is It a useful anti-inflammatory agent? eCAM. 2011; Article ID 307121:1–8.

23. Wolyniak CJ, Brenna JT, Murphy KJ, Sinclair AJ. Gas chromatography-chemical ionization-mass spectrometric fatty acid analysis of a commercial supercritical carbon dioxide lipid extract from New Zealand green-lipped mussel (Perna canaliculus). Lipids. 2005;40(4):355–60.

24. Miller MR, Pearce L, Bettjeman BI. Detailed distribution of lipids in Greenshell mussel (Perna canaliculus). Nutrients. 2014;6(4):1454–74.

25. Wakimoto T, Kondo H, Nii H, Kimura K, Egami Y, Oka Y, et al. Furan fatty acid as an anti-inflammatory component from the green-lipped mussel Perna canaliculus. Proc Natl Acad Sci U S A. 2011;108(42):17533–7.

26. Whitehouse MW, Macrides TA, Kalafatis N, Betts WH, Haynes DR, Broadbent J. Anti- inflammatory activity of a lipid fraction (lyprinol) from the NZ green-lipped mussel. Inflammopharmacology. 1997;5(3):237–46.

27. Mickleborough TD, Vaughn CL, Shei R-J, Davis EM, Wilhite DP. Marine lipid fraction PCSO-524 (lyprinol/omega XL) of the New Zealand green lipped mussel attenuates hyperpnea-induced bronchoconstriction in asthma. Respir Med. 2013;197:1152–63.

28. Pescatello LS, Arena R, Riebe D, Thompson PD. ACSM's guidelines for exercise testing and prescription. 9th ed. Baltimore, MD: Wolters Kluwer - Lippincott Williams & Wilkins; 2014.

29. Sorichter S, Mair J, Koller A, Gebert W, Rama D, Calzolari C, et al. Skeletal troponin I as a marker of exercise-induced muscle damage. J Appl Physiol. 1997;83(4):1076–82.

30. Sorichter S, Mair J, Koller A, Pelsers MM, Puschendorf B, Glatz JF. Early assessment of exercise induced skeletal muscle injury using plasma fatty acid binding protein. Br J Sports Med. 1998;32(2):121–4.

31. Baum K, Telford RD, Cunningham RB. Marine oil dietary supplementation reduces delayed onset muscle soreness after a 30 km run. Open Access J Sports Med. 2013;4:109–15.

32. Pumpa KL, Fallon KE, Bensoussan A, Papalia S. The effects of Lyprinol((R)) on delayed onset muscle soreness and muscle damage in well trained athletes: a double-blind randomised controlled trial. Complement Ther Med. 2011;19(6):311–8.

33. Duke JW, Stickford JL, Weavil JC, Chapman RF, Stager JM, Mickleborough TD. Operating lung volumes are affected by exercise mode but not trunk and hip angle during maximal exercise. Eur J Appl Physiol. 2014;114(11):2387–97.

34. Eston RG, Mickleborough J, Baltzopoulos V. Eccentric activation and muscle damage: biomechanical and physiological considerations during downhill running. Br J Sports Med. 1995;29(2):89–94.

35. Clarkson PM, Nosaka K, Braun B. Muscle function after exercise-induced muscle damage and rapid adaptation. Med Sci Sports Exerc. 1992;24(5):512–20.

36. Watkins MA, Riddle DL, Lamb RL, Personius WJ. Reliability of goniometric measurements and visual estimates of knee range of motion obtained in a clinical setting. Phys Ther. 1991;71(2):90–6. discussion 96–97.

37. Nunan D, Howatson G, van Someren KA. Exercise-induced muscle damage is not attenuated by beta-hydroxy-beta-methylbutyrate and alpha-ketoisocaproic acid supplementation. J Strength Cond Res. 2010;24(2):531–7.

38. Amann M, Dempsey JA. Locomotor muscle fatigue modifies central motor drive in healthy humans and imposes a limitation to exercise performance. J Physiol. 2008;586(1):161–73.

39. Polkey MI, Kyroussis D, Hamnegard CH, Mills GH, Green M, Moxham J. Quadriceps strength and fatigue assessed by magnetic stimulation of the femoral nerve in man. Muscle Nerve. 1996;19(5):549–55.

40. Amann M, Eldridge MW, Lovering AT, Stickland MK, Pegelow DF, Dempsey JA. Arterial oxygenation influences central motor output and exercise performance via effects on peripheral locomotor muscle fatigue in humans. J Physiol. 2006;575(Pt 3):937–52.

41. Willett WC, Sampson L, Stampfer MJ, Rosner B, Bain C, Witschi J, et al. Reproducibility and validity of a semiquantitative food frequency questionnaire. Am J Epidemiol. 1985;122(1):51–65.

42. von Schacky C, Kemper M, Haslbauer R, Halle M. Low omega-3 index in 106 german elite winter endurance athletes: a pilot study. Int J Sport Nutr Exerc Metab. 2014;24(5):559–64.

43. Lembke P, Capodice J, Hebert K, Swenson T. Influence of omega-3 (n3) index on performance and wellbeing in young adults after heavy eccentric exercise. J Sports Sci Med. 2014;13(1):151–6.

44. Warren GL, Lowe DA, Hayes DA, Karwoski CJ, Prior BM, Armstrong RB. Excitation failure in eccentric contraction-induced injury of mouse soleus muscle. J Physiol. 1993;468:487–99.

45. McKune AJ, Semple SJ, Peters-Futre EM. Acute exercise-induced muscle injury. Biol Sport. 2012;29:3–10.

46. Lieber RL, Friden J. Mechanisms of muscle injury after eccentric contraction. J Sci Med Sport. 1999;2(3):253–65.

47. Rodenburg JB, de Boer RW, Schiereck P, van Echteld CJ, Bar PR. Changes in phosphorus compounds and water content in skeletal muscle due to eccentric exercise. Eur J Appl Physiol Occup Physiol. 1994;68(3):205–13.

48. Yu JG, Liu JX, Carlsson L, Thornell LE, Stal PS. Re-evaluation of sarcolemma injury and muscle swelling in human skeletal muscles after eccentric exercise. PLoS One. 2013;8(4):e62056.

49. Kufel TJ, Pineda LA, Mador MJ. Comparison of potentiated and unpotentiated twitches as an index of muscle fatigue. Muscle Nerve. 2002;25(3):438–44.

50. Peoples GE, McLennan PL. Dietary fish oil reduces skeletal muscle oxygen consumption, provides fatigue resistance and improves contractile recovery in the rat in vivo hindlimb. Br J Nutr. 2010;104(12):1771–9.

51. Peoples GE, McLennan PL. Long-chain n-3 DHA reduces the extent of skeletal muscle fatigue in the rat in vivo hindlimb model. Br J Nutr. 2014;111(6):996–1003.

52. Malm C, Yu JG. Exercise-induced muscle damage and inflammation: re-evaluation by proteomics. Histochem Cell Biol. 2012;138(1):89–99.

53. Sorichter S, Puschendorf B, Mair J. Skeletal muscle injury induced by eccentric muscle action: muscle proteins as markers of muscle fiber injury. Exerc Immunol Rev. 1999;5:5–21.

54. Willoughby DS, McFarlin B, Bois C. Interleukin-6 expression after repeated bouts of eccentric exercise. Int J Sports Med. 2003;24(1):15–21.

55. Van der Meulen JH, Kuipers H, Drukker J. Relationship between exercise-induced muscle damage and enzyme release in rats. J Appl Physiol. 1991;71(3):999–1004.

56. Dinarello CA. Role of pro- and anti-inflammatory cytokines during inflammation: experimental and clinical findings. J Biol Regul Homeost Agents. 1997;11(3):91–103.

57. Collins RA, Grounds MD. The role of tumor necrosis factor-alpha (TNF-alpha) in skeletal muscle regeneration. Studies in TNF-alpha(−/−) and TNF-alpha (−/−)/LT-alpha(−/−) mice. J Histochem Cytochem. 2001;49(8):989–1001.

58. Li YP. TNF-alpha is a mitogen in skeletal muscle. Am J Physiol Cell Physiol. 2003;285(2):C370–6.

59. Radak Z, Pucsok J, Mecseki S, Csont T, Ferdinandy P. Muscle soreness-induced reduction in force generation is accompanied by increased nitric oxide content and DNA damage in human skeletal muscle. Free Radic Biol Med. 1999;26(7–8):1059–63.

60. Umegaki K, Daohua P, Sugisawa A, Kimura M, Higuchi M. Influence of one bout of vigorous exercise on ascorbic acid in plasma and oxidative damage

to DNA in blood cells and muscle in untrained rats. J Nutr Biochem. 2000;11(7–8):401–7.

61. Sacheck JM, Milbury PE, Cannon JG, Roubenoff R, Blumberg JB. Effect of vitamin E and eccentric exercise on selected biomarkers of oxidative stress in young and elderly men. Free Radic Biol Med. 2003;34(12):1575–88.

62. Urso ML. Anti-inflammatory interventions and skeletal muscle injury: benefit or detriment? J Appl Physiol. 2013;115(6):920–8.

63. Tenikoff D, Murphy KJ, Le M, Howe PR, Howarth GS. Lyprinol (stabilised lipid extract of New Zealand green-lipped mussel): a potential preventative treatment modality for inflammatory bowel disease. J Gastroenterol. 2005;40(4):361–5.

64. Lemke RA, Peterson AC, Ziegelhoffer EC, Westphall MS, Tjellstrom H, Coon JJ, et al. Synthesis and scavenging role of furan fatty acids. Proc Natl Acad Sci U S A. 2014;111(33):E3450–7.

## 14

The impact of a pre-loaded multi-ingredient performance supplement on muscle soreness and performance following downhill running

Michael J Ormsbee[1,2,3*], Emery G Ward[1], Christopher W Bach[1,2], Paul J Arciero[4], Andrew J McKune[3] and Lynn B Panton[1]

Abstract

The effects of multi-ingredient performance supplements (MIPS) on perceived soreness, strength, flexibility and vertical jump performance following eccentric exercise are unknown. The purpose of this study was to determine the impact of MIPS (NO-Shotgun®) pre-loaded 4 weeks prior to a single bout of downhill running (DHR) on muscle soreness and performance. Trained male runners ($n = 20$) were stratified by VO_{2max}, strength, and lean mass into two groups; MIPS ($n = 10$) ingested one serving daily of NO-Shotgun® for 28 days and 30 min prior to all post-testing visits, Control (CON; $n = 10$) consumed an isocaloric maltodextrin placebo in an identical manner as MIPS. Perceived soreness and performance measurements (strength, flexibility, and jump height) were tested on 6 occasions; 28 days prior to DHR, immediately before DHR (PRE), immediately post (POST) DHR, 24, 48, and 72 hr post-DHR. Perceived soreness significantly increased ($p < 0.05$) post DHR compared to PRE at all time-points, with no difference between groups. Creatine kinase (CK) and lactate dehydrogenase (LDH) increased over time ($p < 0.001$) with no group x time interactions ($p = 0.236$ and $p = 0.535$, respectively). Significant time effects were measured for strength ($p = 0.001$), flexibility ($p = 0.025$) and vertical jump ($p < 0.001$). There were no group x time interactions for any performance measurements. Consumption of MIPS for 4 weeks prior to a single bout of DHR did not affect perceived soreness, muscle damage, strength, flexibility, or jump performance compared to an isocaloric placebo in trained male runners following a single bout of DHR.

Keywords: Eccentric exercise, Muscle damage, Recovery

Background

Exercise induced muscle damage (EIMD) from unaccustomed bouts of eccentric or strenuous exercise has been well documented [1-4]. EIMD promotes an unbalanced ratio of protein breakdown to protein synthesis and is associated with increased muscle soreness, decrements in strength, and impaired muscle function for several days post-exercise [5]. Muscle damage induced by strenuous or unaccustomed downhill running (DHR) initiates biochemical and skeletal muscle morphology changes indicated by localized edema, increased circulating inflammatory markers (cytokines and leukocytes), and increases in indirect markers of muscle damage (creatine kinase (CK), lactate dehydrogenase (LDH)) [3,6].

In parallel with elevated markers of tissue damage following eccentric exercise are decrements in performance measures, including muscular power, maximal contractile force (eccentric, concentric, isometric), and endurance performance [2,7,8]. Previous studies have demonstrated a positive impact on recovery from EIMD through supplementation with whey protein isolate [5], branched-chain amino acids (BCAAs: leucine, isoleucine, and valine) [9,10], leucine only [2], creatine [11,12], and caffeine [13,14]. However, little is known about the effects of multi-ingredient performance supplements (MIPS) [i.e. common MIPS components: protein, BCAAs, creatine, beta-alanine, caffeine, and l-arginine] on the attenuation of muscle damage and repair after EIMD from DHR. Multiple studies

---

* Correspondence: mormsbee@fsu.edu
[1]Department of Nutrition, Food and Exercise Sciences, Florida State University, Tallahassee, FL, USA
[2]Institute of Sports Sciences and Medicine, Florida State University, Tallahassee, FL, USA
Full list of author information is available at the end of the article

have demonstrated beneficial effects following an identical 28-day, pre-exercise supplementation protocol [15-17]. While the improved strength and body composition variables from MIPS supplementation in these studies are promising, a resistance training protocol was used. However, the significantly increased muscle mass and strength gains with MIPS supplementation suggests the MIPS may have elicited improvements via specific ingredients included in the MIPS. Specifically, increased muscle protein synthesis and recovery (i.e. protein, BCAAs, leucine), hydrogen ion buffering (i.e. beta-alanine), ATP resynthesis (i.e. creatine), and/or improved CNS stimulation (i.e. caffeine) are plausible mechanisms of action.

While the aforementioned pre-exercise MIPS supplementation studies are promising [15-17], due to the use of a resistance training protocol, assumptions must be made to draw conclusions about the effects of MIPS on the attenuation of EIMD following a DHR in an endurance population. Therefore, the purpose of this study was to determine the impact of MIPS, pre-loaded 4 weeks prior to- and for 72 hr following a single bout of DHR on muscle damage, soreness, and performance during recovery. We hypothesized that this supplementation protocol would decrease ratings of perceived soreness, improve biochemical markers of muscle damage (i.e. CK and LDH), improve muscle performance of isokinetic and isometric strength, range of motion (ROM), and jump performance greater than an isocaloric placebo in endurance-trained male runners for up to 72 hr post-DHR.

Methods

Participants

Twenty healthy, male endurance-trained runners (maximal oxygen uptake (VO_{2max}) $\geq$ 55 ml/kg/min and an average 20 miles/week of running), ages 18–50 years were recruited to participate in this study (Table 1). Participants were excluded if they had existing diseases (e.g. cardiovascular disease), musculoskeletal disorders, any history of leg injury or any other medical condition

that would be exacerbated by a single bout of DHR, or the regular use of any anti-inflammatory drugs. Participants who were consuming any other dietary or ergogenic supplements were instructed to immediately stop consumption and complete a 4-week washout period before participating in the study (one participant reported use of a generic over-the-counter multivitamin supplement, no other supplement use was reported). All procedures involving human subjects were approved by the Florida State University Human Subjects Institutional Review Board, and written informed consent was obtained prior to participation. Throughout the study, all participants maintained their habitual diet, and were given 24-hr dietary food logs to record their meals the day prior to baseline testing and asked to replicate these meals before all other laboratory visits. Participants ate their last meal at least 6 hr prior to testing and consumed a commercial Chocolate Chip Clif Bar® (240 kcals) 3 hr prior to testing and at least 3 hr from their last meal.

Treatment

The study was a placebo-controlled, double blind protocol with two groups. After baseline testing participants were stratified by VO_{2max}, isometric voluntary contraction strength (60°), and lean mass and assigned to either MIPS (n = 10) or CON (n = 10). MIPS consumed one serving (21 g) of NO-Shotgun® (~72 kcals; 18 g protein; 9.7 g protein hydrolysate matrix including BCAAs; 8.06 g muscle volumizing and power/speed/strength matrix that includes multiple forms of creatine and beta alanine; 376 mg of Redline®energy matrix including caffeine; Vital Pharmaceuticals, Inc., Davic, FL) once per day for 4 weeks prior to the DHR and 30 min prior to all post-testing visits (3 days) with 355 - 473 ml of water. CON consumed one serving (21 g) of an isocaloric, flavor-matched placebo beverage (maltodextrin) once per day for 4 weeks prior to the DHR, as well as 30 min prior to all post-testing visits. All participants received their supplement in identical commercially labeled containers after baseline testing. Participants consumed either MIPS or CON 30 min prior to exercise on all exercise training days, or first thing in the morning on non-training days. Empty containers were collected to verify compliance from all participants.

Experimental overview

Participants reported to the laboratory on 7 different occasions (Figure 1). The first visit included a review of the informed consent document, distribution of the Chocolate Chip Clif Bar®, as well as the measurement of anthropometric values. The second laboratory visit was no later than 1 week from the first visit and was used as the baseline/inclusion testing for participation in the study, including VO_{2max} determination. Subsequent to

Table 1 Participant characteristics (N = 20)

	MIPS (n = 10)	CON (n = 10)
Age (yrs)	24 ± 5	30 ± 10
Height (cm)	178.3 ± 5.6	181.9 ± 7.5
Body Mass (kg)	72.4 ± 8.3	74.4 ± 6.3
Body Fat (%)	9.2 ± 2.6	10.3 ± 3.1
VO_{2max} (ml/kg/min)	61.7 ± 5.3	61.4 ± 4.9

Values are expressed as mean ± SD.
MIPS: Multi-Ingredient Performance Supplement; CON: Control Carbohydrate Placebo; VO_{2max}: Maximal Oxygen Uptake.

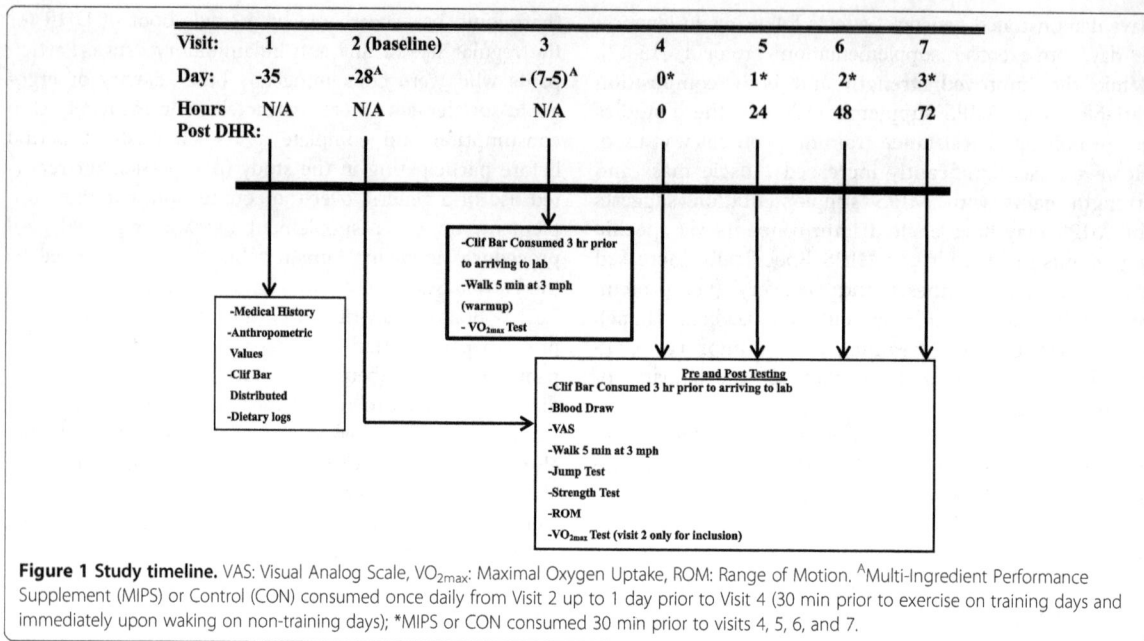

Visit:	1	2 (baseline)	3	4	5	6	7
Day:	-35	-28^A	- (7-5)^A	0*	1*	2*	3*
Hours Post DHR:	N/A	N/A	N/A	0	24	48	72

-Clif Bar Consumed 3 hr prior to arriving to lab
-Walk 5 min at 3 mph (warmup)
- VO$_{2max}$ Test

-Medical History
-Anthropometric Values
-Clif Bar Distributed
-Dietary logs

Pre and Post Testing
-Clif Bar Consumed 3 hr prior to arriving to lab
-Blood Draw
-VAS
-Walk 5 min at 3 mph
-Jump Test
-Strength Test
-ROM
-VO$_{2max}$ Test (visit 2 only for inclusion)

Figure 1 Study timeline. VAS: Visual Analog Scale, VO$_{2max}$: Maximal Oxygen Uptake, ROM: Range of Motion. ^{A}Multi-Ingredient Performance Supplement (MIPS) or Control (CON) consumed once daily from Visit 2 up to 1 day prior to Visit 4 (30 min prior to exercise on training days and immediately upon waking on non-training days); *MIPS or CON consumed 30 min prior to visits 4, 5, 6, and 7.

performance testing on this visit, an incremental treadmill running protocol was employed to determine VO$_{2max}$ using a motor driven treadmill (Woodway®, Waukesha, WI, USA). Expired air was measured breath-by-breath by indirect calorimetry using a metabolic measurement system (Parvomedics Truemax® 2400, Consentius Technologies, Sandy, UT, USA). Prior to the beginning of each test, the gas analyzer was calibrated using ambient air and a gas of a known composition containing 20.9% O_2 and 4% CO_2. The turbine flowmeter was calibrated using a 3-L syringe (Hans Rudolph, Inc., Kansas City, MO, USA).The participant began by walking for 5 min at 3 mph then the speed was increased to 5.5 mph at a 0% grade for 2 min (stage 1). Upon completion of the first stage the speed was increased 1 mph every 2 min until the participant reached the speed of 9.5 mph (stage 5). After the completion of stage 5 the participant maintained a running speed of 9.5 mph and the grade was increased by 2% every 2 min until the participant reached volitional fatigue. Heart rate was monitored using a heart rate monitor (Polar™, Lake Success, NY, USA). Ratings of perceived exertion (RPE) and heart rate were recorded at the end of each stage, as well as when participants reached volitional exhaustion, or requested to stop the test. The test was considered to be a maximal test under 2 conditions: 1) If the participants' VO$_2$ reached a plateau for more than 1 stage (2 min intervals) while intensity continued to increase or 2) Participants exhibited 2 of the following secondary criteria: RPE $\geq$ 19, respiratory exchange ratio (RER) $\geq$ 1.1, or a heart rate within 10 beats/min of the theoretical age

predicted maximum heart rate (220 – age). The researchers provided verbal encouragement during the test to ensure maximal effort.

Upon completion of baseline testing the participants were given instructions on supplementation and instructed to maintain their normal dietary and training patterns for the next 28 days during supplementation. Approximately 3 weeks from baseline testing participants returned to the laboratory under the same pretesting conditions as baseline to perform a VO$_{2max}$ test to determine their intensity (75% of VO$_{2max}$) during the DHR.

A 10 ml venous blood sample was collected and perceived muscle soreness, jump height, isokinetic and isometric strength, and ROM were measured, respectively, during 5 different laboratory visits: baseline (28 days before DHR), immediately before the DHR (PRE), immediately after the DHR (POST), and 24, 48, and 72 hr post-DHR. After the blood draw and muscle soreness was measured, participants walked for 5 min at 3 mph on a motorized treadmill to warm-up prior to any performance measurements (the DHR was only performed during visit 4; See Figure 1). Prior to these visits participants consumed their commercial Chocolate Chip Clif Bar® (given during visit 1) 3 hr before testing and replicated their 24 hr dietary food logs. Participants were asked to refrain from physical activity 48 hr and caffeine, alcohol, and pain medication (i.e. ibuprofen) 24 hr prior to all laboratory testing visits.

Measures

Muscle soreness was measured via a visual analog scale (0–100 mm). Participants rated their level of soreness of the rectus femoris, vastus medialis, vastus lateralis, biceps femoris, gastrocnemius, and gluteus maximus on the right leg by drawing an intersecting line across a continuum line extending from 0 mm (0 = no soreness) to 100 mm (100 = extreme soreness). To help quantify pain, an algometer (Force Ten™ Wagner Instruments, Greenwich, CT, USA) was used with an application of 4 kg of pressure. The midline of the muscle was determined using a tape measure and the algometer was placed at this point with the application of the 4 kg of pressure.

Jump height was assessed using a Vertec vertical jump system (Perform Better, Cranston, RI), recording the best of 5 attempts. The squat jump test was used to assess dynamic explosive force production of the leg extensors. With no restriction on knee angle during the eccentric phase of the knee flexion, participants were instructed to bend down with their knees shoulder width apart and explosively jump, reaching their hand as high as possible during the peak height of the jump to shift the tabs at the top of the Vertec bar. Participants completed 5 jumps with 30 seconds of rest between each jump with the highest measure recorded for analysis.

Isokinetic (5 repetitions, 180°/sec unilateral knee/extension flexion) and isometric (3 repetitions/5 second rest, 60° isometric knee extension/flexion) strength of the dominant leg were determined using the Biodex System 3 (Biodex Medical Systems, Shirley, New York) exercise dynamometer. Each participant was placed in the upright-seated position in the Biodex system, and the seat height and position were adjusted in order to align the instrument's axis of rotation with the participant's knee. Once positioned correctly and secured, ROM was determined along with the weight of the limb. The dominant leg was used for all Biodex testing. Participants were instructed to cross their arms over their chests without holding the restraints or handles. The first test was an isokinetic 180°/sec unilateral knee/extension flexion. Five repetitions of consecutive maximal extension and flexion concentric contractions were performed. Sixty seconds following the isokinetic test, a 60° isometric knee extension/flexion test was performed. The test involved 3 alternating maximal extension and flexion exertions against an immovable arm, with 5 second rest periods between exertions. Continuous verbal encouragement was provided by the research team throughout the duration of all tests. Participants were allowed to view the data reporting screen and all values as they were recorded. The peak torque of the isokinetic and isometric tests for the quadriceps and hamstrings were recorded for later analysis.

Range of motion (ROM) was measured by sit-and-reach assessment using standard testing procedures [18]

(Figure Finder Flex Tester® box; Novel Products, Inc., Rockton, IL, USA). The best of 3 trials was recorded as the final value used for statistical analysis.

Height and weight were measured via the use of a wall-mounted SECA 216 stadiometer and a digital scale (SECA, Hamburg, Germany), respectively. All measurements were taken without shoes and wearing minimal clothing (e.g. running shorts). Body composition was measured non-invasively using the sum of 3 skinfold measurements (chest, abdomen, and thigh), all taken by the same technician, that were used to calculate body fat percentage [19].

Blood (10 mL) was collected via venipuncture of the antecubital vein at baseline testing, PRE, POST, 24, 48, and 72 hr after the DHR. Following the blood collection, serum (BD Vacutainer, no coagulant) was allowed to clot and centrifuged at 3500 RPM at 4°C for 15 min (Sorvall ST16R Multispeed Centrifuge; Thermo Electron Corporation, Needham Heights, Massachusetts). Aliquots (300 μL) were then transferred into microtubes and immediately frozen at −80°C for later batch analysis. Serum CK activity and LDH were analyzed in duplicate using commercially labeled assay kits (BioAssay Systems, EnzyChrom).

Downhill running protocol
Prior to the DHR during visit 4, participants began by warming up for 5 min walking on a level grade at 3 mph. The treadmill grade was then lowered to -5% grade. Participants ran continuously for 60 min at a speed eliciting 75% of their VO_{2max} on a level grade (determined during visit 3) [18]. Heart rate and RPE were monitored continuously and recorded every 10 min during the DHR (data not shown).

Statistical analysis
Sample size was determined using the data from the study by Hoffman et al. [8]. Using an alpha level of 0.05 and power of 80% an effect size of 0.88 was determined. Therefore, a total of 10 participants per group were needed. Participant characteristics and baseline data between groups were analyzed using one-way analysis of variance (ANOVA). Baseline data were also compared to PRE data (after 4 weeks of MIPS or CON) to see if supplementation affected measured parameters by using a 2×2 repeated measures ANOVA. The DHR data were analyzed using a 2 × 5 (group: MIPS or CON × time: PRE, POST, 24, 48, 72 hr) ANOVA with repeated measures. A LSD post-hoc test was used to examine pairwise differences if there were significant main effects. Greenhouse-Geisser analysis was used if the Mauchly's Test of Sphericity was violated. Significance was set at $p < 0.05$. SPSS version 21.0 (SPSS Inc, Cary, NC) was

used for statistical analyses. Data are presented as means ± standard deviations.

Results

There were no significant differences between groups at baseline (Table 1) and no differences were observed for any variable when baseline data were compared to PRE data, with the exception of a significant time effect for an increase in flexibility and vertical jump ($p = 0.005$ and $p = 0.006$, respectively). Supplement compliance was reported to be 100% as verified by collection of empty supplement containers and questioning.

Delayed onset muscle soreness

There were no significant differences in perceived muscle soreness between groups at any time point for any of the muscle groups tested (Table 2). There were, however, significant main time effects for the rectus femoris ($p < 0.001$), vastus medialis ($p = 0.002$), vastus lateralis, ($p = 0.001$), biceps femoris ($p = 0.007$), and gluteus maximus ($p = 0.014$). Perceived muscle soreness was reported to be significantly ($p < 0.05$) greater than PRE in the rectus femoris (24, 48, and 72 hr), vastus medialis (POST, 24 hr), vastus lateralis (POST, 24, 48, and 72 hr), biceps femoris (POST, 24, 48, and 72 hr, and the gluteus maximus (POST, 24, 48 hr) of the right leg in both groups. The mean of all muscle soreness was reported to be significantly greater ($p < 0.05$) than PRE at all time-points (POST, 24, 48, and 72 hr), with no difference between groups.

Performance measurements

There was no significant difference between maximal isometric voluntary contraction strength, maximal isokinetic strength, vertical jump, and ROM, and between baseline and PRE for MIPS and CON (data not shown). However, there was a significant time effect for an increase in ROM ($p = 0.005$) and vertical jump ($p = 0.006$) from baseline to PRE in both groups.

There were no significant group × time interactions for the MIPS and the CON across time for any of the performance measures (Table 3). There were, however, significant time effects for maximal voluntary isometric contraction for extension ($p = 0.001$) and flexion ($p = 0.013$) strength, maximal isokinetic flexion strength ($p = 0.001$), flexibility ($p = 0.025$), and vertical jump height ($p < 0.001$).

Maximal oxygen uptake

There was a significant group × time interaction for VO_{2max} between baseline and 1 week prior to the DHR (MIPS: $61.7 ± 5.3$ to $63.3 ± 5.8$ ml/kg/min; CON: $61.4 ± 4.9$ to $60.4 ± 5.9$ ml/kg/min). When evaluating the within group differences, there were no significant differences in VO_{2max}; however, MIPS had an increase approaching significance ($p = 0.06$) while CON had a non-significant

Table 2 Perceived muscle soreness of the right leg

Variable	Group	Pre DHR (day 0)	POST (day 0)	24 hr post	48 hr post	72 hr post
Gastrocnemius	MIPS ($n = 9$)	$15.7 ± 20.7$	$18.3 ± 19.8$	$17.7 ± 21.4$	$12.8 ± 21.1^c$	$13.1 ± 17.4^c$
	CON ($n = 10$)	$9.3 ± 9.7$	$10.6 ± 10.6$	$16.1 ± 13.1$	$11.4 ± 9.7^c$	$13.0 ± 14.9^c$
Rectus Femoris*	MIPS ($n = 9$)	$11.2 ± 18.5$	$14.7 ± 14.5$	$19.4 ± 15.0^{abde}$	$14.7 ± 15.5^e$	$8.5 ± 10.1^b$
	CON ($n = 10$)	$10.3 ± 9.0$	$14.7 ± 9.6$	$26.1 ± 18.0^{abde}$	$15.8 ± 14.6^e$	$13.5 ± 11.1^b$
Vastus Lateralis*	MIPS ($n = 8$)	$6.6 ± 10.6$	$16.0 ± 15.3^a$	$21.8 ± 19.6^{ab}$	$17.2 ± 17.3^a$	$16.7 ± 21.2^a$
	CON ($n = 10$)	$8.2 ± 5.8$	$14.0 ± 11.2^a$	$19.9 ± 15.6^{ab}$	$19.4 ± 15.7^a$	$11.1 ± 7.9^a$
Vastus Medialis*	MIPS ($n = 8$)	$11.0 ± 14.3$	$24.6 ± 19.7^a$	$34.3 ± 24.8^{abde}$	$20.7 ± 24.8$	$16.6 ± 20.9$
	CON ($n = 10$)	$12.6 ± 10.0$	$16.6 ± 12.3^a$	$26.5 ± 21.0^{abde}$	$21.4 ± 16.9$	$17.0 ± 13.8$
Biceps Femoris*	MIPS ($n = 9$)	$7.3 ± 12.8$	$9.45 ± 11.7^a$	$21.5 ± 17.5^{abe}$	$11.7 ± 17.8^a$	$12.1 ± 14.6^a$
	CON ($n = 10$)	$5.0 ± 4.0$	$10.2 ± 9.4^a$	$19.2 ± 18.9^{abe}$	$13.3 ± 12.0^a$	$7.9 ± 9.8^a$
Gluteus Maximus*	MIPS ($n = 9$)	$6.5 ± 10.2$	$13.6 ± 16.9^a$	$20.2 ± 21.3^a$	$13.2 ± 19.3^a$	$8.5 ± 14.5$
	CON ($n = 10$)	$6.3 ± 6.5$	$9.0 ± 8.6^a$	$10.8 ± 11.7^a$	$6.6 ± 6.7^a$	$8.2 ± 7.7$
Mean Muscle Soreness*	MIPS ($n = 7$)	$66.3 ± 88.1$	$110.9 ± 97.1^a$	$153.3 ± 104.4^{abde}$	$105.9 ± 106.6^a$	$88.6 ± 100.6$
	CON ($n = 8$)	$55.3 ± 40.3$	$74.1 ± 58.6^a$	$114.6 ± 90.5^{abde}$	$86.6 ± 73.3^a$	$74.4 ± 63.2$

Values are expressed as mean ± SD. MIPS: Multi-Ingredient Performance Supplement; CON: Control Carbohydrate Placebo.
*$p < 0.05$, significant time effect.
[a] $p < 0.05$, significantly different from Pre.
[b] $p < 0.05$, significantly from POST.
[c] $p < 0.05$, significantly different from 24 hr.
[d] $p < 0.05$, significantly from 48 hr.
[e] $p < 0.05$, significantly different from 72 hr.

Table 3 Performance measurements (*n* = 10 for MIPS and CON)

Variable	Group	Pre DHR (day 0)	POST (day 0)	24 hr post	48 hr post	72 hr post
MVC Extension (60°) (N·m)*	MIPS	207 ± 52	185 ± 40	199 ± 58[b]	210 ± 49[b]	217 ± 37[bcd]
	CON	196 ± 58	184 ± 50	200 ± 58[b]	205 ± 59[b]	221 ± 64[bcd]
MVC Flexion (60°) (N·m)*	MIPS	116 ± 36[b]	107 ± 31	109 ± 33[b]	117 ± 34[b]	118 ± 26[bc]
	CON	109 ± 30[b]	99 ± 27	108 ± 30[b]	108 ± 28[b]	113 ± 33[bc]
Maximal Isokinetic Extension (180°/sec) (N·m)*	MIPS	149 ± 22[c]	149 ± 23	140 ± 20[a]	151 ± 19[c]	152 ± 18[c]
	CON	143 ± 27[c]	139 ± 18	136 ± 26[a]	140 ± 28[c]	145 ± 32[c]
Maximal Isokinetic Flexion (180°/sec) (N·m)*	MIPS	78 ± 17	77 ± 19	78 ± 16	81 ± 17[ab]	81 ± 18[ab]
	CON	70 ± 22	72 ± 19	79 ± 17	80 ± 20[ab]	82 ± 23[ab]
ROM (cm)*	MIPS	25.1 ± 11.7[c]	25.8 ± 11.3[c]	23.6 ± 12.6[a]	25.7 ± 11.4[c]	25.5 ± 11.3[c]
	CON	20.3 ± 10.6[c]	21.2 ± 10.4[c]	19.6 ± 10.5	19.3 ± 10.1	20.1 ± 10.4[c]
Vertical Jump (cm)*	MIPS	51.3 ± 7.3[c]	52.3 ± 6.6[c]	50.0 ± 18.0	50.0 ± 6.6[bc]	51.0 ± 7.1[cd]
	CON	50.0 ± 14.7[c]	50.2 ± 14.2[c]	47.4 ± 13.4	49.0 ± 13.9[bc]	50.0 ± 13.7[cd]

Values are expressed as mean ± SD.
MIPS: Multi-Ingredient Performance Supplement; CON: Control Carbohydrate Placebo; MVC: Maximal Voluntary Isometric Contraction; ROM: Range of Motion; DHR: Downhill Run; POST: Immediately Post-DHR.
*$p < 0.05$, significant time effect.
[a]$p < 0.05$, significantly different from Pre.
[b]$p < 0.05$, significantly from POST.
[c]$p < 0.05$, significantly different from 24 hr.
[d]$p < 0.05$, significantly from 48 hr.

decrease. The standard error for the flow calibration of the Parvomedics metabolic cart was an average of 0.4%.

Muscle damage markers

There were no significant group × time interactions for either CK or LDH from baseline to PRE ($p = 0.056$ and $p = 0.392$, respectively); however a significant time effect was observed for CK ($p = 0.021$) but not for LDH ($p = 0.079$). There was a significant time effect for both CK and LDH from PRE to 72 hr post-DHR ($p < 0.001$) (See Figures 2 and 3); however no group x time effect for CK or LDH was observed ($p = 0.236$ and $p = 0.535$, respectively). When data from both groups were collapsed, CK levels were significantly elevated from POST to 48 hr when compared to PRE values. LDH levels were significantly elevated POST before returning to PRE values at 24 hr.

Discussion

The main findings of this study were that consumption of MIPS for 4 weeks prior to a single bout of DHR did not attenuate the changes of ratings of perceived soreness, isokinetic or isometric strength, jump performance, or ROM greater than an isocaloric placebo (CON) in highly trained male runners for up to 72 hr post-

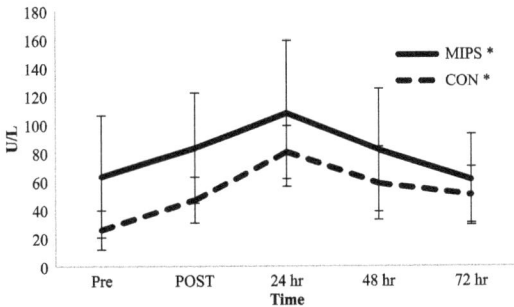

Figure 2 Creatine Kinase measured in serum. Values are expressed as mean ± SD creatine kinase levels. MIPS: Multi-Ingredient Performance Supplement; CON: Control Carbohydrate Placebo; Pre, immediately before downhill run; POST, immediately post-downhill run; 24 hr, 24 hr post-downhill run; 48 hr, 48 hr post-downhill run; 72 hr, 72 hr post-downhill run. *$p < 0.05$, significant time effect.

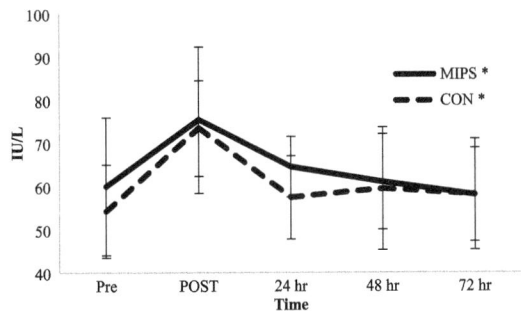

Figure 3 Lactate Dehydrogenase measured in serum. Values are expressed as mean ± SD lactate dehydrogenase levels. MIPS: Multi-Ingredient Performance Supplement; CON: Control Carbohydrate Placebo; Pre, immediately before downhill run; POST, immediately post-downhill run; 24 hr, 24 hr post-downhill run; 48 hr, 48 hr post-downhill run; 72 hr, 72 hr post-downhill run. *$p < 0.05$, significant time effect.

exercise. Therefore, we reject our hypothesis that the MIPS would decrease ratings of perceived soreness, improve biochemical markers of muscle damage (i.e. CK and LDH), improve muscle performance of isokinetic and isometric strength, range of motion (ROM), and jump performance greater than an isocaloric placebo in endurance-trained male runners for up to 72 hr post-DHR.

Delayed onset muscle soreness

Delayed onset muscle soreness (DOMS) generally develops between 24-48 hr after exercise, peaks at 24-72 hr, and subsides 5-7 days post-exercise [20]. Two days after DHR, tenderness, measured by a pressure transducer, was greatest in the gluteus maximus, rectus femoris, vastus medialis, vastus lateralis, tibialis anterior, gastrocnemius and biceps femoris [21]. Our findings confirmed that the greatest amount of perceived soreness was reported during 24 and 48 hr following the DHR with no differences between groups. Therefore, it appears the selected intensity of running downhill at -5% at 75% VO_{2max} was a sufficient enough stimulus to elicit muscle soreness as shown in other studies [6,22]. In an attempt to reduce DOMS and stimulate protein synthesis following strenuous exercise supplementation with protein [22], BCAAs [9,23-25], leucine [2], and creatine [11,26] have been used. Interestingly, acute ingestion of protein (100 g of protein containing 40 g essential amino acids) immediately after a single 30 min bout of DHR had no effect on DOMS during 72 hr of recovery [22]; however supplementation with BCAAs (2.5 g of BCAAs taken both immediately prior to- and during exercise) significantly decreased DOMS from 24 to 72 hr post-endurance exercise [9]. In the present study, no significant difference in perceived soreness was reported between groups, which agrees with others using protein [22], BCAAs [10], leucine individually [2], or creatine [11,26]. The discrepancies could be due to higher individual dosages of each individual supplement in previous studies compared to our MIPS.

Biochemical markers of muscle damage

Our findings of elevated muscle damage markers (CK and LDH) following eccentrically-based exercise support previous research [3,27-29]. Although large variability exists in the response of these muscle proteins to eccentric exercise [30-32], the concurrent elevations in subsequent pain experienced (DOMS ratings) by participants suggest the two are closely linked. Indeed, our findings support this relationship as both mean perceived muscle soreness (Table 2) and CK levels (Figure 2) were significantly elevated POST, 24, and 48 hr post-DHR in comparison to PRE. In addition, LDH levels (Figure 3) were significantly elevated POST and had a tendency to remain

elevated up to 48 hr post-DHR. While the DHR protocol induced muscle soreness and damage a MIPS did not attenuate this response. Our findings agree with others examining the eccentrically-induced CK response to whey protein [5,8,22], BCAAs [10,33], leucine alone [2], caffeine [14], and creatine [11,12], but not others showing a reduction in CK as a result of creatine [12,34] or BCAA supplementation [9,24,35]. Furthermore, our findings corroborate the increased LDH response to whey protein (1.5 g/kg/day of whey protein isolate for 14 days) [5] and caffeine (4.5 mg/kg immediately prior to exercise) [14], but not the reduction of LDH as a result of BCAA supplementation (12 g/day of BCAAs for 14 days and an additional 20 g immediately prior to- and post-exercise) [35]. Again, this is likely due to different dosing of the individual ingredients within the propriety blend of our MIPS and that of other studies as well as differences in supplement timing and training status of the participants in each study.

Performance measurements and range of motion

Decrements in performance measurements of strength (isometric and isokinetic strength) [2,5,6,23], jump height [2], and ROM [11,24,26] following eccentric exercise have been well documented. Across groups, maximal isometric strength was significantly lower at 24, 48, and 72 hr compared to immediately post-DHR. Similarly, isokinetic extension strength decreased compared to baseline at 24 hr post-DHR, returning back to baseline values at 48 hr. Interestingly, isokinetic flexion strength actually improved significantly in both groups at 48 and 72 hr post-DHR compared to baseline, suggesting a possibility of familiarization with the equipment, and/or the absence of any structural damage to the muscle fibers allowing strength to be maintained and even improve throughout the recovery period.

Etheridge et al. reported that participants supplementing with whey protein (100 g of protein containing 40 g essential amino acids) immediately after a single 30 min bout of DHR had significantly greater isometric strength at 48 hr compared to a carbohydrate supplement [22]. Controversy still exists as to whether BCAAs are effective in attenuating strength loss following EIMD. Some studies have shown that BCAAs are only effective in augmenting strength at 48 hr [9,25] after EIMD and only during the flexion phase of the contraction [9] versus placebo. Creatine also shows conflicting results for improving strength performance following EIMD. Despite our findings and others that report no change in 1-repetition maximum after EIMD with creatine use [11,26], Cooke et al. have shown that maximal isometric extension strength of the lower leg from 24 to 96 hr and isokinetic extension strength at 48 hr was significantly greater in the creatine supplementation group (0.3 g/kg/day) compared to that of a carbohydrate placebo [34]. The primary differences between studies appears to be differences in training status as the present study and others [11,26] have shown no effect of creatine supplementation with trained males, while Cooke et al. have shown improvements in strength following EIMD with untrained males [34]. Acute ingestion of protein prior to a single bout of DHR resulted in a [22] maximal voluntary isometric contraction strength that returned to normal more rapidly at 48 hr than that of placebo. Our results do not support this conclusion with the consumption of MIPS. Our findings agree with others showing that BCAA consumption (7.3 g for two days) resulted in no difference in maximal voluntary isometric contraction strength during recovery from exercise [10]. However, the aforementioned study by Etheridge et al. documented improvements in strength and power; though the authors based the intensity of the DHR on age predicted maximal heart rate (220 - age) and used recreationally active males [22].

Jump height has been found to significantly decrease at 24 and 48 hr following EIMD and remain below pre-exercise values for up to 96 hr [2,23]. Similarly, our data show decreased jump height at 24 hr following the DHR compared to all other time points with a return back to baseline values at 72 hr post-exercise, regardless of group. Eccentric exercises have been shown to significantly decrease maximal isometric contraction strength from 24 up to 120 hr compared to baseline values [5,6,9,10,22,23]. These decrements in strength from eccentric exercise are associated with a decreased ROM immediately following [11,26] and up to 96 hr [24] after exercise. ROM was slightly elevated immediately following exercise in the present study, as documented by others [12], but was significantly lower at 24 hr compared to before the DHR and was back to baseline values at 72 hr (Table 3).

As previously mentioned, decreased ROM and strength [11,26] are expected following EIMD. Our results also found a decrease in ROM at 24 hr post-DHR with ROM returning back to baseline values at 72 hr, with no differences between groups. Similarly to the findings of the present study, Nosaka et al. and Rawson et al. demonstrated no improvement in ROM between supplementation or placebo when consuming BCAAs [24] or creatine [11,26].

One interesting finding from the present study was the group x time interaction in VO_{2max} over the 4-week pre-loading period. The supplement group had an increase in VO_{2max} approaching significance at $p = 0.064$ and the CON group had a non-significant decrease in VO_{2max}. The 1.6 ml/kg/min increase likely does not represent a true physiological improvement. These findings should be examined further in future research. Participants were asked not to change their training volume over the 4-week supplementation period. While training logs were not completed, verbal verification was obtained to confirm that the participants did not alter their training regimen. It is plausible that MIPS improved training quality over the 4 weeks and that this was responsible for adaptations that improved aerobic capacity. Therefore, MIPS may not improve performance in recovery but rather impacts other indices of fitness in athletes. However, this is all speculative.

Finally, it is important to note that the indirect markers of muscle damage that were used in the present study may have been limited in terms of their sensitivity, and bias, to identify specific responses to the downhill run and the effects of MIPS. This statement relates to a recent alternative perspective on changes in skeletal muscle in response to unaccustomed eccentric exercise in humans [36-38]. Specifically, these authors argue that the changes following voluntary eccentric exercise do not represent muscle damage, muscle necrosis or inflammation in human skeletal muscle but rather provide evidence for myofibrillar remodeling and adaptation [36-38]. Further, the use of indirect measures and direct antibody visualization of EIMD in previous studies, provides limited and biased information in human eccentric exercise models such as downhill running [36]. Rather, Malm and Yu [36] suggest that researchers should use proteomics to provide a powerful and unbiased protein profiling method for studying skeletal muscle adaptation to eccentric exercise. This is an important methodological issue to consider for future studies.

Conclusions

Our results are consistent with others reporting increases in perceived soreness, CK, LDH and decreases in strength, vertical jump and ROM 24 hr after strenuous DHR exercise. However, the use of a proprietary blend MIPS had no effect on markers of muscle damage, soreness or performance compared to an isocaloric placebo. Despite the supporting body of research documenting results in the attenuation of markers of muscle damage, soreness and improved performance measurements with supplementation, other studies using protein, BCAAs, creatine, and leucine reported similar results to ours. The primary differences between our studies and those with contradicting results appear to be greater individual supplementation dosages than the proprietary blend of individual supplements in the MIPS. In addition, we used trained male endurance runners compared to that of recreationally active or untrained males in similar studies.

Competing interests

This study was supported by product donation from Vital Pharmaceuticals, Inc. (Davie, FL) to MJO. None of the authors had financial or other interests concerning the outcomes of the investigation. The authors declare that they have no competing interests.

Authors' contributions

The study was designed by MJO, AJM, LBP, and EGW; Funding was obtained by MJO; data were collected and analyzed by EGW, LBP, CWB, MJO, and PJA; data interpretation and manuscript preparation were undertaken by EGW, MJO, AJM, PJA, CWB, and LBP. All authors approved the final version of the paper.

Acknowledgements

We would like to thank all the participants who volunteered their time and contributing to this project. We would like to thank Laurin Conlin and Joseph Fraser for assistance with data collection.

Author details

[1]Department of Nutrition, Food and Exercise Sciences, Florida State University, Tallahassee, FL, USA. [2]Institute of Sports Sciences and Medicine, Florida State University, Tallahassee, FL, USA. [3]Discipline of Biokinetics, Exercise and Leisure Sciences, University of KwaZulu-Natal, Durban, South Africa. [4]Human Nutrition and Metabolism Laboratory, Skidmore College, Saratoga Springs, NY, USA.

References

1. Gibala MJ, MacDougall JD, Tarnopolsky MA, Stauber WT, Elorriaga A. Changes in human skeletal muscle ultrastructure and force production after acute resistance exercise. J Appl Physiol. 1995;78:702–8.
2. Kirby TJ, Triplett NT, Haines TL, Skinner JW, Fairbrother KR, McBride JM. Effect of leucine supplementation on indices of muscle damage following drop jumps and resistance exercise. Amino Acids. 2012;42:1987–96.
3. McKune AJ, Semple SJ, Smith LL, Wadee AA. Complement, immunoglobulin and creatine kinase response in black and white males after muscle-damaging exercise. South African J Sport Med. 2009;21:47–52.
4. Proske U, Allen TJ. Damage to skeletal muscle from eccentric exercise. Exerc Sport Sci Rev. 2005;33:98–104.
5. Cooke MB, Rybalka E, Stathis CG, Cribb PJ, Hayes A. Whey protein isolate attenuates strength decline after eccentrically-induced muscle damage in healthy individuals. J Int Soc Sports Nutr. 2010;7:30.
6. Chen TC, Nosaka K, Lin M-J, Chen H-L, Wu C-J. Changes in running economy at different intensities following downhill running. J Sports Sci. 2009;27:1137–44.
7. Chen TC, Nosaka K, Tu J-H. Changes in running economy following downhill running. J Sports Sci. 2007;25:55–63.
8. Hoffman JR, Ratamess NA, Tranchina CP, Rashti SL, Kang J, Faigenbaum AD. Effect of a proprietary protein supplement on recovery indices following resistance exercise in strength/power athletes. Amino Acids. 2010;38:771–8.
9. Greer BK, Woodard JL, White JP, Arguello EM, Haymes EM. Branched-chain amino acid supplementation and indicators of muscle damage after endurance exercise. Int J Sport Nutr Exerc Metab. 2007;17:595–607.
10. Jackman SR, Witard OC, Jeukendrup AE, Tipton KD. Branched-chain amino acid ingestion can ameliorate soreness from eccentric exercise. Med Sci Sports Exerc. 2010;42:962–70.
11. Rawson ES, Conti MP, Miles MP. Creatine supplementation does not reduce muscle damage or enhance recovery from resistance exercise. J Strength Cond Res. 2007;21:1208–13.
12. Santos RVT, Bassit RA, Caperuto EC, Costa Rosa LFBP. The effect of creatine supplementation upon inflammatory and muscle soreness markers after a 30km race. Life Sci. 2004;75:1917–24.
13. Bishop NC, Fitzgerald C, Porter PJ, Scanlon GA, Smith AC. Effect of caffeine ingestion on lymphocyte counts and subset activation in vivo following strenuous cycling. Eur J Appl Physiol. 2005;93:606–13.
14. Machado M, Koch AJ, Willardson JM, dos Santos FC, Curty VM, Pereira LN. Caffeine does not augment markers of muscle damage or leukocytosis following resistance exercise. Int J Sports Physiol Perform. 2010;5:18–26.
15. Ormsbee MJ, Mandler WK, Thomas DD, Ward EG, Kinsey AW, Simonavice E, et al. The effects of six weeks of supplementation with multi-ingredient performance supplements and resistance training on anabolic hormones, body composition, strength, and power in resistance-trained men. J Int Soc Sports Nutr. 2012;9:49.
16. Spillane M, Schwarz N, Leddy S, Correa T, Minter M, Longoria V, et al. Effects of 28 days of resistance exercise while consuming commercially available pre- and post-workout supplements, NO-Shotgun® and NO-Synthesize® on body composition, muscle strength and mass, markers of protein synthesis, and clinical safety markers in. Nutr Metab (Lond). 2011;8:78.
17. Shelmadine B, Cooke M, Buford T, Hudson G, Redd L, Leutholtz B, et al. Effects of 28 days of resistance exercise and consuming a commercially available pre-workout supplement, NO-Shotgun(R), on body composition, muscle strength and mass, markers of satellite cell activation, and clinical safety markers in males. J Int Soc Sports Nutr. 2009;6:16.
18. Thompson WR, Gordon NF, Pescatello LS. ACSM's Guidelines for Exercise Testing and Prescription. 8th ed. Wolters Kluwer/Lippincott Williams & Wilkins; 2010. p. 158.
19. Jackson AS, Pollock ML. Generalized equations for predicting body density of men. 1978. Br J Nutr. 2004;91:161–8.
20. Clarkson PM, Nosaka K, Braun B. Muscle function after exercise-induced muscle damage and rapid adaptation. Med Sci Sports Exerc. 1992;24:512–20.
21. Eston R, Critchley N, Baltzopoulos V. Delayed-onset muscle soreness, strength loss characteristics and creatine kinase activity following uphill and downhill running. J Sports Sci. 1994;12:135.
22. Etheridge T, Philp A, Watt PW. A single protein meal increases recovery of muscle function following an acute eccentric exercise bout. Appl Physiol Nutr Metab. 2008;33:483–8.
23. Howatson G, Hoad M, Goodall S, Tallent J, Bell PG, French DN. Exercise-induced muscle damage is reduced in resistance-trained males by branched chain amino acids: a randomized, double-blind, placebo controlled study. J Int Soc Sports Nutr. 2012;9:20.
24. Nosaka K, Sacco P, Mawatari K. Effects of amino acid supplementation on muscle soreness and damage. Int J Sport Nutr Exerc Metab. 2006;16:620–35.
25. Shimomura Y, Inaguma A, Watanabe S, Yamamoto Y, Muramatsu Y, Bajotto G, et al. Branched-chain amino acid supplementation before squat exercise and delayed-onset muscle soreness. Int J Sport Nutr Exerc Metab. 2010;20:236–44.
26. Rawson ES, Gunn B, Clarkson PM. The effects of creatine supplementation on exercise-induced muscle damage. J Strength Cond Res. 2001;15:178–84.
27. Brancaccio P, Maffulli N, Limongelli FM. Creatine kinase monitoring in sport medicine. Br Med Bull. 2007;81–82:209–30.
28. McKune AJ, Semple SJ, Peters-Futre E. Acute Exercise-Induced Muscle Injury. Biol Sport. 2012;29:3–10.
29. Van de Vyver M, Myburgh KH. Cytokine and satellite cell responses to muscle damage: interpretation and possible confounding factors in human studies. J Muscle Res Cell Motil. 2012;33:177–85.
30. Lee J, Clarkson PM. Plasma creatine kinase activity and glutathione after eccentric exercise. Med Sci Sports Exerc. 2003;35:930–6.
31. Clarkson PM, Ebbeling C. Investigation of serum creatine kinase variability after muscle-damaging exercise. Clin Sci (Lond). 1988;75:257–61.
32. Fridén J, Lieber RL. Serum creatine kinase level is a poor predictor of muscle function after injury. Scand J Med Sci Sports. 2001;11:126–7.
33. Hsu M-C, Chien K-Y, Hsu C-C, Chung C-J, Chan K-H, Su B. Effects of BCAA, arginine and carbohydrate combined drink on post-exercise biochemical response and psychological condition. Chin J Physiol. 2011;54:71–8.
34. Cooke MB, Rybalka E, Williams AD, Cribb PJ, Hayes A. Creatine supplementation enhances muscle force recovery after eccentrically-induced muscle damage in healthy individuals. J Int Soc Sports Nutr. 2009;6:13.
35. Coombes JS, McNaughton LR. Effects of branched-chain amino acid supplementation on serum creatine kinase and lactate dehydrogenase after prolonged exercise. J Sports Med Phys Fitness. 2000;40:240–6.
36. Malm C, Yu J-G. Exercise-induced muscle damage and inflammation: re-evaluation by proteomics. Histochem Cell Biol. 2012;138:89–99.
37. Yu J-G, Liu J-X, Carlsson L, Thornell L-E, Stål PS. Re-evaluation of sarcolemma injury and muscle swelling in human skeletal muscles after eccentric exercise. PLoS One. 2013;8:e62056.
38. Yu J-G, Malm C, Thornell L-E. Eccentric contractions leading to DOMS do not cause loss of desmin nor fibre necrosis in human muscle. Histochem Cell Biol. 2002;118:29–34.

## 15

A nutrition and conditioning intervention for natural bodybuilding contest preparation: case study

Scott Lloyd Robinson[1*], Anneliese Lambeth-Mansell[2], Gavin Gillibrand[3], Abbie Smith-Ryan[4] and Laurent Bannock[1]

Abstract

Bodybuilding competitions are becoming increasingly popular. Competitors are judged on their aesthetic appearance and usually exhibit a high level of muscularity and symmetry and low levels of body fat. Commonly used techniques to improve physique during the preparation phase before competitions include dehydration, periods of prolonged fasting, severe caloric restriction, excessive cardiovascular exercise and inappropriate use of diuretics and anabolic steroids. In contrast, this case study documents a structured nutrition and conditioning intervention followed by a 21 year-old amateur bodybuilding competitor to improve body composition, resting and exercise fat oxidation, and muscular strength that does not involve use of any of the above mentioned methods. Over a 14-week period, the Athlete was provided with a scientifically designed nutrition and conditioning plan that encouraged him to (i) consume a variety of foods; (ii) not neglect any macronutrient groups; (iii) exercise regularly but not excessively and; (iv) incorporate rest days into his conditioning regime. This strategy resulted in a body mass loss of 11.7 kg's, corresponding to a 6.7 kg reduction in fat mass and a 5.0 kg reduction in fat-free mass. Resting metabolic rate decreased from 1993 kcal/d to 1814 kcal/d, whereas resting fat oxidation increased from 0.04 g/min to 0.06 g/min. His capacity to oxidize fat during exercise increased more than two-fold from 0.24 g/min to 0.59 g/min, while there was a near 3-fold increase in the corresponding exercise intensity that elicited the maximal rate of fat oxidation; 21% $\dot{V}O_{2max}$ to 60% $\dot{V}O_{2max}$. Hamstring concentric peak torque decreased (1.7 to 1.5 Nm/kg), whereas hamstring eccentric (2.0 Nm/kg to 2.9 Nm/kg), quadriceps concentric (3.4 Nm/kg to 3.7 Nm/kg) and quadriceps eccentric (4.9 Nm/kg to 5.7 Nm/kg) peak torque all increased. Psychological mood-state (BRUMS scale) was not negatively influenced by the intervention and all values relating to the Athlete's mood-state remained below average over the course of study. This intervention shows that a structured and scientifically supported nutrition strategy can be implemented to improve parameters relevant to bodybuilding competition and importantly the health of competitors, therefore questioning the conventional practices of bodybuilding preparation.

Keywords: Sports nutrition, Physique, Conditioning, Body composition, Fat oxidation, Metabolic health

Background

During bodybuilding competitions individuals are assessed on their physical or 'aesthetic' appearance and are usually required to demonstrate a high degree of muscularity and symmetry, as well as low levels of body fat. Careful attention to nutrition and exercise conditioning is undoubtedly important in facilitating the process of becoming 'competition ready'. Frequently used methods by those preparing for contest include chronic energy restriction, dehydration (water manipulation), sporadic eating and inappropriate use of diuretics and supplements of anabolic steroids and 'fat burners' [1]. These methods pose the risk of adverse health consequences that can be physiological (i.e., decreased bone mineral density [2], metabolic disruption [3], increased cardiovascular strain [4]), hormonal [5,6] and/or psychological (i.e. anger, anxiety, loss of eating control/ binge eating, pre-occupation with food, short temper [1], mood disturbance [6]), in nature. Competitors may also suffer a reduction in their muscular function, strength and power during the preparation phase of competition [6,7],

* Correspondence: scott@guruperformance.co.uk
[1]Guru Performance LTD, 58 South Molton St, London W1K 5SL, UK
Full list of author information is available at the end of the article

as physique-oriented objectives are often placed above exercise performance and health goals.

A case study approach has recently been used to outline effective support strategies for the achievement of body composition and/or performance goals in professional boxing [8], professional jockeying [9], and international-standard women's football [10]. These examples highlight sports (especially boxing and horse riding) where athletes are required to repeatedly manipulate body composition to compete and perform at the highest level, similar to bodybuilding preparation. Despite insightful studies that have documented the physiological changes and dietary practices [6,11,12] that occur during prolonged bodybuilding contest preparation, there have been no case studies that provide a detailed nutrition and conditioning support strategy for the preparation phase of natural bodybuilding competition. Accordingly, we present a 14-week case study demonstrating how a scientifically designed nutrition and conditioning intervention improves body composition, resting and exercise fat oxidation, and muscular strength in an amateur bodybuilding competitor (referred to hereafter as 'The Athlete').

Case presentation
The Athlete
The Athlete was a 21-year-old male amateur bodybuilder who was aiming to compete in his first bodybuilding competition, UK Bodybuilding and Fitness Federation (UKBFF), in the Men's Physique category. He had been undertaking bodybuilding training for two years and had not previously sought any conditioning or dietary advice other than that sourced from the Internet and popular fitness magazines. Furthermore, the Athlete was not on any prescribed medication, was a non-smoker and previously supplemented his diet with whey protein only. In the 3 months prior to the intervention his diet was identical on a daily basis; comprising of four meals and two snacks that were high in carbohydrate and protein and very low in fat (Table 1). In addition to the meals he already consumed, he incorporated one 'cheat meal' approximately every two weeks, which consisted of one large take-away pizza and one serving (~200 g) of ice cream. His conditioning regime consisted of six to seven days per week of resistance training, focusing on individual muscle groups in each session (total nine hours per week).

The Athlete was fully informed of the study aims and potential risks and discomforts following which he provided written informed consent to participate in the study that received full ethical approval from the University of Worcester Ethics Committee.

Goals of the intervention
The primary goals of the support provided were to: (a) achieve the best possible aesthetic appearance in

Table 1 Example of foods consumed by the Athlete before the intervention

Item/description	Amount (g)
Meal 1	
Scrambled egg	150
Oats	40 (dry)
Meal 2	
Chicken breast	170
Broccoli	150
White rice	40 (dry)
Meal 3	
Whey protein	50
Meal 4	
Chicken breast	170
White rice	40 (dry)
Sweet potato	150
Meal 5	
Chicken breast	170
White rice	40 (dry)
Sweet potato	150
Meal 6	
Whey protein	25
Apple	100
Totals	
Energy (kcal)	2128
Carbohydrate (g)	212
Fat (g)	28
Protein (g)	257

preparation for UKBFF; (b) improve resting and exercise fat oxidation; (c) preserve muscular function and strength; (d) maintain a positive mood-state during the 14-week lead in to competition.

Metabolic assessment
Resting Metabolic Rate Assessment (RMR) was determined on six occasions (Familiarization, Baseline, Week 3, Week 8, Week 10 and Week 13) and a graded Exercise Test was completed on three occasions (Familiarization, Baseline and Week 13) to determine rates of fat oxidation during exercise and cardiorespiratory fitness ($\dot{V}O_{2max}$). For all assessments the Athlete reported to the laboratory at 07:00 h following an overnight fast from 10 pm the evening before and having abstained from strenuous physical activity, alcohol and caffeine consumption in the 24 h preceding each visit. The Athlete was asked not to perform any physical activity on the morning of testing, such as brisk walking or cycling to the laboratory, and to consume 500 ml water upon waking to encourage hydration. The

Athlete was fitted with a facemask for both the RMR and Exercise Testing (Combitox, Drager, Jaeger, Nussdorf Traunstein, Germany) and breath-by-breath measurements of oxygen consumption ($\dot{V}O_2$) and carbon dioxide production ($\dot{V}CO_2$) were measured continuously using an online gas analysis system (Oxycon Pro, Jaeger, Wuerzberg, Germany). The gas analyzer was calibrated immediately prior to testing with a known gas concentration (5% CO_2; 16% O_2; 79% N_2 [BOC Gases, Surrey, UK]) and a three-liter calibration syringe (Hans Rudolf, USA) was used to calibrate the volume transducer. Environmental conditions during testing were: humidity $51 \pm 6\%$; temperature $20 \pm 1°C$.

For the RMR Assessment the Athlete was required to lie still on a bed in the supine position for 30 minutes in a dimly lit room. There was no visual or auditory stimulation throughout this period. The Exercise Test was completed ~15 minutes after the RMR assessment. This was based on the protocol described previously by Achten and colleagues [13] with the starting speed and inclination of the treadmill (HP Cosmos, Jaeger, Nussdorf Traunstein, Germany) set at 3.5 km/h and 1%, respectively. The treadmill speed was increased by 1 km/h every three minutes until the respiratory exchange ratio (RER) reached 1.00. At this point the treadmill gradient was increased by 1% every minute until volitional exhaustion. Heart rate was measured continuously throughout testing using a heart rate monitor (Polar FT-1, Finland) and was recorded during the final 30 seconds of each exercise stage.

Calculations

Resting energy expenditure and fat oxidation were calculated during a stable measurement period i.e., a deviation in $\dot{V}O_2$ of <10% of the average $\dot{V}O_2$ between minutes 20–30 (mean ± SD recording period was 5 ± 2 minutes) using the equations of Frayn [14] and a protein correction factor of 0.11 mg/kg/min, as used previously [15,16]. During the Exercise Test $\dot{V}O_2$ and $\dot{V}CO_2$ were averaged over the last minute of each submaximal exercise stage and fat and carbohydrate oxidation were calculated according to the equations of Frayn [14], with the assumption that the urinary nitrogen excretion rate was negligible. $\dot{V}O_2$ was considered as maximal when two of the following three criteria were met; an RER >1.1, heart rate within 10 beats of predicted maximum (calculated as 220-age [17]), or an increase of <2 ml/kg/min in $\dot{V}O_2$ with a further increase in workload. $\dot{V}O_{2max}$ was calculated as the highest rolling 60 second average $\dot{V}O_2$. The results of the Exercise Test were used to create a curve of fat oxidation rate against exercise intensity, expressed as% $\dot{V}O_{2max}$. The maximal rate of fat oxidation during exercise (MFO) was determined by visual inspection i.e., by judging the peak of the curve and its corresponding rate of fat oxidation.

Fat$_{max}$ was defined as the exercise intensity (%$\dot{V}O_{2max}$) that corresponded to MFO, as described previously [18].

Diet and activity recordings

At Baseline, the Athlete was provided with two sets of digital weighing scales (Electronic Kitchen Scale SF 400 and Swees Digital Pocket Weighing Scales); blank four-day diet log and physical activity diaries; and detailed instructions to enable the completion of these at week 3, 6, 10 and 12. The Athlete was instructed to record all consumed food and drink items accurately and in as much detail as possible. The activity diary was based on Bouchard et al. [19] and required the Athlete to record level-of-activity every 15 minutes, using a code from a 12-point scale (provided). The diary was completed over a 24-hour period on each of the four days. The scale ranged from 'sleeping' to 'vigorous exercise' and provided examples of activities at each point to assist the Athlete. To ensure the highest possible level of accuracy in estimations of energy expenditure, he was encouraged to make notes on any sport or exercise performed during the four days sampled. Diet logs were analyzed using Nutritics dietary analysis software (Nutritics v3.06, Ireland).

Daily energy expenditure was estimated using the factorial approach [20]. Here, each of the 12 codes, which had a corresponding metabolic equivalent (MET) value, was assigned a Physical Activity Level (PAL) [21] and a daily PAL was determined by multiplying each of the 12 codes by the total amount of time spent at the activity level. Where he had made notes on a specific sport and exercise activity undertaken during the 4 days, the Compendium of Physical Activities [22] was used to calculate the specific PAL value. Daily energy expenditure was then estimated by multiplying the daily PAL value by the age and sex specific resting metabolic rate (RMR; kcal/d) using height, weight and the World Health Organization (WHO) equation [23]:

$$\text{Energy Expenditure(kcal/d; men} < 30 \text{ years)}$$
$$: \text{Daily PAL value} * RMR(15.4 * \text{body mass[kg]})$$
$$-(27.0 * \text{height[m]}) + 717)$$

Anthropometric assessment

Baseline assessments are shown in Table 2. Height (Stadiometer, Seca, UK), mass (Seca, UK) and body composition using skin-folds and girths (measured by an International Standards for Anthropometric Assessment (ISAK) Certified Anthropometrist) were assessed at Baseline and at Weeks 3, 5, 7, 10, 12, 13 and 14 of the intervention at a standardized time of 07:00 h. Body fat percentage, fat-free mass (FFM) and fat mass (FM) were calculated using updated sex and race/ethnicity specific equations [24]. All skinfold measurements followed the

Table 2 Anthropometric and physiological characteristics at baseline

Characteristic	Value
Age (y)	21
Height (cm)	178.5
Body mass (kg)	86.0
BMI (kg/m^2)	27
Body fat (%)	14
Fat mass (kg)	11.7
Fat-free mass (kg)	74.3
Maximal oxygen uptake (ml/kg/min)	49.0
Maximal rate of fat oxidation (g/min)	0.24
Fatmax (%$\dot{V}O_{2max}$)	21
Resting metabolic rate (kcal/d)	1993

ISAK i.e., measurements were taken on the right hand side of the body in duplicate or in triplicate if the total error of measurement of the first and second measurement was >5%, following which a mean value was obtained.

Additional assessments

The Brunel Mood Scale (BRUMS) [25] was completed at Baseline and at Week 13. Peak torque of the hamstring (flexors) and quadriceps (extensors) of the dominant leg were determined at Baseline and Week 14 at 08:00 h following 24 hours of rest and following meal 1. This was performed on a separate day from RMR and Exercise Testing. A HUMAC NORM Isokinetic Dynamometer (Computer Sports Medicine, Inc. [CSMI], USA) was set up in the seated position, with the adjustments identical on both testing occasions. The Athlete completed three sets of five repetitions of a concentric flexion and concentric extension at 60°/second, with 60 seconds of rest between sets. After 90 seconds of recovery the Athlete completed three eccentric contraction sets of five repetitions flexion and extension at 60°/second, with 60 seconds recovery between sets. For the concentric and eccentric contractions the initial five repetitions of each set were a warm-up, the second set was a familiarization and the final set was performed to maximal exertion. Peak torque values were recorded using the CSMI computer. Prior to isokinetic testing the weight of the limb was weighed to correct for gravity using HUMAC software (CSMI, USA).

The intervention

To encourage a reduction in fat mass, we chose to obtain an energy deficit through a combination of decreased energy intake and increased energy expenditure. Adjustments in nutritional intake and the quantity of exercise performed during the intervention were made to accommodate the target energy deficit, which was set according the rate of body composition change over the period of study.

Diet

Over the 14-week period of study the Athlete followed a set-meal plan comprising of two menus. Menus 1 and 2 were followed on Conditioning and Rest days, respectively and were designed by the authors who are all certified sports nutritionists (CISSN). Table 3 shows example foods and drinks offered by the two menus and Figure 1 shows energy and macronutrient provision over the 14-week period. A set meal plan was provided for two reasons: 1) it allowed the authors to carefully control energy and macronutrient intake; 2) the Athlete favoured this approach, as opposed to receiving macronutrient and calorie targets, as used in other similar case studies [6,11]. Absolute (relative) carbohydrate, fat, and protein intake over the 14 weeks was 100 ± 56 g/d (20 ± 3% energy), 79 ± 17 g/d (37 ± 4% energy) and 212 ± 13 g/d (45 ± 8% energy), respectively. Carbohydrate recommendations focused on low or medium glycemic index (GI) sources to improve satiety [26] and enhance lipolysis [27]. To enhance muscle glycogen restoration and for purposes of improving meal enjoyment, high GI carbohydrates were also recommended [28]. To improve satiety [26] and help retain FFM and augment fat loss whilst in an energy deficit [29] the Athlete was advised to consume high biological value protein such as chicken and eggs and distribute protein intake throughout the day. This 'pulsing' strategy has been found to stimulate daily muscle protein synthesis more effectively than skewing protein intake toward the evening meal [30]. Carbohydrate intake underwent the greatest manipulation over the 14-week period to accommodate the target energy intake (Figure 1). Reducing carbohydrate intake has been suggested as a viable strategy to allow protein intake to remain high in the face of an energy deficit [31]. Fluid suggestions were water, sugar-free cordial and flavored tea that were to be consumed *ad libitum* throughout the day.

Conditioning

The 14-week conditioning programme is presented in Table 4. Briefly; the Athlete completed four resistance-training sessions (RT) during each week of the intervention; targeting each major muscle group on two occasions per week. Each RT consisted of 6–8 exercises performed for 8–10 repetitions and 4–5 sets [32]. A combination of high intensity interval training (HIIT) and low-intensity steady-state (LISS) exercise, that was performed in the overnight fasted state (07.00-08.00 h), was completed with the aim being to up-regulate oxidative enzyme adaptations to enhance fat utilization [33] and help preserve FFM whilst on a carbohydrate restricted diet [34]. Whilst two recent studies [35,36] show that fasted-state training, compared with fed-state training, does not result in greater losses in fat mass when daily caloric deficit is similar, we prescribed fasted-state training based on the Athletes

Table 3 Menus provided on rest and training days during weeks 1–5

Menu 1: Training day		Menu 2: Rest day	
Item/description	Amount (g)	Item/description	Amount (g)
Meal 1		**Meal 1**	
Venison burger	150	Poached egg	150
Poached egg	150	Oats	50 (dry)
Spinach	50	Whey protein powder	30
Meal 2		**Meal 2**	
Whey protein powder	60	Tuna (tinned)	130
Creatine	5	Asparagus	100
Brazil nuts	20	Macadamia nuts	30
Meal 3		**Meal 3**	
Mackerel	150	Chicken breast	150
Brown rice	100	Sweet potato	150
Salad leaves	50	Almonds	20
Avocado	50		
Apple cider vinegar	12		
Meal 4		**Meal 4**	
Turkey breast	155	Salmon fillet	140
White Basmati rice	100 (dry)	White Basmati rice	50
Mushrooms	100	Broccoli	100
Coconut oil	12	**Snack**	
Snack		Chocolate flavored mousse	50
Full-fat cottage cheese	225	Coconut Oil	12
Totals		**Totals**	
Energy (kcal/d)	2413	Energy (kcal/d)	2246
Carbohydrate (g)	137	Carbohydrate (g)	143
Fat (g)	119	Fat (g)	96
Protein (g)	207	Protein (g)	212

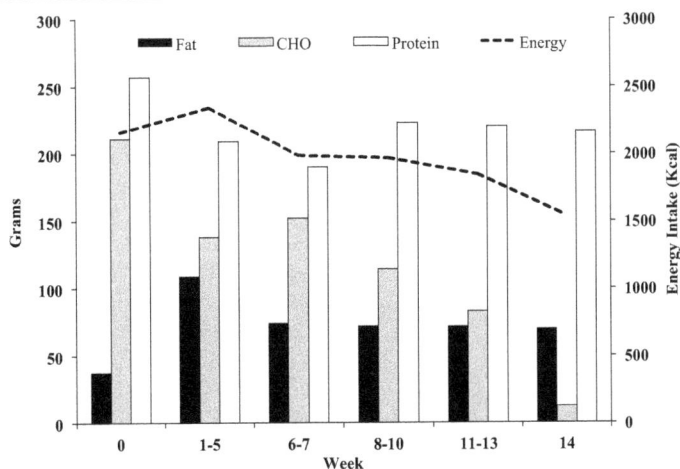

Figure 1 Energy (kcal) and macronutrient (g) intake over the 14-week period of study.

Table 4 Training program undertaken throughout the intervention period

Day (time)	Weeks 1-7	Weeks 8-10	Weeks 11-14
Monday (AM)	Rest	Sprints	Sprints
		10×10–15 sec	10×10–15 sec
Monday (PM)	RT	RT	RT
	Chest and back	Chest and back	Chest and back
Tuesday (AM)	Rest	Rest	Incline walk on treadmill
			40 minutes
Tuesday (PM)	RT	RT	RT
	Legs	Legs	Legs
Wednesday (AM)	Rest	Incline treadmill walk	Incline treadmill walk
		40 minutes	40 minutes
Wednesday (PM)	Rest	Rest	RT
			Shoulders and Arms
Thursday (AM)	Rest	Rest	Incline treadmill walk
			40 minutes
Thursday (PM)	RT	RT	RT
	Shoulders and arms	Shoulders and arms	Shoulders and arms
Friday (AM)	Rest	Incline treadmill walk	Incline treadmill walk
		40 minutes	40 minutes
Friday (PM)	Circuit training	RT	RT
	30 minutes	Legs	Legs
Saturday (AM)	Rest	Rest	Incline treadmill walk
			40 minutes
Saturday (PM)	Rest	Rest	Rest
Sunday (AM)	Rest	Rest	Rest
Sunday (PM)	Rest	Rest	Rest

RT = Resistance Training (the mean duration of each session was 30 minutes).

preference i.e. (i) he found it difficult to perform HIIT and LISS training sessions having eaten in close-proximity (time-wise) to training and (ii) he wanted to consume his morning calories after training, as this gave him something to look forward to. The authors believe these are important practical considerations when prescribing fasted- or fed-state training to athletes.

The number of HIIT and LISS training sessions performed each week was adjusted according to the target energy deficit. In the six weeks prior to competition, "posing practice" was implemented (2–4 times per week), which involved holding isometric contraction of the major muscle groups for 30–60 seconds.

Provision of supplements

Whey protein (Optimum Nutrition, Glanbia Plc, Ireland) and one serving of a high protein (with a high whey and casein content), low carbohydrate snack in the late evening (Muscle Mousse, Genetic Supplements, Co. Durham, UK) was provided. Creatine monohydrate (Optimum

Nutrition, Glanbia Plc, Ireland) was given as 20 g per day for the first five days of the intervention, followed by 5 g per day for 93 days [37].

Evaluation of the intervention and commentary

Recorded energy intake, predicted energy expenditure and energy balance (Figure 2), and anthropometric changes (Figure 3) over the 14-week period are shown. There was a reduction in RMR over the course of the preparation period, which is consistent with previous reports that have shown a decline in RMR during periods of caloric restriction [6,38,39] (Figure 4).

Over the course of the 14-weeks total body mass loss was 11.7 kg's. This equated to an average weight loss of 0.98%/week, which is in accordance with the recommended weekly rate of 0.5-1.0% [40]. The energy deficit was 882 ± 433 kcal/d and this led to a reduction of 6.7 kg's (or 6.8% body fat or 33 mm using sum of 8 skinfolds) and 5.0 kg's, in fat mass and FFM, respectively. It is not uncommon for individuals to lose FFM whilst in a

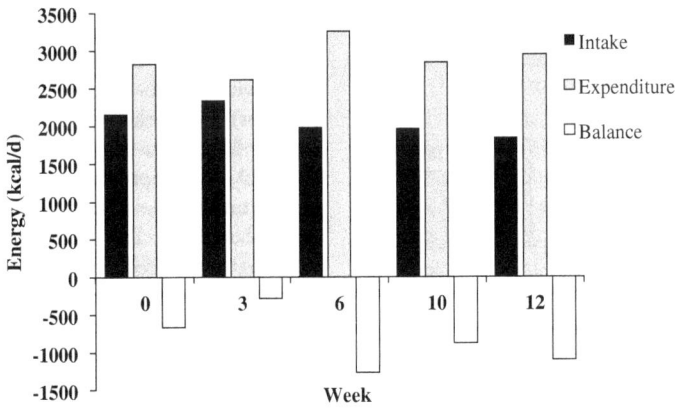

Figure 2 Recorded energy intake and predicted energy expenditure and energy balance.

negative energy balance [8,9]. Resistance training, HIIT, creatine monohydrate supplementation, and high-protein diets have all been reported to promote FFM accretion and prevent FFM loss during energy restriction (for review, see Churchward-Venne, Murphy, Longland, & Phillips [41]), however these strategies were not sufficient to prevent the decline observed in our study.

One potential reason why the Athlete lost FFM in spite of the abovementioned approaches could be because of the size of the energy deficit was larger than that applied by others. For example, one case study observed an increase (albeit only slight, 0.45 kg) in FFM during a period of less severe caloric restriction (mean ± SD energy deficit: −343 ± 156 kcal/d) [10]. A weight loss strategy that is more gradual might have induced a lesser reduction in FFM. For instance, the athlete studied in Kistler et al. [11] dieted at a rate of ~0.7% bodyweight per week and had a higher percentage of FFM loss (32% of total body mass loss) than Rossow et al. (21% of total body

mass loss) [6] where the athlete dieted at a rate of ~0.5% bodyweight per week. The Athlete in this study dieted at a rate of ~1.0% bodyweight per week and had the highest percentage of FFM loss (43% of total body mass loss). This suggests that the rate of weight loss might influence the percentage of FFM loss, even within the 0.5-1.0% bodyweight per week range as previously recommended [40]. Indeed, there is greater potential for loss of FFM as adipose tissue declines. Accordingly, an additional strategy to offset reductions in FFM whilst in energy deficit might be to reduce the size of the energy deficit as competition nears [40]. This strategy would require that the athlete allows sufficient time to reach a desirable level of body fat, such that when competition nears they do not need to place themselves in a large energy deficit to reduce body fat. Furthermore, the Athlete consumed (mean ± SD) 37 ± 4% energy from fat and 20 ± 3% energy from carbohydrate over the duration of the intervention. This is less carbohydrate and more fat (expressed as% energy) than was

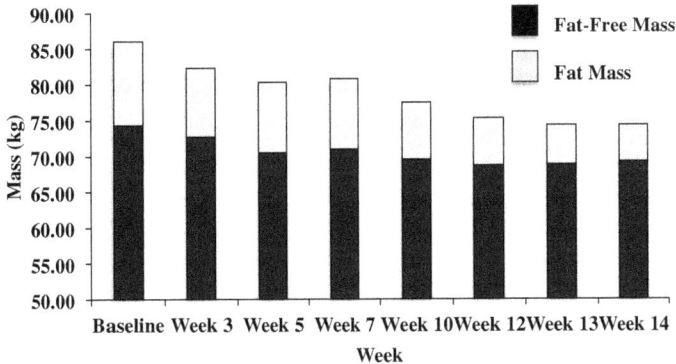

Figure 3 Anthropometrical changes over the 14-week period of study.

improving physiological parameters of health, maintaining a favourable mood state and positively influencing strength. Here, the Athlete consumed four meals and one snack on each day of preparation. The majority of the Athlete's nutrition came from whole foods and there was minimal reliance on dietary supplements, with the exception of those that have only strong scientific evidence in support of their ergogenic effects. Taken collectively, and in contrast to popular myth, our case study shows that it is not necessary to skip meals, neglect specific macronutrient groups, dehydrate or consume a large variety of supplements to adequately prepare for bodybuilding competition. Nevertheless, we acknowledge that 43% of the total body mass lost was FFM, which is not a favourable response. Accordingly, we propose a variety of practical strategies to assist in counteracting this. Whilst the authors appreciate that a limitation of the present study is its sample size of 1, this approach enabled us to accurately document a variety of measures that may not have been possible to acquire using a randomized control trial in a laboratory. As such, we offer this case study as a real-world applied example for other male bodybuilding competitors and coaches seeking to deploy nutrition and training strategies. Finally, the Athlete placed 7th out of 19 competitors, which he and the support team acknowledged as a successful performance given that this was his first time competing as a physique competitor.

Consent

Written informed consent was obtained from the patient for publication of this Case report and any accompanying images. A copy of the written consent is available for review by the Editor-in-Chief of this journal.

Competing interests

The authors declare that they have no competing interests.

Author's contributions

Conception of design and research: SLR, ALM, GG, LB. Implementation of exercise trials and sample collection: ALM. Data analysis: SLR, ALM. Interpretation of results: SLR, ALM, ASR, LB. Drafted manuscript: SLR, ALM. Edited and revised the manuscript: SLR, ALM, GG, ASR, LB. Approved the final version of the manuscript: SLR, ALM, GG, ASR, LB.

Acknowledgements

The authors would like to acknowledge Colin Hill and Mark Corbett (Institute of Sport & Exercise Science, University of Worcester, UK) for assistance during data collection and Dr David Hughes (University California Davis, USA) for his intellectual critique during manuscript preparation.

Author details

[1]Guru Performance LTD, 58 South Molton St, London W1K 5SL, UK. [2]Institute of Sport & Exercise Science, University of Worcester, Henwick Grove, Worcester WR2 6AJ, UK. [3]Ultimate City Fitness, 1-3 Cobb Street, London E1 7LB, UK. [4]Department of Exercise and Sport Science, University of North Carolina Chapel Hill, Office: 303A Woolen, 209 Fetzer Hall, Chapel Hill, NC, USA.

References

1. Andersen RE, Barlett SJ, Morgan GD, Brownell KD. Weight loss, psychological, and nutritional patterns in competitive male body builders. Int J Eat Disord. 1994;18:49–57.
2. Villareal DT, Fontana L, Weiss EP, Racette SB, Steger-May K, Schechtman KB, et al. Bone mineral density response to caloric restriction–induced weight loss or exercise-induced weight loss. A Randomized controlled trial. Arch Intern Med. 2006;166:2502–10.
3. Camps S, Verhoef S, Westerterp K. Weight loss, weight maintenance, and adaptive thermogenesis. Am J Clin Nutr. 2013;97:990–4.
4. Ebert TR, Martin DT, Bullock N, Mujika I, Quod MJ, Farthing LA, et al. Influence of hydration status on thermoregulation and cycling hill climbing. Med Sci Sports Exerc. 2007;39:323–9.
5. Maetsu J, Eliakim A, Jurimae J, Valter I, Jurimae T. Anabolic and catabolic hormones and energy balance of the male bodybuilders during the preparation for competition. J Strength Cond Res. 2010;24:1074–81.
6. Rossow LM, Fukuda DH, Fahs CA, Loenneke JP, Stout JR. Natural bodybuilding competition preparation and recovery: a 12-month case study. Int J Sports Physiol Perform. 2013;8:582–92.
7. Bamman MM, Hunter GR, Newton LE, Roney RK, Khaled MA. Changes in body composition, diet, and strength of bodybuilders during the 12 weeks prior to competition. J Sports Med Phys Fitness. 1993;33:383–91.
8. Morton JP, Robertson C, Sutton L, MacLaren DPM. Making the weight: a case study from professional boxing. Int J Sport Nutr Exerc Metab. 2010;20:80–5.
9. Wilson G, Chester N, Eubank M, Crighton B, Drust B, Morton JP, et al. An alternative dietary strategy to make weight while improving mood, decreasing body fat, and not dehydrating: a case study of a professional jockey. Int J Sports Nutr Exerc Metab. 2012;22:225–31.
10. Robinson SL, Morton JP, Close GL, Flower D, Bannock L. Nutrition intervention for an international-standard female football player. JACSSES. 2014;1:17–28.
11. Kistler BM, Fitschen PJ, Ranadive SM, Fernhall B, Wilund KR. Case study: natural bodybuilding contest preparation. IJSNEM. 2014;24:694–700.
12. Guardia LD, Cavallaro M, Cena H. The risks of self-made diets: the case of an amateur bodybuilder. JISSN. 2015;12:16.
13. Achten J, Venables MC, Jeukendrup AE. Fat oxidation rates are higher during running compared with cycling over a wide range of intensities. Metabolism. 2003;52:747–52.
14. Frayn KN. Calculation of substrate oxidation rates in vivo from gaseous exchange. J Appl Physiol. 1983;55:628–34.
15. Flatt JP, Ravussin E, Acheson KJ, Jequier E. Effects of dietary fat on postprandial substrate oxidation and on carbohydrate and fat balances. J Clin Invest. 1985;76:1019–24.
16. Hall LML, Moran CN, Milne GR, Wilson J, MacFarlane NG, Forouhi NG, et al. Fat oxidation, fitness and skeletal muscle expression of oxidative/lipid metabolism genes in South Asians: implications for insulin resistance? PLoS One. 2010;5:e14197.
17. Fox SMI, Naughton JP, Haskell WL. Physical activity and the prevention of coronary heart disease. Ann Clin Res. 1971;3:404–32.
18. Achten J, Gleeson M, Jeukendrup AE. Determination of the exercise intensity that elicits maximal fat oxidation. Med Sci Sports Exerc. 2002;34:92–7.
19. Bouchard C, Tremblay A, Leblanc C, Lortie G, Savard R, Theriault G. A method to assess energy expenditure in children and adults. Am J Clin Nutr. 1983;37:461–7.
20. Manore M, Meyer NL, Thompson J. Sport nutrition for health and performance. 2nd ed. Champaign, IL: Human Kinetics; 2009.
21. Subcommittee on the Tenth Edition of the Recommended Dietary Allowances, Food and Nutrition Board, Commission on Life Sciences, National Research Council. Recommended dietary allowances. 10th ed. Washington DC, USA: The National Academies Press; 1989.
22. Ainsworth BE, Haskell WL, Whitt MC, Irwin ML, Swartz AM, Strath SJ, et al. Compendium of physical activities: A second update of codes and MET values. Med Sci Sports Exerc. 2011;43:1575–81.
23. Food and Agricultural Organization, World Health Organization, United Nations University. Energy and protein requirements. Report of a joint FAO/

WHO/UNU expert consultation, World Health Organization Technical Report Series. Geneva, Switzerland: WHO; 1985. p. 724.

24. Davidson LE, Wang J, Thornton JC, Kaleem Z, Silva-Palacios F, Pierson RN, et al. Predicting fat percent by skinfolds in racial groups: Durnin and Womersley revisited. Med Sci Sports Exerc. 2011;43:542–9.

25. Terry PC, Lane AM, Lane HJ, Keohane L. Development and validation of a mood measure for adolescents. J Sports Sci. 1999;17:861–72.

26. Halton TL, Hu FB. The effects of high protein diets on thermogenesis, satiety and weight loss: a critical review. J Am Coll Nutr. 2004;23:373–85.

27. Wee SL, Williams C, Tsintzas K, Boobis L. Ingestion of a high-glycemic index meal increases muscle glycogen storage at rest but augments its utilization during subsequent exercise. J Appl Physiol. 2005;99:707–14.

28. Burke LM, Collier GR, Hargreaves M. Muscle glycogen storage after prolonged exercise: effect of the glycemic index of carbohydrate feedings. J Appl Physiol. 1993;75:1019–23.

29. Mettler S, Mitchell N, Tipton KD. Increased protein intake reduces lean body mass loss during weight loss in athletes. Med Sci Sports Exerc. 2010;42:326–37.

30. Areta JL, Burke LM, Ross ML, Camera DM, West DW, Broad EM, et al. Timing and distribution of protein ingestion during prolonged recovery from resistance exercise alters myofibrillar protein synthesis. J Physiol. 2013;591:2319–31.

31. Phillips SM, Van Loon LJC. Dietary protein for athletes: from requirements to optimum adaptation. J Sports Sci. 2011;29:29–38.

32. Helms ER, Fitschen PJ, Aragon AA, Schoenfeld BJ CJ. Recommendations for natural bodybuilding contest preparation: resistance and cardiovascular training. J Sports Med Phys Fitness. 2015;55:164–78.

33. Morton JP, Croft L, Bartlett JD, MacLaren DPM, Reilly T, Evans L, et al. Reduced carbohydrate availability does not modulate training-induced heat shock protein adaptations but does up-regulate oxidative enzyme activity in human skeletal muscle. J Appl Physiol. 2009;106:1513–21.

34. Sartor F, de Morree HM, Matschke V, Marcora SM, Milousis A, Thom JM, et al. High-intensity exercise and carbohydrate-reduced energy-restricted diet in obese individuals. Eur J Appl Physiol. 2010;110:893–903.

35. Schoenfeld BJ, Aragon AA, Wilborn CD, Krieger J, Sonmez GT. Body composition changes associated with fasted versus non-fasted aerobic exercise. JISSN. 2014;11:54.

36. Gillen GB, Percival ME, Ludzki A, Tarnopolsky MA, Gibala MJ. Interval training in the fed or fasted state improves body composition and muscle oxidative capacity in overweight women. Obesity. 2013;21:2249–55.

37. Harris RC, Söderlund K, Hultman E. Elevation of creatine in resting and exercised muscle of normal subjects by creatine supplementation. Clin Sci. 1992;83:367–74.

38. Ravussin E, Burnand B, Schutz Y, Jequier E. Energy expenditure before and during energy restriction in obese patients. Am J Clin Nutr. 1985;41:753–9.

39. Leibel RL, Rosenbaum M, Hirsch J. Changes in energy expenditure resulting from altered body weight. N Engl J Med. 1995;332:621–8.

40. Helms ER, Aragon A, Fitschen PJ. Evidence-based recommendations for natural bodybuilding contest preparation: nutrition and supplementation. JISSN. 2014;11:20.

41. Churchward-Venne TA, Murphy CH, Longland TM, Phillips SM. Role of protein and amino acids in promoting lean mass accretion with resistance exercise and attenuating lean mass loss during energy deficit in humans. Amino Acids. 2013;45:231–40.

42. Garthe I, Raastad T, Refsnes PE, Koivisto A, Sundgot-Borgen J. Effect of two different weight-loss rates on body composition and strength and power-related performance in elite athletes. Int J Sport Nutr Exerc Metab. 2011;21:97–104.

43. Murphy CH, Hector AJ, Phillips SM. Considerations for protein intake in managing weight loss in athletes. Eur J Sports Sci. 2014;1:21–8.

44. Wilson JM, Marin PJ, Rhea MR, Wilson SM, Loenneke JP, Anderson JC. Concurrent training: a meta-analysis examining interference of aerobic and resistance exercise. J Strength Cond Research. 2012;26:2293–307.

45. Rosenkilde M, Nordby P, Nielsen LB, Stallknecht BM, Helge JW. Fat oxidation at rest predicts peak fat oxidation during exercise and metabolic phenotype in overweight men. Int J Obesity. 2010;34:871–7.

46. Isacco L, Thivel D, Duclos M, Aucouturier J, Boisseau N. Effects of adipose tissue distribution on maximum lipid oxidation rate during exercise in normal weight-women. Diabetes Metab. 2014;40:215–9.

47. Kelley DE, Simoneau JA. Impaired free fatty acid utilization by skeletal muscle in non-insulin-dependent diabetes mellitus. J Clin Invest. 1994;94:2349–56.

48. Zurlo F, Lillioja S, Puente EA, Nyomba BL, Raz I, Saad MF, et al. Low ratio of fat to carbohydrate metabolism as predictor of weight gain: study of 24-h RQ. Am J Physiol Endocrinol Metab. 1990;259:650–7.

49. Ellis AC, Hyatt TC, Gower BA, Hunter GR. Respiratory quotient predicts fat mass gain in premenopausal women. Obesity. 2010;18:2255–9.

50. Robinson SL, Hattersley J, Frost GS, Chambers ES, Wallis GA. Maximal fat oxidation during exercise is positively associated with 24-hour fat oxidation and insulin sensitivity in young, healthy men. J Appl Physiol (in press)

51. Almeras N, Lavallee N, Despres JP, Bouchard C, Tremblay A. Exercise and energy intake: effect of substrate oxidation. Physiol Behav. 1995;57:995–1000.

52. Eckel RH, Hernandez TL, Bell ML, Weil KM, Shepard TY, Grunwald GK, et al. Carbohydrate balance predicts weight and fat gain in adults. Am J Clin Nutr. 2006;83:803–8.

53. Pannacciulli N, Salbe AD, Ortega E, Venti CA, Bogardus C, Krakoff J. The 24-h carbohydrate oxidation rate in a human respiratory chamber predicts ad libitum food intake. Am J Clin Nutr. 2007;86:625–32.

54. Smith CF, Williamson DA, Bray GA, Ryan DH. Flexible vs. rigid dieting strategies: relationship with adverse behavioral outcomes. Appetite. 1999;32:295–305.

55. Steen SN. Precontest strategies of a male bodybuilder. Int J Sport Nutr. 1991;1:69–78.

## 16

Pea proteins oral supplementation promotes muscle thickness gains during resistance training: a double-blind, randomized, Placebo-controlled clinical trial vs. Whey protein

Nicolas Babault[1,2,6]*, Christos Païzis[1,2], Gaëlle Deley[1,2], Laetitia Guérin-Deremaux[3], Marie-Hélène Saniez[3], Catherine Lefranc-Millot[3] and François A Allaert[4,5]

Abstract

Background: The effects of protein supplementation on muscle thickness and strength seem largely dependent on its composition. The current study aimed at comparing the impact of an oral supplementation with vegetable Pea protein (NUTRALYS®) vs. Whey protein and Placebo on biceps brachii muscle thickness and strength after a 12-week resistance training program.

Methods: One hundred and sixty one males, aged 18 to 35 years were enrolled in the study and underwent 12 weeks of resistance training on upper limb muscles. According to randomization, they were included in the Pea protein (n = 53), Whey protein (n = 54) or Placebo (n = 54) group. All had to take 25 g of the proteins or placebo twice a day during the 12-week training period. Tests were performed on biceps muscles at inclusion (D0), mid (D42) and post training (D84). Muscle thickness was evaluated using ultrasonography, and strength was measured on an isokinetic dynamometer.

Results: Results showed a significant time effect for biceps brachii muscle thickness ($P < 0.0001$). Thickness increased from 24.9 ± 3.8 mm to 26.9 ± 4.1 mm and 27.3 ± 4.4 mm at D0, D42 and D84, respectively, with only a trend toward significant differences between groups ($P = 0.09$). Performing a sensitivity study on the weakest participants (with regards to strength at inclusion), thickness increases were significantly different between groups ($+20.2 \pm 12.3\%$, $+15.6 \pm 13.5\%$ and $+8.6 \pm 7.3\%$ for Pea, Whey and Placebo, respectively; $P < 0.05$). Increases in thickness were significantly greater in the Pea group as compared to Placebo whereas there was no difference between Whey and the two other conditions. Muscle strength also increased with time with no statistical difference between groups.

Conclusions: In addition to an appropriate training, the supplementation with pea protein promoted a greater increase of muscle thickness as compared to Placebo and especially for people starting or returning to a muscular strengthening. Since no difference was obtained between the two protein groups, vegetable pea proteins could be used as an alternative to Whey-based dietary products.

Trial registration: The present trial has been registered at ClinicalTrials.gov (NCT02128516).

Keywords: Muscle strength, Biceps brachii, Muscle thickness, Feeding, Hypertrophy, Nutralys

* Correspondence: nicolas.babault@u-bourgogne.fr
[1]National Institute for Health and Medical Research, (INSERM), unit 1093, Cognition, Action and Sensorimotor Plasticity, Dijon, France
[2]Centre for Performance Expertise, UFR STAPS, Dijon, France
Full list of author information is available at the end of the article

Background

Amino acids accumulate in the sarcoplasm in the hours following exercise, especially of weight-training type [1]. Such accumulation undoubtedly creates favorable conditions to protein synthesis. Indeed, increased protein synthesis (i.e., muscle hypertrophy) is observed immediately after resistance exercises [2-4] as a result of a positive protein net balance; the difference between muscle fiber catabolism and anabolism. Under these conditions, any nutritional modification that could increase protein accretion in the muscle would maximize resistance training effects by enhancing muscle anabolism. In particular, it has now been well demonstrated that protein consumption after exercise shifts the balance in favor of muscle protein synthesis [5]. Taken altogether, these data clearly demonstrate the great interest of an association between amino acids supplementation and resistance training.

Composition of supplements may play a key role in influencing net protein balance since previous studies have revealed that only essential amino acids (EAA) could stimulate muscle protein synthesis [6]. Furthermore, protein type, and not simply its amino acid composition, can differentially modulate protein synthesis depending on digestion kinetics. For example, in a recent review [1], it was speculated that whey, with high leucine content and rapid digestion kinetic [7], may favor muscle protein synthesis while casein, with a slower digestion kinetic [7], may improve muscle net balance by inhibiting muscle protein breakdown. In addition to increases in muscle mass, functional adaptations, such as strength or fatigue, are also obtained after EAA supplementation [8,9]. For example, Vieillevoye et al. [10] found increases in lower body strength with EAA supplementation while no modification was obtained with placebo.

Different supplements' compositions could easily be obtained with different nutrients. For example, NUTRALYS® is a protein isolate obtained from pea (*Pisum sativum*) containing 85% of proteins and particularly rich in essential branched-chain amino acids (BCAA; leucine, isoleucine and valine) known to play an important role in muscle protein synthesis [11]. Studies have shown that an increased plasma concentration in leucine favors muscle protein synthesis and that its action on muscle mass is potentiated by the presence of other amino acids such as those contained in NUTRALYS® pea protein [12]. Therefore, pea protein could contribute to muscle protein synthesis when taken immediately after an effort. Considered globally, these arguments suggest that pea proteins ingestion might maximize muscle mass gains during resistance training. The aim of the present study was therefore to compare the effects of pea proteins against a reference protein (namely whey proteins which has previously been shown beneficial for muscle mass after resistance training [13,14]) and against placebo. It was hypothesized that pea proteins would be as efficient as the reference protein to increase both muscle thickness and strength.

Methods

Participants – ethics statement

A total of 161 male participants were recruited for the study. All had moderate physical activities (2–6 hours per week). None were engaged in any physical activity aimed at increasing muscle strength and mass for the six months before the experiment. All were healthy and free of injury during the three months preceding the study. The study excluded subjects who had asthma with potentially steroids treatment, consumption of high-protein diet, steroids treatment, current consumption of drugs or during the previous month, consumption of dietary supplement, sports drink, special dietary food or functional food, of any kind, liable or presented as liable to enhance physical performances and especially to increase muscle mass. Moreover, subjects with known hypersensitivity to any of the constituents of the studied products were excluded. Throughout the study, subjects maintained their usual training routine and diet. All gave their written consent after being carefully informed about the experimental protocol. The study was conducted in accordance with the Helsinki Declaration without any deviation from the protocol approved by the East I ethics committee (East I committee, France, number: 2011–47, 9 November 2011). The authors confirm that all ongoing and related trials for this intervention are registered before at the French agency for the safety of health products (AFSSAPS number: 2011-A01211-40) and at ClinicalTrials.gov (NCT02128516).

After inclusion, participants were randomly divided into three experimental groups: Pea (n = 53), Whey (n = 54), and Placebo (n = 54). Table 1 sets out their characteristics. Product randomization was balanced by block sizes of 10. The randomization code was not made available to anyone

Table 1 Subjects characteristic at inclusion

	Pea	Whey	Placebo	Anova (P)
Age (years)	22.0 ± 3.5	22.1 ± 3.6	21.7 ± 3.9	0.860
BMI (kg/m^2)	23.1 ± 2.6	23.0 ± 3.0	22.9 ± 2.5	0.946
Biceps brachii thickness (mm)	25.0 ± 3.6	24.3 ± 3.8	25.4 ± 3.8	0.281
Mean circ. at rest (cm)	32.3 ± 2.5	32.0 ± 3.2	32.2 ± 2.5	0.829
Mean circ. contracted (cm)	33.3 ± 2.6	32.7 ± 3.0	32.9 ± 2.5	0.458
Isometric torque (N.m)	80.8 ± 14.1	78.5 ± 18.3	79.0 ± 14.9	0.731
Concentric torque (N.m)	62.7 ± 12.4	61.8 ± 14.3	64.0 ± 13.4	0.687
Eccentric torque (N.m)	92.3 ± 15.0	88.4 ± 17.8	88.9 ± 16.3	0.425
Arm-curl 1-RM (kg)	27.0 ± 6.3	25.3 ± 5.2	26.6 ± 5.3	0.260

BMI: body mass index; 1-RM: one maximum repetition; circ.: circumference.

involved in conducting or evaluating the study and was released after the blind review and the freezing of the final database. The sample size was calculated *a priori* using Nquery Advisor software (version 6.01) based on the primary criterion (muscle thickness) and allowing for a power >90%. This statistical analysis indicated a minimum of 34 participants per experimental group.

Experimental procedure

The objectives of this randomized, double-blind study conducted with parallel arms, was to evaluate the effects of oral Pea protein supplementation, versus Placebo and versus Whey proteins associated with a 12-week resistance training program, on elbow flexors muscle thickness (main outcome) and muscle strength (secondary outcome). The trial consisted in an inclusion visit (D0), an intermediate 6-week follow-up visit (D42) and a final 12-week visit (D84) (Figure 1). Visits were separated by weight training periods with three sessions per week. Testing sessions were conducted on non-training days

and always at the same time of the day for the same subject. D0, D42 and D84 sessions included measurements of (i) muscle thickness using ultrasonography, (ii) arm circumference and (iii) maximal muscle strength in isokinetic conditions (concentric, isometric and eccentric). After the initial evaluation (D0), each subject was given a batch of products, according to randomization, and began weight training for a 12-week period. The same tests were repeated, in the same order, half-way through and at the end of the training period (D42 and D84, respectively). Tolerance, collected from adverse events and compliance with product intake (determined by counting products not consumed) was evaluated at D42 and D84 too.

Training

All subjects followed the same training routine, three times per week with a rest day between each session. Training was based on three exercises involving the elbow flexor and extensor muscles. The exercises soliciting the flexor muscles were arm curl and lateral pull-down. In the arm curl exercise, subjects sat with weights in their hands with a ~40° trunk/arm angle. They had to flex/extend the forearm over the arm. For the lateral pull-down, subjects sat with a bar in their hands above the head. They had to flex/extend the forearm over the arm with a vertical movement. The exercise soliciting the extensors was the bench press. Subjects were lying on their backs with a bar in their hands with a 90° trunk/arm angle, arms extended, and had to flex and extend their upper limbs vertically. Throughout the training program, the number of sets was progressively increased from 2 to 5 while the number of repetitions was reduced in parallel from 15 to 5 repetitions maximum (RM). The final week, training was composed of three sets of 5 RM in order to preclude any fatigue for the D84 tests. Recovery between sets was 2–3 minutes. The load used for each exercise was regularly adapted during training depending on individuals' maximum load (1-RM, one maximum repetition, evaluated every two weeks).

Dietary supplementation

The three products under study were presented as 45 g sachets of banana-flavored cocoa powder to be diluted in 300 mL of cold water at each intake. The diluted drinks were identical in appearance, texture and taste and were isoenergetic (Table 2). Products were taken twice a day for 12 weeks. On training days, one dose was taken in the morning and the second just after training. On non-training days, one dose was taken in the morning and the second dose in the afternoon. The general food intake was not monitored over the experimental procedure but participants were instructed to maintain their diet habits throughout the experimental protocol.

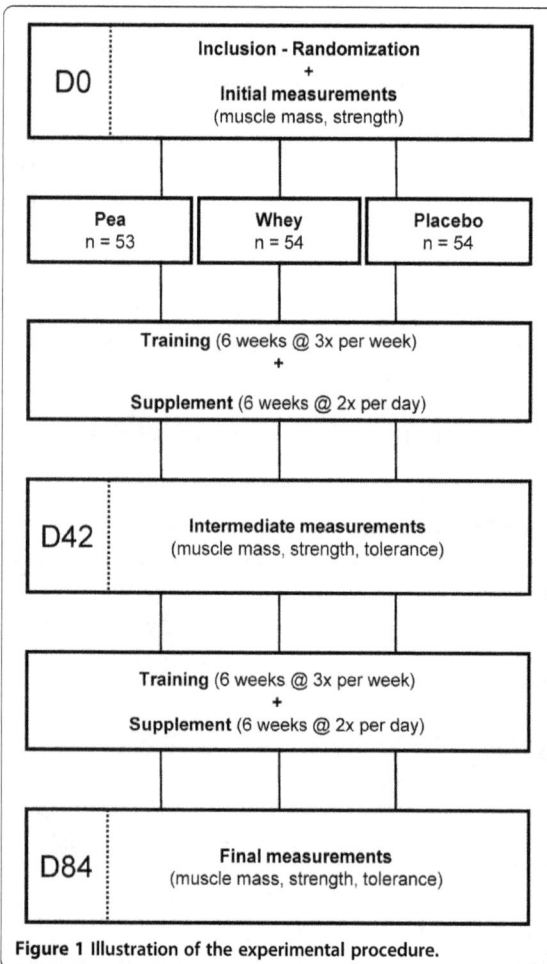

Figure 1 Illustration of the experimental procedure.

Table 2 Nutritional composition of drinks for 100 g of powder

	Placebo	Pea	Whey
Energy value (kcal)	367	387	366
Proteins (g)	3.7	59.2	57
[of which pea or whey protein]	[–]	[55.6]	[53.2]
Carbohydrates (g)	82.5	21.0	20.2
Lipids (g)	1.5	6.3	4.9
Fibres (g)	4.4	5.1	6.7

A dose of powder contained either 25 g of vegetable Pea protein isolate (NUTRALYS®) or 25 g of Whey protein concentrate. The placebo, with no added protein, was composed of maltodextrin. The nutritional composition of each product and the amino acids content of Pea and Whey proteins are shown in Tables 2 and 3, respectively. The other components (fat-reduced cocoa, flavouring, aspartame, salt, silica dioxide) were identical in nature and in quantity in all three products. NUTRALYS® pea protein (ROQUETTE, Lestrem, France) is a vegetable protein isolate from the yellow pea (*Pisum sativum*). Peas are cleaned and ground in a dry process to produce pea flour. Flour is then hydrated and the pea starch and internal fiber are extracted separately. The protein fraction is then coagulated for further purification and, finally, carefully dried in a multi-stage spray dryer. The resulting highly purified pea protein isolate contains 85% protein, 7% fat, 3% carbohydrate, and 5% ash on a dry matter basis.

Table 3 Amino acid composition (g) for 100 g of pea protein or Whey protein

	Pea	Whey
Alanine	3.3	4.1
Arginine	6.6	2.1
Aspartic acid	8.9	8.7
Cystine	0.8	1.9
Glutamic acid	13.2	13.9
Glycine	3.1	1.5
Histidine	1.9	1.5
Isoleucine	3.7	4.9
Leucine	6.4	8.6
Lysine	5.7	7.2
Methionine	0.8	1.6
Phenylalanine	4.2	2.6
Proline	3.4	4.7
Serine	3.9	4.2
Threonine	2.8	5.7
Tryptophan	0.7	1.5
Tyrosine	3.1	2.8
Valine	4.0	4.6

Measurements

Biceps brachii muscle thickness

Right-side biceps brachii muscle thickness was measured in real time using an ultrasound machine (AU5; Esaote Biomedica, Florence, Italy) coupled to a 50 mm probe at a frequency of 7.5 MHz. Subjects were lying supine with arms and legs completely relaxed. The right upper limb was positioned supine with a 45° angle with respect to the trunk. The probe was placed perpendicular to the skin surface at two-thirds of the distance between the acromion process of the scapula and the lateral epicondyle of the humerus [15]. The probe was coated with a water-soluble transmission gel to provide acoustic contact without depressing the dermal surface. Thickness was calculated as the distance between superficial and deep aponeuroses measured at the ends and middle of each 3.8 cm-wide sonograph. Three images were independently obtained for each point. The average value of these nine measures was calculated. To favor reproducibility, probe placement was carefully noted for reproduction during the other test sessions and measurements were always performed by the same operator.

Arm circumference

The circumference of the right arm was measured using a constant tension tape during maximal elbow extension at rest and during a maximal voluntary contraction (with maximal elbow flexion). Three measurements were made (at rest and contracted) along the length of the biceps, namely ¼, ½ and ¾ of the length of the upper arm (distance between the acromion process of the scapula and the lateral epicondyle of the humerus). Averaging was performed to obtain mean values for the circumference at rest and contracted.

Maximal voluntary torque

The maximal voluntary torque was measured on a Biodex (Biodex, Shirley, USA) isokinetic dynamometer during isometric, concentric and eccentric elbow flexions. The right-hand side was tested. Subjects were seated upright with a 95° hip angle. The upper limb was placed horizontally with the elbow rotation axis coinciding with the axis of rotation of the ergometer and aligned with the shoulder axis. The chest, shoulder and forearm were firmly attached to avoid perturbing contributions. Movements were made in the horizontal plan through a 120° elbow range of motion (from 10 to 130°, 0° = full extension). After a standardized warm-up consisting of submaximal contractions, measurements were made in concentric and eccentric conditions at an angular velocity of $60°.s^{-1}$. Subject had to accelerate or resist the ergometer lever arm, respectively. Five maximal voluntary contractions were performed consecutively for each condition. In isometric condition, the position was set at 80° elbow flexion and the subject had to produce a maximal voluntary contraction lasting 5 s. Three isometric contractions were requested with 60 s rest between contractions. Isometric, concentric and eccentric solicitations were presented in a random order and separated by five minutes of passive recovery. These various parameters were recorded for further analysis. The maximum value for each condition was retained for the statistical analysis.

Arm curl 1-RM

The maximum load (1-RM in kg) that could be lifted during elbow flexions was measured during an arm curl movement performed with both arms. For this, the load was progressively increased through successive sets (the first set being considered as warm up). Then, subjects were requested to lift each load only once. Care was taken to lift the load with the largest range of motion (~100 °). One minute rest was permitted between trials. In case of failure, a second try was allowed. The maximal load lifted was considered as the 1-RM. It was regularly evaluated (every two weeks) in order to adjust resistance training intensity.

Statistical analyses

Twenty four subjects left the study early due to personal reasons. At the end of the experimental procedure, 137 subjects were considered for analysis with 47 in the Pea group, 46 in the Whey group and 44 in the Placebo group (see Figure 2 for the CONSORT Diagram). Quantitative variables were presented as mean values and standard deviations. Values were tested using a repeated measures analysis of variances (ANOVA). Groups were used as independent variables and time (D0, D42, and D84) was used as the repeated variable. A sensitivity analysis was also conducted and considered subjects with a 1-RM at inclusion <25 kg (median value of study sample). Sixty eight subjects were considered for this sensitivity analysis. In the case of significant main effects or interactions, Scheffé post-hoc tests were conducted. Qualitative variables (supplementation compliance or adverse effects) were presented as absolute and relative frequencies and were tested by using a Chi square test. Statistics were conducted using SAS software (Ver. 9.2, SAS Institute, Inc., Cary, NC). $P < 0.05$ was taken as the level of statistical significance for all procedures.

Results

General observations

Initial values measured at D0 revealed similar groups for all variables (Table 1). During the experimental protocol, compliance was evaluated through the percentage of products returned by subjects. High average and comparable compliance was observed between groups: 93.4%, 90.8% and 90.7% for Whey, Placebo and Pea groups, respectively ($P = 0.509$). In addition, tolerance to the three products under study was good and comparable in terms of frequency and nature. Of the 161 subjects who took products at least once, three presented an adverse event in the Whey group (7.4%), four in the Placebo group (7.4%) and one in the Pea group (1.9%, $P = 0.370$). Except for two digestive disorders (type diarrhea) in the Placebo group, the adverse effects were all musculotendinous or back pains related to their usual activity throughout the study. All disappeared spontaneously except for an elbow tendinopathy in the Whey group which persisted at the end of the trial but any connection with the product was ruled out.

Muscle thickness and circumference

Results showed a significant time effect for biceps brachii muscle thickness ($P < 0.0001$). Thickness progressively increases with time within each group (Figure 3). Neither group effect nor interaction was obtained. However, when comparing groups, relative increase between D0 and D84 tended towards statistical significance (+15.3 ± 12.7%, +13.4 ± 10.8% and +10.7 ± 8.6% for Whey, Pea and Placebo, respectively; $P = 0.09$). A sensitivity analysis, performed on the weakest participants on muscle thickness increase, highlighted a significant time effect ($P < 0.0001$) and interaction (group × time, $P < 0.01$). Thickness increases between D0 and D84 were +20.2 ± 12.3%, +15.6 ± 13.5%, and +8.6 ± 7.3% for Pea, Whey and Placebo, respectively. A Scheffé test showed a statistically significant difference between Pea and Placebo (absolute difference of the means 2.51 mm IC 95% (0.49; 4.53)) whereas there was no significant difference between Whey and Pea (absolute difference of the means 1.21 mm IC 95% (−0.63; 3.06)) nor between Whey and Placebo (absolute difference of the means 1.29 mm IC 95% (−0.46; 3.05)) (Figure 4).

Mid-training, differences between groups were not statistically significant (Figure 4). Moreover, it can be noted that the increase in the Placebo group (+8.8 ± 7.6% at D42 with respect to D0) was merely maintained with the six additional weeks of training (+8.6 ± 7.3% at D84 with respect to D0), whereas it further significantly increased in the Whey (from +10.7 ± 13.3% to +15.6 ± 13.5%) and Pea (from +13.6 ± 9.0% to +20.2 ± 12.3%) groups.

Changes in the right arm circumference at rest and during maximal contractions showed significant time effect ($P < 0.0001$) and increases over the 12-week period. The average circumference of the right arm at rest increased from 32.0 ± 2.3 cm at D0 to 32.4 ± 2.2 cm at D84 in the Placebo group ($P = 0.005$), from 31.6 ± 3.2 cm to 32.1 ± 3.2 cm in the Whey group ($P = 0.0003$) and from 32.3 ± 2.5 cm to 32.7 ± 2.5 cm in the Pea group ($P = 0.01$). The average circumference of the right arm contracted increased from 32.7 ± 2.2 cm (D0) to 33.7 ± 2.2 cm (D84) in the control group ($P <$

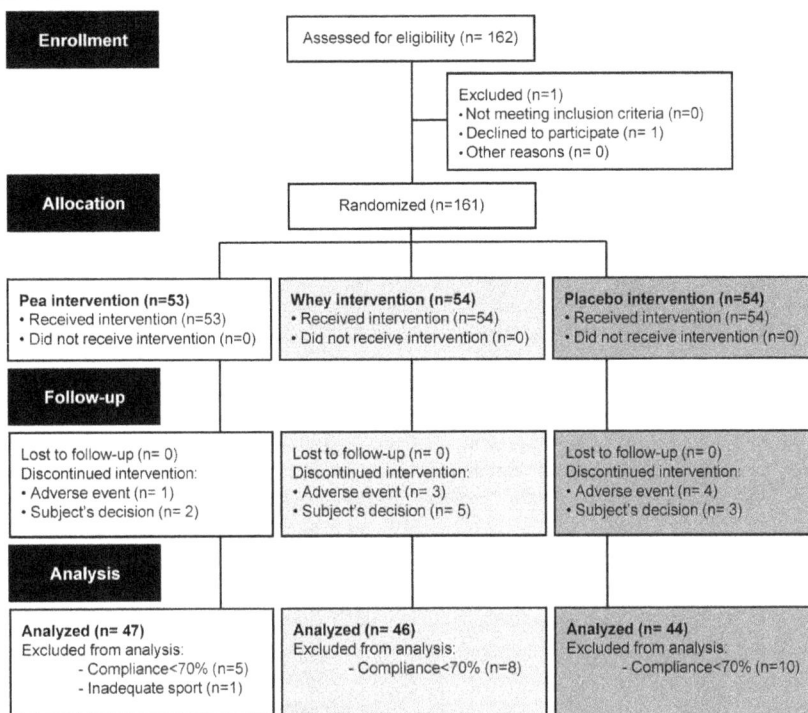

Figure 2 CONSORT diagram outlining participants' inclusion and drop out.

0.0001), from 32.4 ± 2.9 cm to 33.4 ± 3.2 cm in the Whey group ($P < 0.0001$) and from 33.3 ± 2.6 cm to 34.1 ± 2.4 cm in the Pea group ($P < 0.0001$). No difference was observed between the three groups at the end of the trial.

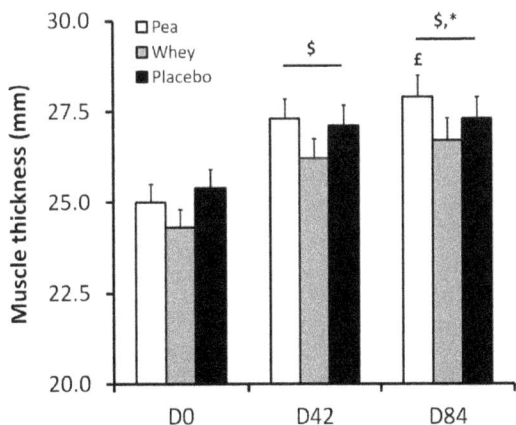

Figure 3 Changes in biceps brachii thickness (mm) during the experimental protocol. $: Significant difference within each group compared with D0 ($P < 0.0001$). £: Tending towards significance compared with D42 for the Pea group only ($P = 0.09$). *: Between group comparison between D0 and D84 approaching significance ($P = 0.09$).

Muscle strength

Maximal load (1-RM) during arm curl and muscle torque during the maximum voluntary isometric, concentric and eccentric contractions increased within each group. Statistical analyses only revealed a significant time effect ($P < 0.0001$). For example, for the Placebo group, the 12-week period produced an increase in the maximal 1-RM strength ($+46.1 \pm 22.4\%$), the maximal isometric ($+20.5 \pm 14.3\%$), concentric ($+15.3 \pm 16.2\%$) and eccentric ($+17.2 \pm 12.5\%$) torque. No significant group effect and interaction (group × time) was observed. For example, the increase in the maximum concentric torque between D0 and D84 was $+8.8 \pm 8.9$ N.m for the Placebo group, $+10.9 \pm 9.9$ N.m for Whey group and $+10.7 \pm 7.6$ N.m for Pea group.

Discussion

The present study aimed to test the hypothesis that a supplementation with pea protein, used in association with resistance training, would be as efficient as Whey protein to increase muscle thickness and strength. The present results showed significant gains in muscle mass as attested by thickness of the biceps brachii in all groups. Differences between groups were observed with the sensitivity study considering participants with the lowest muscle force at the entrance in the protocol. Pea

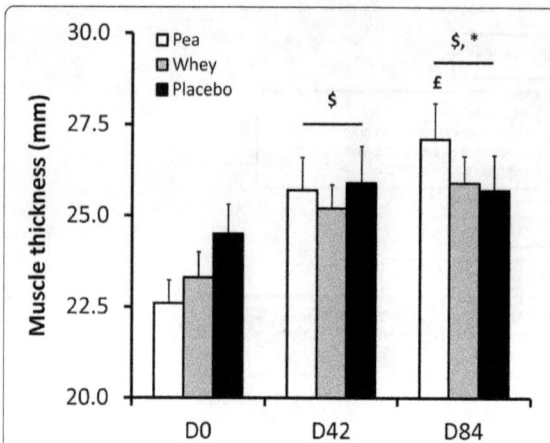

Figure 4 Sensitivity analysis for biceps brachii thickness (mm) during the experimental protocol. Data represent subjects with the 1-RM performance <25 kg at D0. Samples sizes are n = 17, 31 and 20 for the Pea, Whey and Placebo groups, respectively. $: Significant difference within each group compared with D0 ($P < 0.05 – P < 0.0001$). £: Significant difference compared with D42 for the Pea group only ($P < 0.05$). *: Between group comparison between D0 and D84 ($P < 0.05$).

protein group displayed a significantly greater effect than the Placebo on muscle thickness and Whey protein occupied an intermediate position between the other two supplements.

The results obtained on biceps brachii showed an increased muscle thickness with Pea protein. The effects obtained, although greater than those for Whey, do not reach the statistically significant level. The absence of statistical superiority over Whey is not a counter performance for pea protein which is positioned as an alternative to Whey, which, on the contrary, fails in this study to reach the statistical significance level against the Placebo group. Whey was used as a benchmark because most studies have reported a positive effect on muscle hypertrophy in various populations such as young athletes [16-18]. This hypertrophy is supposed to be due to activation of the mTOR (mammalian target of rapamycin) signaling pathway resulting from the simultaneous action of protein ingestion and training [17]. The almost similar supplementation effect of Pea and Whey may be ascribed to the characteristics of both ingredients. Both beverages are particularly rich in essential BCAA (valine, isoleucine and leucine) which play an important role in muscle protein synthesis. A literature review [19] indicated that leucine reportedly stimulates the muscle protein synthesis required to replace muscle protein damaged by resistance exercises. In young adults, protein synthesis is 20% higher after ingestion of leucine, proteins and carbohydrates, compared with ingestion of carbohydrates and proteins with no leucine intake [19]. Moreover, authors reported that consumption of 8 to

11.5 g of EAA containing 2 to 3 g of leucine after exercise may maximize the protein synthetic response [20-22]. In the present study, such content is provided.

The lack of statistical difference between NUTRALYS® and Whey may be attributed to the quite similar amino acids content but also to the kinetic of digestion. Whey protein has a fast kinetic of digestion, bringing rapidly high concentration of amino-acids in plasma after ingestion, but this effect is transient and returns to resting levels within 2-3 h [7]. NUTRALYS® is an intermediate profile fast protein (unpublished observations) and it can be assumed that the amino acid content in blood plasma would increase quickly after ingestion, making it readily and long lastingly available in the body to participate in muscle protein synthesis. In addition, based on Protein Digestibility Acid Corrected Amino Acid Score [23], NUTRALYS® pea protein has shown that it is a high nutritional quality protein with an index of 92.8% out of a maximum 100% [24] corresponding to the values of Whey or casein, while fruit proteins have a mean value of 76% and cereal proteins 59% [25].

Each experimental group underwent 12 weeks of resistance training. As shown previously [26] and as attested by the Placebo group, weight training alone had an impact on biceps brachii thickness. This increase in muscle thickness was obtained during the first six weeks of training. Such result is in general accordance with the literature since muscle architectural changes have been shown to occur between the fourth and eighth weeks of resistance training [27]. Interestingly, beyond six weeks of training, only the groups taking protein supplementations, either Pea or Whey experienced additional increases in muscle thickness. This result suggests that, for a long training period (> six weeks), the association of resistance training and protein consumption is important. It will maintain a positive protein balance (ratio of protein synthesis to degradation in favor of synthesis) and therefore muscle hypertrophy [28].

An increase in muscle thickness, observed here, is fundamental for achieving a gain in strength [29]. However, muscle strength, although improved after the experimental period, was not different between groups. Such result is quite surprising since protein beverages have exacerbated muscle thickness increases and as a consequence should have increased muscle strength gains as compared with the placebo. This lack of difference in muscle strength between groups remains unclear but could be attributed to several factors such as the supplementation characteristics, training type and training status.

Protein was supplemented twice with an intake immediately after the resistance training session. Although debated, such timing may appear as one of the most effective nutrient timing strategies for muscle protein synthesis [11]. As compared to a morning/evening intake group, Cribb and Hayes [30] observed larger muscle mass increases with protein intake before and after training. The best stimulus for protein synthesis appeared to be with protein feeding in close proximity to training sessions [31,32], with feeding recommended within the first two hours post-exercise [2,33,34].

Protein quantity was 50 g.day^{-1} with 25 g after resistance sessions. These doses seem unlikely to be responsible for the lack of difference between groups for muscle strength. Indeed, in a recent review [35], the author recommended the ingestion of 20 g of high quality protein immediately after exercise to maximally stimulate protein synthesis. Therefore, sufficient protein intakes have been proposed here and are likely not responsible for the lack of differences between groups for muscle strength.

It should be remembered that training and supplementation effects are potentiated in subjects exhibiting lower muscle strength at inclusion (1-RM < 25 kg, sensitivity analysis). Such a result is not surprising since training is well known to have larger effects in untrained subjects. For example, greater increases in muscle cross-sectional area have been reported in subjects who had not previously engaged in resistance training in comparison with more accustomed subjects [36]. The effects of amino acids supply may also depend on training status, since greater disturbances in protein turnover (protein synthesis and degradation) are obtained following training in novice than in experienced athletes [37]. Moreover, the expected increase in protein synthesis following exercise appears to be smaller and shorter in trained athletes as compared with untrained subjects [38,39]. Thus, training status may influence muscle performance. Indeed, Vieillevoye et al. [10] found increases in lower body strength with an EAA supplement while no modification was obtained with placebo. Surprisingly, in the same study, strength was similarly enhanced in both groups for the upper body. These authors concluded that supplementation and training adaptations seem to depend on the initial training status; the weaker the subjects, the larger the effect of protein supplementation on muscle strength. Moreover, the present study was conducted in physically active males. It is possible to speculate that, with untrained participants, differences between groups might have been revealed more easily. Furthermore, a plateau, or 'ceiling effect', of the adaptive responses to training is generally observed either for strength gains and muscle protein synthetic response [37,40]. Hence, protein requirements and training stimulus are affected by training status and duration. For instance, greater protein intakes are required during the early stages of intensive bodybuilding training and more particularly in novices [41]. Modification of the training program might also have exacerbated differences between groups for all studied parameters. Training volume [42] concomitant with the load used in terms of 1-RM's percentage [43] are possible parameters.

Conclusions

The present experiment demonstrated that protein supplementation may exacerbate possible adaptations induced by resistance training. The consumption of pea protein promotes gains in biceps brachii thickness and especially in beginners or people returning to weight training. This statistical superiority compared with the Placebo and the comparable results with those obtained for Whey intake make pea protein an alternative to Whey-based dietary products for athletes from different levels and sports. Such proteins should also be of interest in other populations such as elderly to slow down the aging process and maintain muscle mass.

Abbreviations
BCAA: Branched-chain amino acids; EAA: Essential amino-acids; D0: Testing at inclusion; D42: Testing in the middle; D84: Testing at the end; RM: Repetition maximum.

Competing interests
Roquette provided financial support to conduct the study. The funders have no role in the study design, data collection and analysis or preparation of the manuscript. LGD, MHS and CLM, three authors, have an affiliation (employment) to the commercial funders of this research.

Authors' contributions
NB (corresponding author) was responsible for the study design, the execution of the measurements and the writing of the manuscript. CP participated in the execution of the measurements and the writing of manuscript. GD participated in the study design and the writing of the manuscript. LGD participated in the study design and writing of the manuscript. MHS and CLM participated in the study design. FAA participated in the study design, the statistical analysis and the writing of the manuscript. All authors read and approved the final manuscript.

Acknowledgments
The authors would like to thank Mr. Lucas BERTHAIRE for helping with data collection.

Author details
[1]National Institute for Health and Medical Research, (INSERM), unit 1093, Cognition, Action and Sensorimotor Plasticity, Dijon, France. [2]Centre for Performance Expertise, UFR STAPS, Dijon, France. [3]Roquette, Lestrem, France. [4]Chair of Medical Evaluation ESC, Dijon, France. [5]CEN Nutriment, Dijon, France. [6]Faculté des Sciences du Sport, Université de Bourgogne, BP 27877, 21078 Dijon Cedex, France.

References
1. Burd NA, Tang JE, Moore DR, Phillips SM. Exercise training and protein metabolism: Influences of contraction, protein intake, and sex-based differences. J Appl Physiol. 2009;106:1692–701.
2. Phillips SM, Tipton KD, Aarsland A, Wolf SE, Wolfe RR. Mixed muscle protein synthesis and breakdown after resistance exercise in humans. Am J Physiol. 1997;273:E99–107.
3. Biolo G, Maggi SP, Williams BD, Tipton KD, Wolfe RR. Increased rates of muscle protein turnover and amino acid transport after resistance exercise in humans. Am J Physiol. 1995;268:E514–20.
4. Chesley A, MacDougall JD, Tarnopolsky MA, Atkinson SA, Smith K. Changes in human muscle protein synthesis after resistance exercise. J Appl Physiol (1985). 1992;73:1383–8.
5. Rennie MJ, Wackerhage H, Spangenburg EE, Booth FW. Control of the size of the human muscle mass. Annu Rev Physiol. 2004;66:799–828.

6. Tipton KD, Gurkin BE, Matin S, Wolfe RR. Nonessential amino acids are not necessary to stimulate net muscle protein synthesis in healthy volunteers. J Nutr Biochem. 1999;10:89–95.

7. Boirie Y, Dangin M, Gachon P, Vasson MP, Maubois JL, Beaufrere B. Slow and fast dietary proteins differently modulate postprandial protein accretion. Proc Natl Acad Sci U S A. 1997;94:14930–5.

8. Cermak NM, Res PT, de Groot LC, Saris WH, van Loon LJ. Protein supplementation augments the adaptive response of skeletal muscle to resistance-type exercise training: a meta-analysis. Am J Clin Nutr. 2012;96:1454–64.

9. Babault N, Deley G, Le Ruyet P, Morgan F, Allaert FA. Effects of soluble milk protein or casein supplementation on muscle fatigue following resistance training program: a randomized, double-blind, and placebo-controlled study. J Int Soc Sports Nutr. 2014;11:36.

10. Vieillevoye S, Poortmans JR, Duchateau J, Carpentier A. Effects of a combined essential amino acids/carbohydrate supplementation on muscle mass, architecture and maximal strength following heavy-load training. Eur J Appl Physiol. 2010;110:479–88.

11. Stark M, Lukaszuk J, Prawitz A, Salacinski A. Protein timing and its effects on muscular hypertrophy and strength in individuals engaged in weight-training. J Int Soc Sports Nutr. 2012;9:54.

12. Balage M, Dardevet D. Long-term effects of leucine supplementation on body composition. Curr Opin Clin Nutr Metab Care. 2010;13:265–70.

13. Paul GL. The rationale for consuming protein blends in sports nutrition. J Am Coll Nutr. 2009;28(Suppl):464S–72.

14. Tipton KD, Elliott TA, Cree MG, Wolf SE, Sanford AP, Wolfe RR. Ingestion of casein and whey proteins result in muscle anabolism after resistance exercise. Med Sci Sports Exerc. 2004;36:2073–81.

15. Miyatani M, Kanehisa H, Ito M, Kawakami Y, Fukunaga T. The accuracy of volume estimates using ultrasound muscle thickness measurements in different muscle groups. Eur J Appl Physiol. 2004;91:264–72.

16. Hulmi JJ, Lockwood CM, Stout JR. Effect of protein/essential amino acids and resistance training on skeletal muscle hypertrophy: a case for whey protein. Nutr Metab (Lond). 2010;7:51.

17. Farnfield MM, Breen L, Carey KA, Garnham A, Cameron-Smith D. Activation of mtor signalling in young and old human skeletal muscle in response to combined resistance exercise and whey protein ingestion. Appl Physiol Nutr Metab. 2012;37:21–30.

18. Farup J, Rahbek SK, Vendelbo MH, Matzon A, Hindhede J, Bejder A, et al. Whey protein hydrolysate augments tendon and muscle hypertrophy independent of resistance exercise contraction mode. Scand J Med Sci Sports. 2014;24:788–98.

19. Koopman R, Saris WH, Wagenmakers AJ, van Loon LJ. Nutritional interventions to promote post-exercise muscle protein synthesis. Sports Med. 2007;37:895–906.

20. Tang JE, Moore DR, Kujbida GW, Tarnopolsky MA, Phillips SM. Ingestion of whey hydrolysate, casein, or soy protein isolate: effects on mixed muscle protein synthesis at rest and following resistance exercise in young men. J Appl Physiol (1985). 2009;107:987–92.

21. Reidy PT, Walker DK, Dickinson JM, Gundermann DM, Drummond MJ, Timmerman KL, et al. Protein blend ingestion following resistance exercise promotes human muscle protein synthesis. J Nutr. 2013;143:410–6.

22. Burke LM, Winter JA, Cameron-Smith D, Enslen M, Farnfield M, Decombaz J. Effect of intake of different dietary protein sources on plasma amino acid profiles at rest and after exercise. Int J Sport Nutr Exerc Metab. 2012;22:452–62.

23. Boutrif E. Recent developments in protein quality evaluation. Food Nutr Agr. 1991;1:36–40.

24. Yang H, Guerin-Deremaux L, Zhou L, Fratus A, Wils D, Zhang C, et al. Evaluation of nutritional quality of a novel pea protein. Agro Food Industry Hi-Tech. 2012;23:8–10.

25. Schaafsma G. The protein digestibility-corrected amino acid score. J Nutr. 2000;130:1865S–7.

26. Matta T, Simao R, de Salles BF, Spineti J, Oliveira LF. Strength training's chronic effects on muscle architecture parameters of different arm sites. J Strength Cond Res. 2011;25:1711–7.

27. Gondin J, Guette M, Ballay Y, Martin A. Electromyostimulation training effects on neural drive and muscle architecture. Med Sci Sports Exerc. 2005;37:1291–9.

28. Borsheim E, Cree MG, Tipton KD, Elliott TA, Aarsland A, Wolfe RR. Effect of carbohydrate intake on net muscle protein synthesis during recovery from resistance exercise. J Appl Physiol (1985). 2004;96:674–8.

29. Ikai M, Fukunaga T. A study on training effect on strength per unit cross-sectional area of muscle by means of ultrasonic measurement. Int Z Angew Physiol. 1970;28:173–80.

30. Cribb PJ, Hayes A. Effects of supplement timing and resistance exercise on skeletal muscle hypertrophy. Med Sci Sports Exerc. 2006;38:1918–25.

31. Tipton KD, Elliott TA, Cree MG, Aarsland AA, Sanford AP, Wolfe RR. Stimulation of net muscle protein synthesis by whey protein ingestion before and after exercise. Am J Physiol Endocrinol Metab. 2007;292:E71–6.

32. Tipton KD, Rasmussen BB, Miller SL, Wolf SE, Owens-Stovall SK, Petrini BE, et al. Timing of amino acid-carbohydrate ingestion alters anabolic response of muscle to resistance exercise. Am J Physiol Endocrinol Metab. 2001;281:E197–206.

33. Hartman JW, Tang JE, Wilkinson SB, Tarnopolsky MA, Lawrence RL, Fullerton AV, et al. Consumption of fat-free fluid milk after resistance exercise promotes greater lean mass accretion than does consumption of soy or carbohydrate in young, novice, male weightlifters. Am J Clin Nutr. 2007;86:373–81.

34. Rasmussen BB, Tipton KD, Miller SL, Wolf SE, Wolfe RR. An oral essential amino acid-carbohydrate supplement enhances muscle protein anabolism after resistance exercise. J Appl Physiol. 2000;88:386–92.

35. Phillips SM. Dietary protein requirements and adaptive advantages in athletes. Br J Nutr. 2012;108 Suppl 2:S158–67.

36. Ahtiainen JP, Pakarinen A, Alen M, Kraemer WJ, Hakkinen K. Muscle hypertrophy, hormonal adaptations and strength development during strength training in strength-trained and untrained men. Eur J Appl Physiol. 2003;89:555–63.

37. Phillips SM, Tipton KD, Ferrando AA, Wolfe RR. Resistance training reduces the acute exercise-induced increase in muscle protein turnover. Am J Physiol. 1999;276:E118–24.

38. Phillips SM, Parise G, Roy BD, Tipton KD, Wolfe RR, Tamopolsky MA. Resistance-training-induced adaptations in skeletal muscle protein turnover in the fed state. Can J Physiol Pharmacol. 2002;80:1045–53.

39. MacDougall JD, Gibala MJ, Tarnopolsky MA, MacDonald JR, Interisano SA, Yarasheski KE. The time course for elevated muscle protein synthesis following heavy resistance exercise. Can J Appl Physiol. 1995;20:480–6.

40. Alway SE, Grumbt WH, Stray-Gundersen J, Gonyea WJ. Effects of resistance training on elbow flexors of highly competitive bodybuilders. J Appl Physiol. 1992;72:1512–21.

41. Lemon PW, Tarnopolsky MA, MacDougall JD, Atkinson SA. Protein requirements and muscle mass/strength changes during intensive training in novice bodybuilders. J Appl Physiol. 1992;73:767–75.

42. Krieger JW. Single vs. Multiple sets of resistance exercise for muscle hypertrophy: A meta-analysis. J Strength Cond Res. 2010;24:1150–9.

43. Burd NA, West DW, Staples AW, Atherton PJ, Baker JM, Moore DR, et al. Low-load high volume resistance exercise stimulates muscle protein synthesis more than high-load low volume resistance exercise in young men. PLoS One. 2010;5:e12033.

## 17

In a single-blind, matched group design: branched-chain amino acid supplementation and resistance training maintains lean body mass during a caloric restricted diet

Wesley David Dudgeon[*], Elizabeth Page Kelley and Timothy Paul Scheett

Abstract

Background: Athletes and active adults many times have the goal of improving/maintaining fitness while losing weight and this is best achieved by caloric restriction in combination with exercise. However, this poses a risk for lean tissue loss, which can limit performance. Thus, the purpose of this study was to determine the effectiveness of a branched-chain amino acid (BCAA) supplement, in conjunction with heavy resistance training and a carbohydrate caloric-restricted "cut diet" on body composition and muscle fitness.

Methods: Seventeen resistance-trained males (21–28 years of age) were randomized to a BCAA group ($n = 9$) or a carbohydrate (CHO) group ($n = 8$) who both received their respective supplement during the 8 weeks of a prescribed body building style resistance training protocol. Subjects were prescribed a hypocaloric diet (based upon pre-intervention analysis) that was to be followed during the study.

Results: The BCAA group lost fat mass (-0.05 ± 0.08 kg;$p < .05$) and maintained lean mass, while the CHO group lost lean mass (-0.90 ± 0.06 kg; $p < .05$) and body mass (-2.3 ± 0.7 kg; $p < .05$). Both groups increased 1RM squat, but the increase in the BCAA group (15.1 ± 2.2 kg; $p < .05$)was greater ($P < 0.05$) than the CHO group. The BCAA group increased 1RM bench press (7.1 ± 1.6 kg; $P < 0.05$), while the CHO group decreased strength (-3.7 ± 2.3 kg; $P < 0.05$). The only change in muscular endurance was an increase in repetitions to fatigue (5.3 ± 0.2; $p < .05$) in the CHO group.

Conclusion: These results show that BCAA supplementation in trained individuals performing resistance training while on a hypocaloric diet can maintain lean mass and preserve skeletal muscle performance while losing fat mass.

Keywords: Cut diet, Fat mass, Lean mass

* Correspondence: dudgeonw@cofc.edu
Department of Health and Human Performance, College of Charleston, 24
George Street, Charleston, SC 29424, USA

Background

The prevalence of age and lifestyle-induced obesity among adults is increasing rapidly [1]. Thus, many adults engage in intentional weight loss, primarily via reductions in fat mass, to achieve aesthetic, performance, and/or health goals, including reduced risk for chronic disease and disability [2]. Weight loss can be achieved via a reduction in calorie intake in conjunction with the initiation of physical activity [1]. The "cut diet" is a well-known dieting technique in which calorie and carbohydrate restriction reduces carbohydrate stores in the body and increases fat utilization as fuel, which in turn reduces fat mass.

Resistance training is a common training modality that elicits significant muscular and cardiometabolic benefits among both recreational and elite athletes [3]. Resistance training stimulates muscle metabolism for muscle growth and development [4]. When performed regularly, resistance training has been shown to increase strength, muscular endurance, skeletal muscle hypertrophy, as well as result in favorable changes in body composition, including decreases in body fat mass and increases in lean mass, all of which can improve health-related quality of life [4–6].

However, maintaining an energy deficient diet during a period of intense or unaccustomed resistance training may lead to significant losses in lean mass and decrease work output, thus hindering athletic performance, as well as increasing the risk for acute illness and training-related injury [5, 7, 8]. Muscle damage, characterized by increased muscle and whole-body protein turnover and amino acid oxidation during and following exercise, increases the athlete's need for protein intake [9]. Therefore, it is important for athletes and recreationally active adults who engage in higher intensity or resistance training programs, as well as adults at risk for sarcopenia, to maintain a protein intake that can sustain lean body mass for functional and athletic performance, especially during a hypocaloric diet [1, 2].

Insufficient dietary protein intake post-exercise may cause increased protein catabolism, which may result in a negative protein balance and slower muscle recovery [5]. This may lead to muscle wasting (e.g. sarcopenia) and training intolerance [5]. However, dietary protein intake among recreational athletes and adults engaging in intentional weight loss via caloric restriction is often insufficient to avoid muscle wasting [1, 5]. Other susceptible populations include aesthetic athletes, such as dancers, gymnasts, and bodybuilders, and athletes who must meet weight requirement, such as boxers and wrestlers [5]. There is evidence suggesting that preserving muscle mass requires ingesting a sufficient amount of high quality protein [1, 10].

Many athletes and fitness participants consume protein or amino acid supplements to maintain essential amino acid availability and stimulate lean tissue preservation.

The combination of high quality protein and resistance exercise is suggested to have a synergistic effect on muscle mass preservation during intentional weight loss [1]. Nutritional supplements such as branched-chain amino acids (BCAA; valine, leucine, isoleucine) may augment or stimulate skeletal muscle regeneration by suppressing post-exercise protein degradation, therefore leading to greater gains in lean mass [5].

BCAAs are catabolized in the muscle and have been shown to regulate skeletal muscle protein synthesis and muscle recovery [11]. BCAAs may delay fatigue and stimulate muscle protein synthesis leading to post-exercise muscle recovery, allowing consumers to train longer at a higher intensity [5, 8]. Numerous studies have reported the effectiveness of a BCAA supplementation in promoting and regulating protein synthesis and suppressing endogenous protein degradation post-exercise [5, 12, 13]. Shimomoura et al. [12] found that oral ingestion of a BCAA supplement before or after exercise improved the recovery of damaged muscles by suppressing the endogenous muscle-protein breakdown during exercise [12]. Similarly, Norton & Layman [14] found that the consumption of leucine, one of three BCAAs, can turn individuals from a negative to a positive whole body protein balance after intense resistance training exercise [14]. Thus, the use of a BCAA supplement in conjunction with a resistance exercise training regimen may enhance training adaptations in recreational and advanced athletes, and benefit those with or at risk for sarcopenia [15, 16].

However, what is not known is how trained individuals participating in regular resistance training while observing calorically restricted to purposely decrease fat mass respond to BCAA supplementation. Therefore, the purpose of this study was to determine the effectiveness of a BCAA supplement on body composition, metabolism, and muscular fitness in young adult males following a carbohydrate and caloric restricted cut diet while maintaining a vigorous resistance training protocol. A cut diet is utilized to reduce fat mass while maintaining lean muscle mass by restricting calories and carbohydrate intake.

The addition of BCAAs to an athlete's diet may allow the athlete to train longer at a higher intensity and aid in recovery, promoting greater increases in desired outcomes (i.e. strength, endurance, power, body fat, lean mass, etc.) [13]. We hypothesize that daily BCAA supplementation in conjunction with a heavy resistance training protocol and a cut diet will maintain lean body mass and decrease fat mass in resistance-trained males.

Methods
Experimental protocol

For 8 weeks subjects were prescribed a carbohydrate and calorically-restricted diet individually calculated based upon pre-intervention body composition and resting

In a single-blind, matched group design: branched-chain amino acid supplementation...

179

metabolic rate (RMR). It was made clear to subjects that the diet prescription was to be followed for the duration of the study and they were told that no nutritional supplements, other than those supplements provided, were to be ingested. In a single-blind, matched group design, subjects were provided a body building style split resistance training program for 8 weeks (four days/week). Further, subjects were randomized to pre-exercise and post-exercise ingestion of either a BCAA nutritional supplement (Scivation XTend™, Scivation, Inc.) or a carbohydrate based supplement (POWERADE®). All assessments of muscle performance and body composition were completed prior to the initiation of the prescribed diet, first dose of supplement and initiation of resistance training program, and immediately after the conclusion of the 8 week intervention period. Pre and post testing sessions were conducted in the same order and were administered in the Human Performance Laboratory in the Silcox Center at the College of Charleston. Data from another study with similar study methodology have been published, [17] thus what follows is a truncated explanation of study procedures.

Participants

Seventeen males (between the ages of 21 and 28) who self-reported as resistance trained (defined as consistent whole body resistance training for at least 2 years prior to the onset of the study) volunteered for the study. Exclusion criteria included: less than two (2) years of prior resistance training experience, lower or upper extremity surgery within the past year, recent musculoskeletal injury, epilepsy, or another medical condition that would be exacerbated by the consumption of protein. (i.e. excessive consumption of alcohol, diabetes, Lou Gehrig's disease, or branched-chain keto acidura). After signing the informed consent form, subjects completed a Physical Activity Readiness Questionnaire (Par-Q) to ensure that the required health status and physical activity habits for participation in this research were met. The Institutional Review Board of the College of Charleston granted approval of all study procedures.

Body composition assessment

Total body mass was measured on a digital medical scale (Tanita, Tokyo, Japan) and height was measured using a standard medical stadiometer (Seca, Chino, CA). Percent body fat, fat mass, and fat-free mass were determined using hydrostatic weighing.

Muscular fitness assessment

To assess muscular strength, each subject performed a one-repetition maximum (1RM) bench press and a 1RM parallel back squat using the National Strength and Conditioning (NSCA) protocol for a 1RM. Subjects were then asked to complete as many repetitions as possible

at 80 %1RM for the bench press and parallel back squat. Research assistants spotted and supervised all lifts.

Resting metabolic rate

Resting metabolic rate (RMR) was measured (ParvoMedics TrueOne® metabolic cart) following a 45 min period in which participants laid as quiet and motionless as possible under the supervision of a research assistant who ensured the subjects remained awake. Expired air was measured with the use of a plastic canopy, thus preventing the need for a facemask or mouthpiece, which may artificially elevate resting metabolic rate. Participants were instructed to freely inhale and exhale during the 30 min test.

Dietary analyses

Subjects were provided an individualized caloric-restricted diet based on individual data (body mass, body composition, resting metabolic rate, etc.). All subjects, regardless of group, followed the same diet, which was designed by an industry consultant with prior experience consulting with physique athletes during pre-contest preparation. The caloric-restricted diet was designed as an 8 week "cut diet" for reducing body fat, and used a modified carbohydrate-restricted diet approach (percent of total calories for workout days were 30 % carbohydrates, 35 % protein and 35 % fat and for off days were 25 % carbohydrates, 40 % protein and 35 % fat). Each individual's daily caloric and macronutrient intake was determined using the Harris Benedict formula with an activity factor of 1.35 (lightly active individual engaging in light exercise 1–3 days/week) for workout days and 1.125 (sedentary individual) for off days. Subjects were given a diet card (See Fig. 1) for work out days and off days that listed the total caloric goal with three meal options per meal to attain the desired intake. Mean caloric intake and macronutrient composition of the initial 4 week diet for each group are presented in Table 1. The dietary intake needs were re-calculated after 4 weeks of the study to account for any changes in body mass. Subjects were required to maintain the diet provided for them for the entire 8 week study period and weekly interviews with subjects were incorporated to help achieve compliance.

Subjects were screened during recruitment to ensure they were properly motivated and had the required prior experience with resistance training and strictly following a set dietary plan. In addition, subjects met weekly with a research assistant to review their workout cards, adjust loads if necessary and to review their compliance with both the respective supplement and diet plan. An equal number of subjects complained about the restrictiveness of the diet as compare to subjects that reported great satisfaction with the diet. Subjects in both groups followed the same dietary plan, which provided recommendations and substitutions for each meal (See Fig. 1).

Example Meal Plan OFF Days
1604 Calories

Meal 1

# Serv	Meal 1														
5	10.00	Ea	or	335.00	G	Egg Whites	1.25	C	or	285.00	G	NF Cottage Cheese	1.65	C	or	50.00	G	Whey Protein Pwdr
2	2.00	Oz	or	56.70	G	Avocado	12.00	Each	or	17.20	G	Almonds	20.00	Ea	or	1.87	G	Peanuts
1	2.25	Oz	or	64.00	G	Banana	3.50	Oz	or	95.00	G	Blueberries	6.50	Oz	or	184.00	G	Strawberries
1	0.25	C	or	20.00	G	Oatmeal (Dry/Plain)	0.13	C	or	20.00	G	Steel Cut Oats (Dry)	1.25	Tbp	or	15.60	G	Barley (Pearled)(Dry)

Meal 2

# Serv	Meal 2														
4	4.00	Oz	or	113.40	G	Lean Turkey Breast	4.00	Oz	or	113.40	G	Tuna (cnd in H2O)	4.00	Oz	or	113.40	G	Grld Chicken Breast
3	18.00	Each	or	25.80	G	Almonds	3.00	Oz	or	85.05	G	Avocado	6.00	Tsp	or	31.80	G	Peanut Butter
1	3.25	Oz	or	92.00	G	Apple	3.50	Oz	or	95.00	G	Blueberries	0.00	Oz	or	28.25	G	Raspberries

Meal 3

# Serv	Meal 3														
5	5.00	Oz	or	141.75	G	Grld Chicken Breast	3.75	Oz	or	106.25	G	Grld Lean Sirloin	5.00	Oz	or	141.75	G	Grilled Halibut
2	2.00	Oz	or	56.70	G	Avocado	4.00	Tbp	or	60.00	G	Salad Dressing (Light)	12.00	Each	or	17.20	G	Almonds
2	5.50	Oz	or	156.00	G	Steamed Broccoli	6.00	C	or	330.00	G	Chppd LetTomCuc	3.50	Oz	or	100.00	G	Steamed Green Beans
1	2.25	Oz	or	63.80	G	Baked Potato	0.33	C	or	64.35	G	Brown Rice (Ckd)	1.00	Slc	or	32.00	G	Ezekial Bread

Meal 4

# Serv	Meal 4														
4	4.00	Oz	or	113.40	G	Tuna (cnd in H2O)	4.00	Oz	or	113.40	G	Grld Chicken Breast	1.32	C	or	40.00	G	Whey Protein Pwdr
2	12.00	Each	or	17.20	G	Almonds	2.00	Oz	or	56.70	G	Avocado	4.00	Tsp	or	21.20	G	Peanut Butter
2	8.80	Oz	or	250.00	G	Steamed Spinach	3.50	Oz	or	100.00	G	Steamed Green Beans	5.50	Oz	or	156.00	G	Steamed Broccoli
1	0.25	C	or	20.00	G	Oatmeal (Dry/Plain)	0.33	C	or	46.00	G	Whole Grain Pasta	2.00	Oz	or	56.70	G	Baked Sweet Potato

Meal 5

# Serv	Meal 5														
5	3.75	Oz	or	106.25	G	Grld Lean Sirloin	5.00	Oz	or	141.75	G	Grld Chicken Breast	5.00	Oz	or	141.75	G	Grilled Halibut
3	3.00	Tsp	or	13.50	G	Olive/Enova Oil	3.00	Oz	or	85.05	G	Avocado	6.00	Tbp	or	90.00	G	Salad Dressing (Light)
2	8.00	Oz	or	226.00	G	Steamed Asparagus	8.80	Oz	or	250.00	G	Steamed Spinach	6.00	C	or	330.00	G	Chppd LetTomCuc

Fig. 1 Sample dietary card for a subject during an off, non-workout, day. The Harris Benedict formula with an activity factor of 1.35 (lightly active individual engaging in light exercise 1–3 days/week) was used for workout days and 1.125 (sedentary individual) for off days

The subjects were instructed to follow the diet as closely as possible. The subjects were highly motivated to participate in what was described during recruitment as a 'cut diet' designed by a registered dietician who had prior experience helping professional athletes (MMA fighters, boxers, body builders) to lose body fat for a competition. There is no reason to believe that this group of homogeneous subjects experienced with resistance training and following strict diets, would eat dramatically different foods resulting in amino acid profile differences between the two groups.

The principle investigator's prior experience utilizing food records for dietary analyses were not as accurate as desired due to subjects often under reporting foods eaten, portion sizes consumed and omission of foods the subjects felt were not allowed. The little perceived benefit of dietary analyses that confirmed compliance with dietary instructions (in addition to anthropometric outcome measures including changes in body mass, fat mass, lean body mass) did not outweigh the negative tedious aspects of completing dietary records which could have resulted in subjects withdrawing from the study or provided inaccurate data.

Supplementation protocol

Each participant was randomly assigned to either the BCAA supplement group (BCAA; 14 g of a BCAA

Table 1 Sample macronutrient breakdown during workout days and off days for a study subject

		Caloric Intake (Kcal/day)	Protein (g)	Carbohydrate (g)	Fat (g)
Workout Day	BCAA	2456	215	184	96
	CHO	2717	238	204	106
Off Day	BCAA	2046	205	128	80
	CHO	2264	226	142	88

Each individual's daily caloric and macronutrient intake was determined using the Harris Benedict formula with an activity factor of 1.35 (lightly active individual engaging in light exercise 1–3 days/week) for workout days and 1.125 (sedentary individual) for off days

Table 2 Changes in body mass variables before and after 8 week study period

	Age (yrs)	Height (cm)	Body Mass (kg)	Lean Mass (kg)	Fat Mass (kg)
BCAA	24.7 ± 0.6	177.9 ± 4.6	84.3 ± 5.2	72.2 ± 4.7	12.2 ± 0.7
			84.2 ± 4.8	72.6 ± 4.3	11.6 ± 0.7[a]
CHO	23.5 ± 0.6	176.6 ± 5.6	78.3 ± 2.9	67.8 ± 2.5	10.5 ± 0.5
			76.0 ± 2.4[a]	66.9 ± 2.5[a]	9.1 ± 0.7

[a]denotes significant difference ($p < 0.05$) within BCAA and CHO
All subjects were prescribed the same hypocaloric diet and exercise programs. The BCAA group received 28 g of BCAA (14 g prior/during each workout and 14 g post workout) while the CHO group received 28 g of a carbohydrate/electrolyte supplement (14 g prior/during each workout and 14 g post workout)

nutritional supplement containing seven grams of BCAA prior to and following each workout for a total of 14 g of BCAA in 28 g BCAA commercial product) or the carbohydrate nutritional supplement (CHO; 14 g of a carbohydrate based nutritional supplement (POWERADE ®) prior to and following each workout, for a total of 28 g). Thus, subjects in both treatment groups received a 112-calorie dietary supplement at each supplementing time. Neither supplement contained any fat, while the BCAA contained no carbohydrate and the CHO contained only high fructose corn syrup and no protein or amino acids. Each subject was given a 4 week supply of their supplement with specific instructions on how to mix and when to consume. Subjects returned to the lab every 4 weeks to receive additional supplement. Subjects were prohibited from consuming any other nutritional supplements during the study.

Resistance training protocol
All subjects performed a progressive bodybuilding split style resistance-training program 4 days per week for the 8 week study duration. Subjects kept a training log during the training period and returned to the lab after 4 weeks

to have their training logs reviewed. Lack of compliance with the prescript protocol was grounds for dismissal from the study.

Statistical analysis
To determine the effects of the BCAA supplement on body composition and muscular strength, data were analyzed (SigmaSat 3.5) using a *priori* paired and unpaired t-tests to assess changes over time and between group means, respectively. Tukey's Test was used for post hoc analysis. Intraclass correlation coefficients (ICC) were performed to examine the test-retest reliability of the performance tests. The significance level was set at $\alpha = 0.05$. Data are expressed as means ± SE.

Results
Body mass did not change in the BCAA group, but the CHO group did see a significant ($p < 0.05$) reduction in body mass (−2.3 ± 0.7 kg) (see Table 2). Contributing to the change in total body mass was a significant ($p < 0.05$) loss in lean mass (−0.90 ± 0.06 kg) in the CHO group, while the BCAA group showed no change in lean mass. However, the BCAA group exhibited a significant ($p < 0.05$) decrease

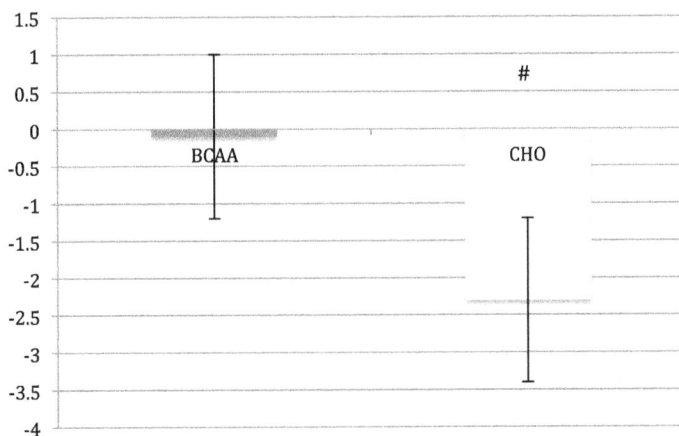

Fig. 2 Change in body mass following 8 week study period as determined by hydrostatic weighing. BCAA group received BCAA product (14 g prior/during each workout and 14 g post workout) while the control group received 28 g carbohydrate/electrolyte mixture at the same times. All subjects followed an individualized hypocaloric diet and resistance training program. # denotes significant difference ($p < 0.05$) within BCAA and CHO

Lean Body Mass Change

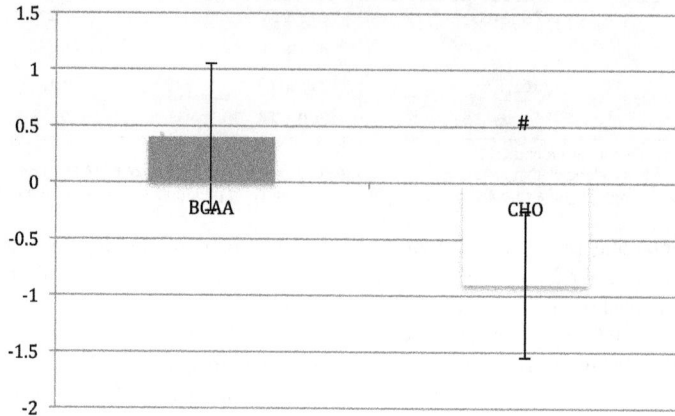

Fig. 3 Change in lean body mass following 8 week study period as determined by hydrostatic weighing. BCAA group received BCAA product (14 g prior/during each workout and 14 g post workout) while the control group received 28 g carbohydrate/electrolyte mixture at the same times. All subjects followed an individualized hypocaloric diet and resistance training program. # denotes significant difference (p < 0.05) within BCAA and CHO

in fat mass (-0.05 ± 0.08 kg) that was not observed in the CHO group (See Figs. 2, 3 and 4).

Both groups significantly ($p < 0.05$) increased lower body strength, but the change in the BCAA group (15.1 ± 2.2 kg) was significantly greater ($p < 0.05$) than the CHO group (4.8 ± 1.8 kg). The BCAA group also significantly increased upper body strength (7.1 ± 1.6 kg; $p < 0.05$), while the CHO group decreased strength (-3.7 ± 2.3 kg; $P < 0.05$), resulting in a significant difference between groups ($p < 0.01$). The CHO group exhibited an increase in repetitions to fatigue (5.3 ± 0.2; $p < 0.05$) on the squat exercise with no changes observed in the BCAA group. Neither group showed a significant change in repetitions to fatigue on the bench press (See Figs 5 and 6).

Finally, the BCAA group decreased RMR (-412 ± 67 kcal/day; $p < 0.05$) from pre to post observation, however this change was not different than the CHO group, who exhibited no change in RMR.

Discussion

The purpose of this study was to examine the effects of BCAA supplementation in conjunction with resistance training and a "cut diet" on indices of muscle performance (strength and endurance) and body composition (fat mass and lean mass) in healthy resistance-trained males. We

Fat Mass Change

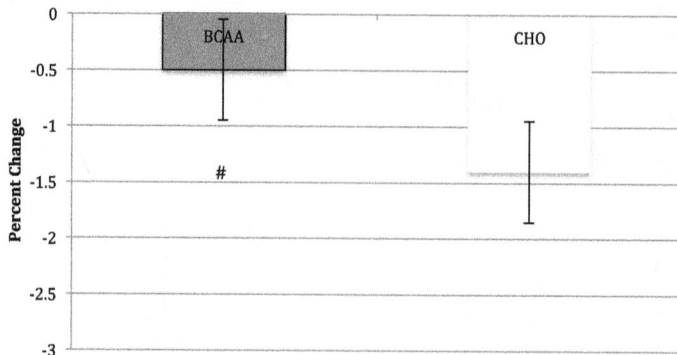

Fig. 4 Change in fat mass following 8 week study period as determined by hydrostatic weighing. BCAA group received BCAA product (14 g prior/during each workout and 14 g post workout) while the control group received 28 g carbohydrate/electrolyte mixture at the same time. All subjects followed an individualized hypocaloric diet and resistance training program. # denotes significant difference (p < 0.05) within BCAA and CHO

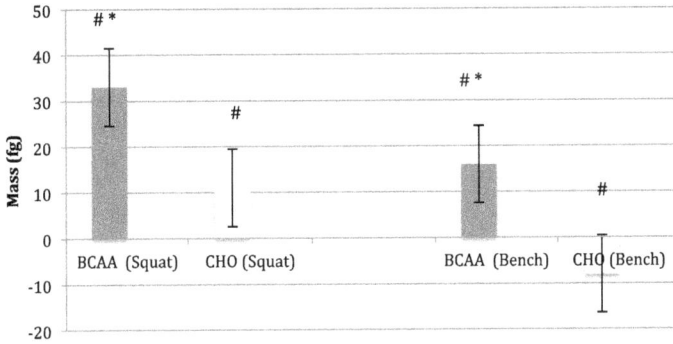

Fig. 5 Change in muscular strength following 8 week study period as determined by 3-RM back squat and bench press. BCAA group received BCAA product (14 g prior/during each workout and 14 g post workout) while the control group received 28 g carbohydrate/electrolyte mixture at the same time. All subjects followed an individualized hypocaloric diet and resistance training program. # denotes significant difference ($p < 0.05$) within BCAA and CHO * denotes significant difference ($p < 0.05$) between BCAA and CHO

hypothesized that a pre- and post-training dose of 14 g of a BCAA supplement would improve muscle performance and decrease fat mass while maintaining lean body mass in resistance-trained males. The findings of this study support our hypothesis, as we demonstrated that 8 weeks of BCAA supplementation, resistance training, and "cut diet" had a preferential positive effect on body composition and muscular performance, compared to a group who consumed carbohydrate instead of BCAA. The observed benefits of BCAA supplementation in conjunction with resistance training and caloric restriction are important for competitive weight class athletes, the aesthetic athlete, recreationally active adults, and others who aim to lose body fat and increase or maintain lean body mass for performance and/or health reasons.

Both BCAA and CHO groups engaged in identical, supervised resistance training programs, and received individualized hypocaloric carbohydrate restricted diets for a duration of 8 weeks. Therefore, changes seen in body composition and muscle performance were likely due to the treatment (BCAA) effects rather than training effects. This is important because protein supplements such as BCAA are relied upon within a variety of populations to maintain or improve muscle mass, aid in muscle recovery, and enhance athletic performance [1, 2]. Whereas there is ample evidence for the attenuation of lean mass during a cut diet in overweight and untrained populations [2, 18, 19], there is a paucity of studies utilizing the unique combination of a resistance training program, isolated BCAA supplement, and cut diet with which to compare our study. Therefore, the results of this study have

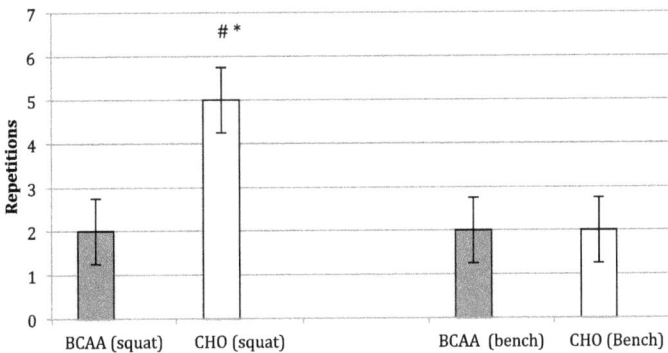

Fig. 6 Change in muscular endurance following 8 week study period as determined by repetitions to fatigue at 80 % of estimated 1-RM on back squat and bench press. BCAA group received BCAA product (14 g prior/during each workout and 14 g post workout) while the control group received 28 g carbohydrate/electrolyte mixture at the same time. All subjects followed an individualized hypocaloric diet and resistance training program. # denotes significant difference ($p < 0.05$) within BCAA and CNO * denotes significant difference ($p < 0.05$) between BCAA and CHO

important implications for expanding understanding for developing nutrition and exercise programs for both athletes and untrained individuals.

Body composition

Both the BCAA and CHO group exhibited changes in body composition, though the groups responded differently to the intervention. The loss in body mass in the CHO group was anticipated; as this is a typical outcome to reduced carbohydrate caloric restriction [20]. While there was a significant decrease in lean mass in the CHO group, there was not a loss of fat mass, though the trend ($p < 0.1$) was strong. This could potentially be due to the presence of high fructose corn syrup (HFCS) in the CHO supplement as HFCS, and other processed carbohydrates such as sucrose, have been associated with fat accumulation [21, 22]. However, it should be noted that the literate is not in agreement that HFCS consumption leads to fat accumulation [23]. The BCAA group showed no change in body mass, due to the maintenance of lean mass in the presence of a significant loss of fat mass. These results differ slightly from a similar study performed by Mourier et al. [24] who found that restricted calorie intake and BCAA supplementation among competitive male wrestlers exhibited a significant reduction in abdominal adipose tissue, compared to high protein, low protein, and control groups [24].

We anticipated that the BCAA group would maintain lean mass at the conclusion of the study, and as anticipated the BCAA group maintained lean body mass, compared to the CHO group who lost lean body mass. These results indicate the effectiveness of the BCAA supplement compared to the carbohydrate placebo at promoting lean mass maintenance. This finding is consistent with other studies that have reported enhanced skeletal muscle protein synthesis and lean muscle maintenance in response to exercise and BCAA supplementation [13, 25].

It is possible that the decreased lean mass in the CHO group can be attributed to a decrease in protein synthesis, due to a reduced calorie diet, coupled with a muscle-damaging resistance training program. It has been shown that BCAA supplementation enhances/promotes myofibrillar protein synthesis and aids in muscle recovery. Some researchers have found that BCAA supplementation post-exercise attenuated the decline in myofibrillar protein synthesis, which is vital in preserving lean mass during weight loss [8, 26]. Thus, the addition of BCAA supplements may have allowed for the maintenance of lean muscle mass because of its potential to enhance lean muscle protein synthesis.

Some studies have indicated a possible dose–response relationship regarding BCAA supplementation and body composition, including a study conducted by Spillane, Emerson, and Willoughby [27]. Subjects were provided

with 9 g/day of a BCAA supplement combined with 8 weeks of heavy resistance training, and found no preferential effect of BCAA supplementation on body composition [27]. However, Mourier et al. [24] found that a high daily dose of a BCAA supplement reduced body fat and spared lean mass in male athletes [22]. Similarly, the 26 g daily ingestion of BCAA product in our study had a beneficial effect of reduced fat mass and lean mass maintenance.

The preservation of lean mass is important for both athletic populations striving to improve athletic performance, and for older or sedentary populations at risk for obesity-related or age-onset obesity or sarcopenia and other age-related diseases [4, 6, 16]. Providing individuals with BCAA can stimulate myofibrillar protein synthesis and in turn preserve lean body mass. Our data suggests that BCAA supplementation may be effective in individuals attempting to lose fat mass while maintaining lean mass.

There is a paucity of studies investigating the use of BCAAs with a hypocaloric diet and resistance training, but some studies attempt to elucidate the connection between some aforementioned factors. In a study investigating a hypocaloric diet in conjunction with increased dietary protein intake, Mettler et al. [25] found that providing a higher percentage of daily caloric intake by protein (35 %) was more effective in maintaining lean body mass during a hypoenergetic diet than 15 % dietary protein intake [25]. However, these researchers sourced protein intake from dietary foods, rather than a supplement such as BCAA.

Coker et al. [2] found that essential amino acids supplementation was effective for preserving lean muscle mass even without exercise [2]. Researchers illustrated that the combination of a protein supplement (whey and essential amino acids) with a calorie restricted diet was more effective than a hypocaloric meal replacement control at concurrently reducing adipose tissue and preserving lean tissue during the caloric restriction-induced weight loss in elderly obese subjects [2]. Similarly, BCAA supplementation was found to provide a beneficial effect on body composition and isometric hand-grip strength, even without a concurrent exercise training protocol [28]. Researchers demonstrated that 30 days of ingesting 14 g of a BCAA supplement significantly lean mass and hand-grip strength in untrained males. However, no control group was provided for this study, making the conclusions as to whether the BCAA supplementation was predominant in improving lean mass and grip strength inconclusive [28].

Metabolism

Eight weeks of resistance training combined with a BCAA supplement and caloric restriction elicited a significant difference in RMR between BCAA and CHO groups, where the BCAA group decreased RMR and the CHO group showed no changes. The amount of lean tissue mass is essential in determining metabolic rate, where a greater amount of lean tissue increases RMR. Lean tissue is more metabolically active than fat tissue, and requires more energy at rest; thus increased energy expenditure can then decrease risk for chronic diseases such as metabolic disease, diabetes mellitus, and cardiovascular disease [6]. Therefore, the insignificant increase in lean mass in the BCAA group would not contribute to a significant change in RMR.

Muscle strength and endurance

Resistance training, provision of adequate amounts of dietary protein, and essential amino acids have all been shown to increase muscle protein synthesis in healthy adults [8], and this is essential to maintaining muscle fitness In this study, the BCAA supplement maintained lean mass while significantly improved participants' 1RM squat and 1RM bench press from pre-test and was more effective than the CHO group, indicating that BCAA supplementation was effective in developing muscular strength in trained subjects during caloric restriction. Similarly, Tsujimoto et al. [29] investigated the effects of BCAA on training volume following 5 weeks of resistance training and daily ingestion of BCAA and found that BCAA supplementation increased maximal strength in bench press and squat exercises [29].

However, a recent study by Spillane et al. [27] utilized a reduced daily dosage of BCAA supplement (9 g/day; 4.5 g pre- and post-exercise, compared to our 28 g per training day) combined with an 8 week resistance-training program [27]. Muscle strength increased with training, but no significant effects were evident between placebo and BCAA groups, indicating the lack of a treatment effect in the BCAA group. The results of this study suggest that there may be a dose–response relationship influencing the effectiveness of a BCAA supplement, where a greater dosage of BCAA induces greater performance benefits [29]. It is unlikely that the training duration of this study influenced results, as Tsujimoto et al. [29] found significant performance benefits with only 5 weeks of resistance training. Further, it may be that in a hypocaloric state the BCAA has a more robust effect [30].

It is difficult to explain the increase in repetitions to fatigue on the parallel squat in the CHO group, with no other changes being observed within or across groups. It was anticipated that on a hypocaloric diet, there would not be any gains in muscular endurance, given the glycolytic nature of the activity [30, 31]. It is possible that the CHO supplementation in the CHO group enhanced glycogen storage, which improved fatigue resistance and in turn resulted in increased repetitions to fatigue. However, our small sample size allows for robust changes in a few subjects to result in significant group improvements. We observed consistent and nearly uniform responses from subjects across the other measures of muscular performance, but in the repetitions to fatigue a couple subjects showed tremendous improvements, thus resulting in a significant group change. Additionally, with human performance testing it is possible these subjects did not perform to their maximal ability during pre-testing data collection for a variety of reasons (fatigue, distraction, lack of effort, etc.).

Though there remains controversy regarding the effectiveness of BCAA supplementation on muscle performance and body composition among both trained and untrained persons, there is a greater amount of consensus regarding the effects of BCAA supplements on muscle damage and recovery, which may in turn inform muscle performance (strength and endurance). Shimomoura et al. [12] found that oral ingestion of a BCAA supplement before or after exercise improved the recovery of damaged muscles by suppressing the endogenous muscle-protein breakdown during exercise (decreasing the release of essential amino acids from exercising muscles) [12]. This in turn may have implications in improved muscle performance and recovery. However Ra et al. [26] found that BCAA supplementation alone was not sufficient to inhibit muscle soreness and damage after a damaging bout of eccentric exercise [26].

Conclusions

The variability in experimental approaches adopted by researchers, and the factors investigated, such as the supplement quantity, treatment duration, timing of ingestion, training status and intensity, and dietary control, make direct comparisons of studies difficult. It is thus difficult to conclusively quantify the benefits of BCAA supplements across populations. However, our data suggest that under hypocaloric conditions, those who participate in heavy resistance training can maintain lean mass and muscular performance by utilizing a BCAA product pre and post workout. Further, while this protocol resulted in a loss of lean mass in the CHO group, the improvement in lower body strength and repetitions to fatigue suggest that minimal CHO supplementation on a cut diet may help to maintain some performance measures.

Competing interests
The authors declare that they have no competing interests.

Authors' contribution
TS designed the study, while data WD, EK and TS completed analysis, interpretation and manuscript preparation. All authors read and approved the final manuscript.

Acknowledgements

Heavy resistance training in combination with reduced caloric intake is a difficult challenge, thus the authors are grateful to our subjects for their cooperation and efforts. The authors would also like to thank Scivation Inc. for providing product and funding for this research. We also want to acknowledge Chuck Rudolf, R.D. for designing the diets for our subjects.

References

1. Verreijen AM, Verlaan S, Engberink MF, Swinkels S, de Vogel-van den Bosch J, Weijs PJ. A high whey protein-, leucine-, and vitamin D-enriched supplement preserves muscle mass during intentional weight loss in obese older adults: a double-blind randomized controlled trial. Am J Clin Nut. 2015;101(2):279–86.

2. Coker RH, Miller S, Schutzler S, Deutz N, Wolfe RR. Whey protein and essential amino acids promote the reduction of adipose tissue and increased muscle protein synthesis during caloric restriction-induced weight loss in elderly, obese individuals. Nut J. 2012;11:105.

3. Hass CJ, Geigenbaum MS, Franklin BA. Prescription of resistance training for healthy populations. Sport Med. 2001;31(14):953–64.

4. Mielke M, Housh TJ, Malek MH, Beck TW, Schmidt RJ, Johnson GO, et al. The effects of whey protein and leucine supplementation on strength, muscular endurance, and body composition during resistance training. J Ex Phys. 2009;12(5):39–50.

5. Kreider RB, Wilborn CD, Taylor L, Campbell B, Almada AL, Collins R, et al. ISSN exercise and sport nutrition review: research and recommendations. J Int Soc Sport Nut. 2010;7:7.

6. Winett RA, Phillips SM. Uncomplicated resistance training and health-related outcomes: Evidence for a public health mandate. Cur Sport Med Reports (ACSM). 2010;9(4):208–13.

7. Garthe, I., Taastad, T., Refsnes, P.E., Koivisto, A. & Sundgot-Borgen, J. Effect of two different weight loss rates on body composition and strength and power-related performance in elite athletes. Int J Sport Nut Ex Met. 2011; 21(2):91–104.

8. Howatson G, Hoad M, Goodall S, Tallent J, Bell PG, French DN. Exercise-induced muscle damage is reduced in resistance-trained males by branched chain amino acids: a randomized, double-blind, placebo controlled study. J Int Soc Sport Nut. 2012;9(1):20.

9. Evans WJ. Muscle damage: nutritional considerations. Int J Sport Nut. 1991;1(3):214–24.

10. Elashoff R, Li Z. A controlled trial of protein enrichment of meal replacements for weight reduction with retention of lean body mass. Nut J. 2008;7:23.

11. Lourad RJ, Barrett EJ, Gelfand RA. Effect of infused branched-chain amino acids on muscle and whole-body amino acid metabolism in men. Clin Sci. 1990;79:457–66.

12. Shimomoura Y, Inaguma A, Watanabe S, Yamamoto Y, Muramatsu Y, Bajotto G, et al. Branched-chain amino acid supplementation before squat exercise and delayed-onset muscle soreness. Int J Sport Nut Ex Met. 2010; 20:236–44.

13. Spillane M, Schwarz N, Willoughby DS. Heavy resistance training and peri-exercise ingestion of a multi-ingredient ergogenic nutritional supplement in males; effects on body composition, muscle performance and markers of muscle protein synthesis. J Sport Sci Med. 2012;13:894–903.

14. Norton LE, Layman DK. Leucine regulates translation initiation of protein synthesis in skeletal muscle after exercise. J Nut. 2006;136(2):533–7.

15. Burke, L.M. Branched Chain amino acids (BCAAs) and athletic performance. Int J Sport Med. 2001;2(3):1–7.

16. Lenz TL. Leucine with resistance training for the treatment of sarcopenia. Am J Lifestyle Med. 2010;4(4):317–9.

17. Dudgeon, W.D., Kelley, E.P. & Scheett, T.P. "Effect of Whey Protein in Conjunction with a Caloric-Restricted Diet and Resistance Training." J Str Cond Res, ePub ahead of Print, Post Acceptance: September 10, 2015

18. Bopp MJ, Houston DK, Lenchik L, Easter L, Kritcevsky SB, Nicklas BJ. Lean mass loss is associated with low protein intake during dietary-induced weight loss in postmenopausal women. J Am Diet Assoc. 2008;108(7):1216–20.

19. Treyzon L, Chen S, Hong K, Yan E, Carpenter CL, Thames G, et al. Effects of branched chain amino acids on training volume, fatigue sensation and muscle soreness in resistance training. Jap J Clin Sport Med. 2008;16(1):59–68.

20. Brehm BJ, Seeley RJ, Daniels SR, D'Alessio DA. A randomized trial comparing a very Low carbohydrate diet and a calorie-restricted Low Fat diet on body weight and cardiovascular risk factors in healthy women. J Clin Endo Met. 2003;88(4):1617–23.

21. Maersk M, Belza A, Stodkilde-Jorgensen H, Ringgaard S, Chabanova E, Thonsen H, et al. Sucrose-sweetened beverages increase fat storage in the liver, muscle, and visceral fat depot: a 6-mo randomized intervention study. Am J Clin Nut. 2012;95(2):283–9.

22. Bocarsly ME, Powell ES, Avena NM, Hoebel BG. High-fructose corn syrup causes characteristics of obesity in rats: Increase body weight, body fat and tryglyceride levels. Pharmacol Biochem Be. 2010;97(1):101–6.

23. Bravo S, Lowndes J, Sinnett S, Yu Z, Rippe J. Consumption of sucrose and high-fructose corn syrup does not increase liver fat or ectopic fat deposition in muscles. Appl Physiol Nutr Metab. 2013;38:681–8.

24. Mourier A, Bigard AX, de Kerviler E, Roger B, Legrand H, Guezennec CY. Combined effects of caloric restriction and branched-chain amino acid supplementation on body composition and exercise performance in elite wrestlers. Int J Sport Med. 1997;18:47–55.

25. Tipton KD, Mettler S, Mitchell N. Increased protein intake reduces lean body mass loss during weight loss in athletes. Med Sci Sport Ex. 2010;42(2):326–37.

26. Ra SG, Miyazaki T, Ishikura K, Nagayama H, Komine S, Nakata Y, et al. Combined effect of branched-chain amino acids and taurine supplementation on delayed onset muscle soreness and muscle damage in high-intensity eccentric exercise. J Int Soc Sport Nut. 2013;10:51.

27. Spillane M, Emerson C, Willoughby DS. The effects of 8 weeks of heavy resistance training and branched-chain amino acid supplementation on body composition and muscle performance. Nut & Health. 2012;21(4):263–73.

28. Candeloro N, Bertini I, Melchiorri G, De Lorenzo A. Effects of prolonged administration of branched-chain amino acids on body composition and physical fitness. Minerva Endocrin. 1995;20(4):217–23.

29. Tsujimoto H, Hamada K, Koba T, Matsumoto K, Mitsuzono R. Effects of branched chain amino acids on training volume, fatigue sensation and muscle soreness in resistance training. Jap J Clin Sport Med. 2008;16(1):59–68.

30. Lima-Silva AE, Pires FO, Bertuzzi R, Silva-Cavalcante MD, Oliveira RSF, Kiss MA, et al. Effects of a low-or a high-carbohydrate diet on performance, energy system contribution, and metabolic responses during supramaximal exercise. Appl Phys Nut Met. 2013;38(9):928–34.

31. Brinkworth GD, Noakes M, Clifton PM, Buckley JD. Effects of a low carbohydrate weight loss diet on exercise capacity and tolerance in obese subjects. Obesity J. 2009;17(10):1916–23.

## 18

The effects of phosphatidic acid supplementation on strength, body composition, muscular endurance, power, agility, and vertical jump in resistance trained men

Guillermo Escalante[1*], Michelle Alencar[2], Bryan Haddock[1] and Phillip Harvey[3,4]

Abstract

Background: Phosphatidic acid (PA) is a lipid messenger that has been shown to increase muscle protein synthesis via signaling stimulation of the mammalian target of rapamycin (mTOR). MaxxTOR® (MT) is a supplement that contains PA as the main active ingredient but also contains other synergistic mTOR signaling substances including L-Leucine, Beta-Hydroxy-Beta-Methylbutyrate (HMB), and Vitamin D3.

Methods: Eighteen healthy strength-trained males were randomly assigned to a group that either consumed MT ($n = 8$, 22.0 +/− 2.5 years; 175.8 +/− 11.5 cm; 80.3 +/− 15.1 kg) or a placebo (PLA) ($n = 10$, 25.6 +/− 4.2 years; 174.8 +/− 9.0 cm; 88.6 +/− 16.6 kg) as part of a double-blind, placebo controlled pre/post experimental design. All participants volunteered to complete the three day per week resistance training protocol for the eight week study duration. To determine the effects of MT, participants were tested on one repetition maximum (1RM) leg press strength (LP), 1RM bench press strength (BP), push-ups to failure (PU), vertical jump (VJ), pro-agility shuttle time (AG), peak power output (P), lean body mass (LBM), fat mass (FM), and thigh muscle mass (TMM). Subjects were placed and monitored on an isocaloric diet consisting of 25 protein, 50 carbohydrates, and 25 % fat by a registered dietitian. Separate two-way mixed factorial repeated measures ANOVA's (time [Pre, Post] x group [MT and PLA] were used to investigate strength, body composition, and other performance changes. Post-hoc tests were applied as appropriate. Analysis were performed via SPSS with significance at ($p \leq 0.05$).

Results: There was a significant main effect ($F_{(1,16)} = 33.30$, $p < 0.001$) for LBM where MT significantly increased LBM when compared to the PLA group ($p < 0.001$). Additionally, there was a significant main effect for LP ($F_{(1,16)} = 666.74$, $p < 0.001$) and BP ($F_{(1,16)} = 126.36$, $p < 0.001$) where both increased significantly more in MT than PLA group ($p < 0.001$). No significant differences between MT and PLA were noted for FM, TMM, VJ, AG, P, or PU.

Conclusion: The results of this eight week trial suggest that the addition of MaxxTOR® to a 3-day per week resistance training program can positively impact LBM and strength beyond the results found with exercise alone.

Keywords: Phospholipid, Muscle protein synthesis, Hypertrophy, Lean body mass, Fat mass

* Correspondence: gescalan@csusb.edu
[1]California State University- San Bernardino, 5500 University Parkway, San Bernardino, CA 92407, USA
Full list of author information is available at the end of the article

Background

Resistance training has been proven to help increase or maintain muscle mass as well as strength for various populations [1]. In an effort to safely maximize the effects of a resistance training program, researchers have investigated the effectiveness of utilizing sports supplements. Sports supplements such as creatine, branched-chain amino acids, and whey protein are among the most commonly researched topics in sports nutrition targeted to improve muscle mass, strength, and/or sports performance [2].

Phospholipids are another class of sports supplement that have been studied for their effect on athletic performance [3]. Phosphatidic acid (PA) is a phospholipid that makes up a small percentage of the phospholipid pool and is a compound formed by two fatty acids and a phosphate group that are covalently bonded to a glycerol molecule through ester linkages [4, 5]. PA is a precursor for the production of other lipids, it can act as a signaling lipid, and it is a major component of cell membranes. Recent research findings have demonstrated a link between PA and muscle protein synthesis [6–9]. A protein kinase known as the mammalian target of rapamycin (mTOR) has been recognized as a critical regulator of muscle protein synthesis [10–16]. Research findings have demonstrated that elevations in amino acids [10, 11], growth factors [12, 13], and energy status [14–16] can increase muscle protein synthesis through an mTOR dependent mechanism. While research has indicated that PA plays a critical role in mTOR signaling, the exact mechanism by which PA stimulates mTOR has not been confirmed. However, it is hypothesized that PA primarily works via direct binding to mTOR [6, 7].

Recent studies demonstrate that a mechanical stimulus, such as resistance training or passively stretching skeletal muscles, can create an increase in the intracellular levels of PA and that an increase in PA contributes to the activation of mTOR-dependent signaling events [7, 8]. It has also been demonstrated that exogenous sources of PA can promote the activation of mTOR signaling [9]. The results of these studies suggest that both mechanical stimuli and the exogenous addition of PA can stimulate mTOR signaling through different pathways that collectively may contribute to a larger effect of mTOR signaling.

Although there has been a significant amount of research performed at the molecular level on the effects of PA on mTOR signaling, more research is needed to fully confirm that mTOR signaling may be stimulated by PA. Conversely, only two studies have investigated the effects of PA supplementation with a resistance training program on human performance. Research performed by Hoffman et al. [17] investigated the efficacy of PA ingestion on lean body mass (LBM), muscle thickness, and

strength in resistance trained men. The authors concluded that the combination of ingesting 750 mg of PA daily during a resistance training program appear to increase strength and lean body mass more than those not taking the PA. Despite these positive findings, two weaknesses of this study were that the subjects were not supervised in their resistance training program and diet was not overseen throughout the study. A more recent study performed by Joy et al. [18] concluded that PA supplementation, as compared to receiving a placebo (PLA), led to significantly increased skeletal muscle hypertrophy, LBM, and maximal strength following a supervised 8-week resistance training program and a customized diet plan.

MT is a dietary supplement that contains 750 mg of PA as the main active ingredient but also contains other synergistic ingredients including L-Leucine, Beta-Hydroxy-Beta-Methylbutyrate (HMB) and Vitamin D3 to deliver mTOR signaling activation. L-Leucine is a branched-chain amino acid that has been shown to have the highest anabolic effect compared to other amino acids on activating protein synthesis and muscle cell growth while decreasing the rate of protein degradation in muscles [19–22]. L-Leucine has also been suggested to have a sparing effect on muscle glycogen and can lead to decreases in proton production [19–22]. HMB is a metabolite of L-Leucine and numerous studies have demonstrated that HMB supplementation combined with resistance training can increase protein synthesis, strength, and lean body mass [20, 23, 24]. It has been suggested that HMB can increase protein synthesis by supporting the integrity of muscle fibers, protecting critical contractile proteins, and improving recovery by attenuating exercise-induced damage in trained and untrained subjects [20, 23, 24]. Despite the positive results reported on the efficacy of HMB, there have also been some contradictory studies [25, 26]. In a review of HMB on exercise performance and body composition across varying levels of age, sex, and training experience, Wilson et al. [27] concluded that conflicting results may be attributed to the variability in humans, inadequate sample sizes, and methodological issues such as the specificity of testing conditions, cases of overtraining, an inadequate training stimulus in experienced participants, limited dependent variables, and short duration experiments. Furthermore, vitamin D3 has also been shown to play an important role on muscle mass and function by enhancing the stimulating effect of L-Leucine and insulin on protein synthesis [28].

The overall purpose of this investigation was to study the effects of the dietary supplement MT in conjunction with a 3-day per week total body resistance training program on muscular strength, muscular endurance, power(P), vertical jump (VJ), agility (AG), lean body mass (LBM), thigh muscle mass (TMM), and fat mass (FM) in resistance trained men.

Methods

Subjects

Initially, nineteen healthy, strength-trained male volunteers signed an informed consent form approved by the Institutional Review Board at California State University, San Bernardino and agreed to participate in this randomized, double-blind, placebo-controlled study. One subject voluntarily withdrew from the study due to time constraints. Eighteen participants completed the trial, where ten (25.6 ± 4.2 years, 174.8 ± 9.0 cm, 88.6 ± 16.6 kg) were randomly assigned to the PLA group and eight (22.0 ± 2.5 years, 175.8 ± 11.5 cm, 80.3 ± 15.1 kg) were randomly assigned to the MT group. The protocol and subject inclusion/exclusion criteria were similar to the study performed by Joy et al. (18).

All participants were required to abstain from consuming any muscle-building supplements (e.g., creatine) for at least 1 month prior to pretest measures, abstain from training outside of the prescribed protocol during the study, be non-smokers, have resistance training experience of no less than one year, and have participated in resistance training at least three days per week for the past six months to be included in this study. Additionally, participants had to be free of any injuries or medical conditions that would prohibit them from participating in a resistance training program. Measures of 1 repetition maximum (1RM) LP, 1RM BP, LBM, FM, TMM, PU, AG, VJ, and P were taken within 7 days prior to, and within 7 days following, the resistance training/supplementation protocol. All resistance training sessions were supervised by certified personal trainers and took place three days per week with 48–72 h between resistance training sessions. Each body part was trained 1–2 times per week following a daily undulating periodization protocol (Table 1). Each participant performed a 5RM for each exercise prior to the first four weeks with the exception of the BP and LP, in which true 1RM values were determined. Five repetition maximum testing was repeated at the end of week 4 for the new exercises.

Strength testing and training

Strength testing and training followed the protocol performed by Joy et al. (18). The 1-RM testing protocol consisted of 1 set of 10–12 repetitions at approximately 50 % 1-RM followed by 1 set of 2–3 repetitions at approximate intensities of 75 and 85 % 1RM. After the final warm-up set, weight was increased in 5–20 lb increments until a 1-RM was attained. Five repetition maximum testing followed an identical pattern; however, intensities were relative to a 5-RM instead of a 1-RM. These RM values were used to calculate the load used

for each exercise for each participant. Training exercises (Table 1) were altered at week 5 to introduce a more novel stimulus. All participants were required to perform a set number of repetitions with their prescribed training load. In the event that a subject reached muscular failure, a certified personal trainer assisted with the completion of the exercise. Strength was assessed via 1RM testing of the LP and BP. In order for a repetition to count as a successful attempt in the leg press, the participant had to reach an angle of 90° at their knee joints as agreed upon unanimously by 3 trained research assistants. In order for a repetition to count as a successful attempt in the bench press, the participant had to touch the barbell to their chest at the bottom of the movement and lock out their arms at the top of the movement as agreed upon unanimously by 3 trained research assistants. Testing for LP and BP strength took place on one day for each subject.

Lean body mass, Fat mass, and thigh muscle mass assessment

A total body DXA (Prodigy™; Lunar Corporation, Madison, WI) scan was performed to measure total body composition as described by Maden-Wilkinsen et al. [29]. Participants laid supine on the scanning bed. The GE Lunar Prodigy computer software was used to provide estimations of total LBM and FM [29]. After total LBM and FM were computed and documented, each participant's dominant thigh was identified as a region of interest using previously reported borders from the femoral neck to the knee joint [29] to determine TMM. Lean mass, FM, and bone mineral content were estimated from the selected region of interest. All DXA analyses were performed by a single certified technician and quality assurance was performed per the manufacturer instructions. In estimating lean mass the typical DXA machine includes not just muscle mass but also connective tissue and the non-mineral components of bone [29]. Bone mineral content (BMC) accounts for approximately 55 % of total bone mass with the rest being made up by protein and water [29]. For this reason, an adjusted lean mass was calculated as follows [29]: Lean mass = total mass - fat mass - (1.82 * BMC). DXA also includes non-adipose components of fat tissue, such as protein, in the lean mass but the contribution this makes is unclear. Hence, no further adjustments were applied [29]. Thigh muscle mass hypertrophy was determined via changes in adjusted thigh lean mass of the dominant thigh as reported by the DXA. Testing for body composition and TMM took place prior to strength testing on the same day.

Vertical jump assessment

Vertical jump (VJ) was assessed by using a Vertec (Vertec2, Sports Imports, Columbus, OH, USA). The participant's

Table 1 Eight-week resistance training protocol

Monday Week 1–4	Monday Week 5–8	Wednesday Week 1–4	Wednesday Week 5–8	Friday Week 1–4	Friday Week 5–8		Monday & Wednesday Repetitions	Friday Repetitions	Monday & Wednesday Rest	Friday Rest
Leg Press	Leg Press	Bent Over Row	Pendlay Rows	Leg Press	Leg Press	Week 1	12	5	45 s	3–5 m
Leg Extension	Safety Bar Squat	Barbell Shrug	Hexbar Shrug	Bench Press	Bench Press	Week 2	10	3	60 s	3–5 m
Leg Curl	Barbell Lunge	Straight Arm Pull Down	Pulldown	Leg Extension	Safety Bar Squat	Week 3	8	2	90 s	3–5 m
Hyperextension	Stiff Leg Deadlift	Australian Row	Decline DB Row	Close Grip Press	Flat DB Press	Week 4	6	1	120 s	3–5 m
Bench Press	Bench Press	Barbell Shoulder Press	DB Shoulder Press			Week 5	12	5	60 s	3–5 m
Incline DB Press	Flat DB Press	Isolated Barbell Military	Upright Row			Week 6	10	3	60 s	3–5 m
Close Grip Bench Press	Cable Cross Over	DB Lateral Raise	Barbell Front Raise			Week 7	8	2	90 s	3–5 m
Cable Rope Extensions	Skull Crusher	DB Bicep Curls	Barbell Bicep Curl			Week 8	6	1	120 s	3–5 m

reach height was measured and recorded by first adjusting the height of the Vertec plastic vanes to be within the subject's reach [30]. The participant stood directly beneath the Vertec and reached as high as possible with their dominant hand without lifting the heels from the floor and touched the highest vane possible [30]. After initial familiarization with the procedures and the Vertec apparatus, the subject warmed-up at a self-selected resistance on a stationary bicycle for five minutes and was allowed to perform several trials of the counter jump procedure with the Vertec [30]. The subjects were instructed to not take any lead-up steps prior to the jump but were allowed to perform a rapid countermovement by quickly descending into a squat while swinging the arms down and back [30]. The rapid countermovement was immediately followed by a maximal jump in which the dominant hand reached to touch the highest possible Vertec vane [30]. Three trials were allowed and the highest was recorded [30]. The vertical jump height recorded was the difference between the highest jump and the reach height [30]. Testing for the VJ took place the day prior to strength testing.

Agility assessment

Agility (AG) was assessed with the pro-agility shuttle [30]. Timing gates (Swift Performance, Speedlight V2 wireless timing system, Walco, Australia) were set up five yards apart and the participant started from the middle timing gate; an upright stance was used and the subject faced forward [30]. The timing gate device randomly sent out a beep to signal the subject to start the agility assessment while simultaneously starting the timer. Upon hearing the beep, the subject turned to the left and sprinted for 5 yards; then turned to the right and sprinted for 10 yards and finally turned back to the left and sprinted for five yards back to the starting point [30]. The lines marking the distance of the timing gates, which were set up with athletic tape on the floor, had to be contacted by each foot [30]. Three trials were performed for the pre-test and post-test and the fastest time was recorded; three minutes of rest was provided between each trial [30]. Testing for AG took place approximately three minutes after VJ assessment was performed.

Muscular endurance

Muscular endurance was assessed with the subject performing standard push-ups (PU) to failure the feet on the floor and the hands shoulder width apart [30]. The starting position was the bottom position of the push-up with the area of the body from the chest to the thighs making contact with the floor [30]. The participant pushed themselves up from the bottom position with the body straight such that a line could be drawn from the shoulder joint to the ankle joint [30]. The participant then lowered their body back to the starting position

and repeated the pattern [30]. The participant continued to exercise at a comfortable rate of 20–30 repetitions per minute until no more PU could be performed with correct form [30]. A push up was counted by a trained research assistant when the participant was in the up position; no resting was allowed between repetitions [30]. Testing for muscular endurance took place approximately three minutes after AG assessment was performed.

Power assessment

Power (P) output was recorded in real time with a Monark cycle ergometer (Monark model 828E, Vansbro, Sweden) that was connected to the Monark Anaerobic test software (Monark 828E Analysis Software 3.0, Monark, Vansbro, Sweden). During the cycling test, the participant was instructed to cycle against a predetermined resistance (7.5 % of body weight) as fast as possible for 10 s [31]. The saddle height was adjusted to the individual's height to produce approximately 10° knee flexion while the foot was in the low position of the central void. A standardized verbal stimulus was provided to the subject. Power output testing took place approximately three minutes after muscular endurance was assessed.

Dietary/Supplement supervision

Prior to the study, participants were required to watch a video made by a registered dietitian specializing in sports nutrition discussing their diet protocols, the diet recording/reporting protocol, and emphasizing the importance of adherence to the diet plan. Two weeks prior to the start of training each participant was provided with an individual meal plan, designed by the dietitian. This meal plan was to be followed throughout the study. Daily caloric need for each participant was estimated via the Harris Benedict equation and was designed to be iso-caloric in nature by adding 55 % more calories to their resting metabolic rate estimation in order to compensate for their moderate activity level of strength training three days per week. The diet consisted of 25 % protein, 50 % carbohydrates, and 25 % fat. Although a sample meal plan was provided for each subject, the dietitian explained in the video that participants could choose any foods they desired as long as the final calorie count and macronutrient breakdown was within the guidelines provided. After the video was watched by the participants, the registered dietitian and principal investigator oversaw the diet logs of the participants throughout the study. All participants were instructed to use the smartphone app MyFitnessPal® to record their nutritional intake and to submit a weekly summary of their diet logs from the MyFitnessPal® website via an email to ensure compliance. Subjects not familiar with the mobile app were instructed by the research team on how to utilize it, but twelve of the eighteen subjects had used this app prior to this study. The use of mobile apps for dietary self-reporting has been previously used in research [32]. The MyFitnessPal® app is a database comprised of over 5 million foods that have been provided by users via entering data manually or by scanning the bar code on packaged goods. Thus, the data themselves are primarily derived from food labels (i.e., Nutrition Facts Panel) derived from the USDA National Nutrient database. The breakdown of dietary intake over the course of the study can be found in the results section.

In addition to the recommended food intake, the MT group received 5 capsules of MT per day per day while the PLA group received 750 mg of rice flour, each delivered in 5 visually identical capsules. A single production lot of both MT and PLA supplements were manufactured in a facility compliant with current Good Manufacturing Practices (cGMP) for dietary supplements (21 CFR 111). Phosphatidic acid purity and potency were analyzed by an ultra-performance liquid chromatograph with triple quadrupole mass spectrometry (LC/MS/MS) methods (Avanti Polar Lipids, Inc., Alabaster, AL). Purity and potency of L-Leucine, HMB and vitamin D3 were analyzed by High Pressure Liquid Chromatography (HPLC) at Micro Quality Laboratories, Inc, Burbank, CA. On resistance training days, participants consumed 3 capsules of their respective supplement 30 min prior to resistance training and 2 capsules immediately following resistance training along with 24 g of hydrolyzed collagen protein powder from beef skin (Peptiplus XB agglomerated, Gelita AG, Eberbach, Germany) mixed with 500 ml water. The protein supplement was provided by the researchers in order to ensure control for post-exercise meals between groups. Furthermore, hydrolyzed collagen protein was chosen as it is an incomplete protein source low in leucine in order to potentially minimize the impact the supplement being studied. On non-resistance training days, participants consumed 3 of their respective supplement pills with breakfast and 2 pills with dinner. In order to ensure compliance, participants were required to return to the laboratory with their empty containers 3 weeks after starting the study in order to receive their next bottle of supplements. Three weeks later, they were required to return to the laboratory again before they received their last bottle of the supplement. Since the dietician/principal investigator had weekly interaction with the participants via email, all participants were monitored for compliance throughout the study. Each subject turned in empty bottles at the designated times and reported taking the supplement as directed.

Product formulations were blinded and coded to both the investigators and the participants so that neither knew which formulation was consumed during the study. Each participant randomly selected a 4 digit participant code that corresponded to a code on their respective bottles. The research team recorded the code on each bottle for each participant; however, the key for each code that determined whether the bottle contained MT or PLA was revealed to the researchers after all the data was collected at the end of the study. Each participant was provided with their supplement bottle (PLA or MT) for 3 weeks on the first Monday and every third Monday thereafter.

Statistical analysis

Separate two-way mixed factorial Repeated Measures Analysis of Variance (time [Pre, Post] x group [MT and PLA] were used to investigate body composition changes (LBM, FM, TMM), strength changes (BP, LP), and other performance changes (PU, P, VJ, and AG). When significant main effects were found, a Tukey post-hoc was conducted to determine where the differences occurred. Data is presented as mean ± standard deviation. All analyses were performed using SPSS version 22 (SPSS, Inc., Chicago, IL). An alpha level was set at $p \leq 0.05$.

Results

There were no significant differences between the MT or the PLA group for any baseline measurement (Table 2). The weekly nutrition logs turned in by the participants to the principal investigator on a weekly basis throughout the study also showed no significant differences in calories consumed (MT: 2709.0 +/− 357.0 Cal vs PLA: 2681.7 +/− 277.8 Cal), carbohydrates consumed (MT: 320.4 +/− 47.8 g vs PLA: 325.9 +/− 34.3 g), protein consumed (MT: 166.5 +/− 22.9 g vs PLA: 158.0 +/− 27.8 g), and fat consumed (MT: 84.7 +/− 26.5 g vs PLA: 82.9 +/− 14.3 g). There was a significant group x time interaction for LBM ($F_{(1,16)} = 33.30$, $p = 0.041$) where the MT group increased LBM to a greater extent (pre: 60.8 ± 9.5 kg; post: 62.7 ± 10.2 kg) when compared to the PLA group (pre: 61.2 ± 9.7 kg; post: 62.0 ± 9.7 kg) (Fig. 1). There was a significant

Table 2 Body composition, strength, and performance baseline measurements

Variable	MT group	PLA group
Lean Body Mass (LBM)	60.8 ± 9.5 kg	61.2 ± 9.7 kg
Fat Mass (FM)	16.6 ± 7.2 kg	23.9 ± 8.1 kg
Thigh Muscle Mass (TMM)	6.43 ± 1.10 kg	6.41 ± 1.45 kg
1-RM Leg Press (LP)	292.6 ± 60.5 kg	306.8 ± 62.5 kg
1-RM Bench Press (BP)	92.0 ± 18.1 kg	98.6 ± 26.5 kg
Power (P)	897.6 ± 178.3 W	854.3 ± 238.7 W
Agility (AG)	5.16 ± 0.34 s	5.45 ± 0.35 s
Vertical Jump (VJ)	62.6 ± 11.1 cm	56.6 ± 10.2 cm
Push-Ups (PU)	31.9 ± 7.6	30 ± 7.2

Data presented as Mean +/− SD. n = 8 for MT and n = 10 for PLA

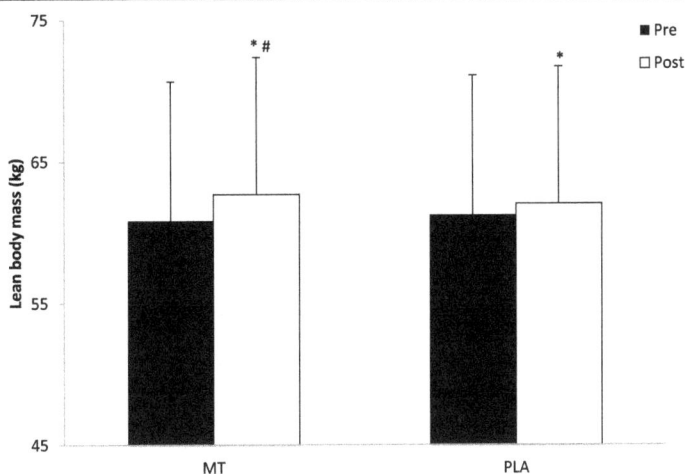

Fig. 1 Changes in Lean Body Mass. All data are reported as mean +/− SD (*denotes significantly different from pre, # denotes significantly different from PLA)

time effect for FM ($F_{(1,16)}$ = 8.64, p = 0.010) where the MT group (pre: 16.6 ± 7.2 kg; post: 15.1 ± 7.8 kg) tended to lose more FM than the PLA group (pre: 23.9 ± 8.1 kg; post: 23.4 ± 8.3 kg) (Fig. 2). Furthermore, there was a significant time effect for TMM ($F_{(1,16)}$ = 5.652, p = 0.030) where the MT group (pre: 6.43 ± 1.10 kg; post: 6.69 ± 1.13 kg) and the PLA group (pre: 6.41 ± 1.45 kg; post: 6.58 ± 1.35 kg) both gained TMM (Fig. 3). Pre versus post individual changes in body weight, body fat percentage, LBM, and FM further illustrate the changes observed in body composition over the course of the study (Table 3).

Pre to post changes in muscle strength were seen in both 1-RM LP and 1-RM BP. There was a significant group x time interaction ($F_{(1,16)}$ = 74.28, p < 0.001) for 1-RM LP where the MT group increased leg strength significantly greater (pre: 292.6 ± 60.5 kg; post: 350. 9 ± 66.9 kg) than the PLA group (pre: 306.8 ± 62. 5 kg; post: 335.9 ± 59.9 kg). Similarly, there was a significant group x time interaction ($F_{(1,16)}$ = 18.69, p < 0.001) for the BP where the MT group increased 1-RM BP significantly greater (pre: 92.0 ± 18.1 kg; post: 107.4 ± 18.6 kg) than the PLA group (pre: 98.6 ± 26.5 kg; post: 105. 5 ±

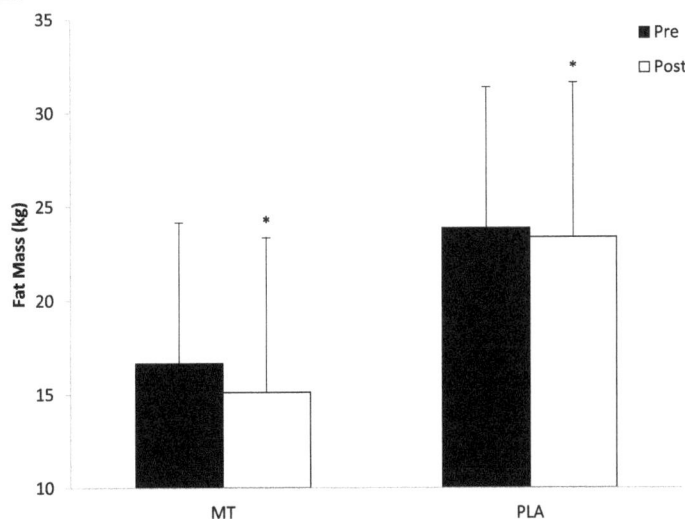

Fig. 2 Changes in Fat Mass. All data are reported as mean +/− SD (*denotes significantly different from pre, # denotes significantly different from PLA)

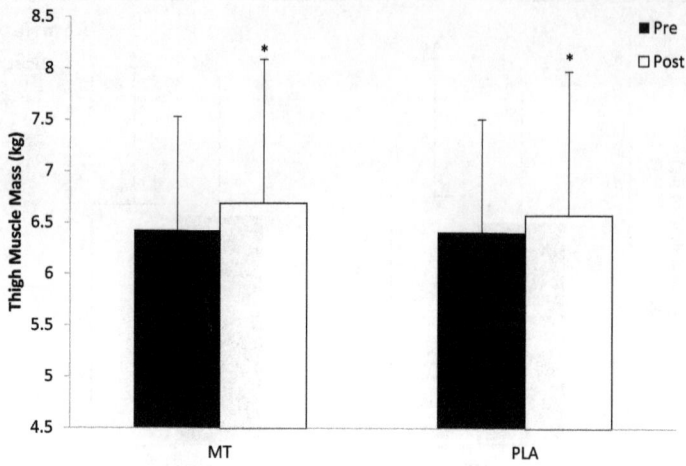

Fig. 3 Changes in Thigh Muscle Mass. All data are reported as mean +/– SD (*denotes significantly different from pre, # denotes significantly different from PLA)

Table 3 Individual changes in body weight, body fat percentage, LBM and FM

	Bodyweight (Kg)		Body Fat %		LBM (Kg)		FM (Kg)	
	Pre	Post	Pre	Post	Pre	Post	Pre	Post
MT								
1	74.6	74.6	24.2	20.9	54.1	56.7	17.3	15.0
2	80.0	80.1	19.1	16.9	62.0	63.6	14.6	12.9
3	60.1	59.6	19.8	18.7	45.8	46.5	11.3	10.7
4	111.3	113.6	30.8	30.2	75.4	77.2	33.6	33.3
5	86.5	82.5	20.6	15.3	66.3	67.2	17.2	12.2
6	70.0	69.6	17.1	12.5	56.2	58.1	11.6	8.3
7	75.0	77.7	21.1	23	56.7	57.4	15.1	17.1
8	85.30	88.6	15	13.2	70.0	74.7	12.4	11.4
MT Mean +/– SD	80.3 +/– 15.1	80.8 +/– 15.9	21.0 +/– 4.8	18.8 +/– 5.8	60.8 +/– 9.5	62.7 +/– 10.2	16.6 +/– 7.2	15.1 +/– 7.8
PLA								
1	93.4	93.6	27.1	25.2	65.3	67.2	24.3	22.6
2	78.1	80.0	26.7	26.4	55.2	56.8	20.1	20.4
3	70.0	69.6	24.3	23.6	51.0	51.1	16.4	15.8
4	81.4	81.8	27.9	27.0	56.7	57.7	21.9	21.4
5	69.6	70.0	26.9	26.0	49.1	50.1	18.1	17.6
6	108.9	110.0	34.4	34.1	68.5	69.8	36.1	36.1
7	86.4	85.9	20.1	19.6	66.0	66.0	16.6	16.1
8	80.2	79.1	21.6	20.2	59.7	59.9	16.4	15.2
9	120.0	120.5	29.1	28.5	81.9	82.6	33.1	32.9
10	98.6	99.1	37.8	37.5	58.7	59.3	35.7	35.6
PLA Mean +/– SD	88.6 +/– 16.6	89.0 +/– 16.8	27.6 +/– 5.3	26.8 +/– 5.6	61.2 +/– 9.7	62.0 +/– 9.7	23.9 +/– 8.1	23.4 +/– 8.3

26.1 kg). Strength changes for the LP and BP can be seen in Figs. 4 and 5, respectively.

Pre to post changes in performance measures were seen between the MT and PLA groups. There was a significant effect for time ($F_{(1,16)} = 43.96$, $p < 0.001$) for PU in the MT group (pre: 31.9 ± 7.6; post: 37.4 ± 7.4) and PLA group (pre: 30 ± 7.2; post 34.8 ± 6.3) where the MT group and the PLA group both performed more PU. Similarly, there was a significant effect for time ($F_{(1,16)} = 20.69$, $p < 0.001$) for P in the MT group (pre: 897.6 ± 178.3 W; post: 989.5 ± 180.0 W) and the PLA group (pre: 854.3 ± 238.7 W; post: 903.6 ± 231.0 W) where MT group tended to produce more P than the PLA group. There were no significant interactions for AG or VJ between groups. Performance changes can be seen in Table 4.

Discussion

The current study investigates the effects of PA on body composition, strength, muscle endurance, AG, P, and VJ in resistance trained males. This study supports the evidence provided by previous researchers [17, 18]. Similar to the studies performed by Hoffman et al. [17] and Joy et al. [18], this investigation provided 750 mg of PA to the experimental group or an identical looking PLA to the PLA group on a daily basis. Also similar to the design of previous researchers [17, 18], each participant received a collagen based protein drink after every workout. In comparison to the first two studies, the supplement (MT) provided to the experimental group in this study had an added proprietary blend of L-Leucine, HMB, and Vitamin D3 to the 750 mg of PA. Furthermore, this investigation examined more fitness parameters including assessments in VJ, AG, and muscular endurance. Table 5 provides a summary of the comparison of the studies on the effects of MT versus PA alone on strength, body composition, thigh hypertrophy, and power.

The effects of PA on strength was reported in this study as well as in previous investigations [17, 18]. In comparison to previous studies on PA [17, 18], significant changes in 1-RM BP were only reported in this study. Although Joy et al. [18] also reported an increase in both the PA and PLA groups in 1-RM BP, the observed differences were not significant ($p = 0.11$). Similarly, Hoffman et al. [17] reported that that the magnitude based inferences were unclear regarding any benefit in upper body strength improvements in those participants consuming the PA. Conversely, the effects of PA on leg strength in this study was similar to that reported by previous researchers [17, 18] where all three studies demonstrated an improvement in lower body strength. Although Hoffman et al. [17] reported that the observed changes lacked a significant group x time interaction between the PA and PLA groups ($p = 0.19$) in their investigation, they stated that the magnitude based inferences on changes observed in 1-RM squat suggest a likely benefit from PA on increasing lower body strength. Similarly, all studies demonstrated an increase in total strength, which was defined by Joy et al. [18] as the sum of 1-RM BP and 1-RM leg strength test.

The effects of PA on body composition was also reported in all three investigations. In comparing the effects of PA on LBM between the three studies, positive significant changes were reported in this investigation as well as in the study performed by Joy et al. [18]. Although Hoffman et al. [17] reported a significant main effect ($p = 0.045$) for LBM, the increase in LBM in the

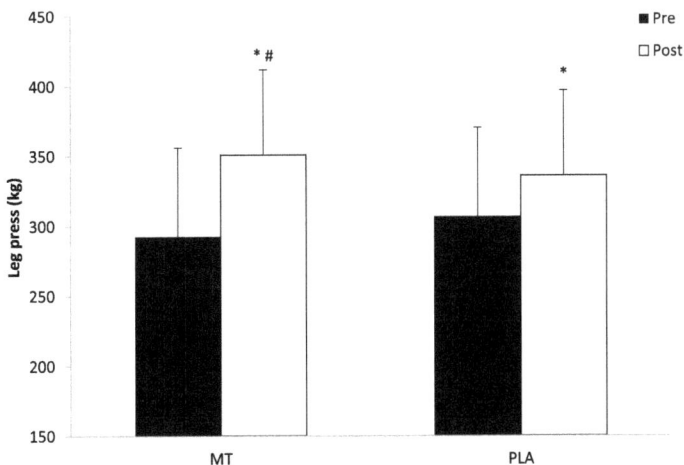

Fig. 4 Changes in Leg Press Strength. All data are reported as mean +/- SD (*denotes significantly different from pre, # denotes significantly different from PLA)

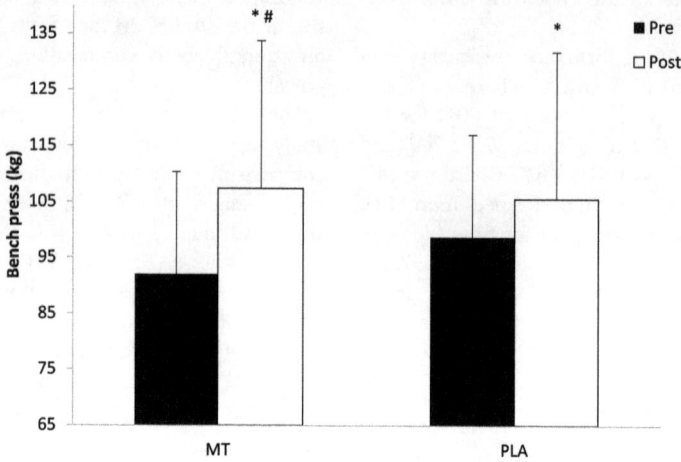

Fig. 5 Changes in Bench Press Strength. All data are reported as mean +/− SD (*denotes significantly different from pre, # denotes significantly different from PLA)

PA group was only reported as a trend ($p = 0.065$) towards significant interaction. The effects of PA on FM was also investigated in all three studies; however, it should be noted that none of the investigations were designed to maximize fat loss as evidenced by the exercise prescription as well as the iso-caloric diet the participants followed. The present study and the study performed by Joy et al. [18] both demonstrated a significant time effect for the PA group and the PLA groups, but the investigation performed by Hoffman et al. [17] reported no significant time effect ($p = 0.95$) or group x time interaction ($p = 0.99$) for changes in FM for the PA or PLA groups.

The effects of PA on thigh hypertrophy also varied between this study and that reported by previous researchers [17, 18]. Part of this variability is likely contributed to the different assessment tools and/or methods used to quantify thigh hypertrophy. The study performed by Hoffman et al. [17] used ultrasonography measurements to measure vastus lateralis fascicle thickness by determining the distance between the subcutaneous adipose tissue and intermuscular interface. Although Joy et al. [18] also used an ultrasound device to measure changes in quadriceps hypertrophy, rectus

femoris cross sectional area was measured as opposed to vastus lateralis thickness. In this investigation, thigh hypertrophy was measured by determining TMM utilizing a DXA machine where the participant's dominant thigh region was identified as a region of interest. The current study and the study performed by Hoffman et al. [17] demonstrated only a time effect for both the PA and PLA groups for thigh hypertrophy. Conversely, the study performed by Joy et al. [18] reported a 22.2 % increase in rectus femoris cross sectional area for the PA group that was significantly greater ($p = 0.02$) than the 13.3 % increase in rectus femoris cross sectional area for the PLA group.

In comparing the effects of PA on P, the results of this investigation were also different than those reported by Joy et al. [18]. Although no significant group x time interactions for P were observed in this study or in the study performed by Joy et al. [18], it should be noted that P increased by 4.2 % more in the MT group as compared to the PLA group in this investigation and that P increased by 0.5 % more in the PLA group as compared to the PA group in the study performed by Joy et al. [18]. Hoffman et al. [17] did not evaluate the effects of PA on P.

Table 4 Changes in performance variables

Performance Variable	MT Group		PLA Group	
	PRE	POST	PRE	POST
Power (P)	897.6 ± 178.3 W	989.5 ± 180.0 W[a]	854.3 ± 238.7 W	903.6 ± 231.0 W[a]
Agility (AG)	5.16 +/− 0.34 s	5.03 +/− 0.39	5.45 +/− 0.35 s	5.31 +/− 0.53
Vertical Jump (VJ)	62.6 +/− 11.1 cm	63.4 +/− 8.6 cm	56.6 +/− 10.2 cm	58.0 +/− 7.2 cm
Push-Ups (PU)	31.9 ± 7.6	37.4 ± 7.4[a]	30 ± 7.2	34.8 ± 6.3[a]

Data are presented as mean +/− SD. $n = 8$ for MT and $n = 10$ for PLA ([a] denotes significant time effect)

Table 5 Comparison on the effects of MT vs PA alone on strength, body composition, and power

Variable	Current Study (Supplement = MT)		Joy et al. (2014) (Supplement = PA only)		Hoffman et al. (2012) (Supplement = PA only)	
	MT % Change	PLA % Change	PA % Change	PLA % Change	PA % Change	PLA % Change
Bench Strength	16.7 % ↑	7.0 % ↑	7.1 % ↑	5.1 % ↑	5.1 % ↑	3.3 % ↑
Leg Strength	19.7 % ↑	9.1 % ↑	22.7 % ↑	14.3 % ↑	12.7 % ↑	9.3 % ↑
Total Strength	19.1 % ↑	8.7 % ↑	18 % ↑	11.7 % ↑	9.1 % ↑	6.6 % ↑
Lean Body Mass	3.1 % ↑	1.4 % ↑	4.0 % ↑	2.0 % ↑	2.6 % ↑	0.1 % ↑
Fat Mass	9.2 % ↓	2.1 % ↓	8.6 % ↓	3.8 % ↓	0 %	0 %
Thigh Hypertrophy	4.0 % ↑	2.7 % ↑	22.2 % ↑	13.3 % ↑	14.8 % ↑	15.5 % ↑
Power	10.2 % ↑	5.8 % ↑	8.2 % ↑	8.7 % ↑	NA	NA

Data are presented as % change between pre and post for the experimental group and placebo group for each variable

This investigation also examined more variables than previous researchers [17, 18]. Although the improvements in these variables with MT appear to be higher than in PLA, they did not reach statistical significance. The lack of significance observed in the performance variables may be largely contributed to the lack of specificity of training in the prescribed training protocol. Since the training protocol prescribed to the participants was a resistance program to gain strength/hypertrophy, these were the variables that were improved by PA.

Some of the more robust effects found in the present study as compared to previous studies [17, 18] could be attributed to the added proprietary blend of L-Leucine, HMB, and vitamin D3 that was provided to the experimental group in addition to the PA. Evidence has demonstrated that if essential amino acids or protein are ingested before or after a workout, the effect of muscle protein synthesis may be magnified [33]. L-Leucine alone has been suggested as an effective supplement in stimulating muscle protein synthesis, even if administered in low dosages [34].

Similar to L-Leucine, an L-Leucine metabolite known as HMB has been shown to stimulate muscle protein synthesis to a similar extent as L-Leucine [20]. HMB has also been found to decrease muscle protein breakdown [20, 24]. In a study performed by Wilkinson et al. [20] investigating the effects of L-Leucine and HMB on human skeletal muscle protein anabolism, it was demonstrated that orally consumed HMB showed fast bioavailability in plasma and muscle and, similarly to L-Leucine, stimulated muscle protein synthesis (+70 % for HMB vs. +110 % for L-Leucine). The study also reported that HMB and L-Leucine both increased mTOR signaling; however, this was more pronounced with Leucine [20]. HMB consumption also reduced muscle protein breakdown by 57 % in an insulin-independent manner [20].

The addition of vitamin D3 to the active ingredient in this study could also potentially contribute to some of the findings. Although systemic review articles have concluded there are conflicting findings on the effect of vitamin D3 on strength [35, 36], it has been suggested that sports dietitians and physicians routinely assess vitamin D status and make recommendations to help athletes achieve a serum 25 (OH) D concentration of $\geq$ 32 and preferably $\geq$ 40 ng·mL [37] as vitamin D3 may improve athletic performance in vitamin D-deficient athletes [38]. Although most studies have looked at the effects of vitamin D3 in the elderly, a study performed on vitamin D3 deficient healthy young adults reported a significant difference between treatment and control groups in grip strength ($p < 0.001$) and calf strength ($p = 0.04$) [39].

Collectively, it is probable that the combination of PA, L-Leucine, HMB, and vitamin D3 used as the active ingredients in this study work synergistically in order to improve LBM and strength beyond the impact of the training program itself. A study recently reported that vitamin D3 has been shown enhance the stimulating effect of L-Leucine and insulin on protein synthesis [28]. Similarly, another study postulated that L-Leucine and HMB enhance muscle anabolism by increasing muscle protein synthesis and reducing muscle protein breakdown through either a different and/or additional mechanism(s) [20]. Furthermore, it has been shown that an increase in intracellular levels of PA via a mechanical stimulus such as weight training and ingestion of exogenous sources of PA can promote the activation of mTOR signaling through different pathways that may collectively contribute to a larger effect of mTOR signaling [7–9]. Thus, the combination of an intense hypertrophy/strength goal oriented training program in conjunction with the ingestion PA, L-Leucine, HMB, and vitamin D3 appears to collectively improve LBM and strength to a greater extent than a hypertrophy/strength training program alone or a hypertrophy/strength training program plus PA alone.

Although the main active ingredient in this study was PA, the proprietary blend of L-Leucine, HMB, and vitamin D3 that was provided as the supplement to the experimental group could be viewed as a limitation as it is difficult to isolate the effects on LBM and strength of each ingredient alone. A second limitation to this study is the lack of participants that completed the study. A larger sample might have led to more statistically significant results. Finally, the lack of a specific training stimulus for the participants to improve VJ, AG, muscular endurance, and P in order to truly assess the effects of MT on these performance variables limited changes in these variables.

Future research on PA and MT is needed to further investigate its efficacy. It is possible that a training program that incorporates specific training for improvements in VJ, AG, muscular endurance, and P output on a cycle ergometer in conjunction with PA (as opposed to a PLA) could significantly improve these performance variables. Furthermore, PA could potentially improve body composition to a greater extent than was observed in these studies. Although diet was controlled in two of the three studies, all participants were provided with an isocaloric diet instead of a hypocaloric diet; it is unknown what would happen if the subjects were on a hypocaloric diet in regards to LBM and FM. Future research on PA could also focus the mechanism of action of the supplement, its effect on other populations (i.e. elderly, highly trained), the absorption profile of orally administered PA, and the safety of PA ingestion. Additionally, future research could investigate if the ingestion of PA, L-Leucine, HMB, and vitamin D3 in specific dosages are collectively more effective at improving LBM and strength than these supplements independently.

Conclusions

MT significantly increased maximum LP strength, BP strength, and LBM as compared to PLA. Although a trend was noted in improvements of AG, TMM, VJ, muscular endurance, P, and FM, the changes observed in the MT group compared to the PLA group were not statistically significant. The findings of this investigation further confirm the studies performed on the potential efficacy of PA for improving lower body strength, upper body strength, and lean body mass.

Availability of data

Raw data can for this manuscript can be found at https://osf.io/6zecp/.

Abbreviations

AG, agility; ANOVA, analysis of variance; BP, bench press; cGMP, current good manufacturing practices; FM, fat mass; HMB, Beta-Hydroxy-Beta-Methylbutyrate; HPLC, high pressure liquid chromatography; LBM, lean body mass; LP, leg Press; MT, MaxxTOR; mTOR, mammalian target of rapamycin; P, power; PA, phosphatidic acid; PLA, placebo; PU, push ups; TMM, thigh muscle mass; VJ, vertical jump

Acknowledgements

The authors would like to thank all of the California State University- San Bernardino volunteers that helped to make this study possible. Furthermore, the authors would like to acknowledge Max Muscle Sports Nutrition (Orange, CA) and Chemi Nutra (Austin, TX) for their support in this investigation.

Authors' contributions

GE was the primary investigator and supervised all study recruitment. All authors worked collectively to design the study. GE, MA, and BH supervised and/or performed the data collection, GE and MA analyzed the data, and MA performed the statistical analysis. GE supervised the manuscript preparation and MA, BH, and PH helped in drafting the manuscript. All authors read and approved the final manuscript.

Competing interests

The investigators disclose that Dr. Phil Harvey is currently the Chief Science Officer for Max Muscle Sports Nutrition and that he developed the MaxxTOR® (MT) supplement while being employed by Max Muscle Sports Nutrition. Furthermore, the funds for this study were provided by Max Muscle Sports Nutrition (Orange, CA) as well as from Chemi Nutra (Austin, TX), which is the patent holder of PA. These funds were used to purchase the necessary supplies, pay research assistants, and pay the investigators a small stipend approved by the CSUSB IRB to conduct their research.

The investigators further disclose that the principal investigator won the Max Muscle MaxxTOR® body transformation challenge in June of 2014 and was awarded $5,000 for winning the contest. The principal investigator currently receives no further compensation for the sale of the product as the money paid in June 2014 was merely for winning the contest. Aside from the stipends reported in the budget approved by the IRB, no investigator will receive any additional compensation from either Max Muscle Sports Nutrition or Chemi Nutra for their involvement in this study. The results of this study are independent and are not be biased despite the relationships mentioned in this section. This product and the use of these supplements is not endorsed by California State University- San Bernardino, California State University- Long Beach, or the University of Phoenix.

Author details

[1]California State University- San Bernardino, 5500 University Parkway, San Bernardino, CA 92407, USA. [2]California State University- Long Beach, 1250 Bellflower Boulevard, Long Beach, CA 90840, USA. [3]Max Muscle Sports Nutrition, 210 West Taft Avenue, Orange, CA 92865, USA. [4]University of Phoenix, San Diego Campus, 9645 Granite Ridge Drive, San Diego, CA 92123, USA.

References

1. Macaluso A, De Vito G. Muscle strength, power, and adaptations to resistance training in older people. Eur J Appl Physiol. 2004;91:450–72.
2. Willoughby DS, Stout JR, Wilborn CD. Effects of resistance training and protein plus amino acid supplementation on muscle anabolism, mass, and strength. Amino Acids. 2007;32:467–77.
3. Jäger R, Purpura M, Kingsley M. Phospholipids and sports nutrition. J Int Soc Sports Nutr. 2007;4:5.
4. Lim H, Choi Y, Park W, Lee T, Ryu S, Kim S, Kim JR, Kim JH, Baek S. Phosphatidic acid regulates systemic inflammatory responses by modulating the Akt-mammalian target of rapamycin- p70 S6 Kinase Pathway. J Bio Chem. 2003;278:45117–27.
5. Andresen BT, Rizzo MA, Shome K, Romero G. The role of phosphatidic acid in the regulation of the Ras/MEK/Erk signaling cascade. FEBS Lett. 2002;531:65–8.
6. Fang Y, Vilella-Bach M, Bachmann R, Flanigan A, Chen J. Phosphatidic acid-mediated mitogenic activation of mTOR signaling. Science. 2001;294:1942–5.
7. You JS, Frey JW, Hornberger TA. Mechanical stimulation induces mTOR signaling via an ERK-independent mechanism: implications for a direct activation of mTOR by phosphatidic acid. PLoS One. 2012;7:e47258.
8. You JS, Lincoln HC, Kim CR, Frey JW, Goodman CA, Zhong XP, Hornberger TA. The role of diacylglycerol kinase zeta and phosphatidic acid in the mechanical activation of Mammalian Target of Rapamycin (mTOR) signaling and skeletal muscle hypertrophy. J Biol Chem. 2013;289:1551–63.
9. Winter JN, Fox TE, Kester M, Jefferson LS, Kimball SR. Phosphatidic acid mediates activation of mTORC1 through the ERK signaling pathway. Am J Physiol Cell Physiol. 2010;299:C335–44.
10. Anthony JC, Yoshizawa F, Anthony TG, Vary TC, Jefferson LS, Kimball SR. Leucine stimulates translation initiation in skeletal muscle of postabsorptive rats via a rapamycin-sensitive pathway. J Nutr. 2000;130:2413–9.

11. Dickinson JM, Fry CS, Drummond MJ, Gundermann DM, Walker DK, Glynn EL, Timmerman KL, Dhanani S, Volpi E, Rasmussen BB. Mammalian target of rapamycin complex 1 activation is required for the stimulation of human skeletal muscle protein synthesis by essential amino acids. J Nutr. 2011;141: 856–62.

12. Dardevet D, Sornet C, Vary T, Grizard J. Phosphatidylinositol 3-kinase and p70 s6 kinase participate in the regulation of protein turnover in skeletal muscle by insulin and insulin-like growth factor I. Endocrinology. 1996;137: 4087–94.

13. Frost RA, Lang CH. Differential effects of insulin-like growth factor I (IGF-I) and IGF-binding protein-1 on protein metabolism in human skeletal muscle cells. Endocrinology. 1999;140:3962–70.

14. Bolster DR, Crozier SJ, Kimball SR, Jefferson LS. AMP-activated protein kinase suppresses protein synthesis in rat skeletal muscle through down-regulated mammalian target of rapamycin (mTOR) signaling. J Biol Chem. 2002;277: 23977–80.

15. Inoki K, Zhu T, Guan KL. TSC2 mediates cellular energy response to control cell growth and survival. Cell. 2003;115:577–90.

16. Hardie DG, Hawley SA, Scott JW. AMP-activated protein kinase–development of the energy sensor concept. J Physiol. 2006;574:7–15.

17. Hoffman JR, Stout JR, Williams DR, Wells AJ, Fragala MS, Mangine GT, Gonzalez AM, Emerson NS, McCormack WP, Scanlon TC, Purpura M, Jäger R. Efficacy of phosphatidic acid ingestion on lean body mass, muscle thickness and strength gains in resistance-trained men. J Int Soc Sports Nutr. 2012;9:47.

18. Joy JM, Gundermann DM, Lowery RP, Jager R, McCleary SA, Purpura M, Roberts MD, Wilson SMC, Hornberger TA, Wilson JM. Phosphatidic acid enhance mTOR signaling and resistance exercise induced hypertrophy. Nutrition and Metabolism. 2014;11:29.

19. Luo JQ, Chen DW, Yu B. Upregulation of amino acid transporter expression induced by L-leucine availability in L6 myotubes is associated with ATF4 signaling through mTORC1-dependent mechanism. Nutrition. 2013;29:284–90.

20. Wilkinson DJ, Hossain T, Hill DS. Effects of leucine and its metabolite beta-hydroxy-beta-methylbutyrate on human skeletal muscle protein metabolism. J Physiol. 2013;591:2911–23.

21. Katsanos CS, Kobayashi J, Sheffield-Moore M, Aarsland A, Wolfe RR. A high proportion of leucine is required for optimal stimulation of the rate of muscle protein synthesis by essential amino acids in the elderly. Am J Physiol Endocrinol Metab. 2006;291:E381–7.

22. Lynch CJ. Role of leucine in the regulation of mTOR by amino acids: Revelations from structure-activity studies. J Nutr. 2001;131:861S–5S.

23. Thomson JS, Watson PE, Rowlands DS. Effects of nine weeks of beta-hydroxy-beta-methylbutyrate supplementation on strength and body composition in resistance trained men. J Strength Cond Res. 2009;23:827–35.

24. Wilson JM, Fitschen PJ, Campbell B, et al. International Society of Sports Nutrition Position Stand: beta-hydroxy-betamethylbutyrate (HMB). J Int Soc Sports Nutr. 2013;0:6.

25. Slater G, Jenkins D, Logan P, Lee H, Vukovich M, Rathmacher JA, Hahn AG. Beta-hydroxy-beta-methylbutyrate (HMB) supplementation does not affect changes in strength or body composition during resistance training in trained men. Int J Sport Nutr Exerc Metab. 2001;11(3):384–96.

26. Kreider RB, Ferreira M, Greenwood M, Wilson M, Grindstaff P, Plisk S, Reinardy J, Cantler C, Almada AL. Effects of calcium B-HMB supplementation during training on markers of catabolism, body composition, strength and sprint performance. Journal of Exercise Physiology online. 2000;3(4):48–59.

27. Wilson GJ, Wilson JM, Manninen AH. Effects of beta-hydroxy-beta-methylbutyrate on exercise performance and body composition across varying levels of age, sex, and training experience: a review. Nutrition and Metabolism. 2008;5:1.

28. Salles J, Chanet A, Giraudet C, Patrac V, Pierre P. Jourdan M.1,25(OH)2-vitamin D3 enhances the stimulating effect of leucine and insulin on protein synthesis rate through Akt/PKB and mTOR mediated pathways in murine C2C12 skeletal myotubes. Mol Mutr Food Res. 2013;57(12):2137–46.

29. Maden-Wilkinson TM, Degens H, Jones DA, Mcphee JS. Comparison of MRI and DXA to measure muscle size and age-related atrophy in thigh muscles. J Musculoskelet Neuronal Interact. 2013;13(3):320–8.

30. NSCA's guide to tests and assessments 1 edition By National Strength & Conditioning Association (U.S.). Todd Miller, editor. 2012. Champaign, IL, USA: Human Kinetics.

31. Smith JC, Fry AC, Weiss LW, Li Y, Kinzey SJ. The effects of high-intensity exercise on a 10-s sprint cycle test. J Strength Cond Res. 2001;15:344–8.

32. Turner-McGrievy GM, Beets MW, Moore JB, Kaczynski AT, Barr-Anderson DJ, Tate DF. Comparison of traditional versus mobile app self-monitoring of physical activity and dietary intake among overweight adults participating in an mHealth weight loss program. J Am Med Inform Assoc. 2013;20: 513–8.

33. Tipton KD, Wolfe RR. Exercise, protein, metabolism, and muscle growth. Int J Sport Nutr Exerc Metab. 2001;11:109–32.

34. Churchward-Venne TA, Burd NA, Mitchell CJ, West DWD, Philp A, Marcotte GR, Baker SK, Baar K, Phillips SM. Supplementation of a suboptimal protein dose with leucine or essential amino acids: effects on myofibrillar protein synthesis at rest and following resistance exercise in men. J Physiol. 2012; 590:2751–65.

35. Stockton KA, Mengersen K, Paratz JD, Kandiah D, Bennell KL. Effect of vitamin D supplementation on muscle strength: a systematic review and meta-analysis. Osteoporos Int. 2011;22:859–71.

36. Muir SW, Montero-Odasso M. Effect of vitamin D supplementation on muscle strength, gait and balance in older adults: a systematic review and meta-analysis. J Am Geriatr Soc. 2011;59:2291–300.

37. Larson-Meyer DE, Willis KS. Vitamin D and athletes. Current Sports Medicine Reports. 2010;9(4):220–6.

38. Cannell JJ, Hollis BW, Sorenson MB, Taft TN, Anderson JJB. Athletic performance and vitamin D. Med Sci Sports Exer. 2009;41(5):1102–10.

39. Gupta R, Sharma U, Gupta N, Kalaivani M, Singh U, Guleria R, Jagannathan NR, Goswami T. Effect of cholecalciferol and calcium supplementation on muscle strength and energy metabolism in vitamin D-deficient Asian Indians: a randomized, control trial. Clin Endocrinol. 2010;73(4):445–51.

## 19

Regulation of mTORC1 by growth factors, energy status, amino acids and mechanical stimuli at a glance

Peter Bond

Abstract

The mechanistic/mammalian target of rapamycin complex 1 (mTORC1) plays a pivotal role in the regulation of skeletal muscle protein synthesis. Activation of the complex leads to phosphorylation of two important sets of substrates, namely eIF4E binding proteins and ribosomal S6 kinases. Phosphorylation of these substrates then leads to an increase in protein synthesis, mainly by enhancing translation initiation. mTORC1 activity is regulated by several inputs, such as growth factors, energy status, amino acids and mechanical stimuli. Research in this field is rapidly evolving and unraveling how these inputs regulate the complex. Therefore this review attempts to provide a brief and up-to-date narrative on the regulation of this marvelous protein complex. Additionally, some sports supplements which have been shown to regulate mTORC1 activity are discussed.

Keywords: mTORC1, Akt, Myostatin, Muscle protein synthesis

Background

The mechanistic/mammalian target of rapamycin complex 1 (mTORC1) has emerged as a key factor in regulation of skeletal muscle protein synthesis (MPS) [1]. mTORC1 is a protein complex comprised of the three core subunits mTOR, Raptor and mLST8 [2] and is regulated by several inputs, such as growth factors, energy status, amino acids and mechanical stimuli. mTOR forms the catalytic center of the two signaling complexes mTORC1 and mTORC2 [3], of which the first is primarily involved in regulation of MPS. Activation of the complex leads to phosphorylation of its two important sets of substrates which are involved in the translation of mRNA to protein. One comprising the eukaryotic initiation factor 4E (eIF4E)-binding proteins 4E-BP1 and 2. 4E-BPs inhibit the formation of the eIF4F complex which facilitates recruitment of the small (40S) ribosomal subunit to the 5' end of mRNA [4]. Therefore, 4E-BPs inhibit mRNA translation initiation and phosphorylation by mTORC1 relieves this inhibition. The other important set of substrates of mTORC1 comprise the ribosomal S6 kinases S6K1 and 2. Phosphorylation of the S6Ks by mTORC1 activates

them and resultingly modulates functions of translation initiation factors [5]. Additionally, S6Ks are thought to promote ribosome biogenesis and thereby increasing the translational capacity of the cell [6].

This manuscript attempts to provide a brief and up-to-date narrative of some important factors which regulate mTORC1 activity at the cellular level. Additionally, some sports supplements which have been shown to regulate mTORC1 activity are discussed.

Regulation by growth factors

Research examining the regulation of mTORC1 by growth factors has mainly focused on the effect of insulin and insulin-like growth factor-1. The insulin receptor (IR) and insulin-like growth factor-1 receptor (IGF-1R) both belong to the class of tyrosine kinase receptors. Activation of either receptor leads to phosphorylation of the insulin receptor substrates (IRS) proteins. This, in turn, exposes binding sites on these proteins which enable interaction with other proteins which contain a Src Homology 2 (SH2) domain. Among the SH2 domain-containing proteins is phosphatidylinositol-3-kinase (PI3K). IRS activates PI3K by associating with the SH2 domain of the kinase [7]. Activated PI3K then phosphorylates inositol phospholipids embedded in the plasma membrane

Correspondence: peter@peterbond.nl
PeterBond.nl, Waterhoenlaan 25, Zeist, Netherlands

on a hydroxyl group located at carbon 3. This gives rise to phosphoinositides, such as phosphatidylinositol (3,4,5)-triphosphate (PIP3). PIP3 interacts with Pleckstrin homology (PH) domain-containing proteins, thereby recruiting these to the plasma membrane. Two important PH domain-containing proteins are 3-phosphoinositide dependent protein kinase (PDK1) and Akt. The interaction of PIP3 with Akt enhances phosphorylation (and thereby activation) of the latter. Additionally, interaction of PIP3 with PDK1 leads to phosphorylation of Akt by PDK1 (Fig. 1).

Akt is considered an important upstream regulator of mTORC1 [8]. The Akt family of proteins comprises the three isoforms Akt1, Akt2 and Akt3. Akt1 and Akt2 are expressed in skeletal muscle, while Akt3 is not [9]. PDK1 phosphorylates Akt1 and Akt2 at residues Thr308 and Thr309, respectively. However, full Akt kinase activity also requires phosphorylation at a serine residue [10, 11], Ser473 and Ser473 on Akt1 and Akt2, respectively. The Rictor-containing mTOR complex mTORC2 is possibly the kinase responsible for phosphorylation of the serine residue [12]. Mechanistic studies commonly measure the phosphorylation status of Akt1 at residues Thr308 and Ser473 in order to assess Akt activity.

Myostatin, a potent negative regulator of skeletal muscle growth [13], has also been found to regulate Akt phosphorylation [14]. Myostatin is a member of the transforming growth factor-β superfamily and a ligand for activin

type II receptors (ActRIIA and ActRIIB). After binding to its receptor, it phosphorylates and activates activin type I receptors [15]. These receptors then phosphorylate and activate the transcription factors Smad2 and Smad3 which then form a heterotrimeric complex by joining with Smad4. After formation, the complex can translocate to the nucleus where it regulates several key genes involved in skeletal muscle growth. Knockout of myostatin in animal models has been found to dramatically increase skeletal muscle fiber size and number [16–18]. In postnatal skeletal muscle, inhibition of myostatin signaling mainly affects fiber size rather than number [19, 20]. Importantly, incubation of human myoblasts with myostatin has been found to reduce Akt phosphorylation at residue Ser473 by 50 % [14]. The reduction of Akt phosphorylation by myostatin might underlie its inhibiting effect on muscle hypertrophy. Recently, researchers discovered that this effect is mediated via the microRNA miR-486 [21]. miR-486 increases Akt phosphorylation, likely by inhibiting phosphatase and tensin homolog (PTEN), a protein which opposes the action of PI3K by dephosphorylating PIP3 to PIP2 [22]. Myostatin negatively regulates the expression of miR-486 at the transcriptional level and therefore inhibits Akt phosphorylation mediated by PI3K.

After Akt is activated it phosphorylates several other proteins. The best researched substrates of Akt are glycogen synthase kinase 3β (GSK3β) [23], proline-rich Akt substrate of 40 KDa (PRAS40) [24], tuberous sclerosis

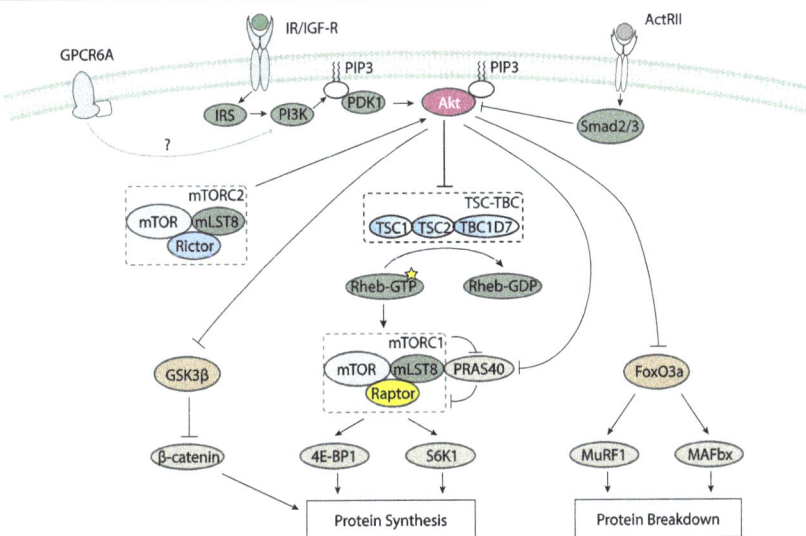

Fig. 1 Regulation of mTORC1 by growth factors. Activation of the IR and IGF-1R leads to phosphorylation of the IRS which subsequently activate PI3K. PI3K generates PIP3 which recruits PDK1 and Akt to the plasma membrane. Akt is then activated by PDK1 and mTORC2. Activated Akt then inhibits several substrates, namely the TSC-TBC complex which functions as a negative regulator of mTORC1, GSK3β which degrades β-catenin, FoxO3a which stimulates MuRF1 and MAFbx and PRAS40 which inhibits mTORC1. Akt activation is also induced by androgens, possibly by enhancing PI3K activity and mediated by GPCR6A. Additionally, Akt activation is inhibited by activation of ActRII receptors through activation of Smad2 and Smad3

complex 2 (TSC2) [25] and forkhead box class O (FoxO) proteins [26]. Both TSC2 and PRAS40 act as negative regulators of mTORC1. TSC2 forms a protein complex with TSC1 and the recently discovered protein TBC1D7 [27]. When the TSC1-TSC2-TBC1D7 (TSC-TBC) complex is formed, it inhibits mTORC1 activity by means of its GTPase-activating protein (GAP) domain [27, 28]. GTP-bound Rheb proteins (Rheb-GTP) activate mTORC1 at the lysosomal membrane [29]. The mechanism for this activation is currently unknown although interaction with the mTOR kinase domain appears to be involved [29]. By virtue of its GAP domain, the TSC-TBC complex can thus regulate the amount of Rheb-GTP and therefore mTORC1 activity. Akt phosphorylates TSC2 at multiple sites (Ser939, Ser981, Ser1130, Ser1132 and Thr1462) in order to inhibit the GAP activity of the TSC-TBC complex towards Rheb-GTP, possibly by dissociating the complex from the lysosome [30]. Moreover, it should be noted that the TSC-TBC complex has the highest affinity for Rheb-GDP rather than Rheb-GTP [30]. This might suggest a mechanism in which the complex acts to prevent the exchange of GDP for GTP in order to keep the Rheb proteins from reloading GTP. Akt further acts by relieving mTORC1 of the inhibition imposed by PRAS40. PRAS40 binds to the mTORC1 subunit Raptor, thereby inhibiting its association with substrates. PRAS40 is phosphorylated at one threonine residue (Thr246) and two serine residues (Ser181 and Ser221) [31]. The threonine residue is phosphorylated by Akt, whereas the serine residues appear to be phosphorylated by mTORC1.

GSK3β is a negative regulator of the Wnt/β-catenin signaling pathway as it forms a complex with other proteins and phosphorylates β-catenin leading to degradation of the molecule [32]. Akt phosphorylates GSK3β, which inactivates the enzyme and thereby stimulates Wnt/β-catenin signaling through removal of its inhibiton. β-catenin seems to play an important role in skeletal muscle hypertrophy by functioning as a transcription factor [33] and inhibition of GSK3β stimulates hypertrophy in C2C12 myotubes [34]. The kinase has also been found to inhibit mRNA translation by blocking the GDP-GTP exhange of eIF2B [35] which is required to form a functional ternary complex for translation initiation [36].

Besides the regulation of anabolic processes through inhibition of GSK3β, PRAS40 and TSC2 activity, Akt is also closely involved in inhibiting protein breakdown by modulating the activity of the FoxO family of proteins. FoxO proteins are key regulators of protein breakdown modulating ubiquitin-proteasome, as well as autophagy-lysosomal proteolytic pathways [37]. Especially the first seems important in muscle protein breakdown and two E3 ubiquitin ligases, muscle atrophy F-box

(MAFbx/atrogin-1) and muscle ring finger 1 (MuRF1) [38, 39], appear to be the two main downstream effectors of FoxO signaling affecting protein breakdown. FoxO proteins are phosphorylated, and thereby inhibited, by Akt [40].

Aside from the regulation of Akt by insulin and IGF-I, some studies [41–46], but not all [47–50], suggest androgens also increase Akt phosphorylation. The large heterogeneity across these studies, such as differences in experimental animal models, differences in the type of androgen used as well as its dosage, timepoint of measurement, among others, might explain why some studies did not find an increase in Akt phosphorylation. Interestingly, one study examining the rapid effects of testosterone in cultured rat myotubes directly implicates the PI3K/Akt/mTORC1 pathway as a mediator of androgens' effect on contractile protein synthesis [46]. Basualto-Alarcón et al., incubated the myotubes with testosterone (100 nM) and performed measurements of total Akt and phosphorylated Akt (at Ser473) 1, 5, 15, 30 and 60 m after incubation. Measurements of α-actin mRNA and protein were taken 6 and 12 h after incubation with testosterone and both were significantly increased, thus indicating an increase in contractile protein synthesis. Indeed, the cross-sectional area (CSA) was significantly increased after 12 h. Moreover, Akt phosphorylation was increased 15 m after incubation. When the authors inhibited PI3K, Akt or mTOR the effect on α-actin was blocked. As such, it appears likely that androgens exert rapid effects by activation of the PI3K/Akt/mTOR pathway. Given that PI3K operates at the cell membrane and that the effect on Akt phosphorylation occured rapidly (after 15 m), it appears highly likely that a cell membrane-localized receptor is involved. Indeed, multiple lines of evidence implicate a cell membrane-localized receptor in the rapid effects of androgens [51]. The G-protein coupled receptor (GPCR) GPRC6A has been shown to mediate a rapid signaling response, including involvement of PI3K, to testosterone [52]. In the experiment by Basualto-Alarcón et al., the addition of the androgen receptor (AR) antagonist bicalutamide blocked the increase in CSA, despite an increase in α-actin protein level. This indicates crosstalk between the intracellular AR and the PI3K pathway activated by testosterone. Strikingly, the intracellular AR has been shown to interact with the p85α regulatory subunit of PI3K in androgen-sensitive epithelial cells, enhancing its activity [53]. However, the addition of bicalutamide to these androgen-sensitive epithelial cells blocked the androgen-induced Akt phosphorylation. This is in contrast with the experiment by Basualto-Alarcón et al., which showed that inhibition of Akt phosphorylation blocked the increase in α-actin protein level, whereas bicalutamide did not affect α-actin protein level, thus suggesting that bicalutamide did not inhibit Akt phosphorylation in this experiment. If bicalutamide also affected Akt phosphorylation in the experiment by Basualto-Alarcón et al., this should therefore be observed in α-actin protein level, but it remained unaltered by addition of bicalutamide. This difference between both studies might be due to the differences in cell lines and AR ligands used. Nevertheless, AR-PI3K crosstalk might, partly, underlie the absence of an increase in CSA with the addition of bicalutamide in the experiment by Basualto-Alarcón et al., despite an increase in α-actin. Additionally, activation of the PI3K/Akt pathway can, in turn, regulate AR activity, since Akt has been shown to post-translationally modify the AR by phosphorylation [54]. Further research might further elucidate the mechanisms through which the cell membrane-localized and intracellular AR regulate mTORC1 activity.

Regulation by energy status

The regulation of mTORC1 by energy status of the cell is less well described than that of growth factors and appears primarily mediated through the AMP-activated kinase (AMPK). AMPK is a heterotrimeric protein comprising a combination of α, β and γ subunits. Currently there are two isoforms known of both the α (α1 and α2) and β (β1, β2) subunits. There are three isoforms known of the γ subunit (γ1, γ2, γ3). The α-subunit functions as the catalytic subunit of the complex, whereas the other two subunits 'sense' the energy status of the cell. The β-subunit can interact with glycogen [55] and the γ-subunit with the nucleotides adenosinetriphosphate (ATP), adenosinediphosphate (ADP) and adenosinemonophosphate (AMP) [56]. The interaction between glycogen and the β-subunit leads to allosteric inhibition of AMPK activity, a decrease in glycogen will

therefore lead to relieve of this inhibition and thus activation of the complex. In sum, the β and γ subunits allow the kinase to measure the energy status of the cell as reflected by its glycogen content and ATP to ADP or AMP ratio. A decrease in glycogen or the ATP to ADP or AMP ratio signals a decrease in available energy to the kinase and activates it. In general, activation of AMPK promotes catabolic pathways in order to recover cellular energy homeostasis and attenuates anabolic pathways to preserve energy (Fig. 2) [56, 57].

Theoretically, the different isoforms of the subunits allows for twelve unique combinations. However, to date only three different combinations have been found in human skeletal muscle: α2/β2/γ1, α2/β2/γ3 and α1/β2/γ1 [58]. The quantitative distribution of these heterotrimeric proteins has been estimated at 15 % α1/β2/γ1, 65% α2/β2/γ1 and 20 % α2/β2/γ3. The three heterotrimers show differential regulation and effects [59]. The α2/β2/γ3 heterotrimer is rapidly activated following physical activity, whereas the other two take far longer to activate. Additionally, only the α1-containing heterotrimer appears to attenuate muscle growth, whereas the α2-containing heterotrimers do not appear to do so [60].

The antagonizing effect AMPK has on muscle growth is mediated, atleast in part, by inhibiting mTORC1 activity. AMPK phosphorylates two residues (Thr1227 and Ser1345) on TSC2 which are important for its activation [61]. TSC2 then acts to inhibit mTORC1 by formation of the TSC-TBC complex as described earlier. Moreover, Raptor, one of the proteins comprising mTORC1, has also been found to be a substrate of AMPK [62]. Phosphorylation of Raptor at residues Ser722 and Ser792 likewise inhibits mTORC1 activity.

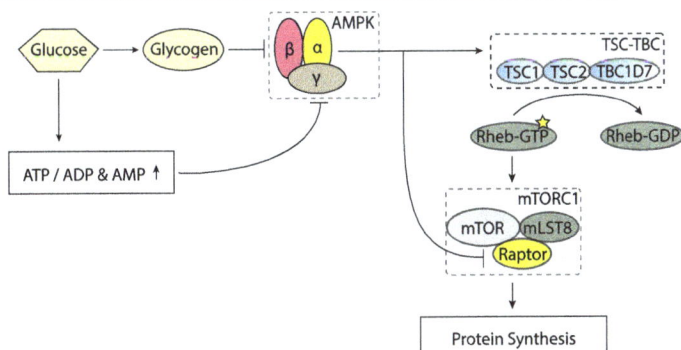

Fig. 2 Regulation of AMPK by energy status. The γ-subunit interacts with the nucleotides ATP, ADP and AMP. A high ATP to ADP and AMP ratio inhibits AMPK, whereas a decrease in the ratio activates the kinase. Interaction of glycogen with the β-subunit allosterically inhibits AMPK activity. Activated AMPK phosphorylates TSC2 at two residues (Thr1227 and Ser1345) which are important for its activation. Moreover, activated AMPK phosphorylates Raptor at two residues (Ser722 and Ser792) which inhibits mTORC1 activity

In sum, the antagonistic effect of AMPK on mTOR is mediated through phosphorylation of TSC2 and Raptor.

Regulation by amino acids

It should come as no surprise that the availability of the basic building blocks of protein control its synthesis. When a cell is deprived of amino acids, mTOR can be found throughout the cytoplasm, whereas addition of amino acids rapidly localizes mTOR to the peri-nuclear region of the cell, to large vesicular structures, or to both [63]. The amino acid-induced locatization is similar to that of Rab7, a late endosome-/lysosome-associated small GTPase. This suggests that amino acids might stimulate mTORC1 activity by localizing it to lysosomal surface where it can be activated by Rheb-GTP. The Ragulator-Rag complex was found responsible for targeting mTORC1 to the lysosomal surface [64]. At the lysosomal surface, mTORC1 associates with Ras-related GTPases (Rags). There are four different Rags: RagA, RagB, RagC and RagD. RagA and RagB (RagA/B) bind to RagC and RagD (RagC/D) to form heterodimeric pairs. Rags, in turn, associate with the protein complex Ragulator which is anchored in the lysosomal membrane. The interaction of Rags with mTORC1 is dependent on their guaninenucleotide binding state. In an amino acid-deprived cell, the RagA/B are bound to GDP, and the RagC/D are bound to GTP. The addition of amino acids induce a nucleotide exchange favoring the GTP bound state of RagA/B and the GDP bound state of RagC/D. The Ragulator, anchored in the lysosomal membrane, associates with Rags, therefore localizing them to the lysosomal membrane. Importantly, the Ragulator functions as a guanine nucleotide exchange factor (GEF) for RagA/B [65], thereby facilitating the exchange of GDP bound RagA/B for GTP bound RagA/B (the active form). The GEF activity of Ragulator is regulated by v-ATPase [65]. v-ATPase consumes ATP in order to pump hydrogens up their concentration gradient into the lysosome in order to maintain its acidic environment. Ragulator is associated with v-ATPase and amino acids induce a conformational change to the protein which then acts to activate Ragulator's GEF activity. As of yet it is unclear how amino acids induce this conformational change, but the signal appears to originate from inside the lysosome due to accumulation of amino acids in its lumen (Fig. 3) [66].

Whereas Ragulator acts as a GEF for RagA/B, the GAP activity towards Rags (GATOR1) complex functions as a GAP towards RagA/B [67]. The GATOR1 complex thus exchanges the GTP for GDP of RagA/B, leading to deactivation of the Rags and subsequently inhibition of mTORC1. Another protein complex dubbed GATOR2 is responsible for inhibiting GATOR1 activity [67] and therefore relieves mTORC1 from its inhibition. The inhibiting effect of GATOR2 on GATOR1 is mediated by Sestrin proteins in response to amino acids [68]. However, it is unknown how GATOR2 mediates its inhibiting effect and how amino acids regulate the complex.

Lastly, there is evidence that the guanine nucleotide binding state of RagC/D is regulated by leucyl tRNA-synthetase (LRS), the enzyme responsible for loading tRNA with leucine. The enzyme acts as a GAP for RagD GTPase, in a leucine depedent manner [69]. However, a later study found that purified LRS did not act as a GAP for any of the Rags [70]. Instead the authors propose that folliculin tumor suppressor (FLCN) and its binding partners act as Rag-interacting proteins with GAP activity for RagC/D, leading to mTORC1 activation. Moreover, leucine specifically appears to regulate mTORC1 through Sestrin2 [71].

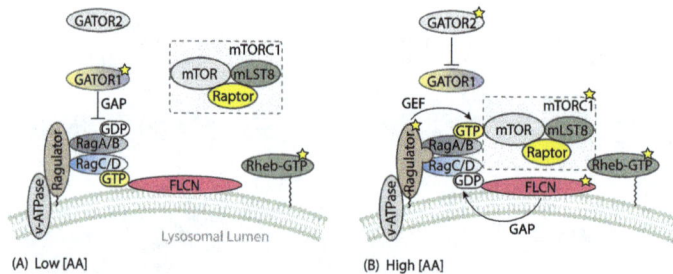

Fig. 3 Regulation of mTORC1 by amino acids. **a** The Rags are found in their inactive state under low amino acid conditions and therefore are unable to recruit mTORC1 to the lysosomal membrane for activation by Rheb-GTP. Ragulator and v-ATPase are in their inactive state, whereas GATOR1 exerts GAP-activity towards RagA/B, ensuring an inactive state of these Rags. **b** An increase in the amino acid concentration triggers a conformational change in v-ATPase and Ragulator, which initiates GEF activity towards RagA/B of the latter. FLCN and its binding partners exhibit GAP activity towards RagC/D and thereby activating them as well. Additionally, GATOR1 its GAP activity is inhibited due to inhibition of GATOR2. These actions lead to the active heterodimer of GTP-bound RagA/B and GDP-bound RagC/D, which then recruit mTORC1 to the lysosomal surface where it can be activated by Rheb-GTP. Figure based on [99]

Regulation by mechanical stimuli

It is well known that physical activity, resistance exercise in particular, increases skeletal muscle mass in healthy persons under most conditions. Currently, two important mechanisms have been identified which regulate mTORC1 by mechanical stimuli. One of these mechanisms shows close resemblance with the PI3K/Akt-pathway in that it leads to dissociation of TSC2 from the lysosomal membrane [72]. Eccentric contractions lead to phosphorylation of TSC2 which leads to the dissociation observed. Since Rheb-GTP, the target of the TSC-TBC complex its GAP activity, is located at the lysosomal membrane, mechanical stimuli effectively prevents the GTP/GDP-exchange. Moreover, mechanical stimuli increase the levels of mTORC1 at the lysosomal membrane, further supporting its activation [72]. The mechanism for this remains uncertain (Fig. 4).

Secondly, mechanical stimuli regulate mTORC1 by regulating levels of phosphatidic acid (PA), a diacylglycerol phospholipid which has been found to directly activate mTORC1 [73]. A twofold effect mediates the stimulating effect of PA on mTORC1: i) displacing the endogeneous mTORC1 inhibitor FK506 binding protein 38 (FKBP38) through competitive inhibition, ii) allosteric activation of mTORC1.

The [PA] is regulated by five classes of enzymes [74]. Three are responsible for the synthesis of PA and two regulate its degradation. A delicate balance between the activities of these enzymes determines cellular PA levels. Glycerol-3-phosphate (G3P), phosphatidylcholine (PC) and diacylglycerol (DAG) are precursors for the biosynthesis of PA. G3P is acetylated twice in order to produce PA. First glycerol-3-phosphate acyltransferase (GPAT) catalyzes the first acetylation reaction, after which

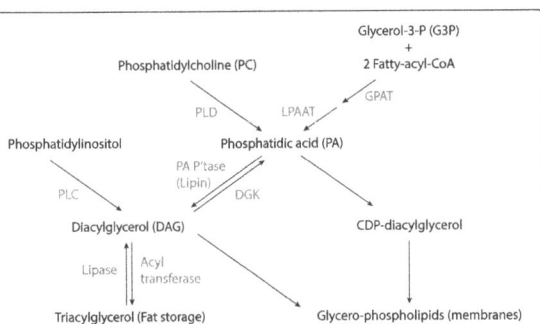

Fig. 4 PA can be synthesized from G3P, PC and DAG. G3P is acetylated twice, requiring fatty-acyl-CoA for its acetylation. First it is acetylated by GPAT and then by LPAAT. PLD is hydrolyzed by PLD to produce PA and DAG is phosphorylated by DGK to produce PA. DAG is derived from triacylglycerols and phosphatidylinositol. PA phosphatase (PA P'tase) is responsible for dephosphorylation of PA to DAG. Various CDP-diacylglycerol synthases produce CDP-diacylglycerol from PA. Figure based on [74]

lysophosphatidic acid acyltransferase (LPAAT) catalyzes the second. PC is hydrolyzed in order to produce PA. This reaction is catalyzed by phospholipase D (PLD). For long it had been assumed PLD was crucial in mediating the mechanical stimuli-induced increase in PA. This assumption was mainly based on experiments which applied the PLD inhibitor 1-butanol, which effectively inhibited mTORC1 activity in several experiments [75]. However, later it was found that not all biological activity induced by 1-butanol could be attributed to its PLD inhibiting effect. Moreover, earlier findings already reported that PLD activity induced by mechanical stimuli poorly correlated with the cellular increase of PA [76]. Recent evidence suggests that the mechanical stimuli-induced increase of PA might be attributed to an increased synthesis from DAG rather than PC. PA is produced from DAG by phosphorylation catalyzed by diacylglycerolkinases (DGK). Many DGKs have been identified and it appears the ζ-isoform is primarily responsible for the mechanical stimuli-induced increase of PA [77].

The regulation of the enzymes responsible for degradation of PA are currently poorly understood.

Sports supplements and mTORC1 signaling

In 2011, Kunkel et al. performed an elegant study to identify a compound which might help against skeletal muscle atrophy [78]. The authors screened for changes in mRNA expression in both human and rodent skeletal muscle during fasting and spinal cord injury. Both fasting and spinal cord injury involve dramatic muscle atrophy over time and this effect is driven by changes in muscle gene expression. The authors therefore hypothesized that pharmacologic compounds with opposite effects on gene expression might inhibit skeletal muscle atrophy. By querying the Connectivity Map [79] with the data they gathered, they identified ursolic acid as a potential pharmacologic compound which might inhibit skeletal muscle atrophy. After identification of the compound they continued to test its effects in mice and found it to reduce muscle atrophy and stimulate muscle hypertrophy. Interestingly, IGF-I mRNA was upregulated in skeletal muscle of the mice treated with ursolic acid. Moreover, Akt phosphorylation was also increased. The researchers also evaluated the effect of C2C12 myoblasts incubated with ursolic acid and found that, on its own, it did not increase Akt phosphorylation. However, in the presence of IGF-I ursolic acid did increase Akt phosphorylation. Similarly, ursolic acid alone did not upregulate S6K1 phosphorylation, but it did enhance IGF-I- and insulin-mediated S6K1 phosphorylation. Later research confirmed these findings and found that ursolic acid stimulates mTORC1 signaling in rat skeletal muscle [80]. This was evidenced by an increase in phosphorylation of Akt (at Thr308, but not Ser473), PRAS40 and S6K1 after resistance exercise.

A recent clinical study also found an improvement in body composition and strength in sixteen Korean men with over 3 years resistance exercise experience who were supplemented ursolic acid compared to placebo [81].

Some evidence suggests that the popular ergogenic aid creatine might also stimulate mTORC1 signaling. In a double-blind placebo-controlled study, participants received either placebo or creatine for 5 days [82]. Muscle biopsies were then taken at rest, immediately after exercise, 24 and 72 h later. The phosphorylation of Akt at Ser473 and Thr308 were determined, as well as the phosphorylation of 4E-BP1 and S6K1. Surprisingly, creatine supplementation decreased Akt phosphorylation at Thr308 in rest, whereas it was unaffected immediately, 24 and 72 h post-exercise. Akt phosphorylation at Ser473 was unaffected at all time points. Similar results were obtained for 4E-BP1 and S6K1 phosphorylation: 4E-BP1 phosphorylation showed a decrease 24 h after training, while it remained unaffected at all other time points and S6K1 phosphorylation remained unchanged at all time points. Nevertheless, MHCIIA mRNA expression showed an increase immediately after exercise and MHC1 mRNA expression showed an increase during rest after creatine supplementation compared to placebo. However, another study with a similar experimental design found an increase in phosphorylated 4E-BP1 24 h after exercise in the creatine group compared to placebo, but found no difference in phosphorylated S6K1 between both groups [83]. Again, no difference was found in phosphorylated 4E-BP1 and S6K1 3 h post-exercise. Notably, an increase in IGF-I mRNA expression was also observed 24 h post-exercise in the creatine group compared to placebo. These results suggest that creatine might activate mTORC1 by increasing IGF-I activity at rest, but does not further potentiate mTORC1 signaling in the hours after exercise. Interestingly, a clinical study also found that creatine supplementation amplified the resistance exercise-induced decrease in serum myostatin [84]. Although no markers of the mTORC1 pathway were measured in this study, it might be that a decrease in serum myostatin might enhance Akt phosphorylation and thus mTORC1 activity.

The mTORC1 signaling pathway is also thought to be involved in the anabolic effects of the leucine metabolite β-hydroxyβ-methylbutyrate (HMB) [85, 86]. In rats fed HMB, mTOR protein expression increased significantly compared to treatment with saline [87]. Moreover, phosphorylated S6K1 also increased significantly in the HMB treated rats compared to the control group. Similar results were obtained in an *in vitro* experiment [88]. C2C12 myoblasts were incubated with proteolysis-inducing factor (PIF, a protein which stimulates proteolysis and inhibits protein synthesis) and addition of HMB increased S6K1 phosphorylation. Notably, in the rat study no differences were found in Akt phosphorylation

between both groups. However, another *in vivo* experiment did find an increase in phosphorylated Akt in differentiated C2C12 myoblasts 10 and 30 m after incubation with HMB, as well as an increase in phosphorylated mTOR 30 m after incubation [89]. These results might seem conflicting, but the measurements in the rat study were taken 15 h to 18 h after HMB supplementation. Thus it might be that the activation of Akt/mTORC1 signaling was short-lived and was therefore missed in the rat study. Interestingly, another leucine metabolite, α-hydroxy-isocaproic acid (HICA), has shown to increase whole lean body mass when compared to placebo in a small sample of soccer players [90]. Rats fed HICA and recovering from hindlimb immobilization also showed a sustained increase in protein synthesis and phosphorylation of S6K1 and 4E-BP1 after 14 days when compared to placebo and leucine [91]. Further research might further clarify the role of mTORC1 signaling in the anabolic effects of these leucine metabolites.

Trimethylglycine (TMG), a methyl derivate of the amino acid glycine and also known as betaine, was recently shown to improve body composition when supplemented to trained athletes [92]. TMG is hypothesized to work as an ergogenic aid by functioning as both an osmolyte as well as a methyl donor in cells [93]. In a small double-blinded crossover trial, participants underwent 2 weeks of supplementation with either TMG or placebo [94]. Before and after the 2-week period, participants performed an acute exercise session. Both before the supplementation period, as well as 10 m before and after exercise, muscle biopsies were taken from the vastus lateralis muscle. Total Akt protein content was significantly increased in the TMG group compared to placebo. There was no difference in phosphorylated Akt and S6K1 in rest, but there was a decrease in phosphorylated Akt and S6K1 after the acute exercise session in the placebo group which did not occur in the TMG group. AMPK phosphorylation at Thr172 was also measured, but there was no difference between both groups. Notably, an increase in circulating growth hormone (GH) and IGF-I concentrations was observed in the TMG group, but not in the placebo group. This makes it appealing to speculate that the increase in circulatory GH and IGF-I underlies the effect of TMG on Akt. However, it should be taken into account that local GH and IGF-I, rather than circulatory, appear to affect skeletal muscle hypertrophy [95]. Nevertheless, an *in vitro* experiment in C2C12 myoblasts showed an increase in IGF-1 receptor protein expression after incubation with TMG [96]. An increase in Akt and myosin heavy chain protein content was also observed. Taken together these observations suggest that TMG activates the IGF-I/Akt/mTORC1 pathway.

A recent study also showed that PA supplementation activated mTORC1 and improved responses in skeletal muscle hypertrophy, lean body mass, and maximal strength to resistance exercise [97]. A sample of 28 resistance trained men received either PA or placebo and took part in an 8 week periodized resistance training program. The PA group showed a larger increase in lean body mass than the placebo group and also the CSA of the rectus femoris muscle showed a larger increase in the PA group than the placebo group. The authors also performed an *in vitro* experiment assessing phosphorylation of S6K1 in C2C12 myoblasts after incubation with two different sources of PA (egg and soy). While both showed a large increase in phosphorylation of S6K1, the soy-derived PA showed the largest increase. As the authors note, the difference might be due to soy and egg derived PA having varying degrees of unsaturated and saturated fatty acid chains which influence its action. A later study carried out both an *in vivo* and *in vitro* experiment to examine the effects of PA on anabolic signaling [98]. In the *in vivo* experiment, male Wister rats received either tap water (CON), PA (PA), whey protein concentrate (WPC) or PA + WPC (PA+WPC) after an overnight fast. Samples were taken after 3 h. Ribosomal protein S6 (rpS6) phosphorylation was increased in the PA and PA+WPC groups compared to the CON group, whereas it was not increased in the WPC group. S6K1 phosphorylation was also only significantly increased compared to control in the PA+WPC group. However, while PA showed an increase in MPS compared to CON, the largest increase in MPS was observed in the WPC group. There was no synergistic effect of PA+WPC in MPS when compared to WPC alone. The authors therefore speculate that combined PA and WPC might alter mTOR pathway activation dynamics, thus shifting MPS levels to the left or right of the sampling point or that PA might interfere with WPC-induced increases in MPS. Future research might clarify this matter. Their *in vitro* experiment in C2C12 myoblasts confirmed that PA increased MPS and mTOR signaling.

Conclusions

In the past few years our knowledge of mTORC1 regulation in skeletal muscle has increased tremendously. This review therefore attempted to provide a brief and up-to-date narrative on its regulation. Energy intake, protein intake, mechanical stumuli, as well as growth factors, have been shown to regulate the mTORC1 complex. All these elements provide signals to muscle cells which are then sensed, transduced and integrated which leads to changes in cellular functions. Ultimately, these signals are sensed by proteins such as cell surface receptors or intracellular kinases. For example, the IR senses the concentration of insulin outside the cell and relays this signal through the PI3K/Akt/mTORC1 pathway, whereas energy availability is directly relayed through AMPK by the nucleotides ATP, ADP and AMP as well as stored glycogen. Finally,

these signals are integrated by the cell in order to respond accordingly by changing cellular functions such as protein synthesis and protein breakdown. mTORC1 plays a pivotal role in integrating several of these signals such as growth factors, energy status, amino acids availability and mechanical stumuli. All these signals together affect the cellular response. Sports supplements might benefit the athlete in optimizing these signals, in addition to resistance exercise training, to maximize muscle hypertrophy. While ultimately clinical trials are required to properly evaluate their effects, they are expensive and sometimes difficult to carry out. For example, it can be challenging to find enough participants which conform the criteria of interest (e.g. young adults with several years of weightlifting experience) to yield enough statistical power. Additionally, strictly controlling all variables, such as dietary intake, can be hard. This is of special concern in studies of several weeks or months of duration. Insights in the mechanistic features of sports supplements might therefore aid clinical trials by providing hypothesizes under which conditions supplements might work best, as well as which combinations of supplements might provide additive effects. Additionally, it might aid in discovering new supplements of interest. The increasing knowledge of mTORC1 regulation therefore helps to refine these matters.

Competing interests
The author declares that he has no competing interests.

Acknowledgements
The author is grateful to Gemma Lahoz Casarramona for drawing the figures. The author would also like to thank the two anonymous reviewers for their feedback as it has greatly improved the quality of the manuscript.

References

1. Adegoke OA, Abdullahi A, Tavajohi-Fini P. mtorc1 and the regulation of skeletal muscle anabolism and mass. Appl Physiol Nutr Metab. 2012;37(3):395–406.
2. Dibble CC, Manning BD. Signal integration by mtorc1 coordinates nutrient input with biosynthetic output. Nature Cell Biol. 2013;15(6):555–564.
3. Huang K, Fingar DC. Growing knowledge of the mtor signaling network. In: Seminars in Cell & Developmental Biology. Elsevier; 2014. p. 79–90. doi:10.1016/j.semcdb.2014.09.011.
4. Sonenberg N, Hinnebusch AG. Regulation of translation initiation in eukaryotes: mechanisms and biological targets. Cell. 2009;136(4):731–745.
5. Ma XM, Blenis J. Molecular mechanisms of mtor-mediated translational control. Nature Rev Mol Cell Biol. 2009;10(5):307–318.
6. Brian M, Bilgen E, Diane CF. Regulation and function of ribosomal protein s6 kinase (s6k) within mtor signalling networks. Biochem J. 2012;441(1):1–21.
7. Myers MG, Backer JM, Sun XJ, Shoelson S, Hu P, Schlessinger J, Yoakim M, Schaffhausen B, White MF. Irs-1 activates phosphatidylinositol 3'-kinase by associating with src homology 2 domains of p85. Proc Natl Acad Sci. 1992;89(21):10350–10354.
8. Bodine SC. mtor signaling and the molecular adaptation to resistance exercise. Med Sci Sports Exerc. 2006;38(11):1950–1957.
9. Wu M, Falasca M, Blough ER. Akt/protein kinase b in skeletal muscle physiology and pathology. J Cell Physiol. 2011;226(1):29–36.

10. Alessi DR, James SR, Downes CP, Holmes AB, Gaffney PR, Reese CB, Cohen P. Characterization of a 3-phosphoinositide-dependent protein kinase which phosphorylates and activates protein kinase bα. Current Biol. 1997;7(4):261–269.

11. Feng J, Park J, Cron P, Hess D, Hemmings BA. Identification of a pkb/akt hydrophobic motif ser-473 kinase as dna-dependent protein kinase. J Biol Chem. 2004;279(39):41189–1196.

12. Sarbassov DD, Guertin DA, Ali SM, Sabatini DM. Phosphorylation and regulation of akt/pkb by the rictor-mtor complex. Science. 2005;307(5712):1098–1101.

13. Rodriguez J, Vernus B, Chelh I, Cassar-Malek I, Gabillard J, Sassi AH, Seiliez I, Picard B, Bonnieu A. Myostatin and the skeletal muscle atrophy and hypertrophy signaling pathways. Cell Mol Life Sci. 2014;71(22):4361–371.

14. Trendelenburg AU, Meyer A, Rohner D, Boyle J, Hatakeyama S, Glass DJ. Myostatin reduces akt/torc1/p70s6k signaling, inhibiting myoblast differentiation and myotube size. Am J Physiol Cell Physiol. 2009;296(6):1258–1270.

15. Lee SJ, McPherron AC. Regulation of myostatin activity and muscle growth. Proc Natl Acad Sci. 2001;98(16):9306–9311.

16. McPherron AC, Lawler AM, Lee S-J. Regulation of skeletal muscle mass in mice by a new tgf-p superfamily member. 1997. http://www.ncbi.nlm.nih.gov/pubmed/9139826, doi:10.1038/387083a0.

17. McPherron AC, Lee SJ. Double muscling in cattle due to mutations in the myostatin gene. Proc Natl Acad Sci. 1997;94(23):12457–12461.

18. Amthor H, Macharia R, Navarrete R, Schuelke M, Brown SC, Otto A, Voit T, Muntoni F, Vrbóva G, Partridge T, et al. Lack of myostatin results in excessive muscle growth but impaired force generation. Proc Natl Acad Sci. 2007;104(6):1835–1840.

19. Whittemore LA, Song K, Li X, Aghajanian J, Davies M, Girgenrath S, Hill JJ, Jalenak M, Kelley P, Knight A, et al. Inhibition of myostatin in adult mice increases skeletal muscle mass and strength. Biochem Biophys Res Commun. 2003;300(4):965–971.

20. Grobet L, Pirottin D, Farnir F, Poncelet D, Royo LJ, Brouwers B, Christians E, Desmecht D, Coignoul F, Kahn R, et al. Modulating skeletal muscle mass by postnatal, muscle-specific inactivation of the myostatin gene. Genesis. 2003;35(4):227–238.

21. Hitachi K, Nakatani M, Tsuchida K. Myostatin signaling regulates akt activity via the regulation of mir-486 expression. Int J Biochem Cell Biol. 2014;47:93–103.

22. Maehama T, Dixon JE. The tumor suppressor, pten/mmac1, dephosphorylates the lipid second messenger, phosphatidylinositol 3, 4, 5-trisphosphate. J Biol Chem. 1998;273(22):13375–13378.

23. Cross DA, Alessi DR, Cohen P, Andjelkovich M, Hemmings BA. Inhibition of glycogen synthase kinase-3 by insulin mediated by protein kinase b. Nature. 1995;378(6559):785–789.

24. Kovacina KS, Park GY, Bae SS, Guzzetta AW, Schaefer E, Birnbaum MJ, Roth RA. Identification of a proline-rich akt substrate as a 14-3-3 binding partner. J Biol Chem. 2003;278(12):10189–10194.

25. Inoki K, Li Y, Zhu T, Wu J, Guan KL. Tsc2 is phosphorylated and inhibited by akt and suppresses mtor signalling. Nature Cell Biol. 2002;4(9):648–657.

26. Tran H, Brunet A, Griffith EC, Greenberg ME. The many forks in foxo's road. Sci Signal. 2003;2003(172):5.

27. Dibble CC, Elis W, Menon S, Qin W, Klekota J, Asara JM, Finan PM, Kwiatkowski DJ, Murphy LO, Manning BD. Tbc1d7 is a third subunit of the tsc1-tsc2 complex upstream of mtorc1. Mol Cell. 2012;47(4):535–546.

28. Li Y, Corradetti MN, Inoki K, Guan KL. Tsc2: filling the gap in the mtor signaling pathway. Trends Biochem Sci. 2004;29(1):32–8.

29. Long X, Lin Y, Ortiz-Vega S, Yonezawa K, Avruch J. Rheb binds and regulates the mtor kinase. Current Biol. 2005;15(8):702–713.

30. Menon S, Dibble CC, Talbott G, Hoxhaj G, Valvezan AJ, Takahashi H, Cantley LC, Manning BD. Spatial control of the tsc complex integrates insulin and nutrient regulation of mtorc1 at the lysosome. Cell. 2014;156(4):771–785.

31. Wiza C, Nascimento EB, Ouwens DM. Role of pras40 in akt and mtor signaling in health and disease. Am J Physiol Endocrinol Metab. 2012;302(12):1453–1460.

32. Ikeda S, Kishida S, Yamamoto H, Murai H, Koyama S, Kikuchi A. Axin, a negative regulator of the wnt signaling pathway, forms a complex with gsk-3β and β-catenin and promotes gsk-3β-dependent phosphorylation of β-catenin. EMBO J. 1998;17(5):1371–1384.

33. Armstrong DD, Esser KA. Wnt/β-catenin signaling activates growth-control genes during overload-induced skeletal muscle hypertrophy. Am J Physiol Cell Physiol. 2005;289(4):853–859.

34. Vyas DR, Spangenburg EE, Abraha TW, Childs TE, Booth FW. Gsk-3β negatively regulates skeletal myotube hypertrophy. Am J Physiol Cell Physiol. 2002;283(2):545–551.

35. Proud C, Denton R. Molecular mechanisms for the control of translation by insulin. Biochem J. 1997;328:329–41.

36. Gebauer F, Hentze MW. Molecular mechanisms of translational control. Nature Rev Mol Cell Biol. 2004;5(10):827–835.

37. Sanchez AM, Candau RB, Bernardi H. Foxo transcription factors: their roles in the maintenance of skeletal muscle homeostasis. Cell Mol Life Sci. 2014;71(9):1657–1671.

38. Bodine SC, Latres E, Baumhueter S, Lai VK-M, Nunez L, Clarke BA, Poueymirou WT, Panaro FJ, Na E, Dharmarajan K, et al. Identification of ubiquitin ligases required for skeletal muscle atrophy. Science. 2001;294(5547):1704–1708.

39. Bodine SC, Baehr LM. Skeletal muscle atrophy and the e3 ubiquitin ligases murf1 and mafbx/atrogin-1. Am J Physiol Endocrinol Metab. 2014;307(6):469–484.

40. Zhang X, Tang N, Hadden TJ, Rishi AK. Akt, foxo and regulation of apoptosis. Biochim et Biophys Acta (BBA)-Mol Cell Res. 2011;1813(11):1978–1986.

41. White JP, Baltgalvis KA, Sato S, Wilson LB, Carson JA. Effect of nandrolone decanoate administration on recovery from bupivacaine-induced muscle injury. J Appl Physiol. 2009;107(5):1420–1430.

42. Yin HN, Chai JK, Yu Y-M, Wu C-AS, Yao YM, Liu H, Liang LM, Tompkins RG, Sheng ZY. Regulation of signaling pathways downstream of igf-i/insulin by androgen in skeletal muscle of glucocorticoid-treated rats. J Trauma. 2009;66(4):1083.

43. Jones A, Hwang DJ, Narayanan R, Miller DD, Dalton JT. Effects of a novel selective androgen receptor modulator on dexamethasone-induced and hypogonadism-induced muscle atrophy. Endocrinol. 2010;151(8):3706–3719.

44. Ibebunjo C, Eash JK, Li C, Ma Q, Glass DJ. Voluntary running, skeletal muscle gene expression, and signaling inversely regulated by orchidectomy and testosterone replacement. Am J Physiol Endocrinol Metab. 2011;300(2):327–340.

45. White JP, Gao S, Puppa MJ, Sato S, Welle SL, Carson JA. Testosterone regulation of akt/mtorc1/foxo3a signaling in skeletal muscle. Mol Cell Endocrinol. 2013;365(2):174–86.

46. Basualto-Alarcón C, Jorquera G, Altamirano F, Jaimovich E, Estrada M. Testosterone signals through mtor and androgen receptor to induce muscle hypertrophy. Med Sci Sports Exerc. 2013;45(9):1712–1720.

47. Hourde C, Jagerschmidt C, Clément-Lacroix P, Vignaud A, Ammann P, Butler-Browne G, Ferry A. Androgen replacement therapy improves function in male rat muscles independently of hypertrophy and activation of the akt/mtor pathway. Acta Physiol. 2009;195(4):471–482.

48. Wu Y, Bauman WA, Blitzer RD, Cardozo C. Testosterone-induced hypertrophy of l6 myoblasts is dependent upon erk and mtor. Biochem Biophys Res Commun. 2010;400(4):679–683.

49. Haren M, Siddiqui A, Armbrecht H, Kevorkian R, Kim M, Haas M, Mazza A, Kumar VB, Green M, Banks W, et al. Testosterone modulates gene expression pathways regulating nutrient accumulation, glucose metabolism and protein turnover in mouse skeletal muscle. Int J Androl. 2011;34(1):55–68.

50. Ma L, Shen C, Chai J, Yin H, Deng H, Feng R. Extracellular signal–regulated kinase–mammalian target of rapamycin signaling and forkhead-box transcription factor 3a phosphorylation are involved in testosterone's effect on severe burn injury in a rat model. Shock. 2015;43(1):85–91.

51. Foradori C, Weiser M, Handa R. Non-genomic actions of androgens. Front Neuroendocrinol. 2008;29(2):169–181.

52. Pi M, Parrill AL, Quarles LD. Gprc6a mediates the non-genomic effects of steroids. J Biol Chem. 2010;285(51):39953–39964.

53. Baron S, Manin M, Beaudoin C, Leotoing L, Communal Y, Veyssiere G, Morel L. Androgen receptor mediates non-genomic activation of phosphatidylinositol 3-oh kinase in androgen-sensitive epithelial cells. J Biol Chem. 2004;279(15):14579–14586.

54. Gioeli D, Paschal BM. Post-translational modification of the androgen receptor. Mol Cell Endocrinol. 2012;352(1):70–78.

55. McBride A, Ghilagaber S, Nikolaev A, Hardie DG. The glycogen-binding domain on the ampk β subunit allows the kinase to act as a glycogen sensor. Cell Metab. 2009;9(1):23–34.

56. Hardie DG, Ross FA, Hawley SA. Ampk: a nutrient and energy sensor that maintains energy homeostasis. Nature Rev Mol Cell Biol. 2012;13(4): 251–62.

57. Jewell JL, Guan KL. Nutrient signaling to mtor and cell growth. Trends Biochem Sci. 2013;38(5):233–242.

58. Birk JB, Wojtaszewski J. Predominant $\alpha 2/\beta 2/\gamma 3$ ampk activation during exercise in human skeletal muscle. J Physiol. 2006;577(3):1021–1032.

59. Mounier R, Théret M, Lantier L, Foretz M, Viollet B. Expanding roles for ampk in skeletal muscle plasticity. Trends Endocrinol Metab. 2015;26(6): 275–286.

60. Mounier R, Lantier L, Leclerc J, Sotiropoulos A, Foretz M, Viollet B. Antagonistic control of muscle cell size by ampk and mtorc1. Cell Cycle. 2011;10(16):2640–2646.

61. Inoki K, Zhu T, Guan K-L. Tsc2 mediates cellular energy response to control cell growth and survival. Cell. 2003;115(5):577–590.

62. Gwinn DM, Shackelford DB, Egan DF, Mihaylova MM, Mery A, Vasquez DS, Turk BE, Shaw RJ. Ampk phosphorylation of raptor mediates a metabolic checkpoint. Mol Cell. 2008;30(2):214–226.

63. Sancak Y, Peterson TR, Shaul YD, Lindquist RA, Thoreen CC, Bar-Peled L, Sabatini DM. The rag gtpases bind raptor and mediate amino acid signaling to mtorc1. Science. 2008;320(5882):1496–1501.

64. Sancak Y, Bar-Peled L, Zoncu R, Markhard AL, Nada S, Sabatini DM. Ragulator-rag complex targets mtorc1 to the lysosomal surface and is necessary for its activation by amino acids. Cell. 2010;141(2):290–303.

65. Bar-Peled L, Schweitzer LD, Zoncu R, Sabatini DM. Ragulator is a gef for the rag gtpases that signal amino acid levels to mtorc1. Cell. 2012;150(6): 1196–1208.

66. Zoncu R, Bar-Peled L, Efeyan A, Wang S, Sancak Y, Sabatini DM. mtorc1 senses lysosomal amino acids through an inside-out mechanism that requires the vacuolar h+-atpase. Science. 2011;334(6056):678–683.

67. Bar-Peled L, Chantranupong L, Cherniack AD, Chen WW, Ottina KA, Grabiner BC, Spear ED, Carter SL, Meyerson M, Sabatini DM. A tumor suppressor complex with gap activity for the rag gtpases that signal amino acid sufficiency to mtorc1. Science. 2013;340(6136):1100–1106.

68. Chantranupong L, Wolfson RL, Orozco JM, Saxton RA, Scaria SM, Bar-Peled L, Spooner E, Isasa M, Gygi SP, Sabatini DM. The sestrins interact with gator2 to negatively regulate the amino-acid-sensing pathway upstream of mtorc1. Cell Reports. 2014;9(1):1–8.

69. Han JM, Jeong SJ, Park MC, Kim G, Kwon NH, Kim HK, Ha SH, Ryu SH, Kim S. Leucyl-trna synthetase is an intracellular leucine sensor for the mtorc1-signaling pathway. Cell. 2012;149(2):410–424.

70. Tsun ZY, Bar-Peled L, Chantranupong L, Zoncu R, Wang T, Kim C, Spooner E, Sabatini DM. The folliculin tumor suppressor is a gap for the ragc/d gtpases that signal amino acid levels to mtorc1. Mol Cell. 2013;52(4):495–505.

71. Wolfson RL, Chantranupong L, Saxton RA, Shen K, Scaria SM, Cantor JR, Sabatini DM. Sestrin2 is a leucine sensor for the mtorc1 pathway. Science. 2015;2674:43–48.

72. Jacobs BL, You JS, Frey JW, Goodman CA, Gundermann DM, Hornberger TA. Eccentric contractions increase the phosphorylation of tuberous sclerosis complex-2 (tsc2) and alter the targeting of tsc2 and the mechanistic target of rapamycin to the lysosome. J Physiol. 2013;591(18): 4611–4620.

73. Yoon MS, Sun Y, Arauz E, Jiang Y, Chen J. Phosphatidic acid activates mammalian target of rapamycin complex 1 (mtorc1) kinase by displacing fk506 binding protein 38 (fkbp38) and exerting an allosteric effect. J Biol Chem. 2011;286(34):29568–9574.

74. Foster DA. Phosphatidic acid and lipid-sensing by mtor. Trends Endocrinol Metab. 2013;24(6):272–8.

75. Hornberger TA. Mechanotransduction and the regulation of mtorc1 signaling in skeletal muscle. Int J Biochem Cell Biol. 2011;43(9):1267–1276.

76. Hornberger T, Chu W, Mak Y, Hsiung J, Huang S, Chien S. The role of phospholipase d and phosphatidic acid in the mechanical activation of mtor signaling in skeletal muscle. Proc Natl Acad Sci USA. 2006;103(12): 4741–4746.

77. You JS, Lincoln HC, Kim C-R, Frey JW, Goodman CA, Zhong XP, Hornberger TA. The role of diacylglycerol kinase ζ and phosphatidic acid

in the mechanical activation of mammalian target of rapamycin (mtor) signaling and skeletal muscle hypertrophy. J Biol Chem. 2014;289(3):1551–1563.

78. Kunkel SD, Suneja M, Ebert SM, Bongers KS, Fox DK, Malmberg SE, Alipour F, Shields RK, Adams CM. mrna expression signatures of human skeletal muscle atrophy identify a natural compound that increases muscle mass. Cell Metabol. 2011;13(6):627–638.

79. Lamb J, Crawford ED, Peck D, Modell JW, Blat IC, Wrobel MJ, Lerner J, Brunet J-P, Subramanian A, Ross KN, et al. The connectivity map: using gene-expression signatures to connect small molecules, genes, and disease. Science. 2006;313(5795):1929–1935.

80. Ogasawara R, Sato K, Higashida K, Nakazato K, Fujita S. Ursolic acid stimulates mtorc1 signaling after resistance exercise in rat skeletal muscle. Am J Physiol Endocrinol Metabol. 2013;305(6):760–765.

81. Bang HS, Seo DY, Chung YM, Oh KM, Park JJ, Arturo F, Jeong SH, Kim N, Han J. Ursolic acid-induced elevation of serum irisin augments muscle strength during resistance training in men. Korean J Physiol Pharmacol. 2014;18(5):441–446.

82. Deldicque L, Atherton P, Patel R, Theisen D, Nielens H, Rennie MJ, Francaux M. Effects of resistance exercise with and without creatine supplementation on gene expression and cell signaling in human skeletal muscle. J Appl Physiol. 2008;104(2):371–378.

83. Deldicque L, Louis M, Theisen D, Nielens H, Dehoux M, Thissen JP, Rennie MJ, Francaux M. Increased igf mrna in human skeletal muscle after creatine supplementation. Med Sci Sports Exerc. 2005;37(5):731–6.

84. Saremi A, Gharakhanloo R, Sharghi S, Gharaati M, Larijani B, Omidfar K. Effects of oral creatine and resistance training on serum myostatin and gasp-1. Mol Cell Endocrinol. 2010;317(1):25–30.

85. Wilson JM, Fitschen PJ, Campbell B, Wilson GJ, Zanchi N, Taylor L, Wilborn C, Kalman DS, Stout JR, Hoffman JR, et al. International society of sports nutrition position stand: beta-hydroxy-betamethylbutyrate (hmb). J Int Soc Sports Nutr. 2013;10(1):6.

86. Albert FJ, Morente-Sánchez J, Ortega Porcel FB, Castillo Garzón MJ, Gutiérrez Á. Usefulness of β-hydroxy-β-methylbutyrate (hmb) supplementation in different sports: an update and practical implications. 2015. http://www.ncbi.nlm.nih.gov/pubmed/26262692, doi:10.3305/nh. 2015.32.1.9101.

87. Pimentel GD, Rosa JC, Lira FS, Zanchi NE, Ropelle ER, Oyama LM, do Nascimento CMO, de Mello MT, Tufik S, Santos RV. b-hydroxy-b-methylbutyrate (hmb) supplementation stimulates skeletal muscle hypertrophy in rats via the mtor pathway. Nutr Metab. 2011;8(11):. http://link.springer.com/article/10.1186%2F1743-7075-8-11, doi:10.1186/ 1743-7075-8-11.

88. Eley HL, Russell ST, Baxter JH, Mukerji P, Tisdale MJ. Signaling pathways initiated by β-hydroxy-β-methylbutyrate to attenuate the depression of protein synthesis in skeletal muscle in response to cachectic stimuli. Am J Physiol Endocrinol Metabol. 2007;293(4):923–931.

89. Kimura K, Cheng XW, Inoue A, Hu L, Koike T, Kuzuya M. β-hydroxy-β-methylbutyrate facilitates pi3k/akt-dependent mammalian target of rapamycin and foxo1/3a phosphorylations and alleviates tumor necrosis factor α/interferon γ–induced murf-1 expression in c2c12 cells. Nutrition Res. 2014;34(4):368–374.

90. Mero AA, Ojala T, Hulmi JJ, Puurtinen R, Karila T, Seppälä T, et al. Effects of alfa-hydroxy-isocaproic acid on body composition, doms and performance in athletes. J Int Soc Sports Nutr. 2010;7(1):8.

91. Lang CH, Pruznak A, Navaratnarajah M, Rankine KA, Deiter G, Magne H, Offord EA, Breuillé D. Chronic α-hydroxyisocaproic acid treatment improves muscle recovery after immobilization-induced atrophy. Am J Physiol Endocrinol Metabol. 2013;305(3):416–428.

92. Cholewa JM, Wyszczelska-Rokiel M, Glowacki R, Jakubowski H, Matthews T, Wood R, Craig SA, Paolone V. Effects of betaine on body composition, performance, and homocysteine thiolactone. J Int Soc Sports Nutr. 2013;10(1):39.

93. Cholewa JM, Guimarães-Ferreira L, Zanchi NE. Effects of betaine on performance and body composition: a review of recent findings and potential mechanisms. Amino Acids. 2014;46(8):1785–1793.

94. Apicella JM, Lee EC, Bailey BL, Saenz C, Anderson JM, Craig SA, Kraemer WJ, Volek JS, Maresh CM. Betaine supplementation enhances anabolic endocrine and akt signaling in response to acute bouts of exercise. European J Appl Physiol. 2013;113(3):793–802.

95. Velloso C. Regulation of muscle mass by growth hormone and igf-i. British J Pharmacol. 2008;154(3):557–68.

96. Senesi P, Luzi L, Montesano A, Mazzocchi N, Terruzzi I. Betaine supplement enhances skeletal muscle differentiation in murine myoblasts via igf-1 signaling activation. J Transl Med. 2013;11(1):174.

97. Joy JM, Gundermann DM, Lowery RP, Jäger R, McCleary SA, Purpura M, Roberts MD, Wilson SM, Hornberger TA, Wilson JM. Phosphatidic acid enhances mtor signaling and resistance exercise induced hypertrophy. Nutrition Metabol. 2014;11(1):1–10.

98. Mobley CB, Hornberger TA, Fox CD, Healy JC, Ferguson BS, Lowery RP, McNally RM, Lockwood CM, Stout JR, Kavazis AN, et al. Effects of oral phosphatidic acid feeding with or without whey protein on muscle protein synthesis and anabolic signaling in rodent skeletal muscle. J Int Soc Sports Nutrition. 2015;12(1):1–11.

99. Bar-Peled L, Sabatini DM. Regulation of mtorc1 by amino acids. Trends Cell Biol. 2014;24(7):400–6.

## 20

Critical evaluation of food intake and energy balance in young modern pentathlon athletes: a cross-sectional study

Leticia Azen Alves Coutinho, Cristiana Pedrosa Melo Porto and Anna Paola Trindade Rocha Pierucci[*]

Abstract

Background: Modern pentathlon comprises five sports: fencing, swimming, equestrian jumping, and a combined event of pistol shooting and running. Despite the expected high energy demand of this sport, there are few studies that provide support for the nutritional recommendations for pentathletes. The purpose of the present study was to evaluate young modern pentathlon athletes with respect to body composition, biochemical profile, and consumption of food and supplements.

Methods: Fifty-six young modern pentathletes aged 13.5 ± 2.4 years participated in the study: 22 adolescent girls and 34 adolescent boys, weight 55.8 ± 13.3 kg, height 1.6 ± 0.1 m, and body fat 21.1 ± 3.1 %. Food consumption was analyzed through a 24-h recall method and food-frequency questionnaire. Assessment of body composition was carried out by checking anthropometric measures (body mass, height, and skinfolds) and using protocols according to participants' age and sexual maturity.

Results: Male participants consumed less energy than the general recommendations for athletes from the American Dietetic Association (2749 ± 1024 kcal vs. 3113 ± 704 kcal, $p < 0.01$), whereas female participants consumed more energy than those recommendations (2558 ± 808 kcal vs. 2213 ± 4734 kcal, $p < 0.01$). Neither young men nor young women followed the carbohydrate intake recommendations for athletes (6.3 ± 2.5 g/kg/day and 6.6 ± 2.2 g/kg/day, respectively). Lipid and protein intakes corresponded to recommendations for both sexes; however, insufficient intakes of calcium, fruits, and vegetables were seen, as well as frequent consumption of baked goods and sugared soft drinks.

Conclusions: Adolescent modern pentathlon athletes presented inadequate eating habits with respect to consumption of carbohydrates and energy. Many participants had insufficient intake of micronutrients, especially calcium. However, future research is needed that is aimed at elucidating the real nutritional demands for good physical performance in this sport and the impact of inadequate eating habits on performance, especially among young athletes who are in the growth-stage years and are exposed to intense physical exercise routines.

Keywords: Adolescents, Sports nutrition, Physical exercise, Body composition, Eating habits

* Correspondence: pierucci@nutricao.ufrj.br
Federal University of Rio de Janeiro/Josué de Castro Nutrition Institute, Av. Carlos Chagas Filho, 373 - Centro de Ciências da Saúde, Bloco J, 2° andar, Cidade Universitária, Ilha do Fundão, RJ 21941-902, Brazil

Background

The modern pentathlon is an Olympic sport that involves five modalities [1]. Modern pentathlon competitions last for about 8 h and include the sequential practice of sword fencing (all against all), 200-m freestyle swimming, equestrian show jumping (horses randomly chosen for competition) and finally, a combined event of pistol shooting (five well-aimed shots at the target) and running (four 800-m run cycle) [1].

In Brazil, the modern pentathlon is still not well known but has a significant role in social projects promoted by the Brazilian Modern Pentathlon Confederation (acronym in Portuguese: CBPM), with a predominance of adolescents among its participants.

The practice of competitive sports by adolescents requires special attention owing to their biological stage in which significant body changes related to sexual maturation and growth take place [2, 3]. Adolescent athletes' nutrition must promote adequate growth and development in addition to meeting the increased nutritional demands of strenuous physical activity. However, studies have shown that the intake of certain quantities of energy and nutrients by young athletes is below recommendations [2, 3].

In general, adolescent athletes often show insufficient intake of calcium, thereby becoming susceptible to low bone density and stress fractures [4]. It has been suggested that track and field athletes consume high amounts of lipids, saturated fats, and mono- and disaccharides whereas their iron intake is usually lower than recommendations, especially in women [5]. Such deficient energy balance and insufficient nutrient intake may impair the growth, health, and physical performance of these athletes. Thus, young athletes constitute a population that is vulnerable to the physiological effects of chronic physical fatigue owing to intense exercise, especially if they have inadequate food consumption.

Recently, Le Meuer et al. [6, 7] evaluated physiological demands during the new combined event (sport shooting and running) among adult modern pentathletes. Their most important finding was that the athletes performed this event close to their VO_2 max. However, there is currently little scientific literature [1] in this area; therefore the metabolic demands of other pentathlon events have not been established.

In the shooting and equestrian portions of the pentathlon, a static form of strength performance with low energy demands can be identified whereas events of a cyclic nature, such as running and swimming, have characteristically high demands on athletes' energy systems [8]. Fencing is a combat sport that is characterized by open skills and a noncyclic type of intermittent load, which requires high levels of agility and athlete concentration [9].

Because neither the metabolic requirements nor nutritional practices of the modern pentathlon have been established, and the required anthropometric profile for this sport is well known, the main purpose of the present study was to critically evaluate food consumption among young pentathletes, considering the general recommendations for athletes of the American Dietetic Association (ADA) [10]. Our hypothesis was that young pentathletes present nutritional inadequacies, especially with respect to intakes of energy, lipids, and micronutrients, and that young men and women have different eating habits, as observed in other studies involving adolescents.

Methods

Subjects

Fifty-six healthy young athletes voluntarily took part in this study. There were 22 adolescent females and 34 adolescent males, all affiliated with the Modern Pentathlon Federation of the State of Rio de Janeiro (FPMERJ, acronym in Portuguese). Participants were chosen by their coach as being diligent in training with the "Penta-Jovem" (acronym in Portuguese) team. The inclusion criteria were as follows: a) having trained for at least 6 months; and b) aged between 10 and 18 years (classified as postpubescent, according to sexual maturity). All adults were excluded.

The research was approved by the Committee of Ethics in Research of Clementino Fraga Filho University Hospital of the Rio de Janeiro Federal University (Protocol No. 90/11) and was carried out as per the norms in Resolution No. 196/96 of the National Health Council, which issues directives and regulations on the use of human beings in research.

Antropometry and sexual maturity

One experienced researcher carried out the anthropometric evaluations. Body mass and height were measured in accordance with the criteria of Gordon et al. [11], using a medical scale with a stadiometer (Welmy™, Brazil) ranging from 0 to 150 kg, with precision 100 g.

Two cutaneous skinfolds (triceps and subscapular) were measured in triplicate on the right side of the body, according to Harrison et al. [12], using an adipometer with 10 g/mm^2 constant pressure (Lange™, USA) and precision 1 mm. A new set of measurements were taken if there was >5 % disagreement in one of the three measurements. The final result was expressed as an arithmetic mean of the three measurements.

Evaluation of athletes' sexual maturity was carried out using the criteria proposed by Tanner, which divides adolescence into five phases, starting at the prepubertal stage (stage 1), going through puberty (stages 2 to 4), and finishing at the postpubertal stage (stage 5).

Evaluation was made by showing participants photos that referred to the adolescent developmental stages of pubic hair growth for both sexes, breast development for adolescent girls, and genital development adolescent boys [13].

Body mass index was calculated with AnthroPlus software of the World Health Organization, and results were compared with the reference distribution [14]. Body density and body fat percentage were estimated using the equation of Slaughter et al. [15].

Biochemical profile

After participants had completed a 12-h fast, a qualified nurse drew blood samples from the antecubital vein. Participants had been instructed not to engage in any physical activity for the 24 h prior to sample collection and to abstain from consuming alcoholic beverages for the previous 72 h. Blood counts and blood lipid profiles were automatically analyzed (Lab Max Plenno Labtest™), as well as glucose (Citometro Cell-Dyn 1700 Abbott™), using Diagnostica™ Labtest kits.

Energy expenditure

To estimate the total energy expenditure (TEE), methods proposed by Iglesias-Gutierrez et al. [16] and Leenders et al. [17] were adapted, considering three components: 1) basal metabolic rate (BMR), calculated using the FAO/WHO/UNU equation [18]; 2) thermic effect of food (10 % of TEE); and 3) energy expenditure (EE) related to routine activities and physical training.

To calculate routine activity EE, athletes or their parents were asked to register participants' daily activities based on the questionnaire proposed by Bouchard et al. [19]. Team trainers recorded data of physical training (duration, distances covered, and intensity of each activity, as per the Rated Perceived Exertion Scale [20]. Metabolic equivalents [21] were used to quantify EE for each physical activity.

Food and supplements consumption

Athletes' food consumption was evaluated by a 24-h recall method (R24h) and food-frequency questionnaire (FFQ) for adolescents. Athletes' use of supplements was registered on a separate form, specifying the type, purpose, manner of use, and origin of the indication.

Quantitative analysis of ingested energy and nutrients (carbohydrates, proteins, lipids, calcium, iron, and vitamins A and C) for each meal reported by participants in the R24h was carried out, by assessing nutritional composition in accordance with the Table of Food Composition of the Brazilian Institute of Geography and Statistics [22] and the nutritional information on food labels for foods not listed in the reference table.

Assessment of the adequacy of macronutrient intake was made based on the publication "Nutrition and Athletic Performance" of the ADA [10]. Dietary reference intake (DRI) [23] values were considered to assess the adequacy of micronutrient intake. Intake was considered inadequate for values less than the estimated average requirement (EAR) or greater than the Tolerable Upper Intake Level.

To interpret results of the FFQ, foods were grouped on the basis of food groups set as healthy food markers in the Consumer Expenditure Survey 2008–2009 [24]. Frequency of consumption categories considered were: once or less per week, two to four times per week, and five times per week or more.

Statistical analyses

The results are expressed in averages (±standard deviation). The normality of the data was checked using the Shapiro–Wilk test. To compare independent data, the t-test was chosen for independent samples, at statistical significance level $p < 0.05$. All analyses were performed using IBM SPSS software™ version 20.0 (Armonk, NY, USA).

Results

Results related to anthropometry and sexual maturity are shown in Table 1. The findings showed that 78.5 % of participants, for both sexes, were in the pubertal developmental stage. Adolescent girls showed a higher body fat percentage in the pubertal and postpubertal stages than their male counterparts.

The assessed laboratory parameters were generally within normal ranges for all athletes in this study. The following average results were observed: hemoglobin 13.5 ± 1.2 g/dl; hematocrit 42.0 ± 3.4 %; glucose 90.4 ± 6.5 mg/dl; total lipids 421.7 ± 71.6 mg/dl; total cholesterol 151.9 ± 25.2 mg/dl; HDL cholesterol 52.4 ± 12.7 mg/dl; LDL cholesterol 83.5 ± 23.1 mg/dl; and triglycerides 79.5 ± 5.1 mg/dl.

Values of estimated EE were determined using records of athletes' physical training routines. The youngest athletes (aged between 10 and 14 years and belonging to the Young E10, Young D, Young C categories) had lower EE values compared with the oldest ones (over 15 years old and belonging to the Young B and Young A categories); these results were based on training three times a week, with older athletes training about 3 h a day and younger ones training about 2 h a day. For athletes in both these age groups, EE tended to increase from Monday through Wednesday, subsequently decreasing through Friday, and increasing again on Saturday (Monday, 619 ± 410 kcal vs. 782 ± 280 kcal; Tuesday, 617 ± 223 kcal vs. 887 ± 231 kcal; Wednesday, 1163 ± 371 kcal vs. 1520 ± 363 kcal; Thursday, 896 ± 275 kcal vs. 1188 ± 268 kcal; Friday, 742 ± 296 kcal vs. 812 ± 264 kcal;

Table 1 Anthropometric profile of modern pentathlon athletes ($n = 56$), according to the stages of sexual maturation and gender, X ± SD

	Male ($n = 34$)			Female ($n = 22$)		
	Prepubescent ($n = 1$)	Pubescent ($n = 27$)	Post pubescent ($n = 6$)	Prepubescent ($n = 2$)	Pubescent ($n = 17$)	Post pubescent ($n = 3$)
Weight (kg)	39.4	58.49 ± 12.5	70.8 ± 9.9	34.6 ± 6.9	49.2 ± 9.9	64.2 ± 6.3
Height (cm)	148.0	163.4 ± 10.3	175.9 ± 7.4	146.0 ± 5.6	155.5 ± 10.7	162.6 ± 3.5
BMI (kg/m²)	18.0	21.68 ± 3.2	22.8 ± 1.9	16.1 ± 1.9	20.1 ± 2.6	24.3 ± 2.4
Body fat (%)	20.0	20.4 ± 8.3	15.5 ± 6.4	16.35 ± 0.7	23.8 ± 6.8	28.4 ± 1.2

BMI body mass index

Saturday, 982 ± 262 kcal vs. 1193 ± 191 kcal, for younger and older athletes, respectively) (Fig. 1).

With respect to supplement intake, 35 (62 %) athletes reported the use of some type of nutritional supplement, but only 6 % used supplements as prescribed by a nutritionist. The majority (46 %) used supplements as suggested by their trainer, emphasizing the fact that 86 % of athletes had not received any professional nutritional counseling.

Energy supplements, hydroelectrolytic supplements, vitamin C, and multivitamins were the most frequently consumed supplements, corresponding to 31 %, 25 %, 19 % and 15 % of the products reported by participants, respectively.

Although the difference between adolescent boys and girls was not significant, Table 2 shows that male athletes tended to have greater energy intake than their female counterparts. However, boys did not reach the estimated TEE, whereas girls had higher energy intake than recommendations. In general, macronutrient intake did not differ between boys and girls, whereas intakes of proteins and lipids were adequate. However, both male

and female athletes consumed fewer carbohydrates ($p < 0.01$) than the average recommendations of the ADA (2009) [10].

Considering the energy intake for each meal as a percentage of the consumed total energy value, it was found that the athletes concentrated their largest intake of energy in the main meals (breakfast, lunch and dinner) with 20 % consumed at breakfast, 7 % with mid-morning snacks, 27 % at lunch, 5 % during physical activity, 15 % after physical activity, 25 % at dinner, and 1 % at supper.

According to the needs of each sex and age group, we evaluated the adequacy of micronutrient intake (Table 3). In general, both male and female athletes showed a high proportion of inadequate vitamin A and C intake. Nearly all athletes consumed inadequate amounts of calcium; however, most athletes of both sexes and in all age groups consumed adequate quantities of iron.

The results of qualitative analysis of participants' eating habits, evaluated by means of an FFQ, are shown in Fig. 2. Legumes were consumed by 95 % of athletes, baked goods by 43 %, and sugared soft drinks by 30 %, all with a frequency of five times a week or more. On

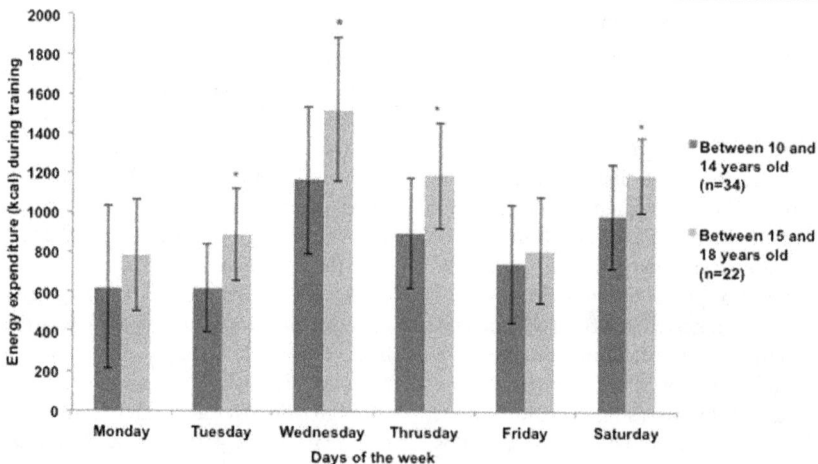

Fig. 1 Weekly energy expenditure (X ± SD) during training performed by modern pentathlon athletes, PentaJovem team, differentiated by age. * Significant difference ($p <0.05$) from the athletes older than 15 years old, t-test for independent sample

Table 2 Intake of macronutrients and energy by modern pentathlon athletes (n = 56), according to gender, X ± SD

Variables	Female (n = 22)		Male (n = 34)	
	ADA (2009) recomendations	Intake	ADA (2009) recomendations	Intake
Energy (kcal)	2213 ± 473[a]	2558 ± 808[b]	3113 ± 704[a]	2749 ± 1024[b]
Protein (g/kg)	1.2–1.7	1.7 ± 0.6	1.2–1.7	1.6 ± 0.5
Carbohydrate (g/kg)	6.0–10.0	6.6 ± 2.2[c]	6.0–10.0	6.3 ± 2.5[c]
Lipids (%VET)	25.0–35.0 %	30.3 ± 6.6	25.0–35.0 %	31.4 ± ± 8.4

[a]Estimated values according to Iglesias-Gutierrez et al. (2005) [16] and Leenders et al. [17]
[b]Significant difference compared to the estimated energy expenditure (p <0.01)
[c]Significant difference compared to the ADA (2009) [10] recommendations (p <0.01), t-test for independent samples

the other hand, 90 % of athletes consumed fish, 87 % ate processed meats, and 74 % consumed vegetables, all with a frequency of once or less per week.

Discussion

For optimal performance in sports, adequate nutrition and physical training are essential factors. There are few scientific studies on this subject that involve pentathletes, so knowledge remains insufficient regarding the physical demands of these athletes and the ideal nutritional habits necessary to improve physical performance. This is the first study of adolescent modern pentathlon athletes to assess body composition, biochemical profile, and consumption of food and supplements.

Body composition is an important indicator of physical fitness and the general health of athletes [8]. The study Claessens et al. [25] among 54 adult female pentathletes (average body weight 61 ± 5.3 kg, body fat 16 ± 2.4 %) revealed an inverse relationship between fat mass and pentathlon performance.

Considering the incompleteness of body mass index data in terms of determining body composition variability and changes in the proportions of fat mass and fat-free mass, it becomes necessary to analyze the body composition of elite pentathletes in the form of component structures. Generally, lower fat mass proportion, greater musculature, and more active mass are required in most sports disciplines [8].

Our research group previously assessed the body composition of elite pentathletes using dual-energy x-ray absorptiometry and found substantial effects of sports activities on anthropometry results [26], especially among men. On the other hand, the optimal body composition for a specific sport discipline is difficult to determine[8].

Cech et al. [8] aimed to describe the current profile of body composition among elite young male and female modern pentathletes. They detected sex differences in that men had a higher proportion of fat free mass (women, 52.6 ± 3.5 kg vs. men, 66.4 ± 3.3 kg) and less fat mass (women, 15.8 + 1.38 % vs. men, 8.8 + 0.7 %). According to the authors, their results were in accordance with the published literature. In the present study, we also observed that adolescent girls had a higher percentage of body fat compared with adolescent boys. However, despite finding higher results for both sexes, our findings could not be compared with those of Cech et al. [8] because body fat was predicted in that study using a different technique (bioelectrical impedance analysis).

Table 3 Average intake of micronutrients and distribution of pentathletes (%) (n =56) on the adequacy of micronutrient intakes, according to gender and age

	Vitamins							Minerals							
	Vitamin A				Vitamin C				Calcium				Iron			
Gender/ Age	Intake (mcg)	<EAR	≥EAR ≤ UL	>UL	Intake (mg)	<EAR	≥EAR ≤ UL	>UL	Intake (mg)	<AI	≥AI ≤UL	>UL	Intake (mg)	<EAR	≥EAR ≤ UL	>UL
Male																
10–13 (n = 13)	551.5 ± 1207.7	92.3 %	–	7.7 %	100.2 ± 120.6	61.5 %	38.5 %	–	312.3 ± 181.5	100.0 %	–	–	11.6 ± 5.5	23.0 %	77.0 %	–
14–18 (n = 21)	870.1 ± 1872.8	80.9 %	14.2 %	4.9 %	76.3 ± 114.8	66.7 %	33.3 %	–	510.5 ± 347.8	95.2 %	4.8 %	–	13.4 ± 5.2	14.3 %	85.7 %	–
Female																
10–13 (n = 12)	1026.3 ± 2508.5	75.0 %	16.7 %	8.3 %	29.6 ± 51.3	83.3 %	16.7 %	–	344.1 ± 243.7	100.0 %	–	–	11.7 ± 8.9	8.3 %	91.7 %	–
14–18 (n = 10)	1248.8 ± 2777.3	70.0 %	20.0 %	10.0 %	117.1 ± 107.6	50.0 %	50.0 %	–	479.2 ± 271.0	100.0 %	–	–	12.4 ± 4.0	10.0 %	90.0 %	–

EAR Estimated Energy Requirement, UL Tolerable Upper Intake Level, AI Adequate Intake

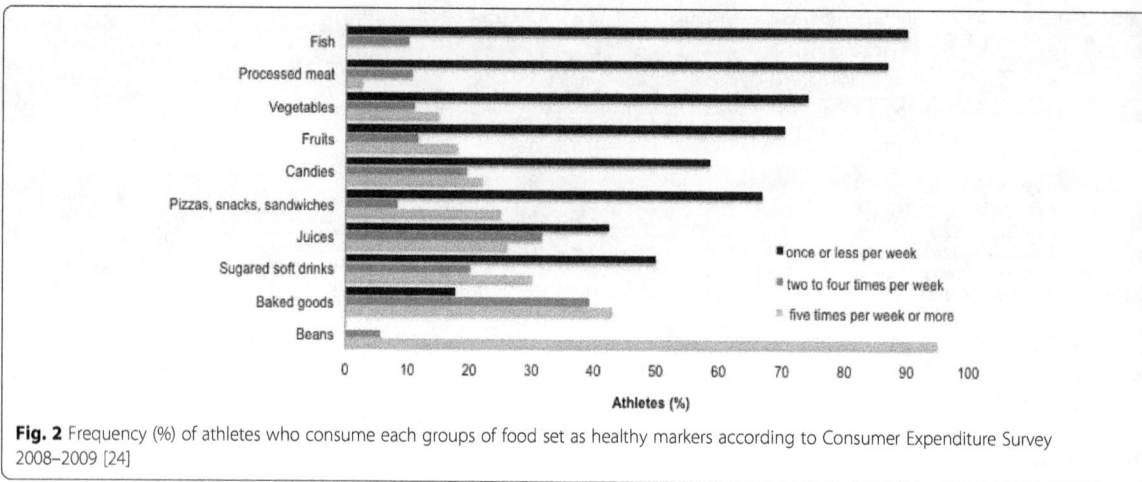

Fig. 2 Frequency (%) of athletes who consume each groups of food set as healthy markers according to Consumer Expenditure Survey 2008–2009 [24]

Nutritional needs during adolescence have a stronger relationship with physiological age than with chronological age and are thus directly proportional to the speed of growth and changes in body composition. Therefore, chronological age alone should not be used as an indicator of adolescent developmental state because individuals of the same age differ in their stages of sexual maturation [27, 28]. In the present study, we confirmed the importance of evaluating the stage of sexual maturity together with an evaluation of body composition, particularly in adolescent girls between 13 and 15 years old who are classified as either pubertal or postpubertal.

Adolescents require special attention during this biological period, which includes noticeable body changes related to sexual maturity and growth. However, it is known that the eating habits of adolescents are frequently inadequate. Adolescents often substitute meals with snacks of low nutritional value [29] and consume insufficient amounts of milk, dairy products, fruits, and vegetables [30–32], as well as large amounts of high energy-density foods that are rich in sodium and sugar, such as soft drinks and fast foods [31, 33, 34].

Our qualitative analysis of participants' eating habits showed that the most frequently consumed foods (five times a week or more) were legumes, baked goods, and sugared soft drinks. Few pentathletes ate vegetables and fruits with this same frequency. Our findings therefore corroborate previous findings demonstrating that young athletes have inadequate nutritional intake levels, particularly with respect to energy, carbohydrates, vitamins A and C, and calcium. However, intakes of lipids, proteins, and iron among this population were adequate.

In the present study, a deficit in total energy intake among adolescent males was verified, different to the findings of Braggion et al. [35], who observed energy

intake below DRI values among both male and female adolescent athletes. Moreover, Kazapi and Ramos [30] observed a greater prevalence of restricted energy intake among female athletes than their male counterparts. According to Panza et al. [36], many athletes who engage in different sports, especially female athletes, usually adopt dietary restrictions as a way to reduce body weight and optimize sports performance. Paradoxically, in this study, female athletes consumed more energy than the recommendations.

Carbohydrates are essential for athletes because they contribute to meeting their specific energy needs, to maintain glycemia and recover glycogen reserves [28]. Furthermore, inadequate carbohydrate intake could result in the use of body protein as an energy source, impairing the growth and development processes in both sexes [37]. Additional studies should be carried out to assess whether insufficient intake of energy and carbohydrates, according to ADA recommendations [10], impairs either the growth or physical performance of young modern pentathletes.

Calcium intakes were below the EAR for both male and female study participants, regardless of age. In surveys carried out in Brazil among adolescent non-athletes [38] and athletes [32, 39, 40], low intakes of calcium according to dietary recommendations were common. Santos et al. [38] reported that given the presence of calcium in many metabolic processes, its deficiency may be noted in several ways, such as muscle numbness, musculoskeletal pains, menstrual cramps, and osteoporosis.

In addition to calcium, dietary iron intake also appears to be inadequate among adolescent athletes [38]. However, in the present study, the average amounts of iron ingested by most athletes of both sexes were in accordance with recommendations [23].

The habit of consuming small snacks by physically active individuals could help meet their energy and nutrient needs, according to Burke et al. [41]. The majority of adolescent athletes in this study concentrated their food intake in the three main meals (breakfast, lunch and dinner). Considering the fact that participants reported a short interval between lunch and the start of training sessions, we suggest an evaluation of using snacks as part of the daily nutritional contribution, mainly during periods of training.

According to Jacobson [42], young athletes normally receive guidance from an unreliable source when it comes to use of supplements, such as from trainers, friends, family, magazines, or television. Our data reinforced these findings; most athletes reported following their trainers' advice and only a few stated that they used supplements in a manner prescribed by a nutritionist. Energy and hydroelectrolytic supplements were the most frequently used among study participants. Vitamin C supplements, multivitamins, and branched-chain amino acids were also mentioned by a smaller number of athletes.

Vigorous and taxing physical activity together with reduced energy availability may cause adverse effects on pubertal development and reproductive function [43]. Therefore, accurate estimation of individual energy needs is needed to establish appropriate dietary guidelines [44]. In the present study, TEE was estimated by predictive equations. However, we believe that errors might exist in the final values obtained; our research group recently suggested that the FAO/WHO/UNU equation [18] tended to overestimate basal metabolic rate measured by indirect calorimetry [44].

The findings of this work can contribute to awareness among young modern pentathletes of the importance of nutrition and the role of each nutrient, for adequate physical performance, muscular recovery, health preservation, and promoting growth and development. Our results will also help sports nutrition professionals in advising adolescent pentathletes.

A main limitation of this study is that we were unable to obtain a homogeneous distribution of athletes at each stage of sexual maturity, so as to more accurately investigate the influence of this variable on eating habits. In addition, the analyses performed here might provide more useful information if conducted using a larger sample size. Further studies will be carried out that are focused on this sport, especially regarding the nutritional demands of athletes during each pentathlon event.

Conclusions

The adolescent modern pentathlon athletes in this study had inadequate eating habits with respect to energy, carbohydrates, and calcium intake. Moreover, the majority of athletes made use of supplements, even without qualified nutritional counseling, and showed qualitative inadequacy in their eating habits, especially with regard to frequent consumption of soft drinks and low consumption of fruits and vegetables.

Competing interests
The authors declare that they have no competing interests.

Authors' contributions
APTRP, CPMP, and LAAC contributed significantly to all aspects of this study, and read and approved the final manuscript.

Acknowledgments
The authors would like to thank FAPERJ for financial support and budgeting, the leaders of the Brazilian Modern Pentathlon Confederation for authorizing our research, and the athletes for their collaboration.

References
1. Kelm J. Modern Pentathlon. In: Caine DJ, Harmer PA, Schiff MA, editors. Epidemiology of injury in olympic sports. Oxford: Wiley-Blackwell; 2010;176–80.
2. Croll JK, Neumark-sztainer D, Story M, et al. Adolescents involved in weight-related and power team sports have better eating patterns and nutrient intakes than non-sport-involved adolescents. J Am Diet Assoc. 2006;106:709–17. doi:10.1016/j.jada.2006.02.010.
3. Volpe SL. Micronutrient requirements for athletes. Clin J Sport Med. 2007;26: 119–30. doi:10.1016/j.csm.2006.11.009.
4. Nattiv A, Armsey TD. Stress injury to bone in the female athlete. Clin Sport Med. 1997;16:197–224.
5. Aerenhouts D, Hebbelinck M, Poortmans JR, et al. Nutritional habits of Flemish adolescent Sprint athlete. Int J Sport Nutr Exerc Metab. 2008;15:509–23.
6. Le Meur Y, Hausswirth C, Abbiss C, Baupi Y, Dorel S. Performance factors in the new combined event of modern pentathlon. J Sports Sci. 2010;28:1111–6. doi:10.1080/0264041.2010.497816.
7. Le Meur Y, Dorel S, Baup Y, Guvomarch JP, Roudaut A, Hausswirth C. Physiological demand and pacing strategy during the new combined event in elite pentathletes. Eur J Appl Physiol. 2012;112:2583–93. doi:10.1007/s00421-011-2235-2.
8. Cech P, Marly T, Maia L, et al. Body composition of elite youth pentatlhetes and its gender diferences. Sports Sci. 2013;6:29–35.
9. Roi GS & Bianchedi D. The science of fencing – Implications for performance and injury prevention. Sports Med. 2008;38:465–81. doi:10.112/08/0006-0465.
10. American Dietetic Association, Dietitians of Canada, and the American College of Sports Medicine. Position stand: Nutrition and Athletic Performance. J Am Diet Assoc. 2009;509–27. doi:10.1016/j.jada.2009.01.005.
11. Gordon CC, Chumlea WC, Roche AF. Stature, recumbent length, weight. In: Lohman TG, Roche AF, Martorell R, editors. Anthropometric standardization reference manual. Champaign, Illinois: Human Kinetics Books; 1988;3–8.
12. Harrison GG, Buskirk ER, Carter JEL, et al. Skinfold Thickness and measurement technique. In: Lohman TG, Roche AF, Martorell R, editors. Anthropometric standardization reference manual. Champaign, Illinois: Human Kinetics Books; 1988;55–70.
13. Chipkevitch E. Avaliação clínica da maturação sexual na adolescência. J Ped. 2001;77:S135–42.
14. Onis M, Onyango AW, Borghi E et al. Development of a WHO growth reference for school-aged children and adolescents. Bull World Health Organ. 2007;85:660–7. doi:10.1590/S0042-96862007000900010.
15. Slaughter MH, Lohman TG, Boileau RA, et al. Skinfold Equations of Body Fatness in Children and Youth. Hum Biol. 1988;60:709–23.
16. Iglesias-Gutierrez E, Garcia-Roves PM, Rodríguez C et al. Food habits and nutritional status assessment of adolescent soccer players. A necessary and accurate approach. Can J Appl Physiol. 2005;30:18–32. doi:10.1139/h05-102.
17. Leenders NYJ, Sherman WM, Nagaraja HN et. al. Evaluation of methods to assess physical activity in free-living conditions. Med Sci Sports Exerc. 2001;33:1233–40. doi:10.1097/00005768-200107000-00024.

18. Food and Agriculture Organization, World Health Organization, United Nations University. Human energy requirements. Food Nutr Technical Report Series. 2004.
19. Bouchard C, Trewblay A, Leblanc C, et al. Method to assess energy expenditure in children and adults. Am J Clin Nutr. 1983;37:461–7.
20. Borg G. Borg's perceived exertion and pain scales. Champaign, IL: Human Kinetics; 1998.
21. Ainsworth BE, Haskell WL, Whitt MC, et al. Compendium of Physical Activities: An update of activity codes and MET intensities. Med Sci Sports Exerc. 2000;32:498–516.
22. Instituto Brasileiro de Geografia e Estatística. Tabelas de composição de alimentos. 5nd ed, Rio de Janeiro, IBGE, 1996.
23. Institute Of Medicine. DRI Dietary Reference Intakes for Calcium and Vitamina D. Washington: The National Academies Press; 2011.
24. Instituto Brasileiro de Geografia e Estatística. Pesquisa de orçamentos familiares 2008–2009. Análise do consumo alimentar pessoal no Brasil. Rio de Janeiro, 2011.
25. Claessens AL, Hlatky S, Lefevre J, Holdhaus H. The role of anthropometric characteristics in modern pentathlon performance in female athletes. J Sports Sci. 1994;12:391–401.
26. Junior SJF, Loureiro LL, Oliva GO, et al. Composição corporal de pentatletas adolescents avaliada com a absortometria radiologica de dupla energia. Rev Educ Fis. 2015;26:465–72. doi:10.4025/reveducfis.v6i3.25203.
27. Colli AS, Silva LEV. Crescimento e desenvolvimento físico. In: Marcondes E, Vaz FAC, Ramos JLA, Okay Y, editors. Pediatria básica: pediatria geral e neonatal. São Paulo: Sarvier; 2002.
28. Vitalle MSS. Crescimento e desenvolvimento físico na adolescência. In: Carvalho ES, Carvalho WB, editors. Terapêutica e prática pediátrica. São Paulo: Atheneu; 2000.
29. Estima CCP, Salles-Costa R, Sichieri R et al. Meal consumption patterns and anthropometric measures in adolescents from a low socioeconomic neighborhood in the metropolitan area of Rio de Janeiro, Brazil. Appetite. 2009;52:735–9. doi:10.1016/j.appet.2009.03.017.
30. Kazapi IM, Ramos LAZ. Hábitos e consumo alimentares de atletas nadadores. Rev Nut. 1998;11:117–24.
31. Leal GVS, Philippi ST, Matsudo SMM et al. Consumo alimentar e padrão de refeições de adolescentes, São Paulo, Brasil. Rev Bras Epidemiol. 2010;13:457–67. doi:10.1590/S1415-790X2010000300009. doi:10.1590/S1415-790X2010000300009.
32. Meyer F, O'Connor H, Shirreffs S.M. Nutrition for young athletes. J Sports Sci. 2007;25:S73–82. doi:10.1080/02640410701607338.
33. Andrade RG, Pereira RA, Sichieri R. Consumo alimentar de adolescentes com e sem sobrepeso no município do Rio de Janeiro. Cad Saude Publica. 2003;19:1485–95. doi:10.1590/S0102-311X2003000500027.
34. Levy RB, Castro IRR, Cardoso LO, et al. Consumo e comportamento alimentar entre adolescentes brasileiros: Pesquisa Nacional de Saúde do Escolar (PeNSE), 2009. Cien Saude Colet. 2010;15:S3085–97. doi:10.1590/S1413-81232010000800013.
35. Braggion GF, Matsudo SMM, Matsudo VKR. Consumo alimentar, atividade física e percepção da aparência corporal em adolescentes. Rev Bras Ci e Mov. 2000;28:15–21.
36. Panza VP, Coelho MSPH, DI PIETRO PF, et al. Consumo alimentar de atletas: reflexões sobre recomendações nutricionais, hábitos alimentares e métodos para avaliação do gasto e consumo energéticos. Rev Nutr. 2007;20:681–92. doi:10.1590/S1415-52732007000600010.
37. Cotugna N, Vickery CE, McBee S. Sports nutrition for young athletes. J Sch Nurs. 2005;21:323–8. doi:10.1177/10598405050210060401.
38. Santos FC, Martini LA, Freitas SN, et al. Ingestão de cálcio e indicadores antropométricos entre adolescentes. Rev Nutr. 2007;20:275–83. doi:10.1590/S1415-5273200700030000.
39. Ferraz AP, Alves MRA, Bacurau RFP, Navarro F. Avaliação da dieta, crescimento, maturação sexual e treinamento de crianças e adolescentes atletas de ginástica rítmica. Rev Bras Nutr Esport. 2007;1:1–10.
40. Ribeiro BG, Soares EA. Avaliação do estado nutricional de atletas de ginástica olímpica do Rio de Janeiro. Rev Nutr. 2002;15:181–91.
41. Burke LM, Slater G, Broad EM, Haukka J, Modulon S, Hopkins WG. Eating patterns and meal frequency of elite Australian athletes. Int J Sports Nutr Exerc Metab. 2003;13:521–38.
42. Jacobson BH, Sobonya C, Ransone J. Nutrition practices and knowledge of college varsity athletes a follow-up. J Strength Cond Res. 2001;15:63–8.
43. Alves C, Lima RVB. Impacto da atividade física e esportes sobre o crescimento e puberdade de crianças e adolescentes. Rev Pal Pediatr. 2008;26:383–91.
44. Loureiro LL, Fonseca S, Castro NGCO, et al. Basal metabolic of adolescent modern pentathlon athletes: agrément between indirect calorimetry and predictive equations and the correlation with body parameters. PLoS One. 2015;16:1–12. doi:10.1371/jornal.pone.0142859.

## 21

Ramadan fasting does not adversely affect neuromuscular performances and reaction times in trained karate athletes

Nidhal Zarrouk[1,5*], Omar Hammouda[2], Imed Latiri[3], Hela Adala[4], Ezzedine Bouhlel[3], Haithem Rebai[5] and Mohamed Dogui[1]

Abstract

Background: The present study aimed to investigate the concomitant effects of Ramadan intermittent fast (RIF) and muscle fatigue on neuromuscular performances and reaction times in young trained athletes.

Methods: Eight karate players (17.2 ± 0.5 years) were tested on three sessions: during a control period (S1: one week before Ramadan), and during the first (S2) and the fourth week of RIF (S3). Dietary intake and anthropometric measurements were assessed before each session. During each test session, participants performed maximal voluntary isometric contractions (MVC) and a submaximal contraction at 75 % MVC until exhaustion (T_{lim}) of the right elbow flexors. Surface electromyography was recorded from biceps brachii muscle during MVC and T_{lim}. Simple (SRT) and choice (CRT) reaction times were evaluated at rest and just after T_{lim} in a random order.

Results: The total daily energy (S2: +19.5 %, $p < 0.05$; S3: +27.4 %, $p < 0.01$) and water (S2: +26.8 %, $p < 0.01$; S3: +23.2 %, $p < 0.05$) intake were significantly increased during RIF. However, neither body mass nor body mass index was altered by RIF ($F_{(2,14)} = 0.80$, $p = 0.47$ and $F_{(2,14)} = 0.78$, $p = 0.48$, respectively). In addition, T_{lim} ($F_{(2,14)} = 2.53$, $p = 0.12$), MVC ($F_{(2,14)} = 0.51$, $p = 0.61$) and associated electrical activity ($F_{(2,14)} = 0.13$, $p = 0.88$) as well as neuromuscular efficiency ($F_{(2,14)} = 0.27$, $p = 0.76$) were maintained during RIF. Moreover, neither SRT nor CRT was affected by RIF ($F_{(2,14)} = 1.82$, $p = 0.19$ and $F_{(2,14)} = 0.26$, $p = 0.78$, respectively) or neuromuscular fatigue ($F_{(1,7)} = 0.0002$, $p = 0.98$ and $F_{(1,7)} = 3.78$, $p = 0.09$, respectively).

Conclusions: The present results showed that RIF did not adversely affect the neuromuscular performances and anthropometric parameters of elite karate athletes who were undertaking their usual training schedule. In addition, neither RIF nor neuromuscular fatigue poorly affects reaction times in elite karate athletes.

Keywords: Ramadan fasting, Strength, Electromyography, Cognitive performance, Reaction time, Karate

Background

Karate is currently considered as one of the most popular martial arts practiced worldwide [1]. It is divided into two competitive disciplines: kata and kumite. Kata consists of prescribed sequences of offensive and defensive techniques and movements, while kumite is a free form of sparring against an opponent. In competitions, kata performers are judged based on specific parameters:

technique, rhythm, power, expressiveness of movements, and kime (i.e., short isometric muscle contractions performed at the end of a technique) [2]. The karate fight (i.e., kumite) requires high technical skills (i.e., kick and punch) with precision and high velocity to adequately execute effective attack and defense techniques [2–4]. In addition, technical performance in karate is considerably saturated by cognitive abilities and efficient attentional processes allowing more time for preparation and organization of motor behavior and ensuring quick and correct responses to visuospatial stimuli [3–7]. Therefore, reaction time, or the elapsed time between the onset of a stimulus and the initiation of a movement response [8], is crucial to achieve a high quality performance in karate

* Correspondence: nidhal.zarrouk@yahoo.com
[1]Research Laboratory: "Medical Imaging Technologies" (LR 12ES06, TIM), Faculty of Medicine of Monastir, University of Monastir, Monastir, Tunisia
[5]Research Unit: "Education, Motricity, Sports and Health" (UR 15JS01), Higher Institute of Sport and Physical Education of Sfax, University of Sfax, Sfax, Tunisia
Full list of author information is available at the end of the article

techniques [2, 3]. Indeed, it has been shown that compared to novices, expert karate athletes reacted faster and/or more accurately in simple reaction time (SRT) [7], choice reaction time (CRT) [5, 6], and identical pictures test [4]. However, though it has been recently shown that reaction time was affected by some factors such as age, gender, number of stimuli and expertise in karate [9], little is known about the effects of neuromuscular fatigue on reaction time and attentional processes. In fact, the majority of the studies investigating acute effects of exercise on cognitive performance have typically incorporated aerobic (e.g., cycling or running) and resistance tasks [10]. Although aerobic and resistance exercises are common modes of exercise and considered as key determinants in achieving top karate performances, isometric exercise (i.e., kime) merits the attention since it represents the most important criterion of proper kata execution [2]. In this context, Del Percio et al. [11] showed that muscle fatigue induced by repeated isometric contractions at 50 % of maximal voluntary contraction (MVC) negatively affects visuo-spatial attentional processes in non-athletes but not in elite karate athletes. Recently, Brown and Bray [12] showed that performing isometric exercise (at 30, 50 and 70 % of MVC) until exhaustion is associated with reduced cognitive performance and that higher intensity of isometric exercise leads to greater performance impairments suggesting that exercising at high intensity levels or to exhaustion results in impaired cognitive performance.

During every day of the Ramadan month, Muslims abstain from food and fluid between dawn and sunset resulting in many effects upon individual's physiology, biochemistry and behavior [13–15]. As major sporting calendars do not consider religious observances, competitive Muslim athletes continue to train and/or compete while undertaking the Ramadan intermittent fast (RIF). Therefore, the absence of food and fluid intake during the training as well as throughout the competition may have significant implications for physical performances. Several studies have investigated the effect of RIF upon physical performance and presented conflicting results (see for review [16]). Indeed, some authors reported significant alterations in neuromuscular performances during RIF [17, 18], while others reported no significant changes [19, 20]. However, successful performance in many sports, especially martial arts, requires not only high physical performances allowing efficient execution of motor behavior but also a high level of cognitive abilities [2, 3]. To the best of the authors' knowledge, few studies have examined the effect of RIF on cognitive function [21, 22], and especially the combined effects of RIF and physical exercise on cognitive performances [23]. In this context, it has been reported that physical performance was not affected by RIF, while psychomotor components (i.e., recognition

reaction time and total reaction time) were affected during the first week of fast in nine male resistance trained athletes [23]. Same, Roky et al. [22] observed slower CRT on the sixth day of Ramadan in ten sedentary subjects. During RIF, Tian et al. [24] found that psychomotor performance and vigilance were enhanced in the morning, however in the afternoon, verbal learning and memory were both impaired in fasted martial arts athletes.

In this way, the topic of neuromuscular fatigue and cognitive performance is of particular interest for training and competing of elite athletes involved in combat sports and especially karate. In addition, the literature reveals that the effect of RIF on neuromuscular and cognitive performances still needs to be explored. Therefore, the aim of the present study was to investigate the concomitant effects of RIF and fatigue on cognitive and neuromuscular performances in trained karate athletes undertaking training schedule during Ramadan. Given that muscle fatigue could impair cognitive performance [12], and that Ramadan fasting resulted in many effects upon individual's physiology, biochemistry and behavior [13–15], we hypothesized that both fatigue and RIF could negatively affect reaction times and neuromuscular performances in elite karate athletes.

Methods
Participants
Ten right-handed male karate athletes of the Tunisian Regional Team, were volunteered to take part in this study. While eight of them (age: 17.2 ± 0.5 years; height: 175.6 ± 4.2 cm) achieved the complete experimental protocol, two athletes were excluded because of injuries during experimental period. They were at least black belt 1st Dan and regularly engaged in 2 h a day, 5 days a week for at least 3 years. All the participants observed the traditional pattern of Ramadan fasting, abstaining from food and fluid from sunrise to sunset. During the study, they were regularly exercising to maintain their physical performance and undertaking their usual training sessions supervised by their coaches. Training sessions have been scheduled from 04:30 pm to 06:30 pm during control period, and after breaking the fast during RIF (i.e., from 09:30 pm to 11:30 pm [25]). The regular training sessions consisted mainly of repeated series of short-term high intensity exercises involving various basic offensive and defensive techniques (i.e., blocking, kicking, punching, displacements), sparring and katas. Some additional flexibility exercises, cardiovascular (i.e., high-intensity intermittent training) and fundamental resistance training (i.e., proprioceptive and balance exercises, core strength, and upper and lower body workout) were incorporated within these sessions. The study design is in accordance with the Declaration of Helsinki

for human experimentation and was approved by the Ethics Committee of the Faculty of Medicine, University of Sousse (Tunisia). A written informed consent was obtained from the participants' parents and participants after receiving a complete verbal description of the protocol.

Experimental design

The study was conducted in Sousse (Tunisia) when Ramadan occurred between 22 August 2009 and 20 September 2009 (sunrise was about 05:30 am and sunset about 07:30 pm, local time). The participants were first asked to report to the laboratory 14 days before Ramadan to become familiar with the testing procedures that they would perform during the experimental sessions.

All the assessments were performed between 04:30 pm and 06:30 pm on three occasions (Fig. 1). The first study session (S1) was performed one week before Ramadan, the second (S2) was performed at the end of the first week of Ramadan, and the third (S3) was performed at the end of the last week of Ramadan. The laboratory temperature was held between 22 and 24 °C, with an average relative humidity of 56 % during the testing periods.

Dietary nutrients intake was recorded for 3 days before each session, including the last meal before the tests. This was completed by interview with the same experienced nutritionist using a 24-h recall method. Dietary records were analyzed for energy intake using Bilnut program (Nutrisoft, Cerelles, France) and values based on the food composition tables published by the Tunisian National Institute of Statistics. The height and body mass of the athletes were determined before each session using

standard calibrated scale and stadiometer. The body mass index (BMI) was then calculated as body mass (in kg) divided by height (in meters squared). During each session, SRT and CRT were evaluated at rest and just after neuromuscular fatiguing exercise in a random order (Fig. 1).

Isometric maximal voluntary contraction

During each test session, participants were seated comfortably on a Scott Bench (Panatta Sports, Apiro, MC, Italy), with the right shoulder flexed to 90°. Velcro straps secured the waist and shoulder to ensure stability and limit extraneous movements. The wrist was placed in a half-supinated position and secured by a wrist cuff using Velcro straps just below the styloid process. The wrist cuff was tightly attached to a load cell (range 0–2500 N; Globus Ergometer, Globus, Codogne, Italy) by an adjustable chain perpendicularly to the forearm. The chain was adjusted in length so that the elbow remained at 90° of flexion during the contraction (0° corresponding to full elbow extension). The position of the elbow was confirmed using an universal goniometer. The signal from the load cell was amplified using a Globus amplifier (Tesys 400, Globus, Codogne, Italy) and fed through an analog-to-digital converter (12 bit) and stored on computer with a sampling frequency of 1000 Hz.

Following a warm-up phase (sub-maximal dynamic elbow contractions) and a series of familiarization contractions (two to three sub-maximal isometric contractions followed by two to three maximal isometric contractions), participants were asked to perform three MVC of the elbow flexors. Each contraction was held for 5-s, and 3-min recovery period was provided between the attempts. All participants were given standard

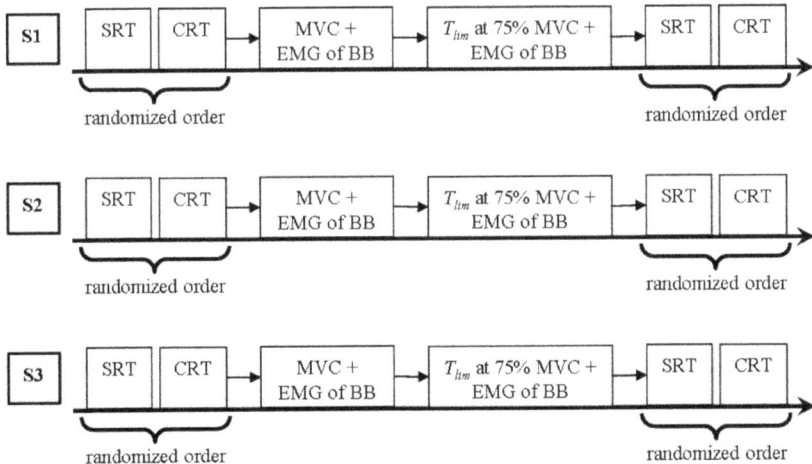

Fig. 1 Experimental design. S1, S2 and S3: one week before Ramadan, the end of the first week of Ramadan, and the end of the last week of Ramadan, respectively; SRT: simple reaction time; CRT: choice reaction time; MVC: maximal voluntary isometric contraction of the elbow flexor; BB: biceps brachial muscle; T_{lim}: isometric sub-maximal elbow flexion contraction until exhaustion

verbal encouragement during each MVC and visual feedback of the produced force was provided. The most forceful contraction of the three values was used for further analysis and considered the reference MVC allowing targets to be set on a visual feedback display for the subsequent endurance tasks fixed at 75 % of MVC.

Isometric muscle endurance

Following a 10-min rest period, the muscle endurance tests were carried out using the same test apparatus described above. Participants were required to maintain an isometric sub-maximal elbow flexion (T_{lim}) at 75 % MVC until exhaustion in accordance to muscle endurance task used by Bigard et al. [17] and Brown and Bray [12] (i.e., 70 % MVC). T_{lim} intensity was chosen according to the suggestion of Brown and Bray [12] who showed greater cognitive performance impairments at higher intensity of isometric contraction (30 vs. 50 and 70 % of MVC).

During the tests, the participants had a visual feedback for their contraction level on a control monitor in order to keep the output force level as close to the designated target force as possible. The endurance test ended if the level of force output appeared to have declined consistently (more than 3-s) to less than 90 % of the target force. Verbal encouragement was provided to the participants throughout the test to maintain the force level. The absolute T_{lim} was calculated as the time from the beginning of force production to the point where the above described 3-s criteria was reached.

Electromyographic measurement and analysis

During both the maximal and sub-maximal test, electromyographic (EMG) activity was recorded from biceps brachial (BB) muscle of the right arm by using bipolar surface electrode (Delsys DE-2.1, Delsys® Inc., Boston, USA). The electrode is fitted with two silver bar contacts measuring 1 cm in length, 0.1 cm in large and with a fixed inter-electrode spacing of 1 cm. After careful preparation of the skin (shaving, abrasion, and cleaning with alcohol), surface electrode was placed parallel to muscle fibers, in accordance with the European Recommendations for Surface Electromyography [26]. The exact electrode position over the BB muscle was carefully measured for each subject and marked on the skin with a waterproof permanent marker to ensure consistent location throughout the experiment. A reference electrode was placed over the collar bone.

EMG signals were amplified (Common Mode Rejection Ratio, CMRR = 92 dB; input impedance > 10^{15} Ω; gain = 1000) using a differential amplifier (Bagnoli-4 EMG System, DelSys Inc., Boston, USA) and filtered to a bandwidth between 20 Hz and 450 Hz, using a band-pass second order Butterworth filter. The signals were analogue-to-digital converted (with 16-bit accuracy in the signal range ± 5 V; Bagnoli-4 EMG System, DelSys Inc., Boston, USA) at a sampling rate of 1000 Hz and stored in a personal computer for subsequent analysis (EMGworks 3.0 DelSys Analysis software, Boston, USA).

The EMG analysis was performed in the time and frequency domains by calculating the root mean square (RMS) and the mean power frequency (MPF). For the best MVC contraction, the EMG signal of BB muscle were analyzed over a 500 ms window centered at the highest generated force to calculate RMS amplitude. The RMS was used to calculate the neuromuscular efficiency (NME = MVC/RMS) during the MVC. For the fatigue task, RMS value and MPF of the power spectrum (512 points, Hanning window processing, Fast Fourier Transform) were calculated for consecutive 5-s windows throughout the whole fatigue task. For each participant and during each session, the changes in EMG parameters (i.e., RMS and MPF) over the entire duration of the T_{lim} were assessed by the absolute slope of the linear regression between EMG activity and time. The coefficient of determination (R^2) was calculated for each of these relationships.

Reaction times

The SRT and the CRT were measured using a "Superlab 4.5" program (Cedrus, San Pedro, USA). These tests measure the reaction time to visual stimuli. The subject sat 0.4 to 0.5 m in front of a computer monitor. After 10 familiarization trials, each participant performed randomly and double-blinded 20 SRT and 32 CRT tests at rest and after neuromuscular fatiguing task. The interval between the appearances of two consecutive stimuli on the monitor varied randomly between 10 and 1500 ms.

When measuring the SRT, the appearance of a white square on the monitor served as a warning signal, and the participant's task was to press the space bar with the right hand (i.e., favored hand) as quickly as possible after the appearance of a black square. For the CRT, four white squares were presented occupying the entire monitor. The participant was then required to react as quickly as possible, pressing the key corresponding to the location of a black square (responding with a letter "A" if the black square appeared at the top left of the screen, "W" if it appeared at the bottom left, "U" if it appeared at the top right, or a letter "N" if it appeared at the bottom right).

Reaction times of less than 150 ms and greater than 800 ms were excluded from analysis to avoid any effects from either anticipation or a temporary lapse of concentration.

Statistical analyses

All data are presented as means ± standard deviation (SD) and were analyzed using Statistica for Windows software (version 6.0, StatSoft, Inc, Tulsa, OK). The reproducibility of SRT, CRT, MVC and T_{lim} measurements was assessed by calculating the intra-class correlation coefficient (ICC) and the standard error of measurement (SEM) between the familiarization session and S1. Once the assumption of normality was confirmed using the Shapiro-Wilk W-test, parametric tests were performed. For all EMG variables, MVC, T_{lim}, anthropometric measures and dietary data, one-way analysis of variance (ANOVA) with repeated measures was used to detect significant differences between the three sessions. For the SRT and CRT data, two-way (Sessions × pre/post exercise) ANOVA with repeated measures was used. When appropriate, the least-significant difference (LSD) post-hoc test was used for multiple pair-wise comparisons. Statistical significance was accepted at $p < 0.05$.

Results

The reproducibility of SRT (ICC = 0.92; SEM = 11.58 ms), CRT (ICC = 0.88; SEM = 10.26 ms), MVC (ICC = 0.98; SEM = 34.60 N) and T_{lim} (ICC = 0.91; SEM = 4.40 s) was high.

Compared to the control values (i.e., S1), total daily energy intake was significantly increased during RIF (S2: +19.5 %, $p < 0.05$; S3: +27.4 %, $p < 0.01$; Table 1). As shown in Table 1, the diet pattern used by our participants during Ramadan showed a significantly greater estimated daily total fat content during the first (+34.9 %, $p < 0.01$) and the last (+46.0 %, $p < 0.001$) week of Ramadan compared to the usual diet (i.e., S1). However, there was no significant difference in the intake of protein over the whole period of the investigation. In addition, although the fractional contribution of carbohydrate to the daily diet was significantly higher before than during Ramadan (S2: −11.1 %, $p < 0.05$; S3: −10.9 %, $p < 0.05$; Table 1), no significant difference of the dietary carbohydrate content in g was found across the three

sessions. Estimated total daily water intake from ingested food and fluids was significantly increased during Ramadan (S2: +26.8 %, $p < 0.01$; S3: +23.2 %, $p < 0.05$; Table 2) compared with before Ramadan (i.e., S1).

As shown in Table 2, neither body mass nor BMI was altered by Ramadan fasting ($F_{(2,14)} = 0.80$, $p = 0.47$ and $F_{(2,14)} = 0.78$, $p = 0.48$, respectively; Table 2).

The ANOVA indicated that there was no significant effect of session for MVC ($F_{(2,14)} = 0.51$, $p = 0.61$; Table 2). The level of RMS activity of the BB during the MVC was also not statistically different between sessions ($F_{(2,14)} = 0.13$, $p = 0.88$; Table 2). Moreover, the NME of the elbow flexor remained similar throughout the experiment ($F_{(2,14)} = 0.27$, $p = 0.76$; Table 2).

Our data also indicate that the T_{lim} during the elbow flexion was not statistically different between sessions ($F_{(2,14)} = 2.53$, $p = 0.12$; Table 2). Table 3 gives an overview of the EMG results during the T_{lim}. For all tests, a significant linear regression was found between EMG parameters (i.e., RMS or MPF) and time. More precisely, we found a positive linear regression for RMS, indicating an increase over time, and a negative linear regression for MPF, indicating a decrease over time. The one-way ANOVA indicated that the slopes coefficients of the RMS ($F_{(2,14)} = 0.71$, $p = 0.51$) and MPF ($F_{(2,14)} = 2.73$, $p = 0.09$) values did not differ between the three sessions.

The two-way ANOVA showed that the isometric submaximal elbow flexion had no effect on SRT ($F_{(1,7)} = 0.0002$, $p = 0.98$; Fig. 2) or CRT ($F_{(1,7)} = 3.78$, $p = 0.09$; Fig. 3) during any of the three sessions. In addition, there was no significant effect of RIF on SRT ($F_{(2,14)} = 1.82$, $p = 0.19$; Fig. 2) or CRT ($F_{(2,14)} = 0.26$, $p = 0.78$; Fig. 3) both at rest and after the isometric muscle endurance task without any significant interaction Sessions × pre/post exercise (SRT: $F_{(2,14)} = 1.14$, $p = 0.35$; CRT: $F_{(2,14)} = 0.48$, $p = 0.63$).

Table 1 Mean values (± SD) of daily dietary intake before Ramadan (S1), in the first week of Ramadan (S2), and in the fourth week of Ramadan (S3)

	S1	S2	S3
Energy (MJ/d)	13.3 ± 2.2	15.9 ± 2.1*	16.9 ± 2.0++
Energy (Kcal/d)	3173.3 ± 531.1	3774.7 ± 527.2*	4042.1 ± 488.9++
Protein (g/d)	108.0 ± 36.7	123.6 ± 21.3	128.0 ± 22.7
Protein (% of energy)	11.9 ± 2.4	12.1 ± 2.1	11.8 ± 1.4
Carbohydrates (g/d)	439.6 ± 78.3	471.1 ± 110.4	495.3 ± 66.9
Carbohydrates (% of energy)	54.1 ± 7.0	48.1 ± 5.5*	48.3 ± 4.7+
Total fat (g/d)	126.8 ± 36.4	171.2 ± 20.2**	185.2 ± 32.2+++
Total fat (% of energy)	34.0 ± 5.8	39.8 ± 5.6**	40.0 ± 5.6++
Fluid intake (l)	1.8 ± 0.6	2.2 ± 0.6**	2.2 ± 0.6+

*, **: significant differences between S2 and S1 at $p < 0.05$ and $p < 0.01$, respectively
+, ++, +++: significant differences between S3 and S1 at $p < 0.05$, $p < 0.01$ and $p < 0.001$, respectively

Table 2 Mean values (± SD) of the anthropometric characteristics, maximal voluntary isometric contraction (MVC), root mean square (RMS) of the EMG signal and neuromuscular efficiency of the biceps brachial muscle during MVC, and absolute endurance time at 75 % MVC (T_{lim}) of elbow flexion obtained from the three sessions: before Ramadan (S1), in the first week of Ramadan (S2), and in the fourth week of Ramadan (S3)

	S1	S2	S3
Body mass (kg)	62.1 ± 7.4	61.8 ± 7.2	61.8 ± 7.1
Body mass index (kg/m^2)	20.1 ± 2.2	20.0 ± 2.1	20.0 ± 2.1
MVC (N)	907.7 ± 230.1	878.4 ± 240.1	870.2 ± 245.9
RMS (mV)	0.7 ± 0.2	0.7 ± 0.3	0.6 ± 0.3
NME	1.4 ± 0.5	1.5 ± 0.5	1.6 ± 0.5
T_{lim} (s)	35.3 ± 16.7	42.5 ± 22.3	29.5 ± 13.2

No difference was observed among the three different sessions

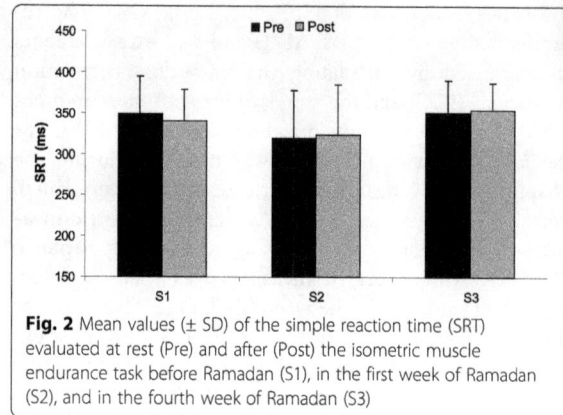

Fig. 2 Mean values (± SD) of the simple reaction time (SRT) evaluated at rest (Pre) and after (Post) the isometric muscle endurance task before Ramadan (S1), in the first week of Ramadan (S2), and in the fourth week of Ramadan (S3)

Discussion

The aim of the present study was to examine the effect of RIF and fatigue on cognitive and neuromuscular performances in trained karate athletes who were undertaking training sessions during Ramadan. The present results showed that RIF did not adversely affect neuromuscular performances and anthropometric parameters. In addition, neither RIF nor neuromuscular fatigue poorly affects reaction times in elite karate athletes.

Similarly to previous studies [27, 28], the present findings showed that estimated total daily energy intake was significantly increased during Ramadan. Yet, other studies have reported a significant decrease [29, 30], or no significant effect [31–34] of RIF on daily energy intake. Obviously, these discrepancies could probably be related to differences in nutritional customs and habits, social and geographical environment of the country where the studies were conducted and the seasonal occurrence of the Ramadan month. In addition, differences in the characteristics of the participants such as sex, age, fitness and individual physical activity may contribute to the inconsistency of the findings across the different studies [29, 33]. The present findings corroborate the common local belief that Muslims tend to overcompensate in terms of food intake during Ramadan fasting. The dietary intake data indicated a larger increase of total fat during Ramadan despite the reduction of meal frequency. In fact, it has been reported that the diet traditionally eaten during Ramadan, in most Muslim countries, tends to be richer in calories and higher in fats, protein and sugars than the normal diet during the other months [13, 30, 33]. Of note, the mean intake composition of carbohydrate and protein throughout the study were within normal values when compared to the recommended dietary allowances (RDA), which are between 45–65 % and 10–35 %, respectively [35]. However, the mean intake composition of fat was higher during RIF (39.8 ± 5.6 % in the 1st week and 40.0 ± 5.6 % in the 4th week) when compared to the RDA values which are between 20 and 35 %. Despite the fact that the total fat intake was significantly higher during Ramadan than the control period, body mass and BMI did not significantly change. This observance could be due to a potential heavier training loads during RIF, and consequently higher energy expenditure. Thus, it is possible that the athletes increased their energy intake during RIF to meet the fuel requirements of higher training loads and promote optimal recovery [25]. Unfortunately, neither training load nor energy expenditure of the participants were monitored. Consequently, the present study is not able

Table 3 Analysis of the relative changes in the values of the root mean square (RMS) and the mean power frequency (MPF) of the EMG signal of biceps brachial muscle across the isometric muscle endurance task tested before Ramadan (S1), in the first week of Ramadan (S2), and in the fourth week of Ramadan (S3)

	RMS						MPF					
	S1		S2		S3		S1		S2		S3	
	R^2	slope	R^2	slope	R^2	slope	R^2	slope	R^2	slope	R^2	slope
Mean	0.665	0.014	0.521	0.009	0.539	0.012	0.952	−1.190	0.873	−0.933	0.939	−1.057
SD	0.278	0.008	0.335	0.008	0.327	0.007	0.071	0.680	0.095	0.623	0.066	0.586

Significant linear regression was found between EMG parameters (i.e., RMS and MPF) and time
Slope: slope of the linear regression between EMG parameters and time
SD standard deviation

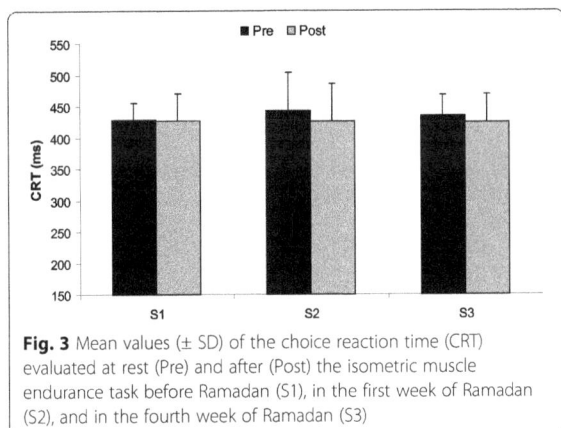

Fig. 3 Mean values (± SD) of the choice reaction time (CRT) evaluated at rest (Pre) and after (Post) the isometric muscle endurance task before Ramadan (S1), in the first week of Ramadan (S2), and in the fourth week of Ramadan (S3)

to provide a precise answer to this suggestion. Another possible explanation that needs to be considered is that the invariability of the body mass could be attributable to a possible increase in the utilization of the ingested fat during RIF. Indeed, Chaouachi et al. [33] reported that energy intake of young elite judo athletes remained constant during Ramadan but observed significant losses in body mass and body fat. The possible increase in fat oxidation during the fasting month is a probable adaptation that is due to the raised concentrations of circulating lipids and low liver glycogen levels that normally occur following several hours of fasting [29, 31, 33].

Otherwise, the present study results show that the maximal force generating capacity (i.e., MVC) and associated EMG amplitude (i.e., RMS) were not different between sessions. In addition, the NME, estimated via the MVC/RMS ratio, was unchanged during Ramadan suggesting that both muscle recruitment and contractility were not altered by the RIF during short-duration maximal skeletal muscle force. In this context, Racinais et al. [19] reported similar results in 11 moderately active Muslim males of various origins living in Qatar. These authors showed that knee extensors and flexors MVC, associated EMG and NME were maintained during Ramadan [19]. Moreover, Waterhouse et al. [20] showed that maximal handgrip strengths of both dominant and non-dominant hands were not different between control days and Ramadan. Furthermore, previous findings on changes of single maximal isometric strength [36] and explosive force [36–40] demonstrated similar observations. In contrast, other studies have shown significant impairments in short-term muscular performances (e.g., MVC, squat jump, countermovement jump, etc.) during RIF [17, 18, 34]. For instance, significant decrements in elbow flexion and knee extension MVC ranged from 10 to 15 % during Ramadan in comparison with control values were observed in fighter pilots [17]. Same, Brisswalter et al. [18] demonstrated that RIF led to an

impairment in knee extensors MVC (−3.75 %) associated with decreased median frequency (−5.6 %) and RMS (−18 %) of the EMG signal from the vastus lateralis muscle. In the other hand, some studies have shown a reduction in both hand-grip strength and 30-s maximal isometric performance associated with a ~5 % body mass loss following a 7-day restricted energy and fluid intake in national-level judo players [41, 42]. Therefore, while the studies of Filaire et al. [41] and Degoutte et al. [42] were conducted with food and fluid restrictions, our results demonstrated higher estimated total daily energy and water intake during RIF which could defend against muscular performance decrements. In fact, it has been suggested that the alteration in energy substrate and metabolism, concomitant with acute hypohydration caused by the RIF could result in a reduced physical capacity to exercise [13, 43]. Otherwise, the present results did not show any session's effect on T_{lim} at 75 % MVC and the manifestations of corresponding EMG parameters over time. It is well known that during submaximal exercise, as performed in the present study (i.e., T_{lim} at 75 % MVC), neuromuscular fatigue induces a decrease in action potential muscle conduction velocity, an increase in motor units synchronization and force loss which can be compensated by recruitment of additional motor units [44]. Consequently, these phenomena may induce an increase in EMG amplitude [45] and a decrease in the MPF of the Power Spectrum Density Function [46], while force or power output remains constant. In accordance with the literature [47, 48], the present findings showed significant positive and negative linear relationships between T_{lim} and both RMS and MPF, respectively. Notably all the participants of the present study took part in regular training sessions including resistance exercise training during Ramadan. Therefore, we speculate that due to the level of physical condition and habitual physical training, athletes were able to maintain their neuromuscular performances during the month of fast. Similar observations in subjects undertaking usual sports activities and training schedule throughout Ramadan have been reported [32, 39, 40]. Indeed, it has been shown that RIF had no adverse effect on moderate exercise in physically active subjects [43], on anaerobic performance in power athletes [32], on aerobic (i.e., Multistage Fitness Test) and anaerobic (i.e., Squat Jump, Counter Movement Jump, and maximal 30 m sprint) performances in elite judo athletes [39], on vertical jump and balance performance in female taekwondo players [40] and on speed, power, agility, passing and dribbling skills in young soccer players [34, 38]. In contrast, other studies have observed a negative effect of RIF on physical performances in competitive professional athletes [18, 34, 37, 49]. From a soccer perspective, Meckel et al. [34] reported a significant decrease in endurance and jumping performances concomitant to a reduced training load when energy intake and sleep duration were unchanged. In addition, Zerguini et al. [37] found significant reductions in agility, dribbling speed and endurance performance in professional soccer players with reduced training during RIF. While these two last studies observed reduced training load, most of the studies have reported that physical performance can be maintained during RIF once training duration, intensity, and loads are maintained compared with the pre-Ramadan period [32, 39]. It is interesting to note that both groups of soccer players in the studies of Zerguini et al. [37] and Meckel et al. [34] were free living, whereas in the study of Kirkendall et al. [38] the players stayed in a residential training camp which could provide a more physically rigorous, rigid, and healthier lifestyle than when free living. In more similar tasks to those used in the present study, Bigard et al. [17] demonstrated that muscular endurance time evaluated in elbow flexors and knee extensors at both 35 and 70 % of MVC in 11 fighter pilots were lower at the end of Ramadan in comparison with the control period (–28 and –22 %, respectively). In addition, Chaouachi et al. [39] showed significant reduction in the 30-s repeated jump test performance and an increased perception of fatigue at the end of RIF. These discrepancies in the literature might partly be related to a potential effect of mood and motivation level of the subjects and the influences of changes in sleep patterns and calorie intake [37]. Interestingly, it has also been suggested that changes in sleep habit may also indirectly impair psychomotor performance and cognitive function [15, 21, 22, 50] via changes in mental alertness, motivation, coordination and mood during RIF [13–15, 22, 51]. The present study results' demonstrated that both reaction times (i.e., SRT and CRT) were unchanged. Unfortunately, neither sleep pattern nor mood and motivation were monitored in the present study. However, we can suggest that the karate athletes have not been suffered from a lack of sleep during Ramadan, as they were in a residential school which could provide a healthier lifestyle than when free living. In fact, Roky et al. [14] demonstrated that subjective alertness, evaluated by a visual analogue scale, decreased at 09:00 and 16:00, and increased at 23:00 during Ramadan. These authors concluded that sleep loss and reduced energy intake were responsible. The role of decreased food intake was supported by observation of improved mood in the evening after fasting had ended [14]. It has been reported that both fluid and food (particularly carbohydrate intake) deprivation, may adversely affect physical and cognitive abilities [52]. However, the present results show that the total daily water and energy intake were increased during RIF, while the dietary carbohydrate content (in g) was unchanged throughout the study. This probably reflects the experience of athletes and coaches, who ensured a compensatory increase of fluid and energy intake during the hours of darkness, when drinking and eating were permitted [25]. These findings may explain, at least in part, the unaltered cognitive performances (i.e., SRT and CRT) in the present study. Consistent with our findings, Gutiérrez et al. [53] demonstrated that perception-reaction time (simple and discriminant) and hand grip strength were unchanged after one day and three days of fasting in eight sportsmen. Regarding RIF, previous studies that have assessed psychomotor performance have reported conflicting results. In fact, while some studies have reported no adverse effects of RIF on psychomotor performance in Muslim athletes [23, 24], other studies have demonstrated that some indicators of psychomotor performance, such as critical flicker fusion [21], daytime alertness [22], irritability [50], memory [51], functional attention [54], continuous attention and reaction time [22, 55] were impaired by RIF in sedentary subjects. It could be argued that fasted athletes have a greater mental and stronger motivation to perform cognitive tasks compared to sedentary subjects [52]. Particularly, Tian et al. [24] examined various aspects of cerebral function in martial arts athletes. These authors found that psychomotor performance and vigilance were enhanced at 9:00, but verbal learning and memory were impaired at 16:00 during RIF, when blood glucose levels were presumably reduced. Lotfi et al. [23] demonstrated that critical flicker fusion and motor reaction time were unchanged during Ramadan observance in nine male resistance athletes, although the recognition reaction time and the total reaction time were impaired only at the beginning and not at the end of Ramadan. Similarly, impairments of critical flicker fusion [21] and choice reaction time [22] have been reported only in the first week of Ramadan suggesting a possible adaptation to intermittent fasting.

Furthermore, the present findings show that the muscle endurance task had no effect on reaction times. In fact, it has been reported that cognitive performance may be maintained, enhanced or impaired depending on the time when it is measured, the physical fitness level of the subjects, the type of cognitive task selected, and the type of exercise that is performed [56]. Regarding muscular exercise, Kroll [57] found no effect of purely muscular fatigue on reaction time. More recently, Del Percio et al. [11] demonstrated that tiredness and muscle fatigue after repeated isometric muscle contractions at 50 % MVC did not affect visuo-spatial attentional processes of elite karate athletes. These authors speculated that brain circuits of reflexive attention are poorly sensitive to the effects of tiredness and muscular fatigue in elite karate athletes, so that they can effectively react to unexpected kicks and/or punches even during the final part of the match characterized by high muscular fatigue [11].

The current study has some limitations that need to be addressed. First, the number of recruited volunteers is relatively low without a control group. Nevertheless, obtaining such a naturally non-fasting group in Muslim countries is somewhat difficult. Second, the present study lacks some details and measurements that would be able to strengthen the interpretation such as the training load monitoring and measurement of the energy expenditure of the athletes. Finally, some parameters (e.g., motivation, alertness, sleep quantity and quality) and factors (e.g., circadian rhythm and time-of-day effect) that we did not assess have been demonstrated to affect physical and cognitive performances during RIF. Therefore, upcoming investigations should take these parameters and factors into consideration.

Conclusions

The present findings did not show any adverse effect of RIF on cognitive and neuromuscular performances in trained karate athletes undertaking training sessions during Ramadan. However, these results need to be confirmed for longer testing procedures (e.g., isometric muscle endurance at 50 or 25 % MVC) which could be more sensitive to intermittent fasting. In addition, further research is needed to assess the effects of RIF on reaction time using more specific stimuli and motor responses with dynamic displays of karate athletes performing offensive and defensive actions [5, 6].

Abbreviations

ANOVA: analysis of variance; BB: Biceps brachii; BMI: body mass index; CRT: choice reaction time; EMG: electromyography; ICC: intra-class correlation coefficient; MPF: mean power frequency; MVC: maximal voluntary contraction; NME: neuromuscular efficiency; RDA: recommended dietary allowances; RIF: Ramadan intermittent fast; RMS: root mean square; S1: first session; S2: second session; S3: third session; SEM: standard error of measurement; SRT: simple reaction time; T_{lim}: submaximal isometric contraction at 75 % MVC.

Competing interests
The authors declare that they have no competing interests.

Authors' contributions
NZ, OH, EB, HR, and MD designed the experiments. NZ, OH, IL, HA, and MD collected and analyzed the data. Data interpretation and manuscript preparation were undertaken by NZ. All authors read and approved the final manuscript.

Acknowledgements
The authors would like to thank all of the volunteers and their coaches, specially Hosni Bouhlel, for their understanding and availability in the completion of this study.

Author details
[1]Research Laboratory: "Medical Imaging Technologies" (LR 12ES06, TIM), Faculty of Medicine of Monastir, University of Monastir, Monastir, Tunisia. [2]Research Laboratory: "Equipe de Physiologie, Biomécanique et Imagerie du Mouvement" (CeRSM, EA 2931), UFR STAPS, Université Paris Ouest Nanterre La Défense, 200 avenue de la République, 92000 Nanterre, France. [3]Research Unit: "Exercise Physiology and Pathophysiology: from the Integrated to the Molecular Biology, Medicine and Health" (UR 12ES06), Faculty of Medicine of Sousse, University of Sousse, Sousse, Tunisia. [4]Research Laboratory: "Sport Performance Optimization", National Center of Medicine and Sciences in Sport (CNMSS), Tunis, Tunisia. [5]Research Unit: "Education, Motricity, Sports and Health" (UR 15JS01), Higher Institute of Sport and Physical Education of Sfax, University of Sfax, Sfax, Tunisia.

References

1. Tan KS. Constructing a martial tradition: rethinking a popular history of Karate-Do. J Sport Soc Issues. 2004;28(2):169–92.
2. Chaabène H, Hachana Y, Franchini E, Mkaouer B, Chamari K. Physical and physiological profile of elite karate athletes. Sports Med. 2012;42(10):829–43.
3. Mori S, Ohtani Y, Imanaka K. Reaction times and anticipatory skills of karate athletes. Hum Mov Sci. 2002;21(2):213–30.
4. Kim HS, Petrakis E. Visuoperceptual speed of karate practitioners at three levels of skill. Percept Mot Skills. 1998;87(1):96–8.
5. Scott MA, Williams AM, Davids K. Perception-action coupling in karate kumite. In: Valanti SS, Pittenger JB, editors. Studies in perception and action II: posters presented at the VIIth international conference on event perception and action. Hillsdale: Erlbaum; 1993. p. 217–21.
6. Williams AM, Elliott D. Anxiety, expertise, and visual search strategy in karate. J Sport Exerc Psychol. 1999;21(4):362–75.
7. Fontani G, Lodi L, Felici A, Migliorini S, Corradeschi F. Attention in athletes of high and low experience engaged in different open skill sports. Percept Mot Skills. 2006;102(3):791–805.
8. Magill RA. Motor learning concepts and applications. 5th ed. Boston: McGraw-Hill; 1998.
9. Coşkun B, Koçak S, Saritaş N. The comparison of reaction times of karate athletes according to age, gender and status. Sci Movement Health. 2014;14(2):213–7.
10. Chang YK, Labban JD, Gapin JI, Etnier JL. The effects of acute exercise on cognitive performance: a metaanalysis. Brain Res. 2012;1453:87–101.
11. Del Percio C, Babiloni C, Infarinato F, Marzano N, Iacoboni M, Lizio R, et al. Effects of tiredness on visuo-spatial attention processes in élite karate athletes and non-athletes. Arch Ital Biol. 2009;147(1–2):1–10.
12. Brown DM, Bray SR. Isometric exercise and cognitive function: an investigation of acute dose–response effects during submaximal fatiguing contractions. J Sports Sci. 2015;33(5):487–97.
13. Leiper JB, Molla AM, Molla AM. Effects on health of fluid restriction during fasting in Ramadan. Eur J Clin Nutr. 2003;57 Suppl 2:S30–8.
14. Roky R, Houti I, Moussamih S, Qotbi S, Aadil N. Physiological and chronobiological changes during Ramadan intermittent fasting. Ann Nutr Metab. 2004;48(4):296–303.
15. Reilly T, Waterhouse J. Altered sleep-wake cycles and food intake: the Ramadan model. Physiol Behav. 2007;90(2–3):219–28.
16. Shephard RJ. The impact of Ramadan observance upon athletic performance. Nutrients. 2012;4(6):491–505.
17. Bigard AX, Boussif M, Chalabi H, Guezennec CY. Alterations in muscular performance and orthostatic tolerance during Ramadan. Aviat Space Environ Med. 1998;69(4):341–6.
18. Brisswalter J, Bouhlel E, Falola JM, Abbiss CR, Vallier JM, Hausswirth C. Effects of Ramadan intermittent fasting on middle-distance running performance in well-trained runners. Clin J Sport Med. 2011;21(5):422–7.
19. Racinais S, Périard JD, Li CK, Grantham J. Activity patterns, body composition and muscle function during Ramadan in a Middle-East Muslim country. Int J Sports Med. 2012;33(8):641–6.
20. Waterhouse J, Alabed H, Edwards B, Reilly T. Changes in sleep, mood and subjective and objective responses to physical performance during the daytime in Ramadan. Biol Rhythm Res. 2009;40(5):367–83.
21. Ali MR, Amir T. Effects of fasting on visual flicker fusion. Percept Mot Skills. 1989;69(2):627–31.
22. Roky R, Iraki L, HajKhlifa R, Ghazal NL, Hakkou F. Daytime alertness, mood, psychomotor performances, and oral temperature during Ramadan intermittent fasting. Ann Nutr Metab. 2000;44(3):101–7.
23. Lotfi S, Madani M, Abassi A, Tazi A, Boumahmaza M, Talbi M. CNS activation, reaction time, blood pressure and heart rate variation during Ramadan intermittent fasting and exercise. World J Sport Sci. 2010;3(1):37–43.
24. Tian HH, Aziz AR, Png W, Wahid M, Yeo D, Png AL. Effects of fasting during Ramadan month on cognitive function in Muslim athletes. Asian J Sports Med. 2011;2(3):145–53.
25. Roy J, Hwa OC, Singh R, Aziz AR, Jin CW. Self-generated coping strategies among Muslim athletes during Ramadan fasting. J Sports Sci Med. 2011; 10(1):137–44.
26. Hermens HJ, Feriks B, Disselhorst-Klug C, Rau G. Development of recommendations for SEMG sensors and sensor placement procedures. J Electromyogr Kinesiol. 2000;10(5):361–74.

27. Gharbi M, Akrout M, Zouari B. Food intake during and outside Ramadan. East Mediterr Health J. 2003;9(1–2):131–40.

28. Lamri-Senhadji MY, El Kebir B, Belleville J, Bouchenak M. Assessment of dietary consumption and time-course of changes in serum lipids and lipoproteins before, during and after Ramadan in young Algerian adults. Singapore Med J. 2009;50(3):288–94.

29. Bouhlel E, Salhi Z, Bouhlel H, Mdella S, Amamou A, Zouali M, et al. Effect of Ramadan fasting on fuel oxidation during exercise in trained male rugby players. Diabetes Metab. 2006;32(6):617–24.

30. Ziaee V, Razaei M, Ahmadinejad Z, Shaikh H, Yousefi R, Yarmohammadi L, et al. The changes of metabolic profile and weight during Ramadan fasting. Singapore Med J. 2006;47(5):409–14.

31. El Ati J, Beji C, Danguir J. Increased fat oxidation during Ramadan fasting in healthy women: an adaptive mechanism for body-weight maintenance. Am J Clin Nutr. 1995;62:302–7.

32. Karli U, Guvenc A, Aslan A, Hazir T, Acikada C. Influence of Ramadan fasting on anaerobic performance and recovery following short time high intensity exercise. J Sports Sci Med. 2007;6(4):490–7.

33. Chaouachi A, Chamari K, Roky R, Wong P, Mbazaa A, Bartagi Z, et al. Lipid profiles of judo athletes during Ramadan. Int J Sports Med. 2008;29(4):282–8.

34. Meckel Y, Ismaeel A, Eliakim A. The effect of the Ramadan fast on physical performance and dietary habits in adolescent soccer players. Eur J Appl Physiol. 2008;102(6):651–7.

35. Rolfes SR, Pinna K, Whitney E. Understanding normal and clinical nutrition. 7th ed. Belmont: Thomson Wadsworth; 2006.

36. Bouhlel H, Shephard RJ, Gmada N, Aouichaoui C, Peres G, Tabka Z, et al. Effect of Ramadan observance on maximal muscular performance of trained men. Clin J Sport Med. 2013;23(3):222–7.

37. Zerguini Y, Kirkendall D, Junge A, Dvorak J. Impact of Ramadan on physical performance in professional soccer players. Br J Sports Med. 2007;41(6):398–400.

38. Kirkendall DT, Leiper JB, Bartagi Z, Dvorak J, Zerguini Y. The influence of Ramadan on physical performance measures in young Muslim footballers. J Sports Sci. 2008;26 Suppl 3:S15–27.

39. Chaouachi A, Coutts AJ, Chamari K, Wong DP, Chaouachi M, Chtara M, et al. Effect of Ramadan intermittent fasting on aerobic and anaerobic performance and perception of fatigue in male elite judo athletes. J Strength Cond Res. 2009;23(9):2702–9.

40. Memari AH, Kordi R, Panahi N, Nikookar LR, Abdollahi M, Akbarnejad A. Effect of Ramadan fasting on body composition and physical performance in female athletes. Asian J Sports Med. 2011;2(3):161–6.

41. Filaire E, Maso F, Degoutte F, Jouanel P, Lac G. Food restriction, performance, psychological state and lipid values in judo athletes. Int J Sports Med. 2001;22(6):454–9.

42. Degoutte F, Jouanel P, Bègue RJ, Colombier M, Lac G, Pequignot JM, et al. Food restriction, performance, biochemical, psychological, and endocrine changes in judo athletes. Int J Sports Med. 2006;27(1):9–18.

43. Ramadan J, Telahoun G, Al-Zaid NS, Barac-Nieto M. Responses to exercise, fluid, and energy balances during Ramadan in sedentary and active males. Nutrition. 1999;15(10):735–9.

44. DeVries HA. Method for evaluation of muscle fatigue and endurance from electromyographic fatigue curves. Am J Phys Med. 1968;47(3):125–35.

45. De Luca CJ, Foley PJ, Erim Z. Motor unit control properties in constant-force isometric contractions. J Neurophysiol. 1996;76(3):1503–16.

46. Lindström B, Karlsson S, Gerdle B. Knee extensor performance of dominant and non-dominant limb throughout repeated isokinetic contractions, with special reference to peak torque and mean frequency of the EMG. Clin Physiol. 1995;15(3):275–86.

47. Merletti R, Roy S. Myoelectrical and mechanical manifestations of muscle fatigue in voluntary contractions. J Orthop Sports Phys Ther. 1996;24(6):342–53.

48. Maïsetti O, Guével A, Legros P, Hogrel JY. SEMG power spectrum changes during a sustained 50 % maximum voluntary isometric torque do not depend upon the prior knowledge of the exercise duration. J Electromyogr Kinesiol. 2002;12(2):103–9.

49. Faye J, Fall A, Badji L, Cisse F, Stephan H, Tine P. Effects of Ramadan fast on weight, performance and glycemia during training for resistance. Dakar Med. 2005;50(3):146–51.

50. Kadri N, Tilane A, El Batal M, Taltit Y, Tahiri SM, Moussaoui D. Irritability during the month of Ramadan. Psychosom Med. 2000;62(2):280–5.

51. Hakkou F, Tazi A, Iraki L. Ramadan, health, and chronobiology. Chronobiol Int. 1994;11(5):340–2.

52. Maughan RJ, Fallah J, Coyle EF. The effects of fasting on metabolism and performance. Br J Sports Med. 2010;44(7):490–4.

53. Gutiérrez A, González-Gross M, Delgado M, Castillo MJ. Three days fast in sportsmen decreases physical work capacity but not strength or perception-reaction time. Int J Sport Nutr Exerc Metab. 2001;11(4):420–9.

54. El Moutawakil B, Hassounr S, Sibai M, Rafai MA, Fabrigoule C, Slassi I. Impact du jeûn du Ramadan sur les fonctions attentionnelles. Rev Neurol. 2007; 163(4):60.

55. Dolu N, Yüksek A, Sizer A, Alay M. Arousal and continuous attention during Ramadan intermittent fasting. J Basic Clin Physiol Pharmacol. 2007;18(4):315–22.

56. Lambourne K, Tomporowski P. The effect of exercise-induced arousal on cognitive task performance: a meta-regression analysis. Brain Res. 2010;1341: 12–24.

57. Kroll W. Effects of local muscular fatigue due to isotonic and isometric exercise upon fractionated reaction time components. J Mot Behav. 1973; 5(2):81–93.

Permissions

The contributors of this book come from diverse backgrounds, making this book a truly international effort. This book will bring forth new frontiers with its revolutionizing research information and detailed analysis of the nascent developments around the world.

We would like to thank all the contributing authors for lending their expertise to make the book truly unique. They have played a crucial role in the development of this book. Without their invaluable contributions this book wouldn't have been possible. They have made vital efforts to compile up to date information on the varied aspects of this subject to make this book a valuable addition to the collection of many professionals and students.

This book was conceptualized with the vision of imparting up-to-date information and advanced data in this field. To ensure the same, a matchless editorial board was set up. Every individual on the board went through rigorous rounds of assessment to prove their worth. After which they invested a large part of their time researching and compiling the most relevant data for our readers.

The editorial board has been involved in producing this book since its inception. They have spent rigorous hours researching and exploring the diverse topics which have resulted in the successful publishing of this book. They have passed on their knowledge of decades through this book. To expedite this challenging task, the publisher supported the team at every step. A small team of assistant editors was also appointed to further simplify the editing procedure and attain best results for the readers.

Apart from the editorial board, the designing team has also invested a significant amount of their time in understanding the subject and creating the most relevant covers. They scrutinized every image to scout for the most suitable representation of the subject and create an appropriate cover for the book.

The publishing team has been an ardent support to the editorial, designing and production team. Their endless efforts to recruit the best for this project, has resulted in the accomplishment of this book. They are a veteran in the field of academics and their pool of knowledge is as vast as their experience in printing. Their expertise and guidance has proved useful at every step. Their uncompromising quality standards have made this book an exceptional effort. Their encouragement from time to time has been an inspiration for everyone.

The publisher and the editorial board hope that this book will prove to be a valuable piece of knowledge for researchers, students, practitioners and scholars across the globe.

List of Contributors

Christopher Brooks Mobley, Carlton D Fox, Brian S Ferguson, Corrie A Pascoe, James C Healy,
Jeremy S McAdam and Michael D Roberts
School of Kinesiology, Molecular and Applied Sciences Laboratory, Auburn University, 301 Wire Road, Office 286, Auburn, AL 36849, USA

Christopher M Lockwood
4Life Research USA, LLC, Sandy, UT, USA

Sarah McKinley-Barnard, Tom Andre and Darryn S. Willoughby
Department of Health, Human Performance, and Recreation, Baylor University, Exercise and Biochemical Nutritional Lab, 76798 Waco, TX, USA

Ibaraki, Japan and Masahiko Morita
Function Research Group, Healthcare Products Development Center, KYOWA HAKKO BIO CO., LTD., 2, Miyukigaoka, 305-0841 Tsukuba

Joseph N Sciberras
Sport Nutrition graduate from the University of Stirling, 74, San Anton Court, Pope John XXIII street, Birkirkara BKR1033, Malta

Stuart DR Galloway
Health and Exercise Sciences Research Group, School of Sport, University of Stirling, Stirling, Scotland

Anthony Fenech and Janet Mifsud
Department of Clinical Pharmacology and Therapeutics, University of Malta, Msida, Malta

Godfrey Grech
Department of Pathology, University of Malta, Msida, Malta

Claude Farrugia and Deborah Duca
Department of Chemistry, University of Malta, Msida, Malta

Roxanne M Vogel
Muscle Pharm Sports Science Institute, Muscle Pharm Corp., 4721 Ironton St. Building A, Denver, CO 80239, USA
Metropolitan State University, Denver, CO, USA

Jordan M Joy, Paul H Falcone, Matt M Mosman and Michael P Kim
Muscle Pharm Sports Science Institute, Muscle Pharm Corp., 4721 Ironton St. Building A, Denver, CO 80239, USA

Jordan R Moon
Muscle Pharm Sports Science Institute, Muscle Pharm Corp., 4721 Ironton St. Building A, Denver, CO 80239, USA
Department of Sports Exercise Science, United States Sports Academy, Daphne, AL, USA

Lucio Della Guardia, Maurizio Cavallaro and Hellas Cena
Department of Public Health, Experimental and Forensic Medicine, Unit of Human Nutrition, University of Pavia, via Bassi 21, 27100 Pavia, Italy

Justin D Roberts
Department of Life Sciences, Anglia Ruskin University, East Road, Cambridge, UK
School of Life & Medical Sciences, University of Hertfordshire, College Lane, Hatfield, Hertfordshire, UK

G Roberts, Michael D Tarpey, Jack C Weekes and Clare H Thomas
School of Life & Medical Sciences, University of Hertfordshire, College Lane, Hatfield, Hertfordshire, UK

Tatiana Ederich Lehnen
Faculdade Sogipa de Educação Física, Porto Alegre, Brazil
Instituto de Cardiologia do Rio Grande do Sul, Av. Princesa Isabel, 395 Santana, 90620-001 Porto Alegre, RS, Brazil

Marcondes Ramos da Silva
Instituto de Cardiologia/Fundação
Universitária de Cardiologia (IC/FUC), Porto
Alegre, Brazil

**Augusto Camacho and Alexandre Machado
Lehnen**
Faculdade Sogipa de Educação Física, Porto
Alegre, Brazil
Instituto de Cardiologia/Fundação
Universitária de Cardiologia (IC/FUC), Porto
Alegre, Brazil

Aline Marcadenti
Instituto de Cardiologia/Fundação
Universitária de Cardiologia (IC/FUC), Porto
Alegre, Brazil
Universidade Federal de Ciências da Saúde de
Porto Alegre (UFCSPA), Porto Alegre, Brazil

Matthaus Marriott
Sport and Health Sciences, College of Life and
Environmental Sciences, St. Luke's Campus,
University of Exeter, Exeter, UK

Peter Krustrup
Sport and Health Sciences, College of Life and
Environmental Sciences, St. Luke's Campus,
University of Exeter, Exeter, UK
Department of Nutrition, Exercise and Sports,
Section of Human Physiology, Copenhagen
Centre for Team Sport and Health, University
of Copenhagen, Copenhagen, Denmark

Magni Mohr
Faculty of Natural and Health Sciences,
University of the Faroe Islands, Jónas Broncks
gøta 25 3rd floor, Tórshavn, Faroe Islands
Center of Health and Human Performance,
Department of Food and Nutrition, and
Sport Science, University of Gothenburg,
Gothenburg, Sweden

**Juha J. Hulmi, Mia Laakso, Antti A. Mero,
Keijo Häkkinen, Juha P. Ahtiainen and
Heikki Peltonen**
Department of Biology of Physical Activity,
Neuromuscular Research Center, University
of Jyväskylä, Rautpohjankatu 8, P.O. Box
35FI-40014 Jyväskylä, Finland

**Wataru Aoi, Yumi Ogaya, Maki Takami,
Sayori Wada and Akane Higashi**
Laboratory of Health Science, Graduate
School of Life and Environmental Sciences,
Kyoto Prefectural University, 1-5 Hangi-cho
Shimogamo, Sakyo-ku, Kyoto 606-8522, Japan

Toru Konishi and Yusuke Sauchi
KOHJIN Life Sciences Company, Ltd., Tokyo,
Japan

Eun Young Park
Laboratory of Food Science, Graduate School
of Life and Environmental Sciences, Kyoto
Prefectural University, Kyoto, Japan

Kenji Sato
Division of Applied Biosciences, Graduate
School of Agriculture, Kyoto University,
Kyoto, Japan

**Elfego Galvan, Ryan Dalton, Kyle Levers,
Abigail O'Connor, Mike Greenwood,
Christopher Rasmussen, Chelsea
Goodenough and Richard B. Kreider**
Department of Health and Kinesiology,
Exercise and Sport Nutrition Laboratory,
Texas A&M University, College Station, TX
77843-4243, USA

Dillon K. Walker and Sunday Y. Simbo
Department of Health and Kinesiology,
Center for Translational Research in Aging
and Longevity, Texas A&M University,
College Station, TX 77843-4243, USA

Nicholas D. Barringer
United States Military-Baylor University
Graduate Program in Nutrition, Joint Base,
San Antonio, TX 78234, USA

Stephen B. Smith
Department of Animal Science, Texas A&M
University, College Station, TX 77843-4243,
USA

Steven E. Riechman
Department of Health and Kinesiology,
Human Countermeasures Laboratory, Texas
A&M University, College Station, TX 77843-
4243, USA

James D. Fluckey
Department of Health and Kinesiology, Muscle Biology Laboratory, Texas A&M University, College Station, TX 77843-4243, USA

Peter S. Murano
Department of Nutrition and Food Science, Texas A&M University, College Station, TX 77843-4243, USA

Conrad P. Earnest
Nutrabolt, Bryan, TX 77807, USA

Jill A. Parnell
Department of Physical Education and Recreation Studies, Mount Royal University, 4825 Mount Royal Gate SW, Calgary, Alberta T3E 6K6, Canada

Kristin Wiens
Department of Behavioral Health and Nutrition, University of Delaware, 026 North College Avenue, Newark Delaware 19716, USA

Kelly Anne Erdman
Sport Medicine Centre, University of Calgary, 2500 University Drive NW, Calgary, Alberta T2N 1N4, Canada

Timothy D Mickleborough, Jacob A Sinex, David Platt, Robert F Chapman and Molly Hirt
Department of Kinesiology, Human Performance and Exercise Biochemistry Laboratory, School of Public Health-Bloomington, 1025 E. 7th St. SPH 112, Bloomington, Indiana 47401, USA

Michael J Ormsbee
Department of Nutrition, Food and Exercise Sciences, Florida State University, Tallahassee, FL, USA
Institute of Sports Sciences and Medicine, Florida State University, Tallahassee, FL, USA
Discipline of Biokinetics, Exercise and Leisure Sciences, University of KwaZulu-Natal, Durban, South Africa

Emery G Ward and Lynn B Panton
Department of Nutrition, Food and Exercise Sciences, Florida State University, Tallahassee, FL, USA

Christopher W Bach
Department of Nutrition, Food and Exercise Sciences, Florida State University, Tallahassee, FL, USA
Institute of Sports Sciences and Medicine, Florida State University, Tallahassee, FL, USA

Paul J Arciero
Human Nutrition and Metabolism Laboratory, Skidmore College, Saratoga Springs, NY, USA

Andrew J McKune
Discipline of Biokinetics, Exercise and Leisure Sciences, University of KwaZulu-Natal, Durban, South Africa

Scott Lloyd Robinson and Laurent Bannock
Guru Performance LTD, 58 South Molton St, London W1K 5SL, UK

Anneliese Lambeth-Mansell
Institute of Sport & Exercise Science, University of Worcester, Henwick Grove, Worcester WR2 6AJ, UK

Gavin Gillibrand
Ultimate City Fitness, 1-3 Cobb Street, London E1 7LB, UK

Abbie Smith-Ryan
Department of Exercise and Sport Science, University of North Carolina Chapel Hill, Office: 303A Woolen, 209 Fetzer Hall, Chapel Hill, NC, USA

Nicolas Babault
National Institute for Health and Medical Research, (INSERM), unit 1093, Cognition, Action and Sensorimotor Plasticity, Dijon, France
Centre for Performance Expertise, UFR STAPS, Dijon, France
Faculté des Sciences du Sport, Université de Bourgogne, BP 27877, 21078 Dijon Cedex, France

Christos Païzis and Gaëlle Deley
National Institute for Health and Medical Research, (INSERM), unit 1093, Cognition, Action and Sensorimotor Plasticity, Dijon, France
Centre for Performance Expertise, UFR STAPS, Dijon, France

Laetitia Guérin-Deremaux, Marie-Hélène Saniez and Catherine Lefranc-Millot
Roquette, Lestrem, France

François A Allaert
Chair of Medical Evaluation ESC, Dijon, France
CEN Nutriment, Dijon, France

Wesley David Dudgeon, Elizabeth Page Kelley and Timothy Paul Scheett
Department of Health and Human Performance, College of Charleston, 24 George Street, Charleston, SC 29424, USA

Guillermo Escalante and Bryan Haddock
California State University- San Bernardino, 5500 University Parkway, San Bernardino, CA 92407, USA

Michelle Alencar
California State University- Long Beach, 1250 Bellflower Boulevard, Long Beach, CA 90840, USA

Phillip Harvey
Max Muscle Sports Nutrition, 210 West Taft Avenue, Orange, CA 92865, USA
University of Phoenix, San Diego Campus, 9645 Granite Ridge Drive, San Diego, CA 92123, USA

Nidhal Zarrouk
Research Laboratory: "Medical Imaging Technologies" (LR 12ES06, TIM), Faculty of Medicine of Monastir, University of Monastir, Monastir, Tunisia

Omar Hammouda
Research Laboratory: "Equipe de Physiologie, Biomécanique et Imagerie du Mouvement" (CeRSM, EA 2931), UFR STAPS, Université Paris Ouest Nanterre La Défense, 200 avenue de la République, 92000 Nanterre, France

Mohamed Dogui
Research Laboratory: "Medical Imaging Technologies" (LR 12ES06, TIM), Faculty of Medicine of Monastir, University of Monastir, Monastir, Tunisia

Imed Latiri and Ezzedine Bouhlel
Research Unit: "Exercise Physiology and Pathophysiology: from the Integrated to the Molecular Biology, Medicine and Health" (UR 12ES06), Faculty of Medicine of Sousse, University of Sousse, Sousse, Tunisia

Hela Adala
Research Laboratory: "Sport Performance Optimization", National Center of Medicine and Sciences in
Sport (CNMSS), Tunis, Tunisia

Haithem Rebai
Research Unit: "Education, Motricity, Sports and Health" (UR 15JS01), Higher Institute of Sport and Physical Education of Sfax, University of Sfax, Sfax, Tunisia

Leticia Azen Alves Coutinho, Cristiana Pedrosa Melo Porto and Anna Paola Trindade Rocha Pierucci
Federal University of Rio de Janeiro/Josué de Castro Nutrition Institute, Av. Carlos Chagas Filho, 373 - Centro de Ciências da Saúde, Bloco J, 2° andar, Cidade Universitária, Ilha do Fundão, RJ 21941-902, Brazil

Index

www.ingramcontent.com/pod-product-compliance
Lightning Source LLC
Chambersburg PA
CBHW061939190326

41458CB00009B/2781